PRENATAL MASSAGE

A Textbook of Pregnancy, Labor, and Postpartum Bodywork

PRENATAL MASSAGE
A Textbook of Pregnancy, Labor, and Postpartum Bodywork

Elaine Stillerman, LMT
New York City, New York

Foreword by Penny Simkin

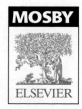

MOSBY

ELSEVIER

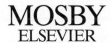

11830 Westline Industrial Drive
St. Louis, Missouri 63146

ISBN: 978-0-323-04253-6

Cover: Mary Cassatt (American, 1845-1926). *After the Bath,* c. 1901. Pastel on paper; 66 x 100 cm.
© The Cleveland Museum of Art, 2003. Gift of J. H. Wade 1920.379

Publishing Director: Linda Duncan
Acquisitions Editor: Kellie White
Associate Developmental Editor: Kelly Milford
Publishing Services Manager: Linda McKinley
Senior Project Manager: Kelly E.M. Steinmann
Designer: Kim Denando

Printed in India

Last digit is the print number: 11

Dedication

For my special boy, Luke, the true love of my life.

For Ersi, my friend, my soul, my guiding light.

Foreword

As you read this book on massage for childbearing women and apply the numerous techniques, you will be reminded, as I have been, of the unique privilege it is to touch and soothe those who are bringing new life into their lives and our world. *Prenatal Massage* is filled with sensitive insight and profound respect for this life-altering time in a woman's life.

This book is divided into four parts, three of which carefully detail the different stages in the childbearing cycle: pregnancy, childbirth, and postpartum. The fourth section about marketing strategies will benefit bodyworkers with much experience and knowledge to help guide you toward a successful practice!

Most important and unique to this textbook is the wide variety of somatic techniques that help bodyworkers provide expectant and new mothers with supportive and nurturing care. Elaine's knowledge, rich experience, and clear instructions benefit all who work with this deserving population.

As I read this book, I was impressed by Elaine's continuing emphasis on the mind-body connection, and I was moved to use this foreword to explore the rapid shifts in the mind-body-baby connection that come during the childbearing year.

The journey through conception, pregnancy, birth, and postpartum is long and full of surprises, as Elaine has carefully explained with rich text, humorous anecdotes, and instructional illustrations. Few women are prepared for the profound emotional shifts and physical changes they experience. They have crossed over into a new world, a new sisterhood. By beginning the cycle of creating new life, they suddenly perceive themselves and are perceived by others in a new and different way. They wonder how they could have lived and worked among pregnant women without any awareness of the mysterious world these women, these *mothers*, inhabited.

Their bodies, guided by unseen hormonal forces, make women into mothers by creating a rich, safe, nourishing place for a baby to grow. Without even realizing it, women are, most of the time, perfect mothers. Merely by breathing, they provide all the oxygen their baby needs. The food they eat meets the needs of two people. As the baby grows, the womb provides everything he needs. Amniotic fluid maintains the baby's temperature and protects him against bumps and blows. It also provides a weightless and buoyant environment that makes it possible for a tiny baby to become strong and coordinated by doing things he would not be able to do outside the womb, like kicking, squirming, and somersaulting. The mother's constant heartbeat, the sloshing sounds of her placenta, her voice and the voices of the father and other loved ones, music, and all the sounds of daily life provide a soothing and interesting soundscape to stimulate the baby. The jiggling caused by the mother's walking or jogging and the big shifts when she lies down or rolls over all contribute to the baby's spatial awareness. She marvels that her body begins making colostrum in late pregnancy and that its constituents change to match the growing unborn baby's nutritional needs. Whenever the baby is born, at whatever gestational age, the colostrum suits the baby's needs.

The mother provides for all of her baby's needs. She is the perfect mother, even though she is only barely aware of all that she is doing for her child. Her body, if not her conscious mind, knows how to do this.

What she is aware of, however, are changes in her size, shape, and weight, and new aches and pains as her body prepares to open and release her baby. Her changing appearance is a source of pride and awe but also of sadness at the loss of her former self. She tires more quickly, even as she continues her usual responsibilities and activities.

She is proud of her baby and fiercely protective at the same time that she holds some doubts about her ability to manage the child's well-being. She becomes more emotional and sensitive to the beauty and kindness in our world but also to misfortune and cruelty. She feels vulnerable for herself and her baby and more dependent on her partner and others. She realizes with some ambivalence that there is no turning back on this journey and may even wonder at times whether it was a good decision to have a baby. But she is unlikely to share such feelings with anyone.

As pregnancy nears its end, the process of labor is set into motion. This textbook elucidates the science and the spirit that work together to start this complex physical phenomenon. Few people realize that it is the baby who initiates labor. When the baby is ready and her lungs are mature, she begins producing a cocktail of hormones and other key substances that prepare her and her mother for their journey through labor and birth and the baby's survival outside the womb. Large amounts of lung liquid (important for lung development) now begin to be reabsorbed to enable the lungs to take over respiration as soon as the baby is born. The baby's "hormone cocktail" passes to the placenta and causes the placenta to produce a different balance of estrogen and progesterone, which makes the uterus more sensitive to the mother's oxytocin. This triggers uterine contractions. Other hormones from the baby cross to the mother's circulation. They increase her production of prostaglandin, which causes the cervix to ripen, efface, and become more ready to dilate with the increasing contractions. In addition, these same fetal hormones reach the mother's pituitary gland and stimulate greater production of oxytocin and prolactin to enhance lactation.

The timing of the onset of labor is perfect about 90% of the time. Labor begins (1) when the fetus is strong and able to breathe on her own, to suckle, and to keep herself warm; (2) when the placenta can no longer support fetal growth; (3) when the mother's uterus is ready to contract, open, and expel the baby and placenta; and (4) when the mother is psychologically ready to welcome and nurture her baby and physically ready to nourish her baby with her colostrum and milk.

In the 10% of births that are true prematurity and postmaturity, factors other than the baby's readiness dictate the onset of labor, such as the mother's health and some inherited tendencies. A negative emotional state can interfere with the onset and progress of labor. Chronic stress or illness in a woman's life sometimes causes labor to begin prematurely. If she is very angry, anxious, or frightened during labor, she produces excessive catecholamines (adrenaline and many others) that slow labor progress by countering the effects of oxytocin and increase her pain by suppressing endorphin production. Excessive catecholamines in labor sometimes indirectly interfere with fetal well-being.

What can be done to ease the mother's emotional state and reduce catecholamine production? As this textbook powerfully and passionately demonstrates, massage and touch, given with the intention to reassure, soothe, and calm the mother, can reverse the negative effects of catecholamines, as can a feeling of physical and emotional safety provided by a nurturing, respectful caregiving staff. The uninterrupted presence, guidance, and empathy of a birth doula has been found to fill the gap of support that is widespread in modern maternity care. Some doulas are also massage therapists who bring their bodywork skills and their additional training in emotional support and physical comfort to laboring women.

If the people and the environment are conducive to her sense of safety and well-being, the mother is free to focus on coping with her contractions. The labor-enhancing effects of oxytocin and endorphins predominate over the catecholamines. But when she feels safe and uninhibited, she unconsciously does what needs to be done to birth her child. She walks, sways, rocks, moans, taps, or strokes rhythmically, repetitively, and instinctually. She repeats the same actions—her ritual—contraction after contraction. Her support people may be a part of her ritual, stroking her and murmuring soothing sounds in her rhythm.

She moans, sighs, and lets her mind go into a reverie state, allowing the part of her that knows how to give birth to take over and guide her body. Women should not be disturbed or interrupted with questions, sounds, or bright lights, especially during contractions. Those around her should respect her privacy when she is in this state.

Then, near the end of labor, her body produces a physiologic surge of catecholamines (called "the fetal ejection reflex")—this time not due to fear or anxiety—to take the woman out of her reverie, alert her, and give her renewed energy and strength to press her baby out of her body. The baby also produces catecholamines during the "stress of being born" that heighten his alertness and help him adapt to the sudden shift from fetus to newborn—clearing his lungs and breathing, maintaining his body temperature, and suckling and digesting colostrum and milk.

Birth heralds yet another massive shift in hormone production, which causes her milk to come in, enables her to awaken whenever her baby needs her, and opens her to deep feelings of love and commitment to the baby. In addition, the physical recovery and her emotional state are largely hormonally driven. Many women are unaware of the dramatic changes that occur almost immediately after childbirth, and Elaine provides comfort measures for this time, helping the transition from pregnant woman to new mother. Women whose babies are healthy, who had a normal birth, who are well-supported, and who get enough sleep tend to recover smoothly over a period of weeks or months. Family, friends, and postpartum doulas can be a helpful resource for any new family, but especially those who are challenged by prolonged recovery or mood disorders. Sometimes, the emotional recovery is delayed by a postpartum mood disorder, such as postpartum depression, anxiety, posttraumatic stress disorder (after a traumatic birth), or others. The mind-body-baby connection may be strained during a mood disorder, and recovery may depend on her getting the right kind of support, counseling, or therapy. Elaine carefully explains the normalcy of recovery and warning signs that require attention from the woman's maternity care provider.

All those who care for childbearing women should try to understand and appreciate the complex connections and the interdependent workings of a woman's mind, body, and baby during the childbearing year. Elaine models just that understanding in this essential book with insight, compassion, and deep respect. *Prenatal Massage: A Textbook of Pregnancy, Labor, and Postpartum Bodywork* is also a beautiful book to scan. The magnificent artwork by master artists in the theme of Mother and Child are coupled with historical pictures that portray childbearing practices of earlier times. In addition, Elaine's personal experiences are richly reported and exhibit a universal humanity shared by so many expectant and new mothers.

What affects the mind also affects the body and the baby. What is good for the baby is good for the mother. By caring for the mother we are also caring for her baby. The effects of our care remain with the mother and baby forever.

What a privilege and what a responsibility.

Penny Simkin, PT
Childbirth educator, doula, doula trainer, birth counselor, and author of numerous books including
The Birth Partner: Everything You Need to Know to Help a Woman Through Childbirth

Note from the Author

Massaging a woman during her pregnancy, labor, and postpartum recovery is a privilege and an honor. You are invited to share a time of her life that is very intimate and personal, and your healing ministrations can impact her experience tremendously. Pregnancy can shape a woman's social and emotional world. Your work can transform a woman who is uncomfortable in her body into someone who celebrates its changes and uniqueness. Massage can minimize the effects of depression, experienced by almost 20% of pregnant women, and replace it with feelings of joyous anticipation.[1,2] You can reverse the harmful effects of stress and promote a healthful in utero environment, and you can replace her feelings of fear and concern about childbirth with those of confidence and ownership.

Ritualistic touch and massage have been a part of the childbearing experience for countless generations in many traditional societies where pregnancy is respected, labor is dignified, and the new mother is revered. In this country, pregnancy and labor are often medically managed while women's rights and choices are often ignored. With all of our technological advances in prenatal medical care that save countless lives, the United States finally established itself in tenth place among the best countries to have a child, according to the listing of the *State of the World's Mothers 2005* by the Save the Children Foundation.[3] However, our infant mortality rates continue to rise.

Many women are seeking alternatives to hospital births when they can. Birthing centers are women and family centered in their approach to birth and offer laboring women countless personal choices and options for their comfort. Other women prefer home birth (which are proven safer than hospital births) as a way to maintain and honor the deeply personal and intimate nature of childbirth. Massage and bodywork have now become restored as an integral part of perinatal health care, whether offered by a massage therapist, through childbirth education classes, or through the loving hands of a midwife or labor doula. The far-reaching benefits of perinatal massage are becoming more recognized and accepted by the general population as well as the medical community. This wasn't always the case, however.

When I attended massage school in New York City in 1978, the curriculum neither mentioned the physiology of pregnancy nor taught the appropriate way to massage pregnant women. Other massage schools across the country—and there were only about a dozen at that time—seemed to reflect similar views by omitting this subject from their courses of study altogether. Since then, there has been a renaissance and new awareness about the benefits of prenatal, labor support, and postpartum recovery massage therapy and bodywork. Many massage schools offer basic prenatal classes to their students and advanced training is available through continuing education programs.

Obstetricians are more appreciative of the stress-reducing benefits of massage and suggest it to their patients. Research is also catching up with this evolving trend. In 1999, the Touch Research Institute published its first study on the benefits of prenatal massage in the *Journal of Psychosomatic Obstetrics and Gynecology.*[4] This study assigned 26 pregnant women to either a massage therapist or a relaxation therapy group. Each woman received two 20-minute sessions each week for 5 weeks. The results indicated that although both groups felt less anxious after the first session and had less leg pain after the first and last sessions, the massage group exhibited reduced anxiety, improved mood, better sleep, and less back pain than the relaxation group. In addition, the massage group experienced fewer labor complications, had lower levels of the stress compound norepinephrine, and had newborns with fewer postnatal complications.

The professional and public appreciation of these benefits is constantly growing. With an average of 4 million babies born annually, women are seeking prenatal and postpartum massage either through referrals from their doctors and midwives or through the recommendations of friends and other pregnant women.

While there is unparalleled interest in prenatal massage, training at massage schools and on the continuing education circuit is inconsistent and sometimes misguided. Some massage schools offer as little as one classroom session of prenatal massage instruction, paying little or no attention to the dynamic physiology of pregnancy, trimester massage considerations, contraindications and precautions of prenatal massage, and how to safely treat high-risk pregnancies. Bodyworkers are treating pregnant women with as little as 3 hours of instruction while others are receiving continuing education credits for home study and video courses that certify them to practice on pregnant women. The ardor these bodyworkers convey about massaging pregnant and postpartum women is certainly understandable, but appropriate training is essential if the work is to be effective and safe.

The massage and bodywork techniques found in this text are varied and are by no means all that the massage practitioner can employ. As you continue your massage education and learn more skills, you can add innovative techniques to your prenatal treatment and make them uniquely yours, provided they honor the dramatically changing physiology and incorporate all of the precautions and contraindications. You may recognize that you have to modify new techniques to conform to the gravida's needs to provide a suitable treatment.

The most fitting and effective way to learn massage and bodywork is in a classroom with a trained instructor guiding you through the hands-on practicum. While this text provides general knowledge of the subject matter, I hope you will use it as a resource in tandem with a professionally certified course of instruction.

Since 1980, when I massaged my first pregnant client, I have recognized the passion, joy, and reverence this deserving population inspires. However, attention must be paid to the appropriateness of the work and the education of the practitioner. That is what I hope this book provides: the understanding and respect of the dynamic changes women undergo during their pregnancies, labor, and postpartum and how to support these changes through every step of their incredible journey to motherhood.

Elaine Stillerman, LMT
New York City, New York

References

1. Bennett, Heather A., Einan, Thomas, R.: Depressive Symptoms among Pregnant Women Screened in Obstetric Settings, *J Women's Health* 13:1, 2004.
2. Tarkan, Laurie: Dealing with Depression and the Perils of Pregnancy, *New York Times*, Jan. 13, 2004.
3. Save The Children: *State of the World's Mothers 2003: The Complete Mothers' Index and Country Rankings*, 2003.
4. Field, T., Hernandez-Reif, M. et al: Pregnant Women Benefit from Massage Therapy, *J Psych Ob Gyn*, 20, 1999.

Preface

More than ever, women are seeking prenatal and postpartum massage either through referrals from their obstetricians and midwives or through the recommendations of friends and other pregnant women. Research proves the efficacy of prenatal massage (*Journal of Obstetrics and Gynecology*, Vol. 19, 1999), and its benefits are widely accepted by the public and in the massage and healthcare community. As massage therapists see more of this population, it is important for our training to be consistent and for attention to be given to the dynamic physiology of pregnancy, trimester massage considerations, contraindications and precautions of prenatal massage, and how to safely treat high-risk pregnancies and women confined to bed rest.

Who will benefit from this book?

Prenatal Massage: A Textbook of Pregnancy, Labor, and Postpartum Bodywork provides massage schools and their students, childbirth educators, doulas, and midwives with a definitive, comprehensive text on the anatomy and physiology of pregnancy along with appropriate massage and bodywork techniques. It also ensures that massage schools, spas, and resorts have an authoritative and definitive text on which they can base their prenatal massage curriculum and appropriate services.

Organization

This comprehensive text details the intricate physiology of pregnancy and appropriate massage techniques for each trimester, following through to labor and postpartum. Most important to this book is the wide variety of somatic techniques that will help bodyworkers provide expectant and new mothers with supportive and nurturing care. The massage and bodywork techniques covered consist of an eclectic assortment of bodywork techniques, including Swedish massage, acupuncture points, myofascial release, trigger point therapy, lymphatic drainage, and reflexology, to name a few. Equally vital to proper care are contraindications and precautions; these are covered, along with an appropriate review of physiology.

The book is written in four units. **Part 1: Pregnancy Massage** explains the benefits of prenatal massage, the physiological and emotional changes of pregnancy, contraindications and precautions of prenatal massage, working with high-risk pregnancies, detailed descriptions of maternal and fetal development for each trimester of pregnancy, and appropriate bodywork techniques to support the changing body. **Part 2: Labor Massage** focuses on the physiology of labor, the benefits of touch during labor, pain control methods and comfort measures to help ensure normal progress of labor, and labor support techniques to keep the laboring woman calm and focused. **Part 3: Postpartum Massage** discusses complications, physiology, and treatment goals. **Part 4: Marketing Strategies** helps massage practitioners establish, maintain, and grow successful practices.

Many women are unaware of the dramatic changes that occur almost immediately after childbirth, and the author carefully explains the warning signs and normalcy of recovery. She also provides information on comfort measures for this dynamic time, helping the client to transition from pregnant woman to new mother. The author's knowledge, rich experience, and clear instructions benefit all who work with this deserving population.

Features

Beautifully illustrated with full-color artwork, technique photographs, and anatomical illustrations, the text will engage the reader as concepts are highlighted visually. Numerous boxes appear throughout the text, highlighting key information and providing clinical tips, and other special boxes provide unique and interesting sidebars on cultural pregnancy customs. Liberal use of case studies throughout gives concepts further clinical relevance. DVD icons, embedded in chapters, indicate when a relevant video clip is available. This interactive tool provides additional content and enhances learning. Perfect for the classroom, each chapter begins with key terms and learning objectives and ends with a series of self-test questions. The book is rounded out by reference lists in each chapter, a comprehensive glossary, and a list of resources.

Ancillaries

The companion DVD bound into this book provides instructional video demonstrating various massage techniques presented in the book. Instructors will also benefit from an Instructor's Resource Manual on Evolve.

Acknowledgments

There are many people who helped make this book a reality. I had the dream team at Mosby: Linda Duncan, Kellie White, Jen Watrous, Kelly Milford, Kim Fons, editors extraordinaire, Elizabeth Clark, April Falast, Sheryl Krato, Kelly Steinmann, Kim Denando, and the entire production team, including Chris Roider from Tybee Studios and Hortencio Gomes from Village Digital. Patrick J. Watson's beautiful and sensitive photographs enhanced the style and feel of the book. My enchanting and adventuresome models were Shalawn Facey, Leslie Reina, Khristopher Reina, and Kristen Plumley and her handsome son Henry Summerville, who proved how beautiful pregnancy and new motherhood can be. Thanks to Cal Watson and Tim Bracy for their help during the photo shoot and Sarah Lavigne for her generous contribution.

I want to personally thank my family and friends who continuously encouraged me and helped me through the rough patches: Robert, Elena, and Ben Stillerman, Kaye Storm, Belle Stillerman and, in spirit, my dad Victor, Dieter Metzger, Peggy and Gary Brill, Liza and Carl Caruso, Margaret Cantrell, Gail Peele, Donna and Sebastian Vos, Leslie Lightfoot, Julie Tupler, Susan Primer, Janet Markovits, Leeor Sabbah, Barbara Messing, Ilana Stein, Judith Halek, the Metropolitan Doula Group, and Dr. Suzanne Lajoie of Downtown Women's Ob/Gyn.

Help and encouragement come in many forms. I must recognize the love, compassion, and patience of Augusta Green, Alice Apolinaris, Cheryl Jones, and Olga Debord who took care of my son Luke so I could write this book.

Much gratitude goes to my colleagues who, year after year, provide me with a nurturing and professional environment where I teach and enrich my professional life: Linda Derick, Sarah Kolej, Steve Kitts, George Kousaleos, Peggy Jenkins, Crystal Loicano, Iris Burman, Janet Gonzalez, Vanessa Hendley, Bev Byers, Mark Sterghos, Kim Mong, Jen Sheshak, Bill Ashmall, Van Delia, Liz Golden, Greg Hurd, Eric Stahlman, Nancy Smith, and Tim Koert.

The commitment of doulas, midwives, and obstetricians who honor and attend to mothers-to-be cannot be overlooked. I acknowledge and applaud these dedicated professionals, those with whom I have personally worked and those who I do not know.

To all my former students who offered me insight, tips, information, and support, I want to say a big "thank you." I hope you continue to find joy and great success in the magical work you do.

But most of all, to all those exquisite pregnant women and new mothers who shared their experiences with me, taught me, and let me into their lives, I want to say that you have enriched my life, humbled me, and shown me the glory and majesty of womanhood.

Elaine Stillerman, LMT
New York City, NY

Table of Contents

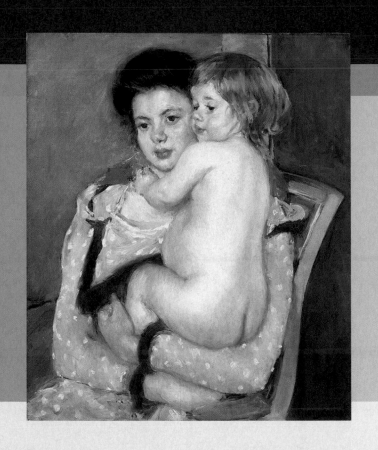

PART ONE

Pregnancy Massage

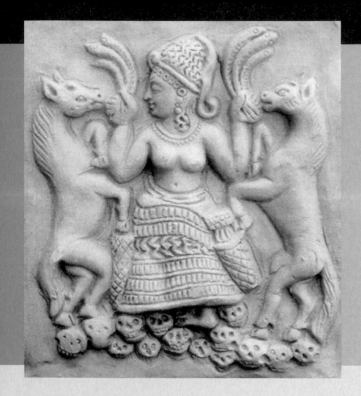

CHAPTER 1

Benefits of Prenatal Massage

Objectives

On completion of this chapter, the student will be able to do the following:

1 Learn the historical relevance of prenatal massage and childbearing practices

2 Recognize the harmful effects of maternal stress during pregnancy

3 Understand how stress affects the developing fetus

4 Recognize the stress-reducing benefits of massage therapy

5 Learn other stress-reducing techniques

6 Recognize the beneficial physiological effects of prenatal massage therapy

7 Learn how massage can control pain

Catecholamines	Midwife	Progesterone
Epinephrine	Neonate	Relaxin
Estrogen	Norepinephrine	Stress
Gravida	Oxytocin	Uterine ligaments
In utero	Physiology	Vertex
Massage	Prenatal	

A Brief History of Childbirth Practices and Prenatal Massage

The role of **massage,** or the manipulation of soft tissue, and bodywork has a long and honorable tradition in a woman's journey to motherhood. Before the advent of modern obstetrics, birth was the domain of women who acted together as care providers, including the **midwife,** or birth attendant, as well as the pregnant woman's friends and family, who supported the laboring woman (Figure 1-1). Massage and touch played an integral part in **prenatal,** or prior to birth, care, particularly during labor.[1] "There is hardly a people, ancient or modern, that do not in some way resort to massage and expression in labor, even if it be a natural and easy one."[1]

The use of massage to correct or prevent breech presentation was practiced by indigenous people for centuries. During labor, if the fetus was not in its preferred head-down or **vertex** position, the laboring woman would lay down on her left side after contractions began and her abdomen would be massaged to examine how the fetus was presenting. If malpresentation was determined, she would turn to the opposite side and rest for a while as the midwife or doctor pressed her abdomen with enough pressure to turn the fetus.[2]

The Tepoztlan of Mexico, the Negritos of the Philippines, the Arikara of North Dakota, and a multitude of other traditional peoples used massage to correct breech presentation.[2] In these cultures, the role of the birth assistant was to physically hold and support the laboring woman and to massage her to speed delivery. Prenatal care among the Nama/Hottentots in Africa, as well as

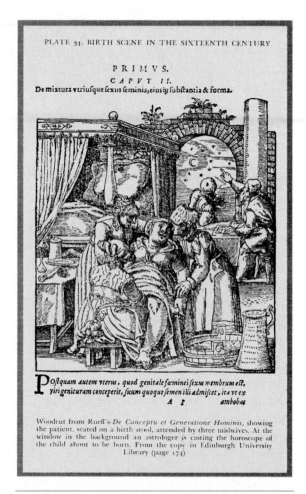

FIGURE 1-1 ■ WOODCUT. Three midwives attending a birth in sixteenth century England. At the window, the astrologer is casting the baby's horoscope. From Rueff J: *De Conceptu et Generatione Hominis,* 1554.

tribal societies in the Gilbert Islands, Java, Japan, and many others, included massage, also referred to as "shampooing."[2]

From ancient times until the eighteenth century, massage was employed during labor by midwives who were almost universally poor,

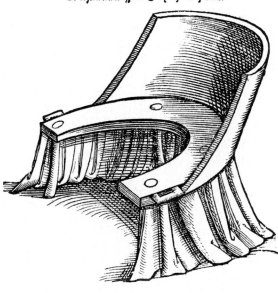

C A P V T II.

De obstetricum officio & apta sedilis forma.

FIGURE 1-2 ■ WOODCUT. Birth stool from 1554 England. (From Rueff J: *De Conceptu et Generatione Hominis,* 1554.)

uneducated but highly skilled women. The midwifery practice included abdominal massage, massage of the legs and back, and massage to correct breech presentation.[3] The first reference to midwives was made in the Old Testament in Genesis 35:17 "And when she (Rachel) was in her hard labor, the midwife said to her, 'Fear not, for now you will have another son.'" Exodus 1:20 says "Therefore God dealt well with the midwives: and the people multiplied, and waxed very mighty."[4]

In Japan, the midwife is known as the Samba, or the woman who massages. In Mexico, the work of the partera is holding and massaging. An English midwifery textbook written in the sixteenth century, *The Sloan Manuscript No. 2463*, teaches the midwife to "anoint her hands with the oil of white lilies and then gently stroke the mother's belly about the navel"[5] (Box 1-1) (Figure 1-2).

The work of midwives during these early times consisted of employing manual skills (massage) and also had a magical, ritualistic component, which created a dualistic atmosphere wherein the midwives were revered for their understanding of the mysteries of life but reviled and feared for their mystical healing abilities. This was never more evident than during the middle ages when hundreds of thousands of women, many of them midwives and healers, were executed by the Church as witches for their healing powers.[6]

In England during the 1700s, as for hundreds of years before, labor was a social event for women.[7] When the expectant mother's labor began, her husband was sent to fetch the midwife (meaning "with woman"),[8] her friends, and her mother. The group of women would help the mother deal with her labor pains and observe the birth. As the midwife took charge of the labor, the expectant mother's friends massaged her, supported her, and helped as best they could. These women were called "god-sibs"[9] (Box 1-2).

In the United States during colonial times, doctors were generally not educated, and women, also without formal training, were the primary health care providers and prominent lay practitioners.[10-13] In 1716, New York City required all midwives to be licensed. These licenses relegated midwives to be servants of the state responsible for social and civil order. By the end of the eighteenth century, it was accepted that midwives had no formal training and since they were largely women, had no intellectual capacity to learn the "modern" obstetrical methods. Wealthy families chose to go to physicians to have their babies, whereas poor women stayed with the midwives.

In 1848, the American Medical Association was founded to uphold medical standards.[13] As the newly burgeoning medical community started gaining power as a political and economic force, birthing practices were taken over by male physicians who called for the abolition of midwifery. Subsequently, the practice of massage during birth fell away as the status and work of midwives was corrupted and usurped by physicians.[3,4]

The first Cesarean section was performed in a Boston hospital in 1894.[10] By 1900, doctors attended nearly half of the births throughout the country and almost all of the births of those women who were wealthy enough to pay them. Midwives assisted the poor who could not afford doctors' fees.[10] In 1938, "twilight sleep" was used in all deliveries. In 1939, it was estimated that 50% of women gave birth in hospitals with 75% from urban areas.[10] By 1950, that number increased to 88%.[10]

In the late 1950s, there was a renaissance in home births attended by midwives and the manual (massage) support that inferred. In 1955, the American College of Nurse-Midwives was created, and in 1956, the La Leche League was founded; these organizations fueled the movement toward more maternal control. During this time, Dr. Ferdinand Lamaze and Dr. Robert Bradley offered women innovative pain-relieving techniques for labor.[10]

By the 1960s, 97% of births in the United States occurred in the hospital.[10] Continuous electronic fetal monitoring was introduced in the 1960s, which was a predictor of the hi-tech birthing practices to come.[10] Conversely, it was during this time that the modern midwifery professional gained strength and power, and in 1970, national certification in nurse-midwifery training and education was formalized.[10]

Feminism became a surging force in the 1970s, and many women's groups promoted gynecological self-care, as well as a move back to midwifery. These groups asserted, contrary to the beliefs of the medical establishment, that childbirth is natural and should not be treated as an illness. They argued that the medical dominance of childbirth needed to be demedicalized and demystified and that hospitalization was not necessary for all births. In 1975, Ina May Gaskin established The Farm in Tennessee with her husband Stephen, where midwives attended all births, and also published the inspirational classic, *Spiritual Midwifery*.

In the 1980s and 1990s, attitudes about maternal control during pregnancy and labor continued to change. In 1980, a new movement reintroduced the time-honored tradition of prenatal massage to massage practitioners, childbirth educators, doulas, and the obstetrical community.[14] As scientific studies continue to validate the beneficial effects of prenatal massage, pregnant women, as well as the once-reticent medical community, are embracing massage as an integral part of their prenatal care.

The Effects of Stress on Pregnancy

Stress has been defined as "any incident in the environment which causes an abrupt change in the mental, physical, or emotional equilibrium of an organism."[15] Pregnancy, for almost every woman,[16] fits that description very well because this is a time of dynamic physical change and contradictory feelings about the pregnancy. Stress and transformation are the hallmarks of pregnancy, and how the pregnant woman, or **gravida,** handles stress can have profound effects on her health and the health of her baby.[17]

Common pregnancy-related physical discomforts, such as nausea and morning sickness, fatigue, swelling, and backaches, can add to maternal stress levels.[18] When pregnancy becomes worrisome and stress builds up to heightened levels, many problems can ensue, among them, fatigue, sleeplessness, anxiety, eating disorders, headaches, and backaches.[18] Long-term exposure to stress can lead to potentially serious health problems such as suppressed maternal immune function, high blood pressure, and heart disease.[18]

Stress and anxiety lead to the elevation of blood **catecholamines,** or stress compounds, that can have negative effects during pregnancy and labor.[17] Catecholamines are predominantly made up of the compounds **norepinephrine** and **epinephrine**, which contribute to homeostatic regulation and are significant in the stress response. Maternal anxiety elevates these levels within the maternal circulation and can slow down the progress of labor. The placental vascular bed is hypersensitive to the constrictive effects of epinephrine that can lead to a failure of labor to progress and decreased placental circulation, thereby inhibiting fetal nutrition. The fetus may exhibit hypoxia with fetal enhancement of catecholamines.[19] These compounds can dampen the effects of hormones, such as **oxytocin**, which is essential for the normal progression of labor.[17] Oxytocin is responsible for more than just muscle contraction, however; it also plays a dominant part in fostering the maternal instinct.[20] Without adequate amounts of oxytocin, there may be an adverse effect on maternal behavior. In addition, stress and anxiety during labor can increase the pain of uterine contractions.[17] Harmful effects of excessive maternal catecholamine levels are as follows:

- Slows labor by dampening effects of oxytocin
- Has an adverse effect on maternal instinct
- Decreases placental perfusion and uterine muscle vasoconstriction, as much as 65%,[21] often leading to fetal hypoxia
- Obstetrical complications[19]

Prenatal stress can have serious consequences for the fetus as well. Since ancient times, it was presumed that the mother's emotional health affected her baby.[22] This belief has been validated by studies that prove maternal stress during pregnancy is associated with increased risk for premature delivery or low birth weight.[23,24]

Studies in rodents and nonhuman primates illustrate that maternal stress can negatively influence the developing fetus and result in delays in motor and cognitive development in their offspring.[25] Mice studies proved that stress creates significant effects on maternal behavior, with stressed dams demonstrating increased levels of aggression.[26] In studies with rhesus macaques, stressed mothers bore infants with lower birth weights, compromised physical growth, delayed neuromotor development, and shorter attention spans.[27,28]

Human studies are understandably sparse. It is generally accepted that first-time mothers, primiparas, are more anxious than second- or third-time mothers, multiparas.[29] The point at which a pregnant woman experiences the highest stress may also be a factor in overall gestational health. Researchers suggested that the earlier in the pregnancy a woman undergoes a major traumatic event, the earlier she is likely to have the baby.[18] Another study[30] concluded that elevated levels of stress in early pregnancy, or extreme concern about labor in midpregnancy,

were associated with diminished mental and psychomotor developmental scores. High levels of maternal cortisol, a stress hormone found in saliva, in late pregnancy are related to psychomotor delays at 8 months postpartum, when the infant has greater awareness and interest in his environment.[30]

Another stress-related hormone produced by the brain and the placenta is corticotrophin-releasing hormone (CRH), which is closely tied to labor. CRH stimulates the body to release prostaglandins that help ripen the cervix and trigger uterine contractions. CRH is also the first hormone released by the brain when a person feels anxious or stressed. High stress, particularly during 18 to 20 weeks' gestation, causes elevated levels of CRH that are linked to preterm labor.[31]

Another important implication associated with stress is that women feeling stressed or anxious are more likely to adopt unhealthy lifestyles and habits. Healthy eating may be discarded, and a woman experiencing stress might reach for a cigarette, alcohol, or drugs to help cope with her anxieties.[32]

Stress can have far-reaching effects during pregnancy and on pregnancy outcome. Since almost no woman goes through this major transition without some stress, it is essential that she receive physical, emotional, and social support to combat these deleterious consequences. Bodyworkers serve their clients best when they are empathetic to the physically taxing and emotionally trying experience expectants mother are going through. Bodyworkers are in a unique position to treat the whole woman and effect change in a supportive, nurturing, and relaxing atmosphere.

Touch Points

Practitioners should always remember that in addition to all the physiological, metabolic and emotional benefits massage provides expectant mothers, one of its most powerful benefits is its ability to reduce stress and minimize the physical, emotional and psychological reactions to stress. By providing a calm, supportive and nurturing environment, practitioners can make a dramatic change in the way of woman feels and experiences her pregnancy.

Bodyworkers should remember these benefits when massaging a mother-to-be. As her levels of stress are reduced, she will experience a much happier, healthier, and enjoyable pregnancy—and she will have her massage practitioner to thank for it!

Harmful effects of stress during pregnancy are as follows:

- Low birth weight and premature labor
- Delayed infant neuromotor development
- Dampened effectiveness of oxytocin
- Prolonged labor or failure to progress in labor
- Uterine vasoconstriction
- Increased labor pain
- Elevated maternal heart rate and blood pressure[29]
- Higher incidences of miscarriage
- Obstetrical complications[33]
- Increase in stress hormones
- Increased likelihood of exhibiting unhealthy lifestyle habits
- Depression

BOX 1-3	*Effects of Stress on Fetal Development*

- Premature labor
- Low birth weight
- High blood pressure and cardiovascular disease later in life
- Cognitive delays, such as autism and autistic spectrum disorders
- Neuromotor delays
- Behavioral problems, such as ADD
- Slowed brain development
- Obesity later in life
- Diabetes later in life
- Hypersensitivity
- Cleft lip and cleft palate

The Effects of Maternal Stress on the Fetus and Neonate

It is important to understand the influence of the maternal temperament on the developing fetus. Prenatal predisposition to stress can profoundly affect the **in utero** environment and may predispose babies to higher risk of disease.[34] If a client is educated about ways to control the stressors in her life, she and her baby will fare a lot better.

As previously noted, preterm labor and low birth weight babies can be a consequence of maternal stress.[35,36] But long-term disabilities and illnesses may plague these babies for the rest of their lives. Animal studies have shown that offspring of stressed mice were smaller than nonstressed animals, and 3 days after birth fewer of them could rotate or right themselves.[37] Maturation was delayed, and these mice exhibited deficiencies in many developmental milestones.[37]

A study with humans showed that anxious pregnant women had increased stress hormones and heart rates that were elevated for longer periods of time than nonstressed mothers. Their fetuses also showed significantly higher heart rates that also stayed high the longest, suggesting a more intense reaction to stress.[34] Low birth weight correlates with high blood pressure in adults and above-average death rates from cardiovascular disease.[34,38,39]

Severe stress during pregnancy has been linked with many other disabilities, such as delayed cognitive development[25]; childhood behavior problems, such as attention deficit disorder (ADD)[41,42] autism, neurodevelopmental disorders, and autistic spectrum disorders[39,43]; hypertension[40]; hyperactivity[40]; diabetes[39]; obesity[39]; slowed brain development[39]; and cleft lip and palate.[44] Obviously, an environment that reduces maternal stress and anxiety and fosters relaxation is essential for a healthy pregnancy and a healthy **neonate** (newborn)(Box 1-3).

Stress-Reducing Benefits of Massage and Bodywork

The time spent with a massage practitioner or bodyworker has profound effects on the expectant woman's **physiological,** or somatic, and emotional reactions to stress. The general adaptation syndrome to stress, as described by Hans Selye,[45] places stress into three categories. The first is the fight or flight response when catecholamines are secreted. The second is the resistance reaction when specific hormonal secretions, such as cortisol, keep the body in active response to the stressor(s) even after the initial stage is over. The third stage is the exhaustion reaction that occurs if the stress has continued for a prolonged period of time.[46] The autonomic nervous system controls and regulates most of the body's systems.[46] Under stress, there is increased activity of the sympathetic nervous system that increases blood pressure, heart rate, and respiration; inhibits blood flow to visceral organs (including the uterus); and helps tense muscles.[46]

Massage has a powerful ability to sedate and restore the nervous system. Proprioceptors of the deeper soft tissues relay messages to the central nervous system about muscle tension and blood pressure.[46] The heat produced by manual manipulation signals both the sympathetic and parasympathetic systems to correct, restore, and balance these self-regulating mechanisms.[46]

The Touch Research Institute has been pioneering studies on the benefits of prenatal massage since the 1990s. One study[47] showed a decrease in anxiety, stress hormones, and obstetrical complications in women who received massages regularly during their pregnancies.

The relaxation provided by a therapeutic massage is further enhanced by the pain-reducing, or analgesic, effect it provides.[46] The release of histamines and local stimulation encourages blood vessels to dilate, waste products and toxins to be reabsorbed and excreted, tissues to be oxygenated, and pain to be diminished.[46] Beta-endorphins and serotonin, a neurotransmitter, are secreted during a massage and work in tandem to inhibit the central nervous system and produce a relaxed and feel-good result.[46,48]

The massage practitioner or bodyworker plays a crucial role in minimizing stress during this turbulent time. The loving, individualized, and nurturing touch that a bodyworker provides has profound effects on how a woman experiences her pregnancy. By creating an environment of acceptance, where there are no judgments, a woman's needs are respected, and her wishes are satisfied, massage practitioners are able to change a time fraught with anxiety into one of eager anticipation and joy.

Other Stress-Reducing Techniques

Massage is certainly one of the most pleasant ways to engender relaxation and reap numerous physiological benefits. There are also a number of other stress-reducing techniques clients can enjoy. Making clients aware of these techniques and discussing which techniques might work best are other ways bodyworkers can nurture and help clients defeat the dangers of stress. Some of these stress-reducing techniques are as follows:

- Meditation[34]
- Visualization and mental imagery[49]
- Prenatal yoga
- Dance classes
- Gentle, modified exercising
- Swimming
- Quiet times of reflection
- Passive relaxation[50]
- Touch and active relaxation[50]
- Education about the normal changes in her body

The Physiological Effects of Prenatal Massage

When clients call for appointments, they will want to know how prenatal massage differs from "regular massage." It is correct to tell them that prenatal massage is regular massage, designed to be safe and appropriate during pregnancy. Bodyworkers can also let clients know that prenatal massage was developed to support and respect the physiological systems that are strained and working overtime to grow the unborn baby.

Massage produces its therapeutic effects through the influences of three categories: reflexive, mechanical, and metabolic.[51,52] Reflexive (indirect) techniques affect the nervous and endocrine systems and the neurochemicals of the body.[51] A reflex is defined as an "involuntary response to a stimulus,"[51] and any kind of bodywork can be called a stimulus. Mechanical techniques use force in varying degrees (i.e., deep or light pressure) to effect changes directly on the body and internally.[51] Metabolic modifications occur within tissue activity that are a result of mechanical and reflex influences.[52] It is also reasonable to assert that the physiological changes that occur after a massage treatment can be caused by any combination of reflexive, mechanical, biochemical, and psychological factors.[53] This is a valuable concept to acknowledge when treating pregnant women, particularly when mechanical methods (i.e., visceral organ massage) often have to be substituted by more appropriate reflexive or other techniques.

The following summations explain how powerful and restorative massage and bodywork can be on the body's systems, although this is merely a glimpse at a complex physiology. The physiology of pregnancy is examined in more detail in Chapter 5.

Musculoskeletal System

The system that carries the greatest burden during pregnancy is the musculoskeletal system. Because of the maladaptive posture the pregnant woman assumes as the baby grows, backaches and muscle soreness are common and are the most common reasons a pregnant client seeks a massage. As her uterus expands and gets heavier, her center of gravity shifts forward[54] and there is greater strain on her weight-bearing joints, particularly her pelvis. The normal lumbosacral curve is increased, and lumbar muscles are compressed. She compensates with an exaggerated anterior flexion of the head (Figure 1-3).

The slight softening and increased mobility of her pelvic joints is normal during pregnancy. This is secondary to the amplified elasticity and loosening of connective and collagenous tissue caused by the increase in steroid hormone circulation, particularly **estrogen**, the female hormone, and **relaxin**, the hormone secreted by the ovaries to soften the pelvic joints in preparation for labor.[54] Peripheral joint laxity also increases in later pregnancy.[55]

An expectant mother's muscles have to hold her upright in this misaligned posture, causing the muscles to become stiff and sore. Her abdominal muscles stretch, weaken, lose tone, and during the last trimester, separate (Figure 1-4).[54,56] This separation, called the diastasis, weakens the abdominal core muscles and exacerbates the lordotic curve.

During pregnancy and at all other times, a therapeutic massage can decrease chronic muscle tension, restore balance to overstretched muscles, release tension in contracted tissues, normalize joint range of motion, and enhance circulation, thereby bringing nutrients to the tissues while reducing waste products and fatigue.[51,57,58]

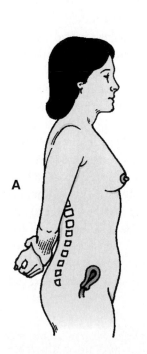
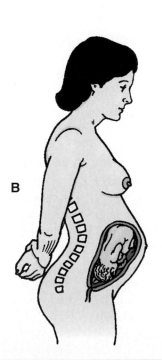
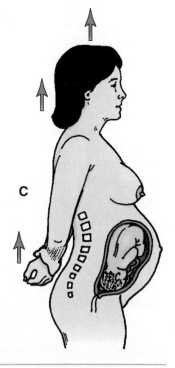

FIGURE 1-3 ■ Postural changes during pregnancy. **A,** Prepregnant posture. **B,** As her uterus expands, her center of gravity shifts anteriorly placing great strain on her weight bearing joints, particularly her pelvis and lower back. The normal lumbosacral curve is exaggerated as the lumbar muscles are compressed. Notice the anterior flexion of her head. **C,** A posterior pelvic tilt and tightened abdominal muscles will shift her weight more evenly. Her neck becomes more aligned with this correction. (From Lowdermilk DL, Perry SE: *Maternity & women's health care*, ed 8, St. Louis, 2004, Mosby.)

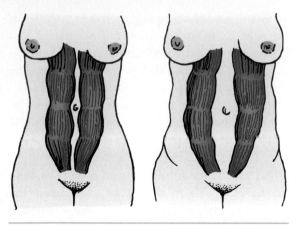

FIGURE 1-4 ■ The separation of the rectus abdominis along the linea alba is called the diastasis recti. This separation weakens core abdominal muscles and contributes to lower back instability. (From Leifer G: *Maternity nursing*, ed 9, St. Louis, 2005, Saunders.)

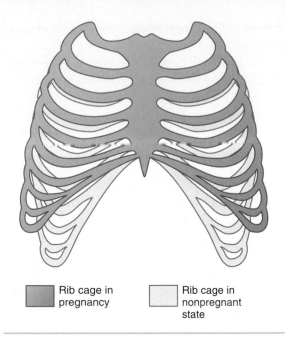

Rib cage in pregnancy

Rib cage in nonpregnant state

FIGURE 1-5 ■ By the end of the third trimester, the pregnant woman's ribcage has expanded 2 to 3 inches anteriorly and laterally. From Fraser D, Cooper M: *Myles' textbook for midwives*, ed 14, Edinburgh, 2003, Churchill Livingstone.

Appropriate prenatal bodywork can reduce the strain and discomfort that is all too common during pregnancy.

Circulatory System

To supply oxygen and nutrients to the developing fetus and expanding uterus, a woman's cardiovascular system undergoes dramatic changes.[59] By the end of the pregnancy, the enlarged uterus exerts considerable pressure on the pelvic veins and the inferior vena cava. Blood pools in her lower limbs with increased pressure below the level of the inferior vena cava.[60] She feels warmer because of her increased blood volume, and her heart has to work harder to pump the additional blood.[61] Other changes to the circulatory system include possible swelling, varicose veins of the legs and vulva, and potential blood clots.

Massage has a tremendous ability to speed up sluggish circulatory (general and local)[52] and lymphatic systems, relieve congested veins,[57] minimize swelling in the extremities, normalize blood pressure,[46] and ease varicose veins. Lymphatic massage, which is very light stroking toward the trunk, is more effective than either passive exercise or electrical muscle stimulation in stimulating lymph flow.[62]

Respiratory System

Backward postural shifting takes place as pregnancy advances, and the compressed respiratory diaphragm, a result of the growing fetus, decreases the space occupied by the lungs at the end of exhalation.[60] The expectant mother's ribcage expands, supporting an increase in tidal volume of air with each inhalation and exhalation (Figure 1-5). In addition, her respiration rate goes up during pregnancy. Breathlessness is common in the last trimester, partially because of weight gain and the increase in basal metabolism.[60]

The relaxation of a therapeutic massage fosters deeper breathing and can often address several respiratory conditions of pregnancy such as dyspnea, or shortness of breath. There is an increase in respiratory activity, partly a result of the reflex influence of massage but also because of the massages' effects in circulating waste products, requiring elimination through the lungs.[52] In addition, internal or tissue respiration is enhanced by massage.[57]

Gastrointestinal System

One of the most common and uncomfortable side effects of hormonal adjustment during pregnancy is nausea or morning sickness, with or without vomiting, which occurs in almost two-thirds of all pregnancies and most often

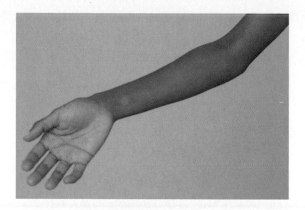

FIGURE 1-6 ■ Stimulating pericardium 6 on both forearms is an effective way to treat morning sickness. The practitioner holds both points for a count of 10, repeating a total of 10 times.

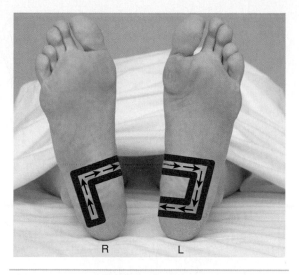

FIGURE 1-7 ■ Stimulating the intestinal reflex points will encourage peristaltic activity of the intestines. All massage on the feet should be light.

in the first trimester.[59] Morning sickness is not an accurate description because this complaint can occur at any time of the day, as well as at any juncture during the pregnancy. Although massage is contraindicated when the client is nauseous or vomiting, one acupuncture point, pericardium 6, a stomach calming point, has been found to be quite effective in reducing the nausea and stomach upset often ascribed to the first trimester (Figure 1-6).

Progesterone, a sex hormone manufactured in the ovaries and placenta that prepares the endometrium for implantation, develops the mammary glands, and supports and maintains the pregnancy, slows down the functioning of all smooth muscle with resultant loss of tone,[59] thus constipation, gas, heartburn, and esophageal reflux are not uncommon.[59] Also, the weight of the uterus compresses the intestines, thereby slowing down bowel function. Through reflex action, massage can encourage the emptying of the intestines by stimulating peristaltic activity (Figure 1-7).

Emotional/Psychological Effects of Massage

A pregnant woman can get more in touch with the changes in her body through the kinesthetic awareness brought about by a massage. As common pregnancy-related discomforts are reduced through massage, the pregnant woman can learn greater acceptance and ownership of her body. Massage can also prepare her physically, emotionally, and mentally for the next step in her journey—labor and the birth of her baby.

The nurturing and respectful touch given by a qualified practitioner helps the expectant mother achieve a sense of peace during this unsettling time. A woman who feels validated and affirmed through someone's loving touch is also more likely to display better parenting skills, be more attentive to her baby, and touch her child in a loving, supportive manner.[63] Considering that most of her prenatal care can be devoid of human touch and rife with technology, massage and bodywork can supplement a pregnant woman's care with a sense of support, intimacy, and wholeness.

Pain Reduction through Massage

When a muscle contracts, it is often accompanied by restricted movement and local circulation[64] (Figure 1-8). The ischemia creates even more pain in an area. Stress and worry, not at all uncommon during pregnancy, aggravate the pain. Because the pregnant woman exhibits continuing muscle imbalance with the growth of the fetus and an anterior shift in the center of gravity, her muscles

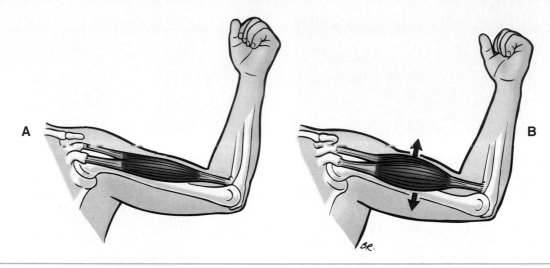

FIGURE 1-8 ■ A contracted muscle has restricted movement and restricted local circulation. **A**, Beginning point. **B**, Contract the muscle by flexing the joint. (From Fritz S: *Mosby's fundamentals of therapeutic massage*, enhanced reprint, ed 3, St. Louis, 2005, Mosby.)

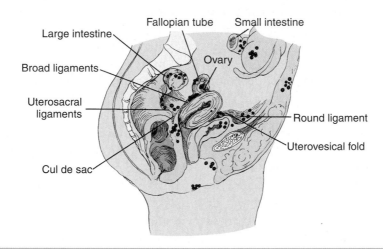

FIGURE 1-9 ■ Uterine ligaments. (From Leifer G: *Maternity nursing: an introductory text*, ed 9, St. Louis, 2005, Saunders.)

often become stiff and sore. Muscle stiffness is exacerbated by the increase in the interstitial fluid she retains.

Low back, pelvic, and **uterine ligament** pain; myofascial restrictions; trigger point pain; swelling; leg and foot soreness; hand weakness; additional body weight; and general muscle fatigue contribute to the client's discomfort and pain level (Figure 1-9). Massage is effective in breaking the pain cycle.[64,65] Touching an area that hurts is an instinctive response to pain. In a professional setting, the relief of pain, as well as the anxiety and stress pain creates, is attained through mechanical and reflex activity.[65] The analgesic effects of massage are derived from improved venous and

lymph circulation, the release of beta-endorphins and serotonin, and the psychological relaxation of a loving touch.

Uterine Ligaments

The uterus is supported by eight ligaments that stretch as the uterus grows, often causing referred anterior or lumbosciatic pain. The two round ligaments stem from the anterosuperior aspect of the uterus and connect at the pubic mons. Pain from these ligaments is often described as a "stitch" on one side. This discomfort can radiate as far as the anterior thigh. The two broad ligaments attach laterally to the internal pelvic walls. Pain in the broad ligaments can be felt in the low back and is often masked as sciatica. Two sacrouterine ligaments attach from the posterior uterus to the posterior pelvic cavity wall and the anterior surface of S2 and S3. Discomfort from these ligaments is often felt as a dull pain in the sacral region and lower back. A single anterior ligament is attached to the bladder, and a posterior ligament anchors the uterus to the rectum; pain from these ligaments can be felt in the lower abdomen and lower back, respectively.

Prenatal Massage Benefits

DVD Some benefits of prenatal massage are:
- Reduces tension, stress, and anxiety
- Supports a healthy in utero environment
- Decreases chronic muscle tension, restores postural balance, normalizes joint range of motion
- Speeds up venous and lymph circulation, brings nutrients to tissues and eliminates waste products, reduces swelling, eases varicose veins, normalizes blood pressure
- Fosters deeper breathing, enhances internal respiration
- Minimizes nausea, stimulates peristaltic activity
- Elevates mood, encourages loving maternal care
- Reduces pain
- Treats the common discomforts of pregnancy
- Prepares the woman physically, emotionally, and mentally for labor

Prenatal massage practitioners can employ other useful adjunctive tools and skills to help their pregnant clientele. Educational materials, a nonjudgmental environment, exercise suggestions, and dietary tips—those within the scope of practice—can provide a more holistic approach to the bodyworker's nurturing hands-on care.

In My Experience...

R was a social worker whose job was to analyze whether foster children should be returned to their biological parents and to report her findings to family court. This was a very stressful job. She was also 9 months pregnant and felt compelled to finalize numerous reports before her maternity leave. She believed she needed more time to make fair decisions but her due date was approaching, and the pressure to complete these reports kept her up nights and impacted her daily life.

R came for massages every other week, and I could see how concerned she was. After each massage, she felt more relaxed but had not successfully figured out a way to complete all those reports in time for her maternity leave. About 2 weeks before her due date, an idea came to her while she was receiving a massage. The solution seemed simple enough, but her stress levels had clouded her thinking. If she could summarize her findings adequately rather than write detailed accounts, this would satisfy the court's requirements and give her more time to finish all of her paperwork.

She admitted that the relaxation from the massage allowed her to think clearly and come up with this working alternative. Her next and last massage before her baby was born was appreciably different. No longer stressed about work, she could enjoy the benefits of the massage with the knowledge that she had done a good job for her clients.

Summary

Massage during pregnancy, labor, and postpartum has a long and honorable tradition. Historical accounts of midwifery and childbearing practices demonstrate the use of manual assistance during labor and birth. Many traditional cultures used massage throughout the childbearing months to maintain optimal maternal and fetal health, prepare the **gravida** (pregnant woman) for labor, and ensure a speedy recovery.

One of the greatest enemies of a healthy pregnancy is stress. Stress not only adversely affects the maternal physiology and emotional experience of pregnancy but also can have harmful effects on the **in utero** environment and fetal growth. Massage is one of the safest and most effective ways to reduce tension, stress, and anxiety.

Additional benefits of prenatal massage include decreasing chronic muscle tension, increasing venous and lymphatic circulation, reducing swelling, easing varicose veins, normalizing blood pressure, and fostering deep breathing. Massage supports the dynamic physical and emotional changes of pregnancy.

References

1. Englemann G: Massage and expression or external manipulations in the obstetric practice of primitive people, *Am J Obstet Dis Women Children* 15:601-625, 1882. Reprinted in *MTJ* 33(3):38-40, 1994.
2. Goldsmith J: *Childbirth wisdom*, New York, 1984, Congdon and Weed.
3. Calvert R: *The history of massage: an illustrated survey from around the world*, Rochester, Vt, 2002, Healing Arts Press.
4. Sullivan N: A short history of midwifery, MidwifeInfo. Available at http://www.midwifeinfo.com/content/view/32/30/. Accessed March, 2002.
5. Brainin K: *Pregnancy and birth*, London, 2005, Active Birth Centre.
6. Achterberg J: *Women as healer*, Boston, 1990, Shambala Publications.
7. Wilson A: The ceremony of childbirth and its interpretations. In Fildes V, ed: *Women as mothers in pre-industrial England: essays in memory of Dorothy McLaren*, London, 1990, Routledge.
8. Willughby P: Observation in midwiferys (ca. 1672), England. In Wilson A, ed: *The making of man-midwifery. Childbirth in England, 1660-1770*, Cambridge, Mass, 1995, Harvard University Press.
9. Culpeper N: A directory for midwives, London, 1675. In Wilson A, ed: *The making of man-midwifery. Childbirth in England, 1660-1770*, Cambridge, Mass, 1995, Harvard University Press.
10. Feldhusen AE: The history of midwifery and childbirth in America: A time line, *Midwifery Today* 53:2000.
11. Rooks JP: *Midwifery and childbirth in America*, Philadelphia, 1998, Temple University Press.
12. Starr P: *The social transformation of American medicine*, New York, 1984, Basic Books.
13. Wertz R, Wertz DC: *Lying-in: a history of childbirth in America*, New Haven, Conn, 1989, Yale University Press.
14. Stillerman E: *MotherMassage: a handbook for relieving the discomforts of pregnancy*, New York, 1992, Dell.
15. Kellogg M: *Mind/body integration—stress management: minimizing negative stress*, Kansas City, 1978, Renascence Project.
16. Leifer M: Psychological changes accompanying pregnancy and motherhood, *Genet Psych Monogr* 95:55-96, 1977.
17. McKay S: *Maternal stress and pregnancy outcome*, Minneapolis, 1980, ICEA.
18. Glynn L, Wadhwa PD, Dunkel-Schetter C, et al: When stress happens matters: effects of earthquake timing on stress responsivity in pregnancy, *Am J Obstet Gynecol* 184(4):637-642, 2001.
19. Fox HA: The effects of catecholamines and drug treatment on the fetus and newborn, *Birth Fam J* 6:1979.
20. Hormonal oxytocin causes artificial mothering in rats, *Brain Mind Bulletin* 5:3, 1980.
21. Gorsuch R, Key M: Abnormalities of pregnancy as a function of anxiety and life stress, *Psychosom Med* 36:352-362, 1974.
22. Ferreira AJ: Emotional factors in prenatal environment. A review, *J Nerv Ment Dis* 141:108-118, 1965.
23. Lou HC, Hansen D, Nordentoft M, et al: Prenatal stresses of human life affect fetal brain development, *Dev Med Child Neurol* 36:826-832, 1994.
24. Pagel MD, Smilkstein G, Regen H, et al: Psychosocial influences on newborn outcomes: a controlled prospective study, *Soc Sci Med* 30:597-604, 1990.
25. Buitelaar JK, Huizink AC, Mulder EJ, et al: Prenatal stress and cognitive development and temperament in infants, *Neurobiol Aging* 24(suppl 1):S53-S60, 2003.
26. Meek LR, Dittel PL, Sheehan MC, et al: Effects of stress during pregnancy on maternal behavior in mice, *Physiol Behav* 72(4):473-479, 2001.
27. Schneider ML: Delayed object permanence development in prenatally stressed rhesus monkey infants, *Occup Ther J Res* 12:96-110, 1992.

28. Schneider ML: The effect of mild stress during pregnancy on birthweight and neuromotor maturation in rhesus monkey infants *(Macaca mulatta)*, *Infant Behav Dev* 15:389-403, 1992.

29. Ascher BH: Maternal anxiety in pregnancy and fetal homeostasis, *JOGN Nurs* 7:18-21, 1978.

30. Van den Bergh BRH: Maternal emotions during pregnancy and fetal and neonatal behavior. In Nijhuis JG, ed: *Fetal behaviour development and perinatal aspects*, Oxford, 1992, Oxford University Press.

31. Hobel CJ, Dunkel-Schetter C, Roesch SC, et al: Maternal plasma corticotrophin-releasing hormone associated with stress at 20 weeks' gestation in pregnancies ending in preterm labor, *Am J Obstet Gynecol* 180:S257-S263, 1999.

32. March of Dimes: *Stress and pregnancy*, 2003.

33. Crandon A: Maternal anxiety and obstetric complications, *J Psychosom Res* 23:109, 1979.

34. Elias M: *Even womb is no haven if mother feels stressed*, USA Today, March 8, 1999.

35. Dunkel-Schetter C: Maternal stress and preterm delivery, *Prenat Neonat Med* 3:39-42, 1998.

36. Copper RL, Goldenberg RL, Das A, et al: The preterm prediction study: maternal stress is associated with spontaneous preterm birth at less than thirty-five weeks' gestation, *Am J Obstet Gynecol* 175:1286-1292, 1996.

37. Meek LR, Burda KM, Paster E: Effects of prenatal stress on development in mice: maturation and learning, *Physiol Behav* 71(5):543-549, 2000.

38. Monk C: Stress during pregnancy can affect fetal heart rate, *J Dev Behav Pediatr* 24(1):32-38, 2003.

39. Huizink A, Buitelaar JK: From postnatal to prenatal determinants of development: a shift of paradigm. Unpublished manuscript, 2004.

40. Sharma VP: Stress during pregnancy can affect a child's health, Mind Publications. Available at http://www.mindpub.com/index.html. Accessed 1996.

41. Van den Bergh BR, Marcoen A: High stress during pregnancy may increase likelihood of behavior problems in child, *Child Dev* 75:1085-1097, 2004.

42. Clements AD: The incidence of attention deficit-hyperactivity disorder in children whose mothers experienced extreme psychological stress, *Georgia Educational Researcher* 91:1-14, 1992.

43. Berersdorf D: Major stress during pregnancy linked to autism. Society for Neuroscience.

44. Hansen D, Lou HC, Olsen J, et al: Serious life events and congenital malformation: a national study with complete follow-up, *Lancet* 356:875-880, 2000.

45. Selye H: *The stress of life*, New York, 1956, McGraw Hill.

46. Fritz S, Grosenbach J: *Essential sciences for therapeutic massage*, ed 2, St. Louis, 2004, Mosby.

47. Field T, Hernandez-Reif M, Hart S, et al: Pregnant women benefit from massage therapy, *J Psychosom Obstet Gynaecol* 290:31-38, 1999.

48. Ironson G, Field T, Kumar A, et al: Relaxation through massage is associated with decreased distress and increased serotonin levels. Paper presented at the Academy of Psychosomatic Medicine meeting, San Diego, 1992.

49. Sears W, Sears M: *The pregnancy book*, Boston, 1997, Little, Brown.

50. Simkin P, Whalley J, Keppler A: *Pregnancy, childbirth and the newborn*, New York, 1991, Meadowbrook Press.

51. Fritz S: *Fundamentals of therapeutic massage*, St. Louis, 2000, Mosby.

52. Kellogg JH: *The art of massage*, Battle Creek, MI, 1929, Modern Medical Publishing.

53. Yates J: *Physiological effects of therapeutic massage and their application to treatments*, Vancouver, BC, 1990, Massage Therapists' Association of British Columbia.

54. Lowdermilk DL, Perry SE: *Maternity & women's health care*, ed 8, St. Louis, 2004, Mosby.

55. Cunningham FG, Gant NF, Leveno KJ, et al: *Williams obstetrics*, ed 21, New York, 2001, McGraw Hill.

56. Tupler J: *Maternal fitness*, New York, 1996, Simon and Schuster.

57. Despard L: *Text-book of massage and remedial gymnastics*, ed 3, London, 1932, Oxford English Press.
58. Muller EA, Schulte am Esch J: Die wirkung der massage auf die leistungsfahigeit von muskeln, *Int Z Angew Physiol* 22, 1966.
59. Leifer G: *Maternity nursing: an introductory text,* ed 9, St. Louis, 2005, Saunders.
60. Hassid P: *Textbook for childbirth educators*, Philadelphia, 1978, Harper and Row.
61. Fraser D, Cooper M: *Myles' textbook for midwives*, ed 14, Edinburgh, 2003, Churchill Livingstone.
62. Ladd MP, Kottke FJ, Blanchard RS: Studies on the effect of massage on the flow of lymph from the foreleg of a dog, *Arch Phys Med Rehabil* 33:604-612, 1952.
63. Rubin R: Maternal touch, *Nursing Outlook* 11:828-831, 1963.
64. Kresge CA: Massage and sports, *The Massage Journal* 45-46, 1985.
65. Jacobs M: Massage for the relief of pain: anatomical and physiological considerations, *Phys Ther Rev* 40:93-98, 1960.

REVIEW QUESTIONS

1 How did midwives in ancient times use massage and touch to facilitate labor and turn breech presentation?

_____

_____

_____

_____

_____

2 How did the practice of massage during birth fall away in the United States during the mid-1800s?

_____

_____

_____

_____

_____

3 How did birthing practices shift from midwives to medical doctors in this country?

_____

_____

_____

_____

_____

4 How and when did the renaissance of midwifery practice come about in this country?

_____

_____

_____

_____

_____

_____

5 When did the reintroduction of prenatal, labor support, and postpartum massage take place in this country?

_____

_____

_____

_____

_____

6 What is the definition of stress?

_____

_____

_____

_____

_____

7 What are the physical sequelae of prenatal stress to the expectant woman and the fetus?

_____

_____

_____

_____

_____

8 Can the maternal emotional health affect her baby's health?

_____

_____

_____

_____

_____

_____

9   How do the catecholamines—stress com-
     pounds—affect maternal hormone levels?

     _____

     _____

     _____

     _____

     _____

10   List the harmful effects of stress on a pregnancy.

     _____

     _____

     _____

     _____

     _____

     _____

11   How does stress slow the progress of labor?

     _____

     _____

     _____

     _____

     _____

     _____

12   List the harmful effects of stress to the fetus and
     neonate.

     _____

     _____

     _____

     _____

     _____

     _____

     _____

13   What are some of the stress-reducing benefits of
     prenatal massage therapy?

     _____

     _____

     _____

     _____

     _____

14   In addition to the numerous stress-reducing
     benefits of prenatal massage therapy, what other
     suggestions can massage practitioners offer their
     clients to minimize stress during pregnancy?

     _____

     _____

     _____

     _____

     _____

     _____

15   What are some of the effects of massage therapy
     on a pregnant woman's musculoskeletal system?

     _____

     _____

     _____

     _____

     _____

     _____

16   What are some of the effects of massage therapy
     on a pregnant woman's circulatory system?

     _____

     _____

     _____

     _____

     _____

     _____

17   What are some of the effects of massage therapy on a pregnant woman's respiratory system? Gastrointestinal system?

_____

_____

_____

_____

_____

_____

18   What are some of the emotional/psychological effects massage may offer a pregnant woman?

_____

_____

_____

_____

_____

19   How can massage help reduce pain?

_____

_____

_____

_____

_____

_____

20   Name and describe the uterine ligaments.

_____

_____

_____

_____

_____

_____

_____

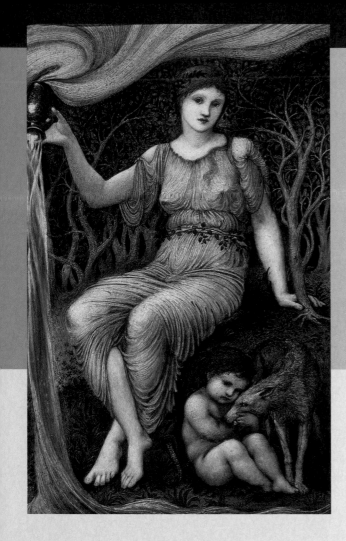

Dispelling the Myths of Prenatal Massage

Objectives

On completion of this chapter, the student will be able to do the following:

1 Understand how a miscarriage occurs
2 Recognize when massage during the first trimester is safe
3 Learn the appropriate touch needed for abdominal massage
4 Understand which massage technique is most effective on feet and legs
5 Teach the client comfortable positions for sleeping and receiving a massage

Key Terms

Acupuncture points	Hormonal imbalances	Nausea
Contraindication	Miscarriage	Placenta
Ectopic pregnancy	Morning sickness	Spontaneous abortion

As with other important milestones in a woman's reproductive cycle, pregnancy is surrounded by misconceptions, old wives' tales, and myths. Many practitioners are given contradictory information about what is safe in the massage of a pregnant client. Some misinformation comes from a simple lack of knowledge, whereas other recommendations are made for legitimate, if unfortunate, liability concerns. When a practitioner is not sure what to do, erring on the side of caution is best and anything that might endanger the client is avoided. However, many attitudes can be reversed once the motives are understood and the science explained. Following are some of the common myths of prenatal massage with an examination of why they exist and how prevailing attitudes can be changed.

The five myths of prenatal massage that will be discussed are as follows:

Myth 1: A massage can cause a miscarriage.

Myth 2: Massage is contraindicated in the first trimester.

Myth 3: The abdomen should never be massaged during the first trimester.

Myth 4: The feet and hands should never be massaged during pregnancy.

Myth 5: A pregnant woman should lie only on her left side during sleep and during massage.

Myth 1

The first myth is that massage can cause a miscarriage. In truth, the abdominal work would have to be extremely deep and rough to dislodge the placenta, and a professional would never practice massage techniques on a pregnant client in this manner.

A **miscarriage** is described as a "spontaneous loss of a pregnancy before the fetus is viable."[1] In general, a fetus is viable at 20 weeks' gestation.[2] An early **spontaneous abortion** is a miscarriage that occurs during the first 12 weeks of gestation,

and a late spontaneous abortion occurs between weeks 12 and 20.[3] About 90% of miscarriages occur within the first 8 weeks of pregnancy.[2]

Miscarriages occur more frequently than once estimated; nearly half of all pregnancies possibly end in miscarriage.[4] With a variety of over-the-counter early pregnancy detection products available, women are finding out early—even a few days after conception—that they are pregnant. What once was considered a late period, complete with cramps and clotting, might be a miscarriage. The five types of miscarriage are as follows[5]:

1. Threatened: Slight cramping and slight to moderate bleeding occur. Bed rest is ordered.

2. Inevitable: Moderate cramping and moderate to severe bleeding occur. Bed rest is ordered.

3. Incomplete: Severe cramping with severe to continuous bleeding and passing of placental or fetal tissue occur. Bed rest is ordered.

4. Complete: No cramping and little bleeding occurs, and the passing of the complete placenta and fetus occurs.

5. Missed: No cramping or fetal movement occurs, and brownish discharge and prolonged retention of tissue are seen. Oxytocin may be prescribed to induce labor.

In nearly half of all cases, the reason for miscarriage is that the embryo was chromosomally abnormal and not viable; this etiology is clearly unrelated to massage.[1,4] Other potential causes of miscarriage also have no connection to receiving a massage. The etiologies of miscarriage include the following[4,6]:

- Embryonic abnormalities or chromosomal defects; embryonic absence
- Genital structural abnormalities in the mother such as retroversion of the uterus, bicornuate uterus, and fibroids
- Maternal infection such as chlamydia, rubella, listeria, ureaplasma, and mycoplasma
- Maternal conditions such as diabetes, renal disease, thyroid conditions, and nutritional deficiencies

- **Ectopic pregnancy**, in which the tissues of the conceptus attach to the fallopian tube instead of the uterine wall
- **Hormonal imbalances** resulting in progesterone deficiency
- Immunological rejection of the fetus, in which antibodies that destroy the fetus are created
- Maternal age (The older the gravida, or pregnant woman, the greater the risk of miscarriage. A 25-year-old woman has an estimated 15% risk of miscarriage, and by the time she is 42 years old, her risk escalates to 50%.)[7]
- Environmental factors such as exposure to firsthand or secondhand smoke, excessive alcohol consumption, and exposure to organic solvents[4,6]

Clearly, massage and bodywork do not factor into any of the causes of miscarriage. The expectant mother who embraces a healthy lifestyle—including massage—is more likely to have a successful pregnancy. Listed below are possible signs of miscarriage in early and late pregnancy; if the client has any of the following symptoms, the massage should not proceed.

Symptoms of miscarriage in early pregnancy include the following:

- Bleeding, bright red or dark brown (Nearly 20% of healthy pregnancies have one or two incidents of light bleeding in early pregnancy called *implantation bleeding* as the embryo implants in the uterus; this is not a threatened miscarriage. However, all bodywork should cease until the bleeding stops and the client has received approval from her health care provider to continue. Bleeding that is similar to a menstrual period or that continues for days is probably a miscarriage.)
- Abdominal pain or cramping
- Lower back, thigh, or pelvic pain

Symptoms of miscarriage in late pregnancy include the following:

- Heavy bleeding, including the passage of clots
- Intense uterine contractions[8]

The process of grieving must be respected regardless of when and how the miscarriage occurs. Repeated miscarriages can be physically and emotionally taxing, and couples who required fertility treatments or artificial reproductive technology must face financial implications as well. A miscarriage leaves the woman without a baby but with postpartum recovery issues. The best care to offer the client is acknowledgment of her loss and a loving, restorative massage (see Chapter 22).

Myth 2

The second myth is that massage is contraindicated during the first trimester. Two lines of reasoning exist for why massage should not be performed in the first trimester.

The first line of reasoning is that most miscarriages occur within the first trimester, so if a practitioner does not give a massage, blame for the miscarriage is avoided. Although the rationale is sound, the science does not support attributing a miscarriage to massage. As discussed, appropriate massage and bodywork do not contribute to any of the etiologies of miscarriage.

The second line of reasoning is that most women suffer from nausea and vomiting during the first trimester, called **morning sickness**, and waiting until the nausea subsides is best. This has validity, but not every woman suffers from morning sickness and not every woman who has morning sickness is affected by it in the morning or even during the first trimester. Massage therapists generally do not treat while the client is nauseous or vomiting. However, the practitioner should be assured that although a woman might suffer the effects of morning sickness at one point during the day, ministrations given at another time can alleviate many of the symptoms the client will experience later (Box 2-1).

Many wonderful suggestions can be offered to help the client minimize the effects of morning sickness such as the following:

- Eat small but frequent meals throughout the day.
- Eat a high-protein meal or snack before bed. (Protein takes the longest to digest, so the client should not wake up with an empty, upset stomach.)
- Eat an umeboshi plum, which can found in health food stores and Asian markets. (In Japan, women eat the fruit of the plum and suck on the pit throughout the day to calm the stomach.)

- Cut up a lemon, place the wedges in a plastic bag, and inhale the lemon scent as needed, to reduce nausea.
- Dilute 1 drop of pure peppermint oil in 8 oz of warm, honey water and drink every hour as needed.
- Try ginger ale, ginger tea, and ginger candies.
- Drink peppermint, spearmint, chamomile, and red raspberry leaf teas.
- Wear "sea bands" on **acupuncture point** pericardium 6 (Figure 2-1).

Clients affected by morning sickness are in the majority, with an estimated 85% to 90% of expectant mothers suffering from it. Morning sickness persists beyond the first trimester in 1 out of 10 pregnant women,[1] but the symptoms most often subside after the first trimester when early pregnancy hormone (human chorionic gonadotrophin [hCG]) levels wane. Morning-sickness theorists disagree on why some women experience morning sickness, but others do not. The reason some women have mild symptoms whereas others develop such severe nausea and vomiting (hyperemesis gravidarum) that they must be hospitalized to prevent dehydration also is not understood. Studies have shown that morning sickness correlates to miscarriage and stillbirth, suggesting that women who experience nausea have fewer miscarriages.[9] One theory speculates a nauseous woman may avoid eating foods that might harm the fetus (see Chapter 14).

Myth 3

The third myth is that the abdomen should never be massaged during the first trimester. The fear is that the practitioner may cause

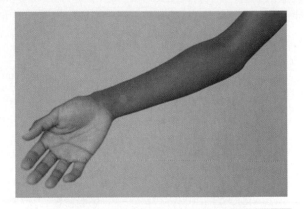

FIGURE 2-1 ■ Stimulating the pericardium 6 acupuncture points on both forearms has been found to be effective in treating morning sickness and nausea. The practitioner should hold both points for a count of 10, repeating a total of 10 times.

a miscarriage by pressing too hard and dislodging the **placenta**—a specialized, vascular, disk-shaped organ for maternal-fetal gas and nutrient exchange. An explanation of the development of the placenta will demonstrate why massage should not be a concern during the first trimester.

About 1 week after conception, a mass of cells called a *blastocyst* implants in the upper part of the uterus. The blastocyst develops small projections called the *chorionic villi* that insinuate into the uterine lining and extract nourishment. At the end of the first month, the chorionic villi penetrate deep into the uterine lining, becoming a primitive placenta (Figure 2-2).[10] (When a woman is carrying twins or multiple fetuses, there may be more than one placenta; generally, fraternal twins have different placentas, whereas identical twins often share the same one.[10]) Although the placenta does not mature fully until the third month, or the end of the first trimester, it is firmly anchored to the uterine walls by a few weeks into the pregnancy. The placenta is deeply entrenched within the endometrium, and only a traumatic shock to the abdomen could cause serious injury.

Because abdominal massage in all trimesters should be gentle, massage cannot cause placental abruption, in which the placenta is separated from the uterine wall. Massage of a pregnant client's abdomen should be extremely light and involve no more pressure than the weight of the practitioner's hands. The practitioner should use an open-handed effleurage in a clockwise

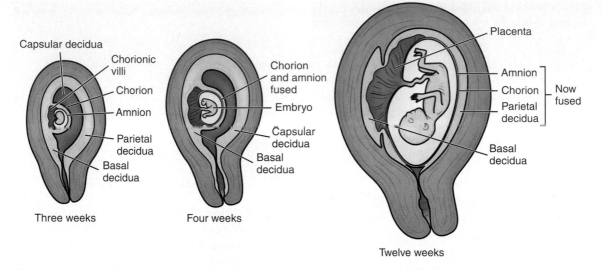

FIGURE 2-2 ■ *Left,* At 3 weeks, the amniotic sac surrounded by chorion and covered with capsular decidua. *Middle,* At 4 weeks, the amnion is in contact with the chorion, and the placenta is embedded in the basal decidua. *Right,* At 12 weeks, the capsular decidua is thinner and atrophied. The chorion is attached to the parietal decidua.

Touch Point

Massage therapy during the first trimester can be a safe and effective way to support the newly pregnant woman. Unfortunately, many spas, resorts, and private offices do not offer massage to women in their first trimester because of the high incidence of miscarriages and nausea—and liability concerns. Considering that appropriate massage is not a contributing factor in miscarriage and that a massage is never performed when a client is nauseous, the remaining reason to avoid first-trimester massage is one of liability. Given the current climate, this is a reasonable concern.

Before one of my trainings, the massage therapists at a renowned golf resort in Georgia did not massage pregnant women in their first trimester. After the training, the administrators reconsidered their former attitude and the resort now offers massage to their first-trimester guests. More spas and resorts may recognize the numerous benefits of this care early in the pregnancy and choose to base their attitudes on science not fear.

direction with a slow, even rhythm; this work will neither cause a miscarriage (see Myth 1) nor dislodge the placenta. Note that permission always should be sought from the pregnant client before massaging her abdomen because this is a very sensitive and emotional area of her body.

If a client is sensitive about skin-to-skin contact, the practitioner's hands should be laid gently on the client's abdomen on top of the sheet. Energetic change can be effected by placement of the practitioner's hands above the client's body within her electromagnetic field. In these ways, the client feels safe and still reaps the benefits of the massage.

Myth 4

The fourth myth is that the feet and hands should not be massaged during pregnancy. Massage on some acupuncture points on the feet, lower legs, and hands is **contraindicated**. Deep, sustained pressure must be avoided in these locations (Figures 2-3 and 2-4). Women generally experience moderate to serious swelling in their feet and legs as pregnancy progresses, and performing lymphatic drainage is always suggested in prenatal massage. Lymphatic drainage will reduce the swelling without damaging sensitive lymph vessels like deeper Swedish massage strokes might do; it is the recommended technique throughout pregnancy and for as long as 3 months postpartum. When working on the feet and legs, the practitioner should remember that the client's blood has an additional clotting factor (fibrinogenic activity) and that deep work might dislodge some emboli.

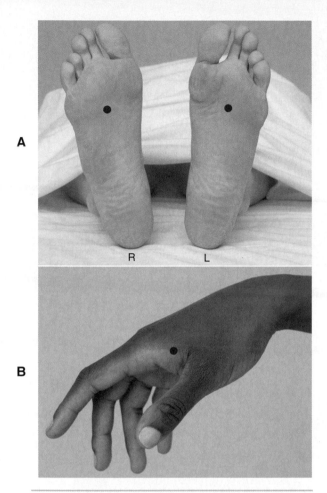

A

B

FIGURE 2-3 ■ **A,** Contraindicated acupuncture point kidney 1 is found on the soles of the feet. **B,** Large intestine 4 is located on the webbing of the thumb.

Myth 5

The final myth is that a pregnant woman should lie only on her left side, whether in bed or on the massage table. Although sleeping on the left side is generally preferred, it is not required and right-side sleeping is sometimes more appropriate. Sleeping on the back is not advised after the first trimester, and when stomach sleeping becomes infeasible as well, the recommended position is known as *sleep on side,* or SOS. This includes the placement of pillows between the woman's knees to keep her legs parallel and prevent pulling on the sacroiliac joint, a pillow under her neck, pillows under her abdomen and lower back if desired, and pillows anywhere else that makes her comfortable.[11]

Women often are encouraged to sleep on their left sides because this position improves blood flow to the placenta,[12] keeps the heavy uterus off the liver, keeps the weight of the growing fetus off the inferior vena cava and aorta, and promotes improved kidney function, which helps to reduce swelling.[11,13] However, a woman's muscles and joints may become sore after she lies on the same side for many months, and it is most important that the expectant mother gets her sleep; for that reason, many care providers also recommend right-side sleeping. Right-side sleeping actually is preferred in cases of heartburn and indigestion because this position allows gravity to empty the stomach at a faster rate,[8] and sometimes the position of the fetus makes right-side lying more comfortable. Sometimes a pregnant woman may sleep on her back with a pillow propping her up and another pillow under her right hip to tilt her slightly to the left.

A pregnant woman should not lie flat on her back after the first trimester because this position can create serious complications such as low blood pressure and a decrease in circulation to the maternal heart and fetus. Decreased circulation occurs when the heavy uterus compresses the larger vessels—the aorta and inferior vena cava. Lying on the back can cause other problems such as backaches, breathing difficulties, digestive disorders such as heartburn, and hemorrhoids. Also, when this position is maintained for too long, the mother often feels short of breath, light-headed, dizzy, faint, and nauseous.[11]

In My Experience...

In my MotherMassage workshop, I address the common myths associated with prenatal massage. The myth that practitioners must avoid abdominal massage during the first trimester is one of the more common misconceptions.

In one of my classes, a student explained that she was told to never massage a pregnant woman's abdomen, particularly in the first trimester. Other students nodded in agreement; they had been taught the same. I explained that as long as the woman gives permission to be touched on her abdomen and the technique is light and appropriate, there is no reason not to provide this soothing touch. I reminded my students that massage does

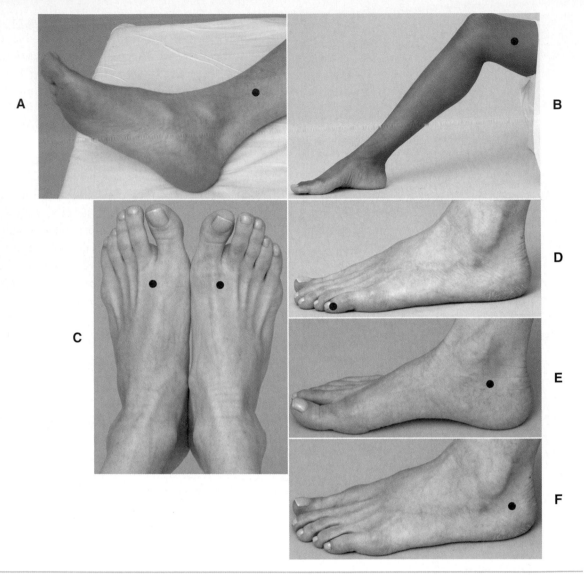

FIGURE 2-4 ■ **A**, Acupuncture point spleen 6, approximately 2 to 3 cm from the anklebone, deep to the tibia, is located on both legs. **B**, Contra-indicated acupuncture point spleen 10 is on the inside of both thighs. **C**, Liver 3 is at the webbing of the big and second toes on both feet. **D**, Bladder 67 is on the outside of the nail of the little toes. **E**, The uterus reflex is located on the inside of the heel. **F**, The ovary reflex is on the outside of both heels.

not cause miscarriage, massage will not create a situation that causes morning sickness when none existed before, and massage will not cause placental abruption.

Summary

Many students approach prenatal massage with misconceptions and misinformation that are fostered by well-intended people who have not studied the anatomy and physiology of pregnancy seriously or who are overly concerned about liability issues. The practitioner must understand the rationale behind these myths and learn the correct approach based on science.

Miscarriage is common during pregnancy but is rarely caused by anything the pregnant women does or avoids doing. By embracing a more healthy lifestyle, such as one that includes bodywork, a woman increases her chances of a successful pregnancy.

Appropriate massage poses no danger during any trimester of pregnancy. This includes gentle abdominal massage and correctly applied foot and leg massage; light lymphatic drainage is the proper technique to use on feet and legs during pregnancy and for as long as 3 months postpartum.

Many women assume that when they are pregnant, they should sleep exclusively on their left sides. Lying on the left side does ease the circulatory burden, but right-side sleeping and back sleeping propped with pillows also can be safe.

References

1. Enkin M, Keirse M, Neilson J, et al: *A guide to effective care in pregnancy and childbirth*, ed 3, Oxford, 2000, Oxford University Press.

2. Lowdermilk DL, Perry SE: *Maternity & women's health care*, ed 8, St. Louis, 2004, Mosby.

3. Gynecology and Obstetrics: Spontaneous abortion (miscarriage). In Beers MH, Porter RS, Jones TV, eds: *The Merck manual of diagnosis*, ed 18, Whitehouse Station, NJ, 2006, Merck.

4. Feldman P, Covington SN: *Facts about miscarriage and the grief it causes*, Minneapolis, 1994, ICEA.

5. Leifer G: *Maternity nursing: an introductory text*, ed 9, St. Louis, 2005, Saunders.

6. Fraser D, Cooper M, eds: *Myles' textbook for midwives*, ed 14, Edinburgh, 2003, Churchill Livingstone.

7. Daly E: *Specialists trying to unravel the mystery of miscarriage,* The New York Times, p F5, F10, February 8, 2005.

8. Sears W, Sears M: *The pregnancy book*, Boston, 1997, Little, Brown.

9. Brody JE: *What could be good about morning sickness? Plenty,* The New York Times, p F7, June 6, 2000.

10. Simkin P, Whalley J, Keppler A: *Pregnancy, childbirth and the newborn*, New York, 1991, Meadowbrook Press.

11. American Pregnancy Association: Sleeping positions during pregnancy, American Pregnancy. Available at http://www.americanpregnancy.org/pregnancyhealth/sleepingpositions.html. Accessed October 2003.

12. O'Malley MO: What's the best sleep position during pregnancy? BabyCenter. Available at http://www.babycenter.com/expert/pregnancy/pregnancysleep/7608.html. Accessed November 2003.

13. Macones G: Sleeping during pregnancy, Kidshealth. Available at http://www.kidshealth.org/parent/pregnancy_newborn/pregnancy/sleep_during_pregnancy.html. Accessed July 2004.

1   What is meant by the term *miscarriage*?

_____

_____

_____

_____

_____

_____

_____

_____

_____

2   Describe when most miscarriages occur and the possible causes.

_____

_____

_____

_____

_____

_____

_____

_____

_____

3   What are some of the symptoms of miscarriage?

_____

_____

_____

_____

_____

_____

_____

_____

_____

4   Is massage safe during the first trimester? Explain some of the misconceptions people hold regarding first-trimester massage therapy.

_____

_____

_____

_____

_____

_____

_____

_____

_____

5   Is it reasonable to massage a pregnant woman while she suffers from nausea or vomiting? When does this nausea usually occur during pregnancy?

_____

_____

_____

_____

_____

_____

_____

_____

_____

6   What are some suggestions for treating morning sickness?

_____

_____

_____

_____

_____

_____

_____

_____

7 Is it ever safe to massage a pregnant woman's abdomen? If yes, describe the techniques that would be used.

_____

_____

_____

_____

_____

_____

_____

_____

8 What is the most effective and appropriate bodywork to use on a pregnant woman's feet and legs? Please describe why this technique is the safest bodywork for her feet and legs.

_____

_____

_____

_____

_____

_____

_____

_____

_____

9 Describe the benefits of lying on the left side during pregnancy.

_____

_____

_____

_____

_____

_____

_____

_____

10 Is it ever safe for a pregnant woman to sleep flat on her back after the first trimester? Why or why not?

_____

_____

_____

_____

_____

_____

_____

_____

11 Can a pregnant woman safely sleep on her right side?

_____

_____

_____

_____

_____

_____

_____

_____

_____

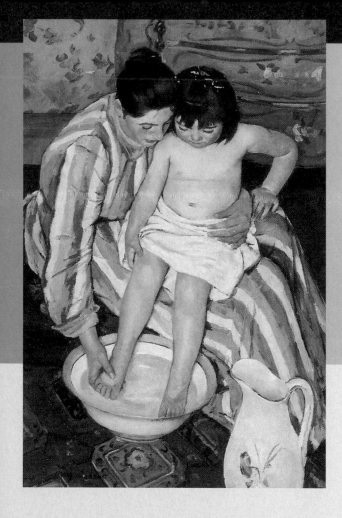

CHAPTER 3

General Prenatal Massage Guidelines

Objectives

On completion of this chapter, the student will be able to do the following:

1 Understand bodywork techniques and determine whether the techniques in use are appropriate for prenatal massage

2 Understand the role the massage practitioner plays during a client's pregnancy

3 Learn the most efficient way to set up the treatment room

4 Drape the client, safely turn the pregnant client on the massage table, and move the client on and off the massage table safely and easily

5 Use effective and proper practitioner body mechanics

6 Understand the most effective way to position clients each trimester

7 Recognize what is suitable pressure during the treatment

8 Allocate time per treatment

9 Understand the importance of pretreatment evaluations

10 Learn which essential oils are safe and which are contraindicated

11 Learn which massage oils are most effective during pregnancy

12 Learn the differences between special treatment tables and pregnancy cushions

13 Learn what additional supplies will be needed for a prenatal practice

Key Terms

Abortifacient	Inferior vena cava	Shiatsu
Active exercise	Ischemic	Side-lying
Acupressure	Joint mobilization	Spindle cells
Anterior tilt	Lomilomi	Strain/counterstrain
Applied kinesiology	Manual lymphatic drainage	Supine
Appropriate	Myofascial release	Swedish massage
Aromatherapy	Passive exercise	Thrombosis
Blood clots	Pitting edema	Time allocation
Body mechanics	Polarity	Toxic
Craniosacral therapy	Posterior pelvic tilt	Toxoplasmosis
Draping	Preeclampsia	Tragerwork
Emmenagogue	Prone	Transverse abdominis
Energy work	Proprioceptive work	Trigger points
Essential oils	Recumbent	Trimester positioning
Golgi tendon organs	Reflexology	Tsubos
Homan check	Reiki	Tui Na

Bodywork Techniques

Hands-on learning is best taught in a classroom setting by an instructor who can guide and correct the students. Thus practitioners can hone their skills more efficiently if the techniques described here are used in conjunction with a professional class.[1]

The somatic practices in this book are varied and eclectic and should be used as a strong foundation for the practitioner's personal techniques. Individual prenatal practices will look and feel different from others because each practitioner's background, training, and continuing education are different. The more techniques practitioners learn, the more effective their prenatal treatments will be.

Appropriate bodywork techniques respect the dynamic physiological changes the pregnant woman undergoes and recognize the specific precautions and contraindications of prenatal massage. Practitioners should analyze their techniques to determine whether certain compensations and changes have to be made to be safe during pregnancy. This could mean that some strokes of a specific bodywork have to be eliminated, adapted, or modified. For example, traditional **Swedish massage** is contraindicated on a pregnant woman's legs after the first trimester because the deep pressure

might damage sensitive anchoring filaments and create more water filtration into the area that needs to be drained.[2] Yet Swedish massage is certainly appropriate on other parts of a pregnant woman's body. Another example is positioning modification. Craniosacral technique, which is very effective during pregnancy and for labor preparation, is usually offered with the client in a **supine** position, or lying on the back, with the upper body only slightly elevated. To use craniosacral therapy during pregnancy, especially in the later stages, the client has to be in a **recumbent** or semisitting position, with her torso at an angle at least 45 degrees and legs and feet elevated. Craniosacral therapy could also be tried with the client on her side. Aestheticians also have to adjust their chairs when giving a facial to a pregnant woman in late pregnancy by sitting her more upright.

Appropriate prenatal massage and bodywork techniques are as follows:

- **Applied kinesiology** evaluates body function through dynamic muscle testing.[3]
- **Craniosacral therapy,** developed by Dr. John E. Upledger, is a gentle manipulation that locates and corrects imbalances in the craniosacral system, which is made up of the brain, spinal cord, cerebrospinal fluid, dural membrane, cranial bones, and sacrum. The effect of this system is realized to a large

extent by the body's innate healing and self-correcting abilities.[4]

- **Energy work,** such as **Polarity** therapy and **Reiki,** work with the human energy biofield to encourage balance.[4]
- **Joint mobilization** takes each joint through its full range of motion to locate resistance. The joint is moved opposite the tightness until there is a release.[4]
- **Lomilomi** is an ancient Hawaiian technique brought to westerners' attention by Aunty (a term of affection and respect) Margaret K. Machado. She calls lomilomi "the loving touch—a connection between heart, hands, souls with the source of all life."[5]
- **Manual lymphatic drainage,** a specific form of physiotherapy used to empty and decompress lymph pathways, supports the immune system and encourages toxin removal.[6] This light stroking can always be used on a pregnant woman's legs even during the first trimester and for at least 3 months postpartum. It is advisable to employ lymph drainage protocol on her hands and arms if they are swollen, or if she has carpal tunnel syndrome.
- **Myofascial release** uses slow, stretching movements to evaluate and relieve fascial restrictions.
- **Passive** and **active exercises** help relax and strengthen muscles and joints by activating stretch receptors. Passive movements are performed by the bodyworker as the client relaxes. Active exercises require the client's participation.
- **Proprioceptive work** helps to balance and strengthen the muscles by relaxing hypertonic muscles and strengthening hypotonic muscles. The work is primarily done with the neuromuscular **spindle cells** found within muscle tissue and the **Golgi tendon organs** in the tendons close to the musculotendinous junction.[3]
- **Reflexology** uses various methods of touch to stimulate specific points on the hands or feet that reflex to particular organs, to maintain optimum health and restore energy throughout the body.[4]
- **Shiatsu,** or **acupressure,** is an ancient technique of traditional Chinese medicine (TCM)

that presses on particular points, called **Tsubos,** to release stagnated energy thought to create "dis-ease." This **ischemic** compression is never done on a pregnant woman's legs after the first trimester and for at least 3 months postpartum.

- **Strain/counterstrain** is a technique designed to relieve muscle dysfunction and pain. A position of relief is found and held for 90 seconds. This technique was developed by Dr. Lawrence Jones.[3]
- **Swedish massage** increases circulation, brings nutrition to muscles, encourages a more rapid absorption of waste products, and relieves pain and discomfort. The strokes of Swedish massage are effleurage, pétrissage, friction, tapotement, and vibration.
- **Tragerwork,** developed by Dr. Milton Trager, is a way of teaching movement reeducation and neuromuscular release. Dr. Trager's approach is one of educating the client rather than treating her.[4]
- **Trigger point release** compresses the trigger points, which are highly sensitive areas within muscles, ligaments, tendons, and fascia, that can cause referred pain elsewhere in the body. Dr. Janet Travell, who pioneered trigger point injection therapy, described trigger points as "…a small, hypersensitive region from which impulses bombard the central nervous system and give rise to referred pain."[4] Trigger point therapy was popularized by Bonnie Prudden.
- **Tui Na,** an ancient system of bodywork, uses a variety of techniques, such as grasping, rolling, pressing, rubbing, vibrating, pushing, squeezing, twisting, tapping, and dragging, to treat injuries of the soft and connective tissues and balance qi energy.

The Role of the Massage Practitioner

The changes in an expectant woman's body, especially a first time mother, can create excitement, confusion, exhilaration, fear, concern, worry, and joy all at the same time. The bodyworker is in a unique position to be nonjudgmental, supportive, and nurturing during this special time. A practitioner's ministrations can promote deep relaxation, minimize the deleterious effects of stress, and reduce tensions and anxieties.[7] Hands-on care can relieve the common discomforts of pregnancy, prepare the client for labor, speed up labor, and promote a faster postpartum recovery.[8] Massage and bodywork also encourage more kinesthetic awareness and greater acceptance of her ever-changing body.

In addition, practitioners can educate clients on childbearing choices and provide resources for others they may not know. Practitioners can also refer them to other professionals, including traditional medical professionals and those who practice complementary medicine, who can help them during the prenatal and postpartum stages. Bodyworkers provide a safe haven where women with all sorts of emotional needs can feel free to express themselves.

The nurturing environment massage provides can be unlike any other care a pregnant woman receives during her pregnancy and recovery. Appropriate touch gives these deserving women the unconditional physical and emotional support they need to ensure a healthy and happy birth outcome.

Treatment Room Set-up

The treatment room should be a well-ventilated space with adequate, soft lighting. The decor of the room is up to you, but a few helpful tips can make the room more agreeable for pregnant clients. Because working memory declines during pregnancy and postpartum[9] (it does come back), the treatment room should be set up in such a way that will help women remember to take their things with them when they leave. Everything should be kept together to make it easier for the client and practitioner to scan the room after treatment to make sure nothing has been left behind. One area should be allocated for clothing, shoes, and jewelry. Hooks with hangers can be placed on the wall for clothing. A waist-high shelf for shoes will make it easier for her to reach them without having to bend down. Another shelf with a small dish or hooks could be used for jewelry. A chair in this dressing area allows the client to sit while

she dresses or undresses. Any rugs in the treatment room and bathroom should be secured firmly to the underlying padding and floor to prevent any accidents.

Correct Draping and Client Turning

The massage table should be covered with one full-sized sheet and another full-sized sheet folded at the foot of the table (Figure 3-1). A large towel should be placed on the foot of the table. If the client is going to be in a **side-lying** position, a pillow should be placed under the sheet at the head of the table. Once the client is on the table, she should be covered with the folded sheet and the towel. The towel

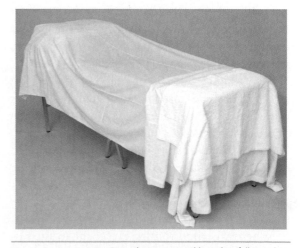

FIGURE 3-1 ■ Cover the massage table with a full-size sheet and place a second folded sheet at the foot of the table.

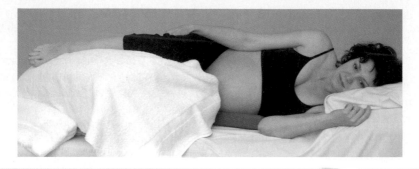

FIGURE 3-2 ■ Pillows between the client's knees should be high enough that her legs are parallel. Her hip, knee, and ankle should be on the same horizontal level to prevent pulling on the ligaments of the sacroiliac joint and developing a sore lower back.

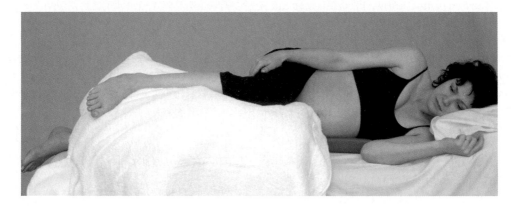

FIGURE 3-3 ■ An alternative to having her legs parallel is to place her top leg forward on pillows. Her hip, knee, and ankle should be on the same horizontal plane.

is used to cover her breasts when her abdomen is massaged and to secure the sheet in place. Any robe or cover she may be wearing should be removed.

Pillows of various sizes are placed between her knees and ankles, under her head, under her abdomen, at the small of her back, and in front of her chest or anywhere that makes her feel more comfortable. The pillows between her knees should be high enough that her legs are parallel (Figure 3-2). Some women prefer to have just the top leg supported by pillows (Figure 3-3). Three landmarks should be on the same level: hip, knee, and ankle. In this position, her sacroiliac joint stays neutral and her back will not hurt. (Many clients sleep with pillows between their knees and still wake up with a sore back because the pillows are not high enough and the weight of her leg pulls on the sacroiliac joint.)

When it is time to turn the client to the opposite side, all extra pillows should be removed. The practitioner can hold the sheet and towel and then ask her to turn face down on her hands and knees. If her wrists or hands are painful or weak, she can roll on her elbows and knees (Figure 3-4). The client should not roll onto her abdomen but should assume a **posterior pelvic tilt,** which is a preferred position of the pelvis that elongates the lumbar spine and shortens the over-stretched abdominal muscles as she turns. When she lies on the other side, all pillows can be replaced.

If the client is on the table in either a **prone,** or face up, or **supine** position, she should be **draped** (or covered) so she is lying between the sheets with a towel securing the top sheet. Pillows should be appropriately placed. In early pregnancy, a prone position can be comfortable, but some women have sensitive breasts. A rolled towel placed under her shoulders provides enough elevation to relieve the pressure on her breasts. In a supine position, particularly as the pregnancy advances, the client

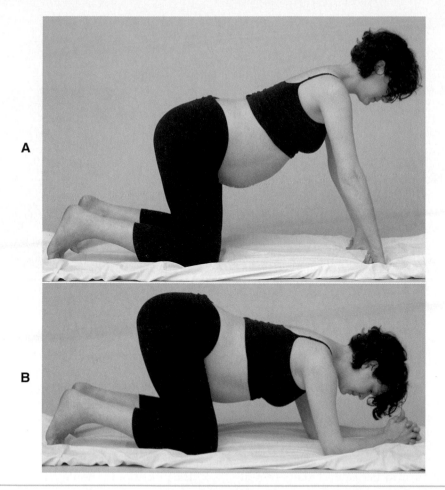

FIGURE 3-4 ■ **A**, To turn the client on the massage table, she should turn face down onto her hands and knees. **B**, If her wrists or hands are painful, she can roll on her elbows and knees. She can do a posterior pelvic tilt in this position. She should avoid rolling directly on her abdomen.

must be in a semisitting or **recumbent** position, slightly tilted to the left. This keeps the uterus off the larger abdominal blood vessels, the aorta and interior vena cava. Pillows placed under her legs and feet should raise them above heart level. This encourages lymphatic drainage and eases the pressure on the lower back. A wedge under her right hip, tilting her slightly to the left, relieves pressure on the abdominal vessels.

Moving the Client on and off the Table Safely and Easily

A step stool (which should be cleaned regularly) will make moving on and off the massage table easier for those women who feel ungainly and clumsy, which is a very common feeling during pregnancy. The client should know where the stool is placed once the massage is over so she does not miss her step or trip over it.

It is very important to keep the client's lumbar spine and pelvis stabilized while getting on and off the massage table and while changing positions on the table. The woman should recruit her **transverse abdominis** muscle, which is the most intrinsic abdominal muscle, by pulling her navel in toward her spine as she makes these transitions (see Chapter 5 for a detailed description of the transverse abdominis muscle). As the client lies down on the table, she should pull in her abdominal muscles.

After the treatment is over, all of the pillows and wedges should be moved out of the way. The sheet around her feet should be removed and all excess lubrication should be wiped off her feet.

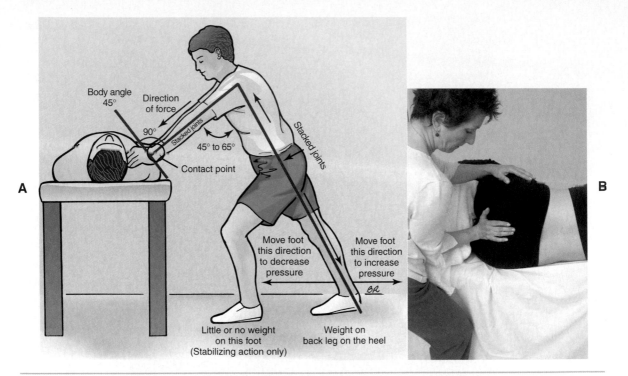

FIGURE 3-5 ■ **A,** The practitioner should bend the knees slightly as weight is shifted from back leg to front leg for the massage. The practitioner's strength comes from the legs not the upper torso. (From Fritz S: *Mosby's fundamentals of therapeutic massage,* enhanced reprint, ed 3, St. Louis, 2005, Mosby.) **B,** To perform an effective sacral lift without straining, the practitioner should lean into the client and lean against the massage table. The practitioner's strength comes from legs and abdominal core muscles. Arms and the upper torso should be relaxed.

The client can turn to her side (if she is not already on her side) and take a deep breath. As she inhales, she will pull her transverse abdominis muscle in toward her spine and can then push herself up slowly with her hands and sit on the edge of the table for a few seconds so her blood pressure can stabilize. If she needs assistance, the bodyworker can stand in front of her and help her up from the side-lying position by supporting her shoulders.

Practitioners should make sure that pregnant and postpartum clients never "jack-knife" on or off the table because this will compromise lower back stability.

Practitioner Body Mechanics

The treatment table should be at a comfortable height for the practitioner. When the client is in a side-lying position, the table may be raised a notch or two because the direction of the massage strokes is horizontal rather than vertical.

The practitioner should be relaxed and should breathe normally. As the practitioner stands at the side of the treatment table, knees should be bent slightly so weight can be shifted from the back leg to the front leg for the massage. A practitioner's strength comes from the legs and not the upper torso. To get a stronger pressure, the practitioner bends the elbows into the body and leans into the stroke (Figure 3-5, **A**). When the massage allows, practitioners can face and lean into the table with knees still slightly bent, continuing to shift their weight from leg to leg. Shoulders, arms, and hands of the bodyworker should all stay relaxed. Recruiting the transverse abdominis muscle can help the practitioner maintain core stability.

For clients in late pregnancy, bodyworkers will perform pelvic tilts and sacral lifts to help clients elongate the lumbar spine and to relieve congestion in the pelvic floor. These techniques require a lot of strength on the part of the practitioner, and proper **body mechanics** are essential to accomplish them effectively (Figure 3-5, **B**).

As previously mentioned, practitioners should use their legs as the base of their force, stabilizing their core muscles and keeping their arms relaxed. Wrists should be as neutral as possible, and other parts of the hands and arms, such as fists, pisiform bones, knuckles, or forearms, can be alternately used.

When a practitioner uses circular kneading or friction with the thumbs, they should be held as close to the midline of the hands as possible. The saddle joint can take a beating over the years from constant use and thumbs should be protected. Carpal tunnel syndrome, de Quervain's syndrome, numbness, and tingling are also the bane of bodyworkers who use poor body mechanics. Practitioners should keep their heads back and chins down in a more neutral position to ensure hand longevity.

Trimester Positioning

Trimester positioning is the appropriate placement of the pregnant client on the massage table. Because client safety and comfort are paramount during the treatment, the client's position at all times should avoid uterine compression of the larger abdominal vessels, the aorta and **inferior vena cava.** This would naturally occur as the uterus begins to take on some bulk during the second or third trimesters with a singleton and perhaps earlier on with multiples.

During the first trimester, prone, supine, side-lying, and sitting positions are all safe. In early pregnancy, a **prone** (lying face down) position is still comfortable; however if the woman's breasts are tender, a rolled towel can be placed under her shoulders to elevate her chest and relieve pressure. A bolster or pillows can be placed under her ankles to relax the muscles of her legs and enhance circulation.

In a supine position, the client should be semi-sitting or recumbent and tilted slightly to the left (which keeps the uterus off the larger abdominal vessels). Her cervical spine should be supported with a pillow, and her legs and feet should be elevated above heart level with bolsters, cushions, or pillows. Her feet should be the same height as her knees to ease the pressure on her lower back, encourage circulation and lymph drainage, ease

varicose veins, and reduce swelling, although swelling usually is not a concern in the first trimester. Pillows should be placed between her knees and ankles (legs parallel to each other) and under her neck, which will provide a comfortable side-lying position.

During the second trimester, the woman's body starts to assume a pregnant shape with a visible swelling in the abdomen, larger breasts, shortened lower back muscles, and an anterior pelvic tilt. At this time, prone positioning directly on the treatment table is uncomfortable and not recommended. With the use of modular bodyCushions, however, prone positioning can be safely offered. The side-lying position should be augmented with pillows, bolsters, or cushions between her legs, with her hips, knees, and ankles on the same horizontal level, and under her cervical spine (see Figure 3-2). Other women prefer pillows placed under the forward top leg, with the bottom leg extended behind her (see Figure 3-3). The pillows should still be high enough that her hip, knee, and ankle are on the same horizontal plane to keep from straining the sacroiliac joint. Some women also like to hold a pillow or small rolled towel in front of their chests, and others feel more secure with a small wedge or hand towel rolled in the small of their backs. Whatever makes the client feel safe and comfortable is in order.

In a supine position, the woman's torso should be elevated at an angle between 45 and 70 degrees so she is semisitting and all abdominal weight is off the great abdominal vessels (Figure 3-6). Once she is 18 to 20 weeks pregnant, supine (flat) positioning must be avoided. A small wedge or pillow can be placed under her right hip to tilt her slightly to the left. Additional pillows can be under her cervical spine if necessary. More wedges or pillows can also be placed under her legs to elevate them. Knees and feet should be on the same horizontal plane to relieve lower back pressure and encourage lymph drainage and venous blood flow to relieve the pressure on varicose veins and hemorrhoids.

Sitting at the head or foot of the table is also a comfortable position at any time during the pregnancy. A wooden stool or a stool with wheels that lock can be used, with a pillow on the stool to add comfort. A larger pillow can go in front of the client's abdomen and under her

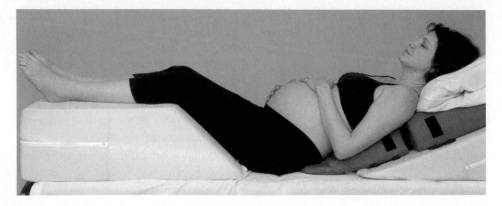

FIGURE 3-6 ■ In a semisitting or recumbent position, elevate the client's torso—from her hips—at an angle no less than 45 degrees and no more than 70 degrees. Some women also like a gentle tilt to the left side, which can be achieved by placing a small wedge under her right hip.

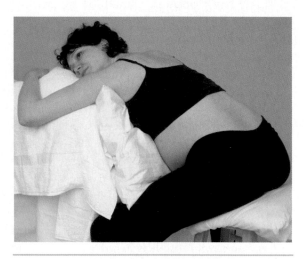

FIGURE 3-7 ■ In a sitting position, enough pillows should be placed under her head so she can comfortably lean over without straining her neck. A pillow can be placed in front of her abdomen for extra support and on the stool if necessary.

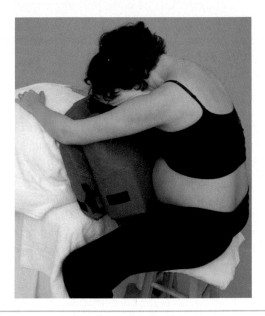

FIGURE 3-8 ■ A face cradle makes a sitting massage very comfortable and prevents hyperflexion of the neck.

chest. An adequate amount of pillows can be put on the table so she can comfortably lean over without straining her neck (Figure 3-7). A face cradle, a headrest, or the bodyCushions can also be used (Figure 3-8).

By her third trimester, a woman's center of gravity moves anteriorly with shortened lower back muscles and an exaggerated lordotic curve. This **anterior tilt**, or displacement of the pelvis anteriorly, is caused by the forward shifting of her center of gravity and further impedes femoral absorption resulting in sore, achy, and swollen legs and feet. Side-lying positioning, as described previously, is very comfortable at this time. The use of the bodyCushions for prone positioning is also

recommended if the client feels comfortable and the practitioner uses them appropriately. In a supine position, as previously mentioned, care must be taken to avoid any compression of the great abdominal vessels, so placing a wedge under the client's right hip and tilting her to the left is suggested. Her torso (from her hips) must be supported at an angle between 45 to 70 degrees and her legs and feet should be adequately elevated. Sitting massage (not to be confused with chair massage tables that are unsupportive during pregnancy, do not conform to the pregnant contour, and do not provide lymphatic drainage) is also safe and comfortable for the pregnant woman in her third trimester who cannot use the massage table. Pillows and supports should be well placed to provide maximum relaxation.

The Amount of Pressure to Use during Treatment

A client's needs may be different each time she comes for treatment and bodyworkers may have to adjust their touch. Pregnancy is not a pathological condition, and the pressure used should be to the pregnant woman's comfort level. Practitioners can continue to use firm pressure and deep tissue techniques (except on the legs and abdomen) on women who are used to receiving deep bodywork. Although fibrinogenic activity does not start until the early second trimester, it is still important to massage her legs and feet using light lymphatic drainage pressure even during early pregnancy. It is also a good idea to advise clients before treatment that the leg massage is going to be light.

If there is swelling in her hands or if she suffers from carpal tunnel syndrome or de Quervain syndrome, the arm and hand massage should start with light lymphatic drainage to help reduce swelling.

As the pregnancy advances, weight-bearing structures are going to be particularly sore and sensitive. Although the release of trigger points and myofascial restrictions are important, care must be taken to start each of the deep techniques lightly and then get progressively deeper following her breathing.

Allocating Treatment Time

Time allocation is the amount of time spent massaging a body part during the massage. Each time a client comes in for an appointment, her body will have changed. Pregnancy is not a static condition; this is one of the exciting aspects of working with this population. The pregnant woman may have had a growth spurt that has placed more stress on her lumbar spine and hip joints. The fetus may have started descending, and symptoms may now be primarily those of the lower digestive tract and lower back instead of the upper digestive tract. These changes indicate that each time a client comes for treatment another assessment of her needs must be done.

The majority of the massage time should be spent treating those areas that need the most work. During the first trimester, the hour-long massage can be evenly spread among all major body parts. Special attention can be paid to treating her fatigue, morning sickness, tender breasts, and hormonal balancing.

During the second trimester, most women feel energized and are content with how their body looks and feels. Many of the symptoms of the first trimester have subsided, and there is a joyfulness and vitality about their pregnancy. There is also an accompanying growing discomfort in her back, legs, hips, and pelvis as her posture starts to shift anteriorly. She may experience breast tenderness, swelling in the extremities, and respiratory and digestive disorders.

The third trimester is fraught with conflicting emotions and physical discomforts. As the fetus gets bigger, postural shifting creates aches and soreness throughout the woman's supporting musculature and myofascia. During this time of maximal fetal growth, the woman's abdominal muscles weaken and separate to accommodate the expanding uterus; this accommodation is called the *diastasis recti*. Increased interstitial fluid carried by weakened vessels promotes swelling of her legs, feet, and sometimes hands. Digestive disorders, such as constipation, heartburn, and hemorrhoids, add to her abdominal pressure. As labor gets closer, some women experience increased levels of stress and anxiety.

Work on the pregnant woman's weight-bearing joints and relief of edema should be the focus of the final trimester. Myofascial tilts, sacral lifts, and lymphatic drainage are helpful during this time. This is also the time to encourage her to use proper body mechanics to reduce additional strain and to recruit her transverse abdominals to support her lumbar spinal segment.

Pretreatment Evaluations

Before each treatment the client's current condition should be evaluated to ensure that she is a candidate for massage. The bodyworker should explain the importance of these pretreatment evaluations so the client is aware of what is being done.

Evaluation 1

The first assessment comes from TCM and is to be used only as an evaluation of the health of the pregnancy not a determinant for treatment. According to the Chinese ancient healers, the arch of the foot can be subdivided into nine equal segments, each representing one of the 9 months of pregnancy. If the health of the pregnancy changes at any time, a change in complexion of the foot, a contusion, a hardening, redness, or clear skin change will show on both feet during the month the change occurs. This change does not tell the practitioner if the problem is maternal or fetal nor does it explain what the problem may be. The only purpose this evaluation serves is to give an overview of the general health of the pregnancy (Figure 3-9).

If a bilateral change in skin tone or complexion on the woman's arches is seen, the bodyworker should find out whether the client has new shoes that might be causing an irritation to her feet. A pregnant woman's feet often grow. The medial arch often drops, so skin friction from a new pair of shoes is not uncommon. If this is not the explanation, the practitioner can then simply ask, without alarming the client, how she is feeling. Since many fetal problems are maternally asymptomatic, she may admit to feeling fine. If, however, the problem is maternal, she may mention that she does not feel right. She should be advised to mention this to her care provider at the next prenatal check-up. The practitioner should take care to not alarm the client, but correct use of this tool can provide an overall check on her pregnancy.

Evaluation 2

Before each treatment, the practitioner should assess whether a client's normal swelling has become an unhealthy condition such as preeclampsia. **Preeclampsia** is a condition characterized by swelling of the face and hands, high blood pressure, excessive fluid retention, and protein in the urine. If left untreated, it can cause serious maternal and fetal health problems.[10] **Pitting edema** usually indicates that the swelling is not normal and her

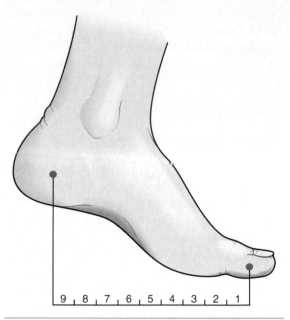

FIGURE 3-9 ■ According to traditional Chinese medicine, the arch of the foot can be subdivided into 9 equal segments that represent the 9 months of pregnancy. A change in the skin may indicate a change in the health of the pregnancy at the month it occurs. This pretreatment evaluation offers practitioners an overview of the general health of the pregnancy but should never be used or interpreted as a diagnosis.

kidneys are unable to filter the blood toxins. Massage is contraindicated when pitting edema is present.

The test for pitting edema is performed on both of her legs just above the ankle and is shown in Figure 3-10. The practitioner should press a finger into the area and slowly count to 5. If the indentation does not fill in within 10 to 30 seconds, or if the ischemic region has not become red again, the massage should not begin and the client should contact her care provider. Swelling during pregnancy is normal, particularly in advanced pregnancy, but pitting edema may indicate a serious problem that requires immediate attention.

Evaluations 3 and 4

By late pregnancy, venous stasis contributes to the potential of **blood clots** or **thrombosis** forming in the lower extremities. Two evaluations must be performed to check for the presence of any clots. Before placing the pillows between a client's legs in a side-lying position, the bodyworker should

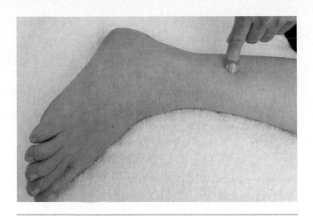

FIGURE 3-10 ■ To test for pitting edema, the practitioner presses above the client's ankle for a count of 5. If the impression does not disappear after 10 to 30 seconds, do not massage.

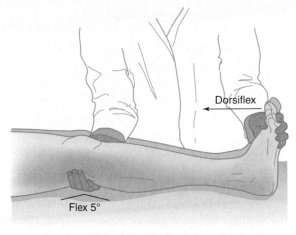

FIGURE 3-11 ■ The Homan sign or check is performed before each massage to test for the presence of blood clots in the calf. The client's knee should be flexed 5 degrees and her foot gently dorsiflexed. If she experiences pain in her calf, do not massage. This evaluation should be performed on both legs. (From Leifer G: Maternity nursing: an introductory text, ed 9, St Louis, 2005, Saunders.)

lightly run his or her hands up and down the backs of the client's legs, feeling for any localized swelling, heat, redness, warmth, muscle contraction, or sensitive dermatomes. The skin above the site of the thrombosis will be tender.

The other assessment involves passively dorsiflexing the client's feet to test for the presence of thrombi in her calves. This examination, the **Homan check** or **Homan sign**[11] is shown in Figure 3-11. If the client tests positive on either of these tests, the practitioner should not proceed with the massage and the client should contact her care provider immediately.

Aromatherapy: The Use of Essential Oils

Many practitioners enjoy using **aromatherapy**, or the use of essential oils, in their work, and many clients reap the benefits. However, during pregnancy, a woman's sense of smell is enhanced[12] and some clients develop an aversion and heightened sensitivity to certain aromas. It is advisable to ask clients how they feel about the use of aromatherapy. It is also a good idea to wait until the second trimester before adding essential oils to massage oil[13] and to dilute it to one-half the dose (2 to 3 drops) to 10 ml carrier oil when doing so.[14]

Essential oils must be pure and not tainted with any preservatives that might be contraindicated during pregnancy. Practitioners should know the source of the essential oils.

Essential Oils that Are Safe During Pregnancy

Although essential oils should never be added to your lubricant when treating a pregnant client, the following list includes some herbs and oils that are safe after the first trimester. The practitioner should confirm that the sources of these **essential oils** are all natural and that the oils are pure.[14] Some beneficial carrier oils and creams for the following oils are jojoba oil, Shea butter, and cocoa butter:[13-15]

- Bergamot (*Citrus bergamia*)—Use only in late pregnancy. Avoid direct sunlight. Bergamot eases depression, reduces stress, and enhances sleep.
- Cypress (*Cupressus sempervirens*)—Use diluted only. Cypress enhances circulation and relieves tension.
- Geranium (*Pelargonium graveolens*)—Use only in late pregnancy. Geranium improves circulation and respiration and relieves anxiety, stress, and depression.
- Grapefruit (*Citrus paradisi*)—Avoid direct sunlight. Grapefruit helps remove excess fluid and treats depression and stress.
- Juniper (*Juniperus communis*)—Use only in late pregnancy. Avoid use in a client with high blood pressure. Juniper relieves muscle soreness, anxiety, and stress.

- Lavender (Lavandin) *(Lavandula x burnatii)*—Use only in late pregnancy. Lavender treats emotional imbalances and stress and provides muscle pain relief.
- Lemon (Lemon Yellow) *(Citrus limonum)*—Use only when highly diluted. Avoid direct sunlight. Lemon may irritate sensitive skin, but it enhances digestion and circulation, relieves nausea, and promotes mental clarity.
- Mandarin (Red or Green) *(Citrus reticulate)*—Mandarin treats stretch marks and enhances digestion and circulation.
- Neroli (Orange Blossom) *(Citrus aurantium)*—Neroli nourishes skin, heals scars and stretch marks, and has antianxiety properties.
- Orange (Sweet) *(Citrus aurantium)*—Orange increases circulation, relieves stress and tension, and is uplifting.
- Peppermint *(Mentha piperita)*—Use in late pregnancy only. Avoid use in clients with high blood pressure. Peppermint must be diluted. It treats nausea and joint and muscle pain, eases mild depression, and makes an excellent foot massage lotion.
- Petitgrain (Bergamot or Mandarin) *(Citrus aurantium bergamia* or *citrus reticuata)*—Petitgrain is relaxing and stress-relieving.
- Roman chamomile *(Anthemis nobilis)*—Use in late pregnancy only. It acts as an antiinflammatory and treats tension, headaches, migraines, and insomnia.
- Rose *(Rosa centifolia)*—Use after the second trimester. "The queen of essential oils," rose is used for skin care, treats grief or a broken heart, and relieves stress, anxiety, and depression.
- Rosewood *(Aniba rosaeaodora)*—Rosewood is good for scars and wrinkles and is uplifting.
- Spearmint *(Mentha spicata)*—Use only in late pregnancy. Spearmint eases headaches, relieves depression, and is calming.

Contraindicated Herbs and Oils

Box 3-1 includes herbs and oils that need to be avoided during pregnancy. Many of them are **abortifacient** oils and may cause a miscarriage, whereas others are **emmenagogues**, which are herbs that stimulate menstruation. The rest of the herbs and oils are either irritating or **toxic** (poisonous) or contain compounds with hormone-like properties. Although there is no conclusive evidence on the effects of these oils and herbs, it would be wise to avoid them during pregnancy. Another word of caution: essential oils should never be taken orally or swallowed during pregnancy.[16] Those herbs normally used for cooking purposes can be used in small amounts.[15-17]

Specialized Treatment Tables, Pillows, and Cushions

Professional consumer items are also starting to appear in the market place as prenatal massage gains in popularity. Tables with cut-out holes and specialized pillows and cushions are now available for practitioners to use with their pregnant clients. Practitioners must make sure these items are safe and comfortable for their clients.

As previously mentioned, during the first trimester, pregnant clients can be safely positioned prone, supine, side-lying, semisitting, or sitting. Once the client's pregnancy starts to show, prone positioning may be uncomfortable without proper support because of a potential increase in intrauterine pressure, exacerbating the lordotic curve, and lack of support of the suspended uterine ligaments. Supine positioning is a concern once there is substantial anterior weight to the uterus. Supine positioning in latter stages of pregnancy can dangerously compress the major abdominal vessels, thereby elevating maternal blood pressure and causing fetal hypoxia.

Tables with cut-out holes and enlarged foam pillows with contours to facilitate prone and supine positioning are not recommended. In a prone position, the tables with cut-outs do not encourage a posterior pelvic tilt to elongate the lumbar spine but will compress the lower back instead. The table offers no support of the uterine ligaments and may increase intrauterine pressure when sufficient force is applied to the client's lower back and pelvis. Breast tenderness is compounded on these tables, and the abdominal hole only accommodates

BOX 3-1 *Herbs and Oils Contraindicated in Pregnancy*[16]

Almond (bitter) (Amygdalus communis amara)
Aniseed (Pimpinella anisum)
Angelica (Angelica archangelica)
Basil (Sweet or Sanctum Tulsi) (Ocimum basilicum, Ocimum sanctum)
Bay leaves (Laurus nobilis)
Birch (Betula alleghaniensis)
Black pepper (Piper nigrum)
Blessed thistle (Carbenia benedicta)
Boldo leaf (Peumus boldus)
Buchu (Barosma betulina)
Calamus (Calamus aromaticus)
Camphor (Cinnamomum camphora)
Cassia (Cinnamomum cassia)
Chamomile (Blue, Roman, Wild) (Tanacetum annuum, Anthemis nobilis, Ormenis multicolis)
Cinnamon (Bark, Leave, Cassia) (Cinnamomum verum, cassia)
Clary sage (Salvia sclarea)
Clove (Eugenia caryophyllata)
Black cohosh (Cimicifuga racemosa)
Blue cohosh (Caulophyllum thalictroides)
Cottonwood (Gossypium herbaceum)
Couchgrass (Agropyrum repens)
Crampbark (Viburnum opulus)
Elecampane (Inula graveolens)
Fennel (Foeniculum vulgare dulce)
Fenugreek seed (Trigonella foenum-graecum)
Fir (Douglas) (Pseudotsuga Douglasii)
Ginger (Zingiber officinalis)
Ginseng (Panax quinquefolius)
Golden seal (Hydrastis Canadensis)
Horseradish (Cochlearia Armoracia)
Hyssop (Hyssopus officinalis)
Jaborandi leaf (Pilocarpus jaborandi)
Jasmine (Jasminum officinale and sambac)

Juniper (Juniperus communis)
Lemongrass (Cymbopogon citrates)
Marjoram (Sweet) (Origanum marjorana)
Melissa (Melissa officinalis)
Motherwort (Leonurus cardiaca)
Mugwort (Artemisia vulgaris)
Mustard (Brassica)
Myrrh (Commiphora myrrha)
Nightshade (Black, Deadly) (Solanum nigrum, Atropa belladonna)
Nutmeg (Myristica fragrans)
Oregano (Corydothymus capitatus)
Parsley seed (Petroselinum sativum)
Pennyroyal (Mentha pulegium)
Peppermint (Mentha piperita)
Pine (Sea, Cembra) (Pinus pinaster, pinus cembra)
Rosemary (Cineol, Highland, Verbenone) (Rosmarinus officinalis, officinalis ct. verbenone)
Rue (Ruta graveolens)
Sage (Salvia officinalis)
Sassafras (Sassafras officinale)
Savine (Sabina cacumina)
Savory (Summer, Winter) (Satureia hortensis, Montana)
Shepherd's purse (Capsella bursa-pastoris)
Southernwood (Artemisia abrotanum)
Stinging nettle (Urtica urens)
Tansy (Tanacetum vulgare)
Thuja (Thuja occidentalis)
Thyme (Field, Thymol, Linalol and Thuyanol) (Thymus serpyllum, zygis, linalol, thuyanol)
Valerian (Valeriana officinalis)
Vervain (Verbena officinalis)
Wintergreen (Gaultheria procumbens)
Wormseed (Chenopodium anthelminticum)
Wormwood (Artemisia absinthium)

those women who happen to conform to the size and shape of the cut-out.

Enlarged foam pillows are also problematic because they are clumsy and require constant raising and lowering of the massage table to suit a pregnant or nonpregnant client. In a prone position, use of an enlarged pillow encourages swelling by situating the feet below the level of the heart. It does not encourage a posterior pelvic tilt and is unsupportive of the growing uterus. In addition, one size does not fit all. Turning is extremely awkward on an enlarged foam pillow. In a supine position, the narrow shape encourages medial shoulder rotation, further shortening the pectorals.

The position that optimizes correct postural alignment and offers safe, uncompromised comfort is the best position for the pregnant client. The bodyCushion system is a modular set of contoured cushions that effectively and safely support the pregnant woman throughout her pregnancy in the prone, side-lying, and supine positions.

With the client in a prone position, wedges are placed under her chest and pelvic cushions are used

The uterine ligament attachments have not changed since humans were quadripedal. Women who experience round ligament pain get quick relief by getting on their hands and knees. In a prone position on the cushions, uterine ligaments are activated in their correct placement. The effects of relaxin allow the ligaments to stretch as the pregnancy advances. This would pose a problem if her uterus were not adequately supported, if she were not in proper alignment, or if she were in a joint-stressed position. Proper placement of the cushions and wedges avoids these complications.

to provide a posterior pelvic tilt that elongates and decompresses the lumbar spine. In the face-down position, the recesses within each cushion softly cradle the uterus and the ligaments are not suspended without support (Box 3-2). The prone position also offers other wonderful benefits for the pregnant woman, including promoting optimum fetal position, occiput anterior, and encouraging a breech position to turn to a vertex position; relief of abdominal pressure, sciatica, and lower back pain; increased intestinal peristaltic activity and lymphatic absorption, and ease of hemorrhoid pain and varicose veins and spider veins. In addition, the fetus rests on the maternal anterior abdominal wall allowing circulation to infiltrate usually congested regions of her lower extremities (Figure 3-12).

Prone cushion positioning is not recommended for those women with severe nasal or sinus congestion, esophageal reflux, heartburn, or nausea (massage is contraindicated with nausea). This positioning also is not recommended for women who are clinically obese, experiencing a high-risk pregnancy, or not comfortable in this position. In these instances, side-lying, semisitting (supine), or sitting massage positions are preferred.

Supine positioning using the bodyCushion system requires an additional wedge and bolster to adequately elevate the pregnant client's torso, particularly in the latter stages of pregnancy. It is also suggested that a wedge be placed under a client's right hip to tilt her slightly to the left, thereby avoiding compression of the abdominal vessels. The angle of her torso should be between 45 and 70 degrees from her hips, and her legs should be raised above her heart.

Side-lying is extremely comfortable with these cushions. All the pressure is taken off her shoulders and hips because the cushions lift her off the table.

Additional Supplies for the Prenatal Practice

Additional supplies that will need to be purchased to adequately supply a prenatal practice are as follows:

- Double the amount of sheets, particularly flat sheets
- Extra towels of various sizes, including additional hand towels to use as rolls and small wedges
- Two or three extra-large wrap-around robes for the client who has to use the bathroom during the massage

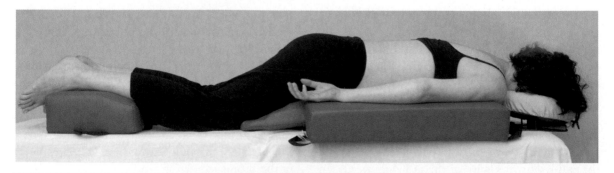

FIGURE 3-12 ■ Prone positioning on the bodyCushion System is safe and comfortable for most pregnant women throughout their pregnancies.

- One size fits all slippers, rubber thongs, or skid-proof socks to protect the client's feet and prevent her from slipping
- A box of nursing pads
- A box of large sanitary napkins for the postpartum client and panty liners for the pregnant client
- Water and cups
- Extra pillows of various sizes to adjust the client's position
- Snack foods for the client with gestational glucose intolerance or for the client who has missed a meal or a snack
- Medicated wipes such as Tucks
- A wooden stool without wheels for sitting massage or a stool with wheels that lock securely
- Tissues
- Ice packs (if you do not have a refrigerator, an ice pack that gets cold when the beads are ruptured is ideal)
- Hair clips for long hair or to secure the sheet in a sitting massage
- Step stool (which must be kept oil-free)
- Alcohol or baby wipes to clean excess lubrication from the feet
- High-density foam wedge for supine positioning (preferable to numerous pillows that can move) 8½-inches high × 18½-inches wide × 22-inches long
- High-density foam leg bolster for supine positioning to enhance lymphatic drainage and promote a posterior pelvic tilt 10-inches high × 18-inches wide × 18-inches long at the top and 28-inches long at the base

In My Experience...

When Florence was in the fourth month of her pregnancy, I noticed bilateral red marks on her feet and asked how she was feeling. Florence had an effervescent personality, was full of energy, and reported feeling terrific. At 7 months, she was screened for **toxoplasmosis** (a protozoan parasite associated with uncooked and undercooked meats, dog and cat feces, contact with infected soil, and frequent consumption of uncooked vegetables outside the home). Fetal risks include intrauterine death, low birth weight, enlarged spleen and liver, jaundice and anemia, hydrocephalus, significant cognitive motor and neurological function delays, and seizures.[18] Her test came back positive. Carriers are asymptomatic, so it made sense that she never felt any effects. However, the test indicated that the fetus was affected early on in the pregnancy, just after the first trimester—when the marks appeared on Florence's feet.

I had no idea whether Florence or her fetus was affected when I saw the marks, and I certainly could not determine what the problem was, but it did show up on her feet when the problem occurred.

Summary

The massage and somatic practitioner has a unique role in the lives of pregnant clients. Massage offers relief from most of their common complaints and is emotionally nurturing. Practitioners can provide information and educational materials about the choices made during pregnancy. Bodyworkers play an active role during a very personal, intimate time in a woman's life, and the impact of bodywork can be the difference between an experience fraught with stress, pains, and concerns or one filled with positive reinforcement, relief from aches and pains, and joyous anticipation.

Essential to a successful prenatal massage practice is the understanding that whichever type of bodywork is used, practitioners must adhere to the dynamic principles of prenatal anatomy and physiology and respect the precautions and contraindications of appropriate touch. Draping the client, turning the client on the massage table, moving the client on and off the treatment table, setting up the treatment room, and maintaining proper alignment and body mechanics are important aspects of working with this special population.

Client safety and comfort are major concerns when it comes to positioning the client for each trimester. Pregnant women should never be placed in a supine position at any stage during their pregnancies but particularly after the first trimester. Although the left side-lying position proves to be the safest way to place a client on the massage table, using adequate pillows, wedges, and cushions can offer comfortable semisitting or recumbent treatment options.

Care must be taken when using essential oils during pregnancy. It is advisable to avoid using them in the first trimester and use only a few safe, nontoxic oils in later pregnancy. Practitioners must also know their source to ensure purity of the oils.

References

1. www.MotherMassage.Net.
2. Zuther J: Traditional massage therapy in the treatment and management of lymph edema, *Massage Today*, p 24, June 2002.
3. Walther DS: *Applied kinesiology*, vol 1, Pueblo, Colo, 1981, Systems DC.
4. Stillerman E: *The encyclopedia of bodywork*, New York, 1996, Facts On File.
5. Bogardus S: Aunty Margaret revisited, *Massage and Healing Arts* 6:30, 1986.
6. *Complete decongestive physiotherapy: an innovative and logical approach to lymphedema*, Lymphedema Services, New York.
7. Field T, Morrow C, et al: Massage reduces anxiety in child and adolescent psychiatric patients, *J Am Acad Child Adol Psych* 31:125-131, 1992.
8. Kitzinger S: *The complete book of pregnancy and childbirth*, New York, 1981, Alfred Knopf.
9. James C, Casey P, Huntsdale C, et al: Memory in pregnancy, *JPOG* 20(2)1999.
10. Sears W, Sears M: *The pregnancy book*, New York, 1992, Little, Brown.
11. Leifer G: *Maternity nursing: an introductory text*, St. Louis, 2005, Saunders.
12. Coad J: *Anatomy and physiology for midwives*, St. Louis, 2001, Mosby.
13. Rapp F: Aromatherapy: ease the discomforts of pregnancy, *The Arom'Alchem Newsletter* 2001.
14. SunSpirit Aromatherapy: *Pregnancy care and essential oils,* Ballina, Australia.
15. Oshadhi: *Singles therapeutic essential oil guide*, Petaluma, Calif, 2000, Oshadhi.
16. Essential Oils Company: *Pregnancy and the use of essential oils in aromatherapy*, Portland, Ore.
17. Grieve M: *A modern herbal*, New York, 1971, Dover Publishing.
18. Baril L, Ancelle T, Goulet V: Risk factors for toxoplasma infection in pregnancy: a case-control study in France, *Scand J Inf Dis* 31:305-309, 1999.

REVIEW QUESTIONS

1 What is meant by "appropriate" bodywork for prenatal, labor, and postpartum massage?

_____

_____

_____

_____

2 List and describe at least 6 bodywork techniques that are safe and appropriate for prenatal massage.

_____

_____

_____

_____

_____

3 If a client in a semirecumbent or semisitting position starts to feel dizzy, light-headed, short of breath, faint, or nauseous to what position should she be turned to relieve these symptoms?

_____

_____

_____

_____

4 To stabilize her lumbar spine and pelvis while the client gets on and off the treatment table, what muscle should she recruit and how does she do this?

_____

_____

_____

_____

5 During pregnancy, what is the direction of massage strokes: mostly horizontal to elongate or vertical to compress?

_____

_____

_____

_____

_____

6 Describe the client's positioning options during each trimester. Is it ever safe to place a pregnant woman flat on her back in the supine position?

_____

_____

_____

_____

_____

7 In a semisitting or recumbent position, at what angle should her torso be elevated?

_____

_____

_____

_____

_____

8 What is the advantage of placing her feet elevated at the same level as her knees?

_____

_____

_____

_____

_____

9   Should aromatherapy and essential oils be avoided during the first trimester?

_____

_____

_____

_____

_____

10   Describe the amount of pressure you can use during your prenatal massage.

_____

_____

_____

_____

_____

11   What is the importance of the pretreatment evaluations?

_____

_____

_____

_____

_____

12   What is the test for pitting edema? If the test is positive, what does the massage practitioner do?

_____

_____

_____

_____

_____

13   How do you test for the presence of blood clots on the entire leg?

_____

_____

_____

_____

_____

14   The practitioner should feel the client's legs to search for what symptoms that could indicate the presence of a blood clot?

_____

_____

_____

_____

_____

15   What is the Homan check? What does the practitioner do if the client tests positive on either or both blood clot evaluations?

_____

_____

_____

_____

_____

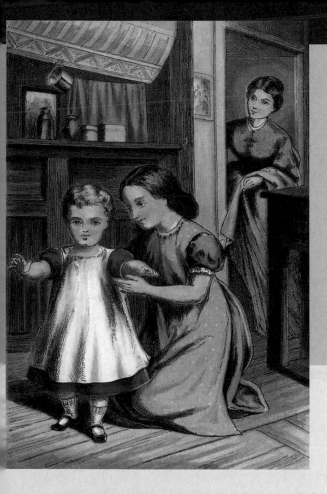

CHAPTER 4

Emotional and Psychological Effects of Pregnancy

My Baby Brother

"O dear Mamma, where are you gone?
Come, see the baby stand alone;
And only think—indeed, 'tis truth—
I can just feel a little tooth.

"Look at his pretty shining hair,
His cheeks so red, his skin so fair;
His curly ringlets, just like flax;
His little bosom, just like wax.

"I think he's growing very wise;
Now don't you think so?" Julia cries:
Then to the cradle off she ran,
To kiss the little baby-man.

Anon.

Objectives

On completion of this chapter, the student will be able to do the following:

1 Understand the emotional impact pregnancy can have on a woman

2 Recognize the signs of depression during pregnancy

3 Learn the different cultural concerns and attitudes about pregnancy

4 Learn how a woman's changing body image can affect the pregnancy

5 Appreciate how pregnancy can affect your client's family and friends

6 Understand sexuality during pregnancy

7 Learn the effects of childhood abuse on pregnancy and pregnancy outcome

8 Recognize the significance of spousal abuse or domestic violence during pregnancy

Antidepressants	Emotional adjustment	Sexuality
Body image	Emotional lability	Sexual intercourse
Cultural differences	Mood disorders	Spousal abuse
Depression	Mood swings	Weight gain
Domestic violence	Psychological adjustment	

The Emotional Impact of Pregnancy

The day a woman learns she is pregnant, her life changes and she is often swept away on a wave of disparate and conflicting feelings. One minute she is overjoyed at the news and prospect of a child, then suddenly these feelings are replaced with doubts about the wisdom of this decision or her ability to get through it. The emotional ups and downs of pregnancy are completely normal and understandable. Life is going to change for her and her partner (if she has one) and her body will make all the biological adaptations it needs to sustain the pregnancy without her active participation.

Settling into the mind set of becoming a mother and countenancing the idea of the pregnancy is called *cognitive restructuring*.[1,2] A woman's ability to accept the pregnancy is reflected in her emotional responses.[3] Most women eventually embrace the idea of a child, including the 25% of women who became pregnant as a result of contraceptive failure.[4]

Emotional lability, or the uncontrollable, unpredictable changes in mood, is part of the early pregnancy experience.[3] Irritability, tears, anger, stress, and uncertainty alternate with elation, happiness, and excitement. The increased levels of estrogen and progesterone play a large role in this emotional roller coaster ride and the pregnant woman's **emotional** and **psychological adjustments**.[3,5]

During the first trimester, a woman's body is adjusting to many extreme changes. She is feeling tired and often short of breath as her hormone levels increase to sustain the pregnancy. Nausea and vomiting is often ascribed to the first trimester. This condition, often referred to as *morning sickness* (although it can occur at any time of the day), is associated with elevated levels of hCG (human chorionic gonadotrophin). HCG levels start to diminish between 60 to 90 days after conception, at which point the nausea subsides. Breast tenderness and changes, frequent urination, and changes in her reproductive system (increased vaginal secretion, vaginal and cervical color changes to a bluish tone, and a softer cervix) make her feel more different than she actually looks.[6,7]

By the second trimester, weeks 13 to 25 of fetal life, the client's early symptoms have generally subsided and she feels more energetic and confident. Her pregnant silhouette is starting to show, and a first time mother should feel fetal movement between weeks 18 to 22. This connection with her child enhances her feelings of motherhood and makes the pregnancy more real. Her partner becomes more involved and interested in the pregnancy.[6] Since the risk of miscarriage is very low after 12 weeks, her feelings of eager anticipation accompanied by more relaxation about the pregnancy are apparent.[7]

By the end of the third trimester, most women look forward to the end of the pregnancy and the discomforts they are experiencing. They often spend a lot of time thinking about the birth and become concerned about labor. As labor draws near, sleeplessness, insomnia, and general fatigue add to increased stress and anxiety. The pregnant woman often feels unattractive and undesirable because of weight gain and physical discomforts.[5] Once again, feelings of ambivalence may surface; she may be sad that the pregnancy is over but glad to be rid of the aches and pains, as well as anticipating and fearing labor and the stress of becoming a family.

Massage practitioners can best serve their clients by being sensitive to and understanding the spectrum of feelings a pregnant woman has.

A practitioner's job is to be supportive and reassuring, not judgmental, of all she is feeling. Stress can have a major impact on birth outcome and can slow labor, so one of a practitioner's major treatment goals is to reduce stress and needless worry. When concerns are serious enough to warrant additional or different types of care, the practitioner's role is to provide appropriate referrals so the client can get the help she needs.

Depression during Pregnancy

The startling number of clinically depressed pregnant women dispels the idea that all pregnancies are happy and wanted (Figure 4-1). Symptoms may appear in early pregnancy, between weeks 10 to 14, in 6% of women who have never been diagnosed with **depression**, which is defined as an intensive and pervasive mood disorder with sadness and emotional lability.[8] Another study cited almost 20% of pregnant women screened as being depressed.[9] On average, it is estimated that 10% to 20% of pregnant women are depressed.[10] Women who suffer from prenatal depression are

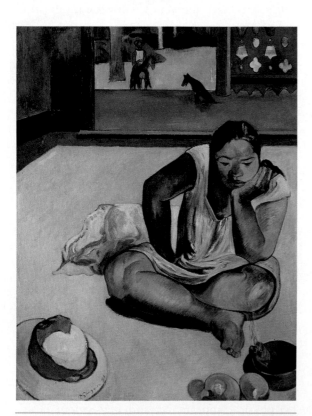

FIGURE 4-1 ■ The Brooding Woman, Paul Gauguin, 1848-1903. (Reprinted by permission of the Worcester Art Museum.)

also at greater risk of developing postpartum depression, so proper help, whether psychological counseling or medication, is essential.

Mood disorders or **mood swings** are normal during pregnancy, but depression can be triggered by a number of factors such as the following[10]:
- Preexisting depression
- Family history
- Unwanted or unplanned pregnancy
- Marital or financial problems
- A significant life change such as a death of a close relative or friend or a new job
- Medical problems
- Complicated pregnancy
- History of miscarriage

Hormonal factors are generally considered to be a major cause of prenatal depression, but other situations may also contribute to this serious problem.

A practitioner should look for some warning signs and indicators. Diagnosing depression is not within the scope of a bodyworker's practice, but because almost 1 of 5 clients will suffer from depression, it is important to be aware of the signs. Depression is most common in the first trimester and final weeks of pregnancy. Signs of depression are the following[10]:
- Difficulty concentrating
- Extreme agitation and anxiety
- Extreme irritability
- Insomnia or difficulty getting restful sleep
- Fatigue
- Binge eating or loss of appetite
- Loss of interest and pleasure in activities once enjoyed
- Exaggerated mood swings
- Depression and sadness that will not go away
- Thoughts of hurting self or others

If a practitioner suspects a client is depressed, it is important to refer her to someone who can help her through this rough time. If left untreated, the symptoms could escalate. In addition to counseling, some women might need **antidepressants** or other medications during their pregnancies to help them cope (Box 4-1). For some of these women, the risks of forsaking their medication during pregnancy may be far greater to both mother and fetus than the drugs themselves.[9]

Depression can also have a tremendous impact on birth outcome and neonate well-being. A group

There are four categories and other agents of anti-depressant drugs that can be prescribed by doctors during pregnancy to treat depression. Some of them demonstrate risk or potential risk to the fetus, but benefits outweigh the possible dangers. This list in not intended to be definitive or appropriate for massage therapists to discuss with their clients.

Selective Serotonin Reuptake Inhibitors
 Citalopram (Celexa)
 Fluoxetine (Prozac)
 Fluvoxamine (Luvox)
 Paroxetine (Paxil)
 Sertraline (Zoloft)

Tricyclics
 Amitriptyline (Elavil)
 Amoxapine (Asendin)
 Clomipramine (Anafranil)
 Desipramine (Norpramin)
 Doxepin (Sinequan)
 Imipramine (Tofranil)
 Nortriptyline (Pamelor)
 Protriptyline (Vivactil)

Quadricyclics
 Maprotiline (Ludiomil)
 Mirtazapine (Remeron)
 Monoamine Oxidase Inhibitors
 Phenelzine (Nardil)
 Tranylcypromine (Parnate)

Other Agents
 Bupropion (Wellbutrin) IR and SR
 Nefazodone (Serzone)
 Trazodone (Desyrel)
 Venlafaxine (Effexor)

Data from Keltner N, Folks D: *Psychotropic drugs*, St. Louis, 2001, Mosby.

of 1- to 3-month-old infants born to depressed teenage mothers were treated with either 15 minutes of massage or rocking twice a week for 6 weeks. Those infants who received massage had heightened alert and awake states, cried less, and had lower salivary cortisol levels, indicating less stress. Over the 6-week trial, the massaged group gained more weight, showed enhanced emotional and social development, had improved soothability, and decreased levels of stress hormones.[11]

Differences in Cultural Concerns and Attitudes

Culture has been defined as "a unified set of values, ideas, beliefs and standards of behavior shared by a group of people; it is the way a person accepts, orders, interprets and understands experiences throughout the life course."[12] Another perspective states "Culture is an integrated dynamic set of values, beliefs and practices shaped by close ties, teachings and common interactions from conception and throughout the lifespan."[13]

Within a practice, massage practitioners will be working with women from many cultures who follow their own cultural customs and beliefs. It is helpful to understand some of these distinctive perspectives of pregnancy and childbirth to provide the best care possible.

The language barrier or speech styles can be different among diverse peoples. Some cultures speak softly, whereas others are rather loud, and it is important for the practitioner to learn to appreciate the differences in communication styles.[3]

Another important difference is how cultures view personal space and the idea of touch. This is particularly relevant for the somatic practitioner. If a client has booked a massage, a practitioner may assume that touch would not be a problem. But this is not always the case. Some cultures believe that touch can spread disease, whereas others are more reticent or bashful about physical contact.[3,14]

The role of the family has important significance during pregnancy in some cultures. For instance, social class and cultural beliefs can affect how involved the father or other female family members may be during childbirth. Other cultures emphasize and prefer that the first child born into the family be a son. This can have a tremendous impact on the mother's feelings about her pregnancy, particularly if she learns the gender of the child in advance.

Culture and ethnicity can affect **body image,** which is a person's subjective concept of his or her physical appearance, and perception; health and dietary habits during pregnancy; and attitudes and acceptance of the pregnancy. There may

BOX 4-2   *Traditional Cultural Concerns and Attitudes Toward Pregnancy*

Cultural differences are comparative distinctions between different ethnicities. Every attempt is made to avoid stereotyping these cultures. These are traditional beliefs within the cultures and subcultures but not necessarily universally practiced.

Hispanic
   Pregnancy wanted soon after marriage.
   Women wait until late pregnancy before receiving prenatal care.
   Expectant mother is influenced by the older women in her family and her husband's family.
   Air conditioning or cool circulated air is considered dangerous.
   Milk is avoided because it is believed to cause large babies and hard births.
   Unsatisfied food cravings are believed to create birthmarks.
   Many predictions are made about the baby's gender.
   It is common for the pregnant woman to use herbs to treat common discomforts.

African-Americans
   Economic status affects pregnancy acceptance.
   Late prenatal care is often associated with lower income women.
   Believe that taking a photograph during the pregnancy will cause a stillbirth.
   Believe that raising both arms above her head will cause umbilical cord strangulation.
   Feel most distorted at 9 months but no change in awareness of abdomen after the birth.

Hawaiian
   Consider pregnancy natural and healthy.
   Prenatal care often includes ethnic healers and community leaders.

Asian-Americans
   Joyous time for pregnant woman.
   Pregnancy is regarded as a natural process.
   Feel more comfortable under the care of female health care providers.
   Avoid soy sauce during pregnancy to prevent dark baby.
   Believe that inactivity or too much sleep can cause a hard labor.
   Avoid drinking milk or eating milk products to prevent stomachaches.

Europeans and North Americans
   Prefer medical attention to ensure healthy outcome.
   Major emphasis is on early prenatal care and prenatal tests.
   Birth is technologically driven.
   Options of a wide variety of childbirth education classes and techniques.

Native Americans
   Pregnancy is normal and natural.
   Prenatal care generally received during late pregnancy.
   Use herbs for medicines.

Data from Lowdermilk DL, Perry SE: *Maternity & women's health care*, ed 8, St. Louis, 2004, Mosby; Mayberry LJ, Alfonso DD, Shibuya J, et al: *J Perinat Neonatal Nurs* 13(1):15-26, 1999; Harris R: *Br J Med Psychol* 52(4):347-352, 1979.

be myths, traditions, customs, and old wives' tales within different cultures.[15] Practitioners must respect and honor these beliefs to make clients feel welcome, safe, and nurtured (Box 4-2).

Body Image

Many women delight in the changes that are going on within their bodies, whereas others are not so happy about putting on the additional weight and how they look. A woman's appearance and how she feels about it can affect her attitude about the pregnancy. Women have to recognize that the weight they gain, which may be undesired, is necessary to support the pregnancy.[16] The current recommended weight gain for a woman carrying a singleton is 25 to 35 lbs and a woman carrying twins can add an extra 10 lbs.[16] Too much **weight gain** is healthy for neither mother nor fetus and too little could lead to premature labor and delivery (Box 4-3).

As a pregnant woman's body shape changes and she starts to feel more uncomfortable, clumsy, and ungainly, she may have a difficult time accepting these dramatic changes. Some women may feel that they are ugly or fat, which can create a negative attitude about the pregnancy.[17] It is important for the bodyworker to respect the pregnant woman's feelings, without denying how she feels, while encouraging her that all the changes she undergoes are necessary for the pregnancy and reminding her that she does have some control over how her body looks and feels. She can eat well, exercise regularly, receive regular massages, and share her feelings with other pregnant women so she can learn first hand that she is not alone.

Other women feel absolutely beautiful, are radiant, and truly enjoy being pregnant. There is no right or wrong way to feel during pregnancy. Massage practitioners can support, acknowledge, and

Touch Points

A woman's body image can affect her pregnancy. Because this is a society that covets thinness, many pregnant women think they are fat and unattractive. Although the practitioner must never deny a client's feelings, a little humor can get her to see things a bit more light-heartedly. After all, her body is doing exactly what it needs to do to support her and her growing baby and it is only a temporary condition.

BOX 4-3	Weight Gain during Pregnancy
Baby	7-9 pounds
Uterus	2 pounds
Placenta	1-2 pounds
Amniotic fluid	1-2 pounds
Breast enlargement	2-3 pounds
Extra blood and fluid	6-8 pounds
Extra maternal fat	6-9 pounds
TOTAL GAIN	25-35 pounds

Data from Sears W, Sears M: *The pregnancy book*, Boston, 1997, Little, Brown.

educate their clients in the hope that negative feelings can turn into more accepting, positive ones.

Many women feel that their bodies seem to take on a life of their own, and they experience less control over many bodily functions such as urinary incontinence, heartburn, and hemorrhoids. It is important to reassure the client that this is only temporary and that relief for these common discomforts is available. Chapter 14 includes massage techniques to relieve common discomforts.

Another aspect of a pregnant woman's body image is her mobility and awkwardness. Dropping things, being clumsy, and feeling exceptionally ungraceful is concomitant with her advancing pregnancy. Exercise and activity should continue, although some activities have to be modified or moderated as pregnancy advances.[17]

Since the massage practitioner's work is intimate by nature, clients must be urged to feel relaxed and accepting of their bodies by reassuring them that their bodies are doing what is necessary to support and sustain the pregnancy. Practitioners can work with them to establish a more positive and self-accepting attitude by understanding how they feel and making them feel more comfortable within their bodies.

How Pregnancy Affects the Partner and Family

The partner also goes through many stages of adjustment towards parenthood.[18] He or she might experience ambivalent feelings about the pregnancy and parenthood and may have conflicting feelings about their relationship as the mother's focus turns inward. Open and honest communication can help avert any misunderstandings and is a helpful way for both partners to get the support they each need from each other.

In older, more traditional societies, men acted out the ritual couvade, which means that he acted out pregnancy and birth-related behaviors. This ritual served to establish his new status as an expectant father and acknowledged his relationship to the mother and child.[3] In more modern times, however, some expectant fathers report feeling similar physical symptoms during their partner's pregnancy such as weight gain, nausea and vomiting, heartburn, cravings, abdominal bloating, and cramps. This is called the Couvade, or fathering, syndrome. For some men, appropriate psychotherapy is necessary.

Partners go through phases of adjustment during the pregnancy. The first phase is called the *announcement phase*. It begins when the pregnancy is confirmed and can last for a few days up to a few weeks. During this phase, the partner has to accept the fact of the pregnancy. For some men this is easy, for others it is not, particularly if this was an unplanned or unwanted pregnancy. If the latter is the case, some men find the inevitable life changes difficult to accept and engage in extramarital affairs or abuse their partners.[19]

The second phase is called the *adjustment* or *moratorium phase*. During this phase, partners adjust to the reality of the pregnancy. They often are actively involved in childbirth classes and become more philosophical about life and relationships with family members. This can last for a short period of time or until the end of the pregnancy.[3,17]

The final phase is called the *focusing phase*. This begins in the last trimester and manifests as the partner begins to feel like a father and gets involved with the pregnancy and his relationship with the child. He is interested in his role during labor and takes an active part with any older children and household modifications.[3,17]

There are also specific ways a man can be involved in the pregnancy. These styles are called the *observer style, expressive style*, or *instrumental style*. In most instances, the observer is happy about the pregnancy but is reluctant or culturally reticent about participating in the pregnancy. Some men need more time to adjust to the idea of fatherhood, whereas others become more self-involved.

The partner who exhibits tremendous interest and strong emotional response is participating in the expressive style. These men are sensitive to their partners' needs and often share emotional and physical symptoms (Couvade syndrome).

The instrumental style of acceptance is the person who wants to perform as the manager of the pregnancy. They feel responsible for the outcome of the pregnancy and are quite protective of their partners.

Just as pregnant clients need to discover and explore their feelings on their own, there is no right or wrong way for their partner to feel. Cultural shaping and personalities may determine how the father fits in, but each man has to come to his style in his own time and in his own way.[20,21]

Older children may have a difficult time adjusting to the idea of sharing the spotlight. Sometimes a child may feel jealous and as if they are being replaced by the newborn. This can add additional stress to the family.

The response of the older child varies with age. A very young child, perhaps 1 year old, has little cognition of the changes that are about to take place. A 2-year–old child, however, is much more aware of his mother's changing body and physical discomforts. The novelty of his mother's appearance may frighten him, and these youngsters often revert to more infantile behavior patterns.

A preschooler has more of an understanding of what is going to happen and often likes to hear the fetal heart beat or touch the baby moving.

School-age children take a more clinical interest and might want to know how this came about. They role play mothers and fathers and enjoy helping prepare for the baby's arrival.

Young adolescents concerned with their own sexuality might have a difficult time adjusting to the idea of their parents as sexual beings. Older teenagers, into their own lives and less concerned with parental behavior, are more of a help than a hindrance.[3]

Grandparents, especially first timers, are usually excited about the news and want to help in any way they can. But becoming grandparents also foreshadows their own mortality, so the pregnancy can be a double-edged sword.

It is inevitable that pregnancy affects all relationships by redefining them. Friendships can also change. Those friends who are also parents are generally quite supportive, whereas those who do not have children think that the friendship might end once the baby is born. The friendship may not end, but it does change.

Sexuality during Pregnancy

Sexuality is the state of being sexual or having sexual desire (libido), and **sexual intercourse** is the act of making love. In most instances, sexuality, sexual intercourse, and orgasms are not contraindicated during pregnancy for the healthy woman.[22] A woman with a history of repeated miscarriages, a threatened first-trimester miscarriage, impending second-trimester miscarriage, or bleeding and abdominal pain during the third trimester should be very cautious about sexual intercourse or orgasm and should discuss this with her care provider.[22]

The partner should avoid blowing into the woman's vagina during oral sex, particularly in the last few weeks of the pregnancy when the cervix is slightly dilated. An air embolism could occur if air penetrates between the uterine wall and the fetal membranes and enters the mother's blood system through the placenta.[22]

Positioning can be problematic for some, humorous for others (Figure 4-2). A position that avoids direct pressure on the woman's breasts and abdomen is recommended. Condoms should also be worn if there is a risk of sexually transmitted emotional intimacy in their relationship with their partners during pregnancy, it does not necessary translate into increased sexual habits, although physical satisfaction is slightly increased.[31,32]

If sexual intercourse is contraindicated because of physical problems that might put the woman at high risk for premature birth, or for any other reason, cuddling, gentle stroking, and massaging are alternatives that can be equally intimate and satisfying.[33]

Clients Who Are Survivors of Childhood Physical or Sexual Abuse

In the United States, it is estimated that 1 out of 3 women have been physically or sexually abused before their eighteenth birthday. For men, the numbers are one 1 out of 6 before the age of 18.[34] These might actually be conservative figures. Chances that a massage practitioner will be working with a survivor of childhood abuse are very high. The health implications and labor outcome for a pregnant woman are significant. In 1994, almost half of the pregnancies (49%) were unplanned and unwanted or happened before the woman wanted to conceive.[35] Half of these ended in abortion, and the chances of complications or poor infant outcome for the other half was appreciably higher than a planned pregnancy.[35] Many studies have looked into the link between childhood abuse and pregnancy in adolescents, but one study explored the ramifications of childhood abuse and pregnancy in adults. Almost 2 out of 3 women reported that they had been exposed to abuse or family dysfunction with almost one-third reporting sexual abuse. Nearly half (45%) reported their first pregnancy was unplanned, and this was linked to childhood exposure to abuse.[35]

Childhood abuse has far-reaching implications for pregnancy and labor (Box 4-4). Studies suggest that past or current abuse often results in poor maternal and fetal outcomes. Practitioners working with survivors have to learn to recognize the signs of abuse, know how to take care of these women, and recognize the importance of referring them to the appropriate therapeutic environment where they can receive counseling.

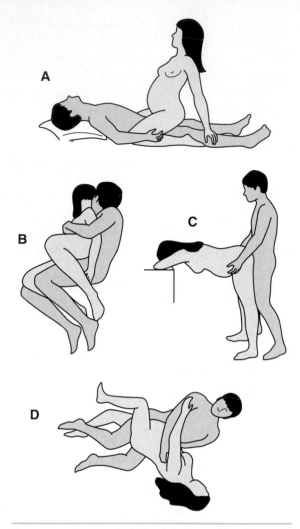

FIGURE 4-2 ■ Gentle lovemaking is safe and enjoyable during pregnancy. **A,** Female superior. **B,** Side by side. **C,** Rear entry. **D,** Side-lying, facing each other. (From Lowdermilk DL, Perry SE: *Maternity & women's health care*, ed 8, St. Louis, 2004, Mosby.)

infections such as herpes, human immunodeficiency virus (HIV), or any other infections.

Sexual desire generally decreases during pregnancy; a sensuous touch and caressing might be more appropriate at times.[23] Fatigue and weakness are popular reasons for avoiding sexual intimacy.[24-27] Interest in sex often increases in the second trimester and is concomitant with the decrease in first-trimester nausea and an increase in energy. There is also an increase in the blood supply to the pelvis that can feel like sexual arousal.[28] During the third trimester, women generally feel more unattractive and have less sexual desire, with reduced frequency and satisfaction.[23,29,30] Whereas most women seem to experience greater

> ### BOX 4-4 *The Sequelae of Abuse during Pregnancy and Labor*
>
> 1. Increase in spontaneous abortions from abuse: 75% versus 19% occurring naturally
> 2. More preexisting maternal illnesses
> 3. More illnesses and complications during pregnancy than nonabused women, such as pregnancy-induced hypertension, gestational diabetes, premature labor
> 4. Failure of labor to progress
> 5. Average of 6 hours longer labors, particularly during stage one of labor
> 6. Need for higher doses of Pitocin
> 7. Increased use of pain medication
> 8. Higher instances of narcotic use during postpartum recovery
> 9. Higher rates of Cesarean sections

Data from Benedict M, Paine LL, Paine LA, et al: *Child Abuse Negl* 23(7):659-670, 1999; Gifford DS, Morton SC, Fiske M, et al: *Obstet Gynecol* 95(4):589-595, 2000; Schei B, Samuelson SO, Bakketeig LS: *Scand J Soc Med* 19 (1), 26-31, 1991; Jacobs JL: *J Child Sexual Abuse* 1(1):103-112, 1992; Tidy H: *Modern Midwife* 17-19, July, 1996; Hobbins D: *J Obstet Gynecol Neonatal Nurs* 33:485-497, 2004.

Signs of Possible Abuse

It is of the utmost importance that the revelation of abuse comes directly from the client and is not prompted or suggested by the practitioner in any way. Signs of possible abuse could be as follows[36,37]:

1. Unexplained bruising on the body, often on areas normally hidden by clothing, such as abdomen, breasts, thighs, or arms
2. Unexplained cuts, burns, or welts
3. Hyperventilation or breath holding when a certain body part is touched
4. Recoiling from touch in certain areas or not permitting touch
5. Drug and alcohol abuse
6. Feelings of isolation
7. Low self-esteem
8. Depression and crying
9. Eating disorders
10. Rejection of own body and poor body image
11. Changes in appetite
12. Fear of abusive person or family member

As labor approaches, women naturally become more concerned and stressed, particularly if this is a first time pregnancy. Clients may articulate irrational concerns about the impending birth. For some women, the intimacy of the bodywork helps her to recall past abuse as labor draws near. Other women may start to hyperventilate or hold their breath during the treatment, whereas others do not want to be touched in certain areas such as the abdomen, buttocks, or thighs. Individually, these reactions to touch may not mean anything significant, but when added together, these signs might indicate a history of physical or emotional trauma. During the treatment, certain memories might surface and there may be an emotional component to them. The best way to work with someone having a "flashback" or who is remembering past trauma is to stop the massage and make certain the client is appropriately draped. The client should open her eyes and concentrate on her breathing until she is emotionally stable. Making the room a bit brighter will also help her come out of her reveries.

It is important that the practitioner recognize any revelations as part of a healing process. The practitioner must validate the client's feelings and understand that in addition to the physical and emotional care the massage provides, the client also needs to see a mental health care practitioner or therapist who can work with her. This therapy will help pave the way for an optimal birth outcome.

Domestic Violence during Pregnancy

Domestic violence, or **spousal abuse,** is physical, emotional, or psychological mistreatment by the husband or domestic partner. According to the American Medical Association, in 1995 almost 1 out of 4 (23%) of all pregnant women were victims of domestic abuse in this country.[38] A few years later, in 1997, that number edged closer to 25%.[39] Domestic violence affects women of all ages, cultures, and socioeconomic backgrounds.[39] Signs of domestic violence include the same signs in the previous list and the following[40]:

1. Delay in seeking prenatal care
2. Unexplained bruising on breasts or abdomen

3. Continuation of unhealthy lifestyle, including smoking and alcohol or substance abuse
4. Recurring psychosomatic illnesses
5. No participation in prenatal education classes

Spousal or domestic violence during pregnancy is not limited to the United States. Industrial countries report a 3.4% to 11% rate of abuse during pregnancy, whereas developing countries (where numbers are available) report 3.8% to 31.7%.[41] China reports 11.7% of physical and sexual abuse occurring during the antenatal, prenatal, and postpartum periods. Those women abused prior to the pregnancy were more likely to be abused during pregnancy.[42] In Canada, 25% of women suffered abuse from current or previous partners. Twenty-one percent of those women abused were pregnant, with 40% reporting that the abuse started during the pregnancy.[43] In Norway, almost 7.5% of pregnant women experienced spousal violence.[44]

Spousal abuse can take the form of physical, sexual, emotional, or financial mistreatment and can obviously injure the fetus as well as the mother. Fetal fractures, infection, and rupture of the uterus are all possible effects of physical abuse in addition to elevated maternal stress levels and depression, intensified chronic illnesses, isolation leading to poor prenatal care, and inadequate nutrition. Premature labor, blunt trauma to the abdomen, hemorrhaging with or without placental separation, premature rupture of the membranes, low fetal birth weight, miscarriages, stillbirths, and increased stress hormones in the fetus are also possible complications of abuse. Stress from abuse may also prevent a woman from eating well or giving up bad habits like smoking, alcohol, or drugs.[39,45-47] Homicide has surpassed cardiovascular disorders, automobile accidents, and falls as the leading cause of death during pregnancy.[48] Those women who are able to leave their abusive relationships have higher murder rates than those who stay in the abusive household[49] (Box 4-5).

In many cases, the spouse is very controlling and may make it impossible for the woman to seek help. The abused woman may be terrified of reprisals from her partner, unaware of viable options available to her, or extremely embarrassed. Whatever the case, the practitioner must

---

BOX 4-5   *Abuse Hotline*

An abused woman can be referred to the National Coalition Against Domestic Violence's hotline at 1-800-799-SAFE (7233), or the American Institute on Domestic Violence. They offer a detailed listing of state by state organizations and can be reached at 505-973-2225 or e-mail at info@aidv-usa.com.
    For immediate help, dial 911.

---

be sensitive to these feelings and the client's needs. It is imperative to remain nonjudgmental and ultimately supportive. It could be a matter of life or death.

In My Experience...

Linda came to me when she was 6 months pregnant with her first child. She kept her underpants on, which is not unusual for many pregnant women who feel cleaner wearing them, and asked me not to massage her abdomen or thighs. When I massaged her upper extremities, I noticed bruises all around her arms that fit the pattern of a hand. I avoided direct pressure to those bruises and gently asked her about them. "I'm clumsy," was her anxious reply.

Whenever she came in for her appointment, she had fresh bruises on her arms. One day, after telling me the same story again, she broke down and cried, confessing her husband was beating her. I stopped the massage and listened to her story. He was an angry man, often screaming at her and blaming her for everything, and the pregnancy escalated his aggression. She felt trapped and unsure what to do.

I helped her get in touch with an agency and a social worker who eventually helped her leave safely. She had her baby with the help of a doula and divorced her husband within months of the birth.

A few years later she came back again for another series of massages. She had happily remarried and was pregnant again.

Summary

Pregnancy can have a tremendous impact on a woman's life and can be a defining experience for her, her family, and her friends. Practitioners are often quick to assume that all pregnancies are joyful occasions, and although many pregnancies are wanted and planned, a pregnant woman's emotions can run the gamut from celebration to panic and concern. Depression is common during pregnancy, and every attempt must be made to help her cope during this stressful time.

Massage practitioners meet people from all walks of life, and it is important to recognize and appreciate the different cultural mores and customs of pregnancy.

Her partner may also express conflicting feelings of impending fatherhood. Men have many different ways and styles of accepting and dealing with the pregnancy and their new roles as parents.

As the pregnancy continues and her body grows, a woman's attitude about her body can have a strong impact on the pregnancy and birth outcome. She needs to learn that these changes are normal adaptations to the pregnancy and that appropriate bodywork can help reduce and alleviate many of the common discomforts she experiences.

The dynamics of the couple can shift, grow, and change in many ways during the pregnancy, including sexual intercourse, which is considered safe for most healthy pregnancies. Couples have to work together to find a mutually satisfying way to please each other.

Survivors of childhood physical and sexual abuse and those pregnant women currently living in abusive households need special care and attention. A massage practitioner's goal is to encourage clients to find safety, peace, and self-acceptance by treating them respectfully and with care. The scope of practice of a bodyworker does not include psychological counseling, so these clients must be referred to those practitioners who work with abused patients. The referrals can be lifesaving for clients.

References

1. Mercer R: *Becoming a mother*, New York, 1995, Springer.
2. Lederman R: *Psychosocial adaptation in pregnancy*, New York, 1996, Springer.
3. Lowdermilk DL, Perry SE: *Maternity & women's health care*, ed 8, St. Louis, 2004, Mosby.
4. Sable M: Pregnancy interventions may not be a useful measure for research on maternal and child health outcomes, *Family Planning Perspectives* 31(5):249-250, 1999.
5. University of Iowa Health Care: *Emotions during pregnancy*, Iowa City, IA, 1997, University of Iowa.
6. Simkin P, Whalley J, Keppler A: *Pregnancy, childbirth and the newborn*, New York, 1991, Meadowbrook Press.
7. Bolane JE: *With child*, Waco, TX, 1999, Childbirth Graphics.
8. Pederson C: Medical management of postpartum psychiatric disorders, *Psychiatric Nursing Inst. Presentation*. Chapel Hill, NC, 1998.
9. Tarkin L: *Dealing with depression and the perils of pregnancy*, The New York Times, p F5, January 13, 2004.
10. Depression during pregnancy, Pregnancy-info. Available at http://www.pregnancy-info.net/depression_during_pregnancy.html. Accessed March, 2006.
11. Field T, Grizzle N, Scaphoid F, et al: Massage therapy for infants of depressed mothers, *Infant Behav Devil* 19:1009-1114, 1996.
12. Thomas N: The importance of culture throughout all of life and beyond, *Holist Nurs Pract* 15(2):40-46, 2001.
13. Willis W: Culturally competent nursing care during the perinatal period, *J Perinate Neonatal Nurs* 13(3):45-49, 1999.
14. Johnson J, Bittorf JL, Balneaves LG, et al: South Asian women's views on the causes of breast cancer: images and explanations, *Patient Educe Conus* 37(3):243-254, 1999.
15. Mayberry LJ, Alfonso DD, Shabby J, et al: Integrating cultural values, beliefs, and customs into pregnancy and postpartum care: lessons learned from Hawaiian public health nursing project, *J Perinate Neonate Nurs* 13(1):15-26, 1999.
16. Sears W, Sears M: *The pregnancy book*, Boston, 1997, Little, Brown.
17. Leifer G: *Maternity nursing: an introductory text*, ed 9, St. Louis, 2005, Saunders.

18. Diemer G: Expectant fathers: influence of perinatal education on stress, coping and spousal relations, *Res Nurs Health* 20: 281-293, 1997.

19. Martin S, Mackie L, Kupper LL, et al: Physical abuse of women before, during and after pregnancy, *JAMA* 285(12):1581-1584, 2001.

20. May K: A typology of detachment and involvement styles adopted during pregnancy by first time expectant fathers, *Western J Nurs Res* 2:445-453, 1980.

21. May K: Three phases of father involvement in pregnancy, *Nurs Res* 31:337-342, 1982.

22. Cunningham FG, Gant NF, Leveno KJ, et al: *Williams obstetrics*, ed 21, New York, 2001, McGraw Hill.

23. Barclay LM, McDonald P, O'Loughlin JA: Sexuality and pregnancy: an interview study, *Aust NZ J Gyn* 34:1-7, 1994.

24. Bick DE, MacArthur C: The extent, severity and effect of health problems after childbirth, *Br J Midwifery* 3:27-31, 1995.

25. Striegel-Moore RH, Goldman SL, Garvin V, et al: A prospective study of somatic and emotional symptoms of pregnancy, *Psychol Wom Quart* 20: 393-408, 1996.

26. Glazener CMA: Sexual function after childbirth: Women experience persistent morbidity and lack of professional recognition, *Br J Obstet Gynaecol* 104:330-335, 1992.

27. Lumley J: Sexual feelings in pregnancy and after childbirth, *Aust NZ J Obstet Gynaecol* 18:114-117, 1978.

28. *Sex during pregnancy*, University of Michigan Health System, 2004, McKesson Provider Technologies.

29. Hyde JS, DeMamater JD, Plant EA, et al: Sexuality during pregnancy and the year postpartum, *J Sex Res* 33:143-151, 1996.

30. Kumar R, Brand HA, Robson KM: Childbearing and maternal sexuality: A prospective survey of 119 primiparae, *J Psychosom Res* 25:373-383, 1981.

31. Adams WJ: Sexuality and happiness ratings of husbands and wives in relation to first and second pregnancies, *J Fam Psychol* 2:67-81, 1988.

32. Snowden LR, Schott TL, Await SJ, et al: Marital satisfaction in pregnancy: Stability and predictions of change, *J Marriage Fam* 52:21-29, 1990.

33. *Sex during pregnancy*, San Francisco Children's Hospital, 2002, University of California.

34. Thompson RG, Smith C: *Trauma touch therapy*, Lakewood, CO, 1995, Colorado School of Healing Arts.

35. Dietz PM, Spitz AM, Anda RF, et al: Unintended pregnancy among adult women exposed to abuse or household dysfunction during their childhood, *JAMA* 282: 1359-1364, 1999.

36. de Benedictis T, Jaffee J, Segal J: Domestic violence and abuse types, signs, symptoms, causes and effects. In *Help guide*: Santa Monica, CA, 1996, Rotary Club of Santa Monica and Center for Healthy Aging.

37. Rice MJ: *One voice: assessment and intervention standards of domestic violence*, Santa Clara, CA, 1998, Concept Media.

38. Shea CA, Mahoney M, Lacey JM: Breaking through the barriers to domestic violence intervention, *Am J Nurs* 97(6):26-33, 1997.

39. The problem of physical abuse in pregnancy, Cyberparent. Available at http://cyberparent.com/abuse/pregnancy. htm, Accessed 1997.

40. Dietz P: Delayed entry into prenatal care: effect of physical violence, *Obstet Gynecol* 90:221-224, 1997.

41. Campbell J, Garcia-Moreno C, Sharps P: Abuse during pregnancy in industrialized and developing countries, *Violence Against Women* 10:770-789, 2004.

42. Guo SF, Wu JL, Qu CY, et al: Physical and sexual abuse of women before, during and after pregnancy, *Int J Gynaecol Obstet* 84(3):281-286, 2004.

43. Hodges K: Wife assault: The findings of a national survey, *Juristat* 1(9): March 1994.

44. Schei B, Samuelson SO, Bakketeig LS: Does spousal physical abuse affect the outcome of pregnancy? *Scand J Soc Med* 19(1):26-31, 1991.

45. Goodwin T, Breen M: Pregnancy outcome and fetomaternal hemorrhage after non-catastrophic trauma, *Am J Obstet Gynecol* 162:665-671, 1990.

46. Newberger E, Barkham S, Liberman E, et al: Abuse of pregnant women and adverse birth outcome, *JAMA* 267:2370-2372, 1992.

47. Bohn D, Hotz K: Sequelae of abuse: Health effects of childhood sexual abuse, domestic battery and rape, *J Nurse Midwifery* 41(6):442-456, 1996.

48. Horon IL, Cheng D: Enhanced surveillance for pregnancy-associated mortality—Maryland, 1993-1998, *JAMA* 285:1455-1459, 2001.

49. Decker M, Martin S, Moracco K: Homicide factors among pregnant women abused by their partners: Who leaves the perpetrator and who stays? *Violence Against Women* 10:498-515, 2004.

1   Describe some possible emotional reactions a woman might experience on learning that she is pregnant.

_____

_____

_____

_____

_____

2   How common is depression during pregnancy? What are some of the contributing factors of depression during pregnancy?

_____

_____

_____

_____

_____

3   What are some signs of prenatal depression a massage practitioner should look for?

_____

_____

_____

_____

_____

4   Does prenatal depression have any impact on birth outcome and neonate well-being?

_____

_____

_____

_____

_____

5   What are some of the cultural concerns and attitudes of pregnancy that massage practitioners should understand about their clientele?

_____

_____

_____

_____

_____

6   Describe how the pregnancy can affect a woman's body image.

_____

_____

_____

_____

_____

_____

7   How can a pregnancy affect the partner and other members of her family?

_____

_____

_____

_____

_____

_____

8   What is couvade?

_____

_____

_____

_____

_____

9   What are the phases of adjusting to the pregnancy?

_____

_____

_____

_____

_____

_____

_____

10   Before the age of 18, how common is sexual or physical abuse against girls? Against boys?

_____

_____

_____

_____

_____

_____

11   Does childhood abuse have any affect on the woman's pregnancy, labor, and postpartum? Please describe.

_____

_____

_____

_____

_____

_____

_____

12   What is the leading cause of death during pregnancy in the United States?

_____

_____

_____

_____

_____

_____

_____

13   How common is spousal abuse during pregnancy?

_____

_____

_____

_____

_____

_____

_____

14   What are some of the sequelae of abuse during pregnancy to the pregnancy and labor?

_____

_____

_____

_____

_____

_____

15   What are common signs of possible abuse?

_____

_____

_____

_____

_____

_____

_____

_____

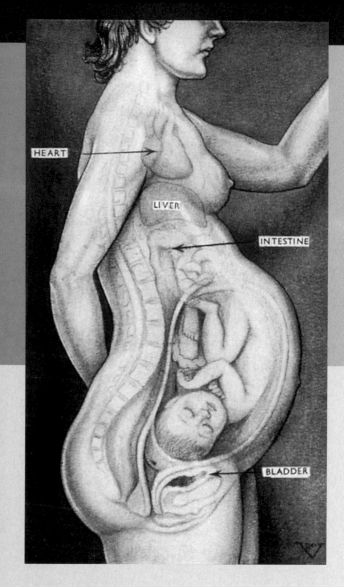

HEART

LIVER

INTESTINE

BLADDER

CHAPTER 5

The Physiology of Pregnancy

Objectives

On completion of this chapter, the student will be able to do the following:

1   Learn the basic facts about conception and early fetal development

2   Recognize the signs of early pregnancy

3   Understand the physiological changes and adaptations during pregnancy to the musculoskeletal system, including abdominal core muscles

4   Demonstrate appropriate prenatal exercise, body mechanics, and back care

5   Understand the physiological adaptations of the cardiovascular system that support maternal metabolism, the increased needs of the pregnancy, and fetal growth

6   Recognize the symptoms of thromboembolism and preeclamptic conditions

7   Understand the changes and adaptations during pregnancy to the respiratory, gastrointestinal, urinary, reproductive, endocrine, neurological, and integumentary systems

8   Understand the changes and adaptations during pregnancy to visceral organs, metabolism, and the five senses

Abdominal muscles
Adaptations
Blastocyst
Cardiovascular system
Cervix
Chorionic villi
Clotting factor
Coagulating factor
Conception
Conceptus
Diastasis

Embryo
Endocrine system
External obliques
Fetus
Fibrinogenic activity
Gastrointestinal system
Implantation
Integumentary (skin) system
Internal obliques
Linea alba
Metabolism

Musculoskeletal system
Neurological system
Rectus abdominis
Reproductive system
Respiratory system
Senses
Urinary system
Uterus
Vagina
Visceral organs
Zygote

The Physiology of Pregnancy

The tremendous changes that occur to maternal physiology begin at **conception** (union of sperm and egg resulting in fertilization; formation of the one-celled **zygote**). Even before the pregnancy is confirmed, a woman's body begins to prepare for pregnancy and labor. Fatigue is very common in early pregnancy as her body is affected by the hormonal and physiological changes.[1] Another common symptom, which many women recognize as a confirmation of the pregnancy, is nausea or morning sickness,[1] although the nausea can occur at any time during the pregnancy. Other common symptoms are listed in Box 5-1.[1,2]

After conception, a large amount of activity and growth is taking place within the woman's body. Once the sperm has penetrated the egg, fertilization take place within one of the fallopian tubes. After only 1 week, the **conceptus** implants into the lining of the **uterus** (the womb) (Figure 5-1). It is not at all uncommon for a woman to experience a slight amount of bleeding called **implantation** bleeding. The conceptus, or **blastocyst,** which means "sprout pouch," divides into hundreds of cells.[1] The uterus starts to form a rudimentary placenta and starts to produce human chorionic gonadotrophin (hCG). This hormone is necessary to sustain the uterine lining and encourages its growth by increasing levels of estrogen and progesterone.[1] As the placenta grows, more amounts of hCG are released into the maternal blood supply. By week 2, sufficient amounts of hCG in her urine confirm the pregnancy.

BOX 5-1 Early Signs of Pregnancy

Late or missed period
Unusually light period
Fatigue
Nausea or vomiting
Light staining or spotting
Aversion to certain foods and odors
Breast soreness or tenderness
Abdominal cramping and bloating
Frequent urination
Food cravings
Increase in normal vaginal discharge
Moodiness

From Sears W, Sears M: *The pregnancy book*, Boston, 1997, Little, Brown; Ting RY, Brant H, Holt K: *The complete mothercare manual*, New York, 1987, Prentice Hall.

After 3 weeks since conception, the menstrual period has been missed and the woman may feel different and aware of certain physical changes. Her ovaries no longer ovulate, and her pituitary gland ceases menstruation. The blood supply to her uterus has increased to establish a thicker lining to nourish the fertilized egg **(zygote)**. There is a softening in the **cervix** (the lowest and narrowest, or "neck," end of the uterus) and uterus, and by the fourth week, finger-like projections, called the **chorionic villi,** surround the mass of cells and help it attach to the lining of the uterus.[3]

At the end of 3 weeks, the **embryo** has evolved from a single cell into millions of cells that are already coded to become one of three differentiating types of cells that make up the nervous

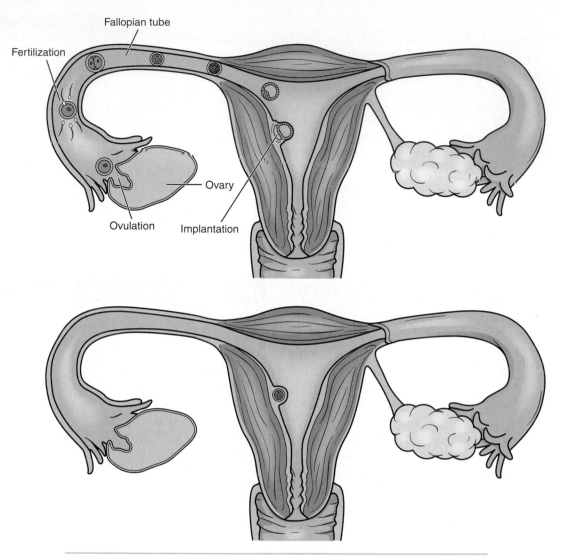

Fallopian tube

Fertilization

Ovary

Ovulation   Implantation

FIGURE 5-1 ■ After 1 week, the conceptus, called an embryo, implants into the lining of the uterus.

system, **integumentary (skin) system** (including hair), **gastrointestinal system** (the digestive and elimination system of the body), **musculoskeletal system** (muscles, bones, and joints), circulatory system, and genitourinary system (Figure 5-2).[1] By the end of the third week of conception, a primitive heart begins to beat and circulate blood.[1]

By the end of the first month of conception, most women know they are pregnant. Pregnancy can be confirmed by either a blood test, urine test, or an internal examination at the doctor's office or some women use a home pregnancy test. Various cultures identify different signs of pregnancy[4,5] (Box 5-2).

The pregnant client may be told an estimated due date (which was formerly referred to as "estimated date of confinement"[3]). This date is an arbitrary date and is calculated from the first day of the last menses, or 266 days from the presumed date of conception, because pregnancy lasts approximately 280 days, or 40 weeks.[2,3] However, the majority of births, as many as 85%, occur within 38 to 42 weeks, so clients need to recognize that 2 weeks on either side of the estimated due date is normal[2] (Box 5-3). Traditional cultures also have different ways to calculate the due date[6-11] (Box 5-4).

During the first 3 months, the **fetus** (the embryo after 12 weeks' gestation) has undergone rapid and vitally important changes; an umbilical cord and its three blood vessels are formed; a

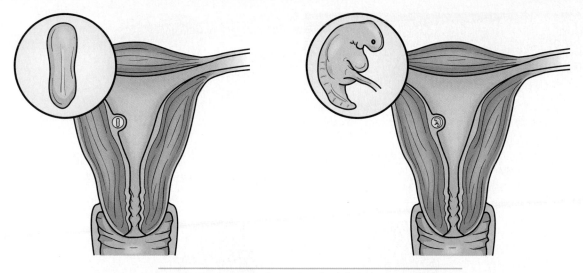

FIGURE 5-2 ■ Embryo at 3 weeks *(left)*. Embryo at 4 weeks *(right)*.

BOX 5-2 *Various Cultural Signs of Pregnancy*

Various cultures identify different signs as a confirmation of pregnancy. The Negritos of the Philippines notice darkening in a woman's armpits, inner flexes of their elbows, and behind their knees, as well as color changes on their abdomen, groin, and thighs.

The Vietnamese notice oozing from the breasts when squeezed.

Midwives in Morocco establish pregnancy by palpating heat and swelling of her veins and noticing sweat glands around her nipples and a change in the coloring of her face.[4]

The Japanese use traditional Chinese medicine methods to ascertain a pregnancy. They took a woman's pulses and note that "The hand of woman belongs to the region of lesser yin. When the motion of her pulse is great she is with child."[5]

BOX 5-3 *Calculating the Due Date*

Traditional societies had different ways to calculate the due date. Most of these cultures did little to prepare for the birth because they believed that the baby would be born when it was ready. However, they did have reasonable approaches to calculating the expected time. Among the North American Kwakiutl tribe, the expectant woman counted 10 complete moon cycles after the date of her last menses. The child was usually born at the full moon of the last month.[6] Ancient Greeks and Romans also regarded pregnancy as a 10-month cycle with calculations based on their 28-day month.[7]

The full moon was a reference point for many other people. For instance, the Tiwi of Australia followed the moon cycle once pregnancy was established, and the Banyankole of Uganda had most births occurring at the full moon.[2,8] The Native American Navajo believed that birth would happen when the moon was straight overhead.[10] In Japan, high tide suggested an easier birth.[11]

---

rudimentary spine is being formed along the outer rim of the fetus' body; arm buds emerge from the body; the heart divides into chambers; blood is pumped into major vessels; the heartbeat has regulated; spots for the ears and eyes are formed on the head; lobes of the brain and spinal cord grow; and future **visceral organs** (organs within the abdominal cavity) start to develop (Figure 5-3).

Changes and Adaptations to the Musculoskeletal System

The physiological changes of pregnancy are mediated by an increase in steroid hormones that are initially secreted by the ovaries and subsequently by the placenta. In early pregnancy, hormonal changes regulate a pregnant woman's physical **adaptations** (changes and modifications the body makes as a result of the pregnancy). In later pregnancy, postural alterations and shifting are caused by the increased size and bulk of the uterus and by the relaxation of the joints.[12-14] Her center of gravity shifts forward, which results in an anterior pelvic tilt and increased lumbar spine compression. The natural anterior lordotic curve is exaggerated because of progesterone, relaxin, and the weight of the gravid uterus on the intravertebral discs

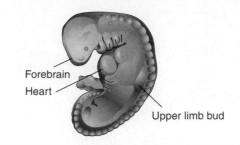

FIGURE 5-3 ■ Embryo at 1 month. (From Leifer G: *Maternity nursing: an introductory text*, ed 9, St. Louis, 2005, Saunders.)

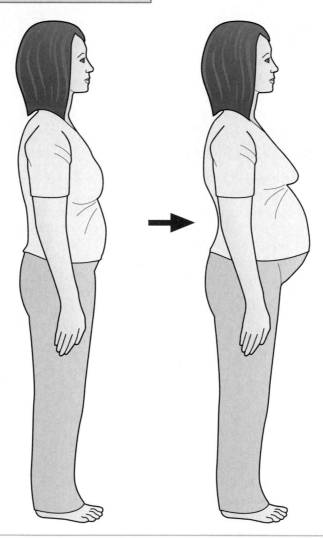

FIGURE 5-4 ■ Posture on the left is early pregnancy. The posture on the right, with its exaggerated lumbar curve, is later pregnancy.

(Figure 5-4).[14] Large breasts and stooped shoulders exacerbate lumbar, dorsal, and cervical curves.[13] In this position, the supporting pelvic ligaments, particularly those of the lumbosacral, symphysis pubis, and sacroiliac joints, are overstressed. Ligaments of the pelvis that are overstressed and cause further weakening of pelvic integrity are as follows:

Sacrum and ilium ligaments
   Anterior sacroiliac (Figure 5-5)
   Posterior sacroiliac (Figure 5-6)

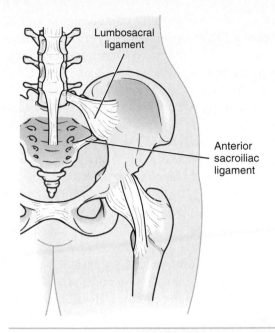

FIGURE 5-5 ■ Lumbosacral and anterior sacroiliac ligaments.

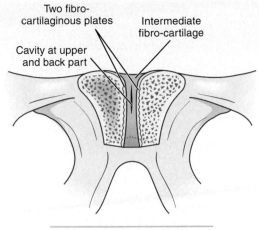

FIGURE 5-7 ■ Symphysis pubis.

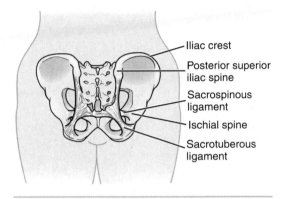

FIGURE 5-8 ■ Sacrotuberous and sacrospinous ligaments.

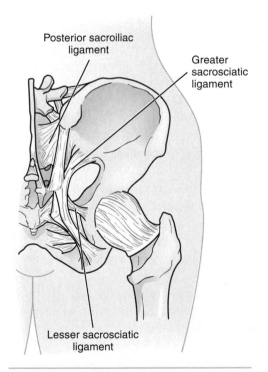

FIGURE 5-6 ■ Ligaments of the sacrum and ischium.

Sacrum and ischium (see Figure 5-6).
   Greater sacrosciatic (posterior)
   Lesser sacrosciatic (anterior)
Sacrum and coccyx
   Anterior sacrococcygeal
   Posterior sacrococcygeal
   Lateral sacrococcygeal
   Interposed fibrocartilage
   Interarticular
Symphysis pubis (Figure 5-7)
   Anterior pubic
   Superior pubic
   Posterior pubic
   Subpubic
   Interpubic disc[15]
Lumbosacral and iliolumbar (see Figure 5-5)
Sacrotuberous (Figure 5-8)
Sacrospinous (see Figure 5-8)

To make room for the growing uterus, a pregnant woman's rib cage expands anteriorly and laterally as much as 2 to 3 inches. This expansion often creates a strain in the midback at the rib attachments and causes discomfort around the rib cage. This strain can be relieved by gently stretching one or both arms overhead.[16] A woman's hips widen and laterally rotate to accommodate

BOX 5-5 *Dairy-Free Calcium-Rich Foods*

Pregnant and nursing women need at least 1300 mg of calcium per day. The foods listed contain approximately 300 mg of calcium.

Fish
1 cup canned herring, oysters or mackerel
3 oz sardines, smelt
4½ oz Coho salmon
5½ oz pink salmon
7 oz Chinook salmon
¾ lb fresh oysters*
2 cups oyster stew

Legumes
2 tofu cakes
1 cup raw black, garbanzo, pinto, or soy beans†

Seeds and Nuts
¼ cup sesame seeds
3 oz almond meal
1 cup almond, Brazil nuts

Vegetables
1-1½ cups cooked dark leafy greens such as collard greens, kale, lamb's quarters, dandelion greens, turnip greens, spinach

Flour
1 cup low fat soy flour

Seaweed
3 Tbsp Irish moss
100 gm each: agar agar (400 mg calcium), hijiki (1400 mg calcium), dulse (560 mg calcium), kombu (800 mg calcium), nori (260 mg calcium), wakami (1300 mg calcium)

Miscellaneous
1½ oz blackstrap molasses

*Eating raw seafood is not recommended during pregnancy.
†Cooking destroys some of the calcium.

From Stillerman E: *MotherMassage: massage during pregnancy professional manual*, New York, 1997.

her widening pelvis. To maintain an erect posture, and because of the hypertension in their hamstrings caused by their anterior pelvic tilt, some women hyperextend their knees and their medial arches may flatten. Most women complain of backaches after the fifth month.[14]

As the lordotic curve develops, there is a compensatory adaptation in the cervical spine as the pregnant woman's neck protracts and compresses the lower cervical vertebrae. Hand and arm weakness, aching, and numbness may be a result of the traction on the median and ulnar nerves.[13,17] By pregnancy's end, the symphysis pubis and sacroiliac joints become wider and many women adopt a waddling gait and walk with their upper backs arched and their shoulders laterally rotated.[14] Extra stress is placed on the ligaments as muscles of the midback and lower back shorten and are subject to strain and discomfort. In the last trimester, pressure of the heavy uterus on nerves and blood vessels often creates numbness or tingling on the lower extremities. Leg cramps (calf and thigh) usually occur in the second half of the pregnancy. They may also be related to calcium/phosphorus metabolism and increased neuromuscular compression and irritability. Excessive dairy products elevate phosphate levels, and a diet full of a wide variety of calcium-rich foods with limited dairy intake is advisable (Box 5-5). Almost 10% of all pregnant women experience restless legs syndrome right after getting into bed. Although the cause is not clear, it may be associated with anemia.[18]

Estrogen and relaxin affect the composition of cartilage and ligamentous structures, particularly the pelvis, allowing them to soften and loosen in preparation for labor (Box 5-6). The joints of pelvis become hypermobile, resulting in additional lumbar instability and muscle and ligament strain and pain.[14]

As the uterus expands, the pregnant woman's **abdominal muscles** stretch, weaken, lose tone, and separate, adding to lumbar instability and increased lower back pain. Stretching of the round ligament may cause additional lower back discomfort.[14]

The different intrinsic (I) and extrinsic (E) muscles and joints that are most strained during pregnancy are as follows:
Upper back (Figures 5-9 and 5-10)
    Longus capitis (I)
    Longus colli (I)
    Splenius capitis (I)
    Semispinalis capitis (I)
    Semispinalis cervicis (I)
    Scalenes (I)
    Sacrospinalis (E) (erector spinae)
    Trapezius (E)
    Levator scapulae (E)

BOX 5-6 *Relaxin*

Relaxin is a hormone that originates in the corpus luteum of the ovaries and placenta and helps remodel and loosen the connective tissues of the pelvic girdle, soften the cervix, and suppress uterine contractions. In addition to enlarging the dimensions of the pelvis for childbirth, relaxin promotes greater elasticity to predominantly collagenous fibers of the uterine ligaments, permitting them to stretch as the uterus grows, and fascial softening of the muscles, making room for the large uterus. Effects of this hormone can be felt as early as 10 weeks, resulting in joint instability, particularly in weight-bearing structures, and softening all connective tissue. Lower back pain or sciatic pain in early pregnancy may result from a laxity in the sacroiliac ligaments, weakening joint integrity and compressing the sciatic region. The body produces maximum amounts of relaxin between weeks 38-42, in time for labor.

Data from Lowdermilk DL, Perry SE: *Maternity & women's health care*, ed 8, St. Louis, 2004, Mosby; Coad J: *Anatomy and physiology for midwives*, St. Louis, 2001, Mosby.

Rhomboids (E)
Sternocleidomastoid (E)
Lower back (Figure 5-11)
    Iliocostalis lumborum (I)
    Longissimus thoracis (I)
    Sacrospinalis (E) (erector spinae)
    Quadratus lumborum (E)
    Gluteus medius (E)
    Gluteus maximus (E)
Trunk (Figure 5-12)
    Pectoralis major (E)
    Pectoralis minor (I)
    Rectus abdominis (E)
    Internal and external obliques (I)
    Transverse abdominis (I)
    Diaphragm (I)
    Serratus anterior (E)
Hip and pelvis (Figure 5-13)
    Flexors (E)
    Psoas major (I)
    Psoas minor (I)
    Iliacus (I)
    Lateral hip rotators (I): piriformis, quadratus femoris, obturator internus, obturator exterus, gemellus superior, gemellus inferior
Legs (Figure 5-14)
    Gastrocnemius (E)
    Soleus (I)
    Peroneus (E)
    Hamstrings (E)

Pelvic floor muscles (I) (Figure 5-15)
    Ischiocavernosus
    Pubococcygeus
    Levator ani
    Iliococcygeus
    Sphincter ani
    Ischiococcygeus
    Bulbospongiosus
    Superficial transverse perineal
    Deep transverse perineal
Affected joints (Figure 5-16)
    Hip
    Intervertebral and facet joints (especially lumbar spine)
    Lumbosacral
    Sacroiliac
Symphysis pubis[20,21]
    Transverse abdominis

As previously mentioned, the abdominal muscles stretch, weaken, lose tone, and separate during late pregnancy and this adaptation contributes to back instability, muscle pain, and weakness. The anterior abdominal wall is made up of four pairs of muscles: the **rectus abdominis** (Figure 5-17), **external oblique** (Figure 5-18), **internal oblique** (Figure 5-19), and the transverse abdominis (Figure 5-20).

The rectus abdominis is a long, flat muscle that has its origin at the costal cartilages of ribs 5 to 7, the xiphoid process, and the sternum. It inserts at the pubic crest and symphysis pubis. The **linea alba**, a sheath of connective tissue, separates the rectus into right and left sides. It is this tendon-like structure that separates in advanced pregnancy (Box 5-7).

The rectus flexes the vertebral column and is assisted by the external and internal obliques and the psoas major and minor. When both sides of the recti are weak, which occurs with the presence of the **diastasis** (separation along the linea alba), it results in a decreased ability to flex the spine and an increased difficulty in performing a posterior pelvic tilt.

The external obliques are the most superficial and largest of all the abdominal muscles. They originate at the external surfaces of the ribs 5 to 8 (anterior fibers) and ribs 9 to 12 (lateral fibers) and insert into the linea alba, inguinal ligament, anterior superior spine, and pubic tubercle into the external lip of the anterior half of the iliac

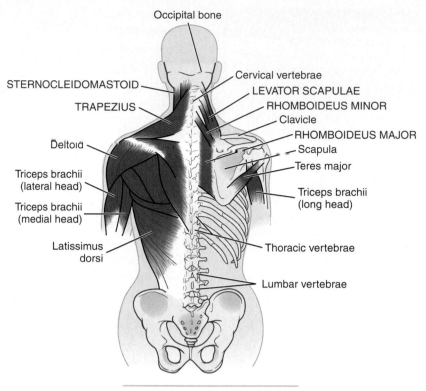

FIGURE 5-9 ■ Muscles of the back.

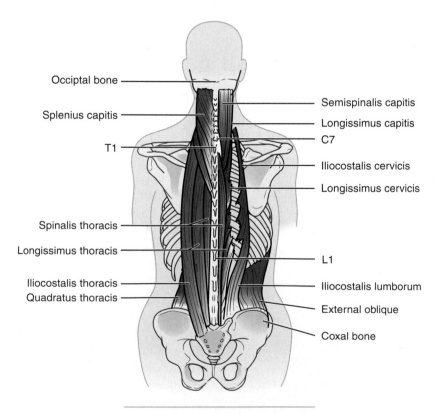

FIGURE 5-10 ■ Intrinsic back muscles.

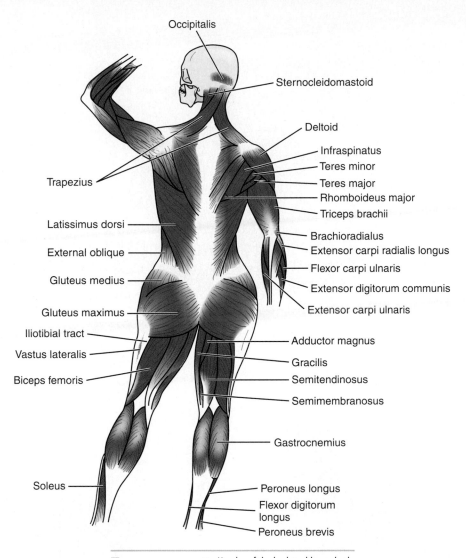

Occipitalis

Sternocleidomastoid

Deltoid

Infraspinatus

Teres minor

Teres major

Rhomboideus major

Triceps brachii

Trapezius

Brachioradialus

Extensor carpi radialis longus

Latissimus dorsi

Flexor carpi ulnaris

External oblique

Extensor digitorum communis

Gluteus medius

Extensor carpi ulnaris

Gluteus maximus

Adductor magnus

Iliotibial tract

Gracilis

Vastus lateralis

Semitendinosus

Biceps femoris

Semimembranosus

Gastrocnemius

Soleus

Peroneus longus

Flexor digitorum longus

Peroneus brevis

FIGURE 5-11 ■ Muscles of the back and lower back.

crest. Bilateral action flexes the vertebral column. Unilaterally, they rotate the spine. The lower anterior fibers of the internal obliques originate at the later two-thirds of the inguinal ligament and iliac crest. They insert with the transverse abdominis into the pubic crest and linea alba. The lower fibers compress and support the lower abdominal viscera in conjunction with the transverse. The lateral fibers originate in the middle one-third of the intermediate line of iliac crest and thoracolumbar fascia. Insertion is at the inferior borders of the ribs 10 to 12 and linea alba. Bilaterally, the obliques flex the spine and unilaterally they rotate the vertebral column.

The deepest of the abdominal muscles is the transverse abdominis. Origin is the inner surfaces of the cartilages of the lower six ribs, thoracodorsal fascia, anterior internal lip of the iliac crest, and lower one-third of the inguinal ligament. It inserts at the linea alba, pubic crest, and pectin of the pubis. It flattens the abdominal wall, compresses the abdominal viscera, eases a bowel movement, stabilizes the linea during lateral trunk flexion, supports the pelvic floor muscles, and stabilizes the lumbar spinal segment. It is known as the "girdle" of the body. During pregnancy, a strong transverse muscle supports the heavy uterus, minimizes the diastasis, stabilizes the lower spine, and facilitates labor.[16,20-25]

All abdominal muscles increase intraabdominal pressure and with the diaphragm, act as a girdle to keep the internal organs in place.[16]

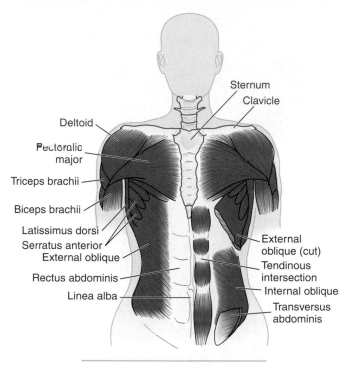

FIGURE 5-12 ■ Muscles of the trunk.

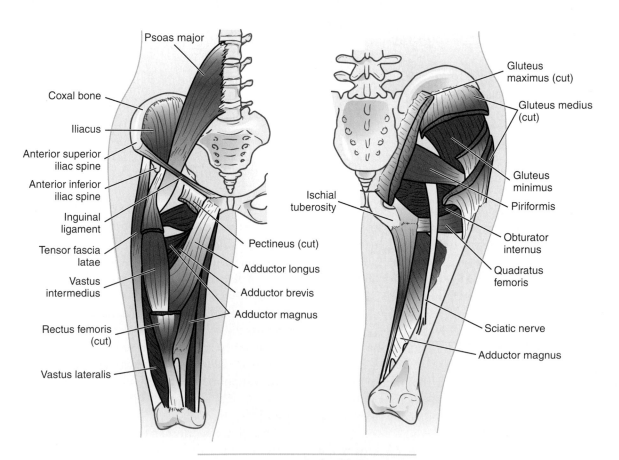

FIGURE 5-13 ■ Muscles of the hip and pelvis.

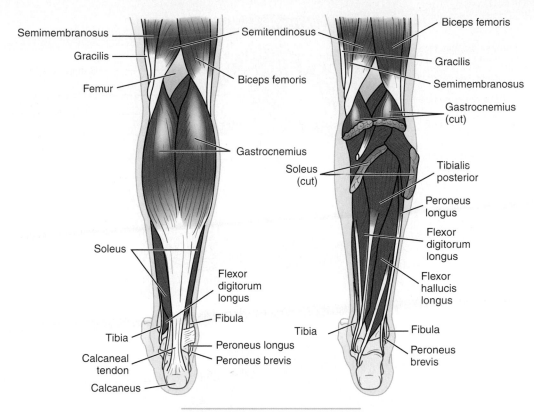

FIGURE 5-14 ■ Muscles of the legs.

Weakness in the transverse abdominis muscle results in a protruding abdominal wall and encourages a separation, or diastasis, of the recti bellies. Lower back instability, muscular imbalance, and back pain are common during pregnancy and can be minimized if the transverse abdominis muscle is recruited during daily activities and strengthened during exercise.[26,27] Relaxin and progesterone soften the collagen fibers in fascia, tendons, aponeuroses, and the linea alba, making these tissues more elastic and less supportive of the large uterus.[28] Examining the common attachments of the overlying muscles, contracting the transverse muscle pulls the linea alba inward, thereby making the diastasis smaller. During exercise, rotation exercises should be avoided because this movement pulls on the linea alba and further enlarges the diastasis.[29]

Proper Prenatal Exercises

Exercises that concentrate on recruiting the transverse abdominis muscle are the most effective ways of strengthening the abdominal wall, encouraging lower back stability, decreasing the diastasis recti, and minimizing the common discomforts

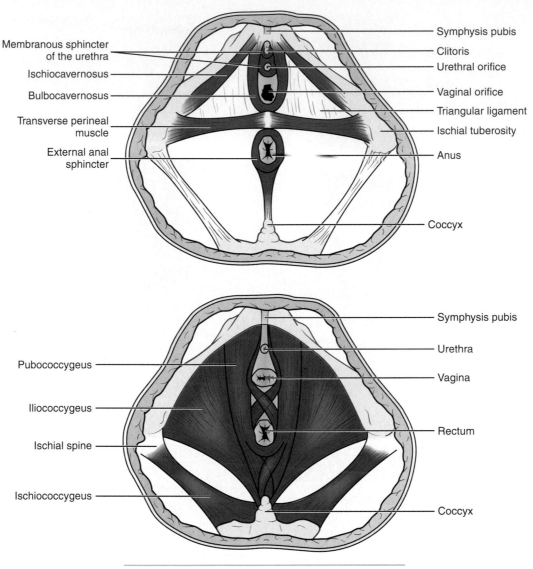

FIGURE 5-15 ■ Pelvic floor muscles (pubococcygeal muscles).

of pregnancy associated with poor posture. Sit-ups, curl-ups, crunches, and any movements that involve twisting should be avoided. These exercises push the head forward even more than it already is, create trigger points in the shoulders and upper back, weaken the transverse by bulging the abdominal muscles outward, and can lead to urinary incontinence because of the additional pressure on the pelvic floor (Figure 5-21).[23] The twisting motion can have a shearing effect on the linea alba.[29]

These exercises should begin as early in the pregnancy as possible. Even during the first trimester, when many women experience fatigue and shortness of breath, these simple exercises can maintain muscle tone, make postpartum recovery easier and faster, make the abdominal muscles more effective during labor, and control backaches. During the second and third trimesters, women should not lie flat because of the concern of supine hypotension.[22,30] Many of these exercises can be performed very effectively sitting or half-lying. The main goal is to use the transverse by pulling the belly in toward the spine, thereby shortening the overstretched abdominals (Figure 5-22). Appropriate prenatal exercises are as follows:

■ Pelvic tilting can be done lying down, standing, or kneeling. While recruiting the transverse, the pelvic tilt shortens the

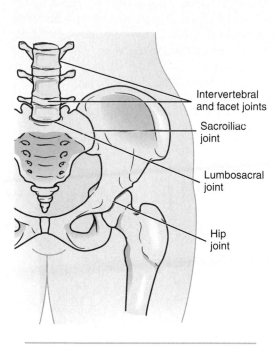

FIGURE 5-16 ■ Affected lumbar and pelvic joints.

Intervertebral and facet joints

Sacroiliac joint

Lumbosacral joint

Hip joint

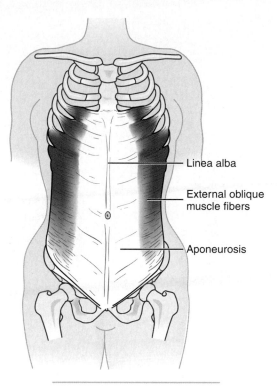

FIGURE 5-18 ■ External oblique.

Linea alba

External oblique muscle fibers

Aponeurosis

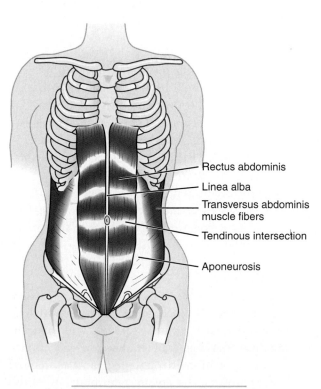

FIGURE 5-17 ■ Rectus abdominis.

Rectus abdominis

Linea alba

Transversus abdominis muscle fibers

Tendinous intersection

Aponeurosis

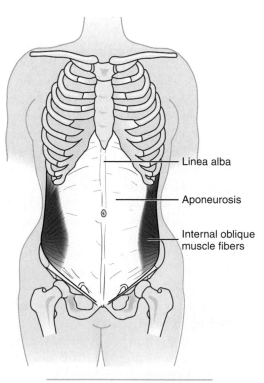

FIGURE 5-19 ■ Internal oblique.

Linea alba

Aponeurosis

Internal oblique muscle fibers

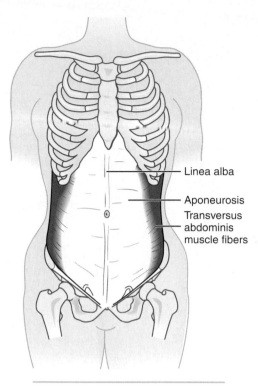

FIGURE 5-20 ■ Transversus abdominis.

Linea alba
Aponeurosis
Transversus
abdominis
muscle fibers

BOX 5-7   *Linea Alba*

The linea alba is positioned between the medial borders of the rectus bellies. It is formed by an aponeuroses of both obliques and the transverse muscle. It is composed of mostly collagenous fibers that are under hormonal influence during pregnancy. Relaxin allows the fibers to widen as the uterus grows. This separation is called the diastasis and is responsible for much of the lower back instability and weakness

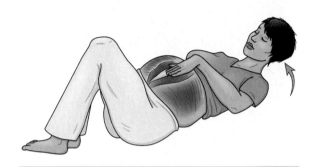

FIGURE 5-21 ■ To test for a diastasis, the client is palpating across her linea alba, feeling for the recti bellies. The number of fingers that can fit into the separation indicates how wide it is. Normal linea alba separation is ½ finger width. Practitioners can test for the diastasis by running their fingers gently across the linea alba from above the symphysis pubis to the xiphoid process. The separation is greatest above and below the umbilicus.

abdominal muscles and elongates the compressed lumbar spine. The client should breathe normally, hold the pose for 10 seconds, and repeat up to ten times (Figure 5-23).

■ Five floor abdominal elevators are done when the client imagines that relaxed abdominal muscles are at the "first floor," muscles pulled halfway toward the spine are the "third floor," and pulled in all the way to the spine is the "fifth floor." As the client sits in a chair or cross-legged on the floor, she takes a deep breath and exhales slowly. During the exhalation, she should bring her navel all the way to her spine (fifth floor). She should hold at the fifth floor and count out loud to 30 while continuing to breathe normally and then repeat 5 more times to complete one set. She should gradually work up to 50 sets a day.

■ Contracting is done as the client sits in a chair or cross-legged on the floor and takes a deep breath. She brings her belly halfway back toward her spine (third floor)

as the starting position. From the third floor, she pulls back to her spine (fifth floor) and counts out loud (exhalation) with each contraction to 25, which is one set. She should practice this several times throughout the day until she can easily do sets of 100 throughout the day. Once she becomes proficient at this, she can advance this exercise by starting at the fourth floor and pulling back to the spine.[22]

Back Care

Proper exercises and postural support are essential elements in promoting back stability and minimizing back stiffness, soreness, and pain. The massage treatment can eradicate trigger points, increase nutrition to tightened muscles, remove waste products, and enhance flexibility. All of this can be undone, however, if the client reverts back

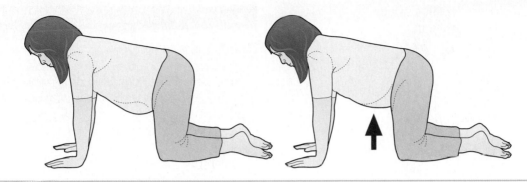

FIGURE 5-22 ■ Pulling the abdomen in toward the spine works the transverse abdominis muscle. The wrists should be neutral if there is pain in the hands. (From Fraser D, Cooper M: *Myles' textbook for midwives*, ed 14, Edinburgh, 2003, Churchill Livingstone.)

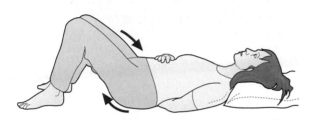

FIGURE 5-23 ■ Pelvic tilt in a lying position. Rotating the pelvic posterior shortens the overstretched abdominals and stretches the compressed muscles of the lower back. (From Fraser D, Cooper M: *Myles' textbook for midwives*, ed 14, Edinburgh, 2003, Churchill Livingstone.)

to her poor postural habits. Part of the practitioner's work, therefore, is to bring to her attention all she can do to maintain proper body mechanics to support her back.

Back Care and Body Mechanics

If the client does revert to habitual poor body mechanics and postural shifting, the effects of the massage will be short-lived. It is important to instruct her about proper body mechanics and make her aware of conscientiously changing her posture. Some techniques that may be helpful are as follows:

- While sitting, the chair should support her back and thighs. A small pillow, cushion, or towel can be placed at the small of her back for additional support. The addition of a footstool encourages further posterior pelvic tilting. She should avoid crossing her legs. To stand, she should slowly inch forward on the chair, recruit her transverse abdominis toward her spine, and push up with her arms and her legs.

- While standing, she should remember to recruit her transverse abdominis muscle by pulling it back to her spine. Her breathing remains normal. She should avoid wearing high heels and keep her shoulders relaxed.
- While getting up from a lying position (i.e., the massage table or bed), she should turn to one side, bend her knees, bring her abdominal muscles to her spine, and slowly push up with her arms. She should never "jack-knife" up.
- Lifting should be avoided during pregnancy, but this is not always possible. Toddlers want to be held, and some household activities require lifting. With her abdominals pulled back towards her spine, she should bend her knees, bring the object close to her body, and keep her back straight. She must use her legs and not her back, and twisting movements should be avoided (Figure 5-24).[16]

Changes and Adaptations to the Cardiovascular System

One of the most dramatic physiological adaptations occurs within the **cardiovascular system** (the circulatory system made up of the heart, veins, arteries, and blood). These changes support normal maternal metabolism, the increased needs of the pregnancy, and provide for fetal growth. The increase in blood volume is commensurate with the woman's weight, the number of previous pregnancies and births she has had and whether this is a single or multiple birth.[31] The elevation of blood volume supports the uterus (because

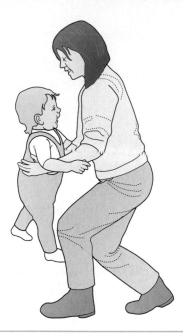

FIGURE 5-24 ■ Correct lifting is performed by pulling in the abdominal muscles, bringing the object close to the body, bending the knees, keeping the back straight, and using the legs to lift. (From Fraser D, Cooper M: *Myles' textbook for midwives*, ed 14, Edinburgh, 2003, Churchill Livingstone.)

> ### BOX 5-8   *Iron-Rich Foods*
>
> In addition to the prenatal vitamin that contains additional iron, women should eat a wide variety of wholesome foods to protect themselves from anemia. Vitamin C, folic acid, and calcium enhance iron absorption. Phosphates found in diet drinks decrease iron assimilation.
>
>   Liver, lean meats, organ meats
>   Eggs
>   Whole grains, cream of wheat, 2 Tbsp wheat germ
>   Cooked greens: spinach, beans, dandelion greens, kale and
>   soybeans
>   Prunes, raisins, apricots
>   Almonds (easiest to digest as a butter)
>   1 Tbsp blackstrap molasses
>   Herbs rich in iron are dandelion, yellow dock

From Stillerman E: *MotherMassage: massage during pregnancy professional manual*, New York, 1992, Dell.

as much as 10% of maternal cardiac output is redirected to the uterus by the third trimester), protects the mother and fetus against harmful effects of compromised venous return in erect or supine positions, counterbalances the effects of increased arterial and venous flow, increases perfusion to other vital organs, especially the kidneys, and compensates for maternal blood loss at birth, which averages 500 to 600 ml for a vaginal birth and 1000 ml for a Cesarean delivery.[12,31] Blood volume increases begin by the sixth week of pregnancy and continues through the end of the pregnancy, with an average volume increase of 30% to 50%. This level generally peaks between weeks 16 and 28 and remains elevated until after week 30. There is a slight decrease to about 20% by week 40 because of the heavy uterus obstructing the vena cava.[31-33] Blood volume for a multiple pregnancy is greater than for a single pregnancy.[34]

Women feel much warmer as a result of this increased blood volume and associated peripheral vasodilatation. A pregnant woman must remember to drink adequate amounts of water, about 8 to 12 glasses daily, to prevent dehydration that

contributes to miscarriage or premature birth. She also does not require heavy blankets during massage treatment because she is so warm. Covering her with a light sheet should be sufficient to maintain modesty while keeping her comfortable.

All blood components increase as a result of the additional blood volume. This increase is comprised of additional serum protein, neutrophils, enzymes, plasma, platelets, **clotting factor** (to prevent hemorrhaging during and after labor), albumin, and white and red blood cells. Plasma levels increase to 1000 ml by early pregnancy, and the red blood cell count is elevated to 450 ml, or about 20% to 30%[13,31,35] Because plasma levels are increased earlier in the pregnancy than the red blood cells, hemoglobin and hematocrit values drop. A pregnant woman must supplement her daily intake of iron through either prenatal vitamins or through food sources to avoid iron deficiency anemia (Box 5-8). A pregnant woman is considered anemic if her hemoglobin values decrease to 10 gm/dl or less, or if hematocrit levels decrease to 35% or less.[13] If not enough iron is available, the fetus leaches iron from maternal stores. This ensures adequate levels of fetal hemoglobin even when mother is iron-deficient. This deficiency might contribute to preterm labor and late spontaneous abortion if it gets serious enough.[31] During the second trimester, white blood cell count increases from a prepregnancy

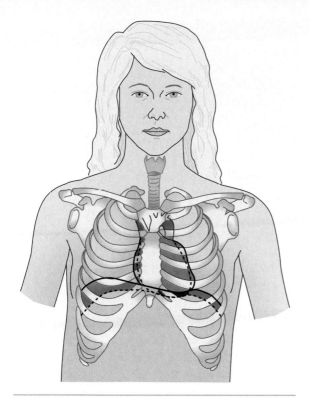

FIGURE 5-25 ■ The solid line demonstrates changes in the heart, lungs, and thoracic rib cage positions during pregnancy. (From Fraser D, Cooper M: *Myles' textbook for midwives*, ed 14, Edinburgh, 2003, Churchill Livingstone.)

is compressed by the enlarged uterus (Figure 5-25).[13,31] Since the heart is so much larger, it is easier to hear and diagnose cardiac irregularities. These changes reverse after the pregnancy.

Between weeks 14 and 20, a pregnant woman's resting pulse increases about 10 to 15 beats per minute and stays elevated until the end of pregnancy. Palpitations and arrhythmias, caused by premature atrial contractions and premature ventricular systole, may result. Almost 90% of women develop a slight systolic murmur that lasts until the first week postpartum.[16] This is not a problem in healthy women, but those women with preexisting cardiac problems should be under the supervision of a medical doctor.[13]

Blood pressure can be affected by stress and the client's position. During pregnancy, blood pressure generally lowers by 10%.[16] Brachial pressure is highest when she is sitting and lowest when she is side-lying. Supine positioning can cause dangerous hypotension, called supine hypotensive syndrome or aortocaval compression, as the fetus and heavy uterus compress the vena cava.[12] After 4 to 5 minutes in a supine position, a reflex bradycardia occurs and heart production is halved. Women feel faint, dizzy, short of breath, or nauseous. Turning her to her left side will decrease the symptoms and return cardiac output to normal (Figure 5-26).[33] Systemic blood pressure declines slightly with the greatest difference in diastolic pressure.[31] During early pregnancy, blood pressure stays the same and then slowly decreases by about week 20. After 20 weeks, maternal blood pressure increases and should be the same as early pregnancy.[33,36]

level of 4300 to 4500/ml to 5000 to 12,000/ml and peaks during the third trimester to as high as 16,000/ml.[31]

There is slight cardiac hypertrophy, as much as 12%, to accommodate the increase in blood-volume, and the maternal heart is pushed upward and rotated toward the left as the diaphragm

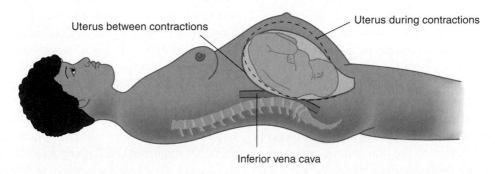

FIGURE 5-26 ■ Supine positioning can create a hypotensive syndrome as the weight of the fetus compresses the vena cava. Maternal blood pressure will rise and oxygen will be cut off to the fetus. (From Leifer G: *Maternity nursing: an introductory text*, ed 9, St. Louis, 2005, Saunders.)

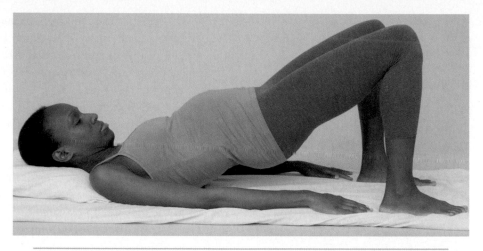

FIGURE 5-27 ■ Elevating the hips can reduce the pressure on vulval varicosities and hemorrhoids.

Blood flow to the lower extremities is slowed during the last few weeks of pregnancy.[37] The combination of sluggish venous return and increased venous pressure and the increased pressure in the veins of the legs, vulva, rectum, and pelvis often leads to edema, varicose veins of the legs and vulva, and hemorrhoids.[33] To ease varicosities and hemorrhoids, these helpful techniques can be followed:

- Lymphatic drainage can be performed on the legs to ease lymph congestion and reduce swelling.
- The client's legs and feet can be elevated frequently to reduce swelling.
- For vulval varicosities and hemorrhoids, the client's hips can be raised to enhance postural venous drainage (Figure 5-27). The client should also raise her trunk for short periods to bring the weight of the uterus upward.
- Client should lie on her left side to encourage circulation.
- Client should be urged to do Kegel exercises (voluntary contracting and relaxing of the sphincter muscles of the pelvic floor).[31]

Although the uterus is the main recipient of increased blood flow, there is increased circulation to her kidneys, skin, and lungs. Blood flow to the kidneys enhances the elimination of waste products.[38] Increased blow flow to the skin and mucous membranes is responsible for the rapid growth of hair and nails.[37] There is a 20% increase of blood to the breasts throughout the pregnancy. Some women notice this by how large their breasts become and by heat and tingling sensations in early pregnancy.

hCG and prolactin, the nursing hormone, suppress maternal immune response. This decreases the white blood cells' ability to fight infection, particularly viral infections. This decrease in immune function starts in the tenth week and remains at this level until the baby is born.[39]

To protect the mother from hemorrhaging at labor, there is an increase in **coagulating factors (fibrinogenic activity)** VII, VIII, IX, X, and fibrinogen and a decrease in anticoagulants or fibrinolytics.[13,40,41] This activity continues throughout the first few months of postpartum. By the end of the first trimester, there is a 50% increase in the synthesis of plasma fibrinogen.[42] The decrease in anticoagulants along with vasodilation contributes to a five to sixfold increase in the risk of thromboembolism in pregnancy.[40,43] Blood clots may also develop because of the weight of the uterus slowing femoral and iliac circulation, sluggish blood flow, greater blood volume, and higher levels of progesterone relaxing smooth muscle fibers. Blood clots can form in any vein but are more prevalent in the deep veins where blood flow is restricted and generally more stagnant. During pregnancy, the veins that might harbor these thromboemboli or deep vein thromboses are the iliac, femoral, and saphenous veins of the inner thigh and calf (Figure 5-28).[43]

If clots do aggregate within the deeper vessels, the client's legs might feel sore and achy, but these clots do not pose any major health threat.

The bodyworker must recognize the potential danger when massaging the legs of a pregnant woman, even in her first trimester, and always assess the legs for clots before beginning the treatment and use appropriate, light lymphatic drainage all times.

By the third trimester, pregnant women have 40% more interstitial fluid that translates into more swelling in the lower extremities. Restricted femoral and iliac circulation, the weight of the uterus, myofascial restrictions of the pelvis, and gravity all work against lymph reabsorption. For most of these women, swelling is not a problem, although it understandably contributes to stiff and sore legs and fatigue. But for 25%, this swelling can be problematic. The swelling is considered to be pitting edema if a small depression remains after finger pressure is applied to the swollen area (Figure 5-29); massage is contraindicated. This assessment tests for preeclampsia, which can be very dangerous to mother and fetus (Box 5-9).

When the upper torso, hands, face, or entire body becomes swollen in the first or second trimester, the pregnant woman may have a preeclamptic condition known as gestational edema proteinuria hypertensive (GEPH) syndrome. The client's face looks very swollen and bulbous, and the swelling prevents her from making a strong fist throughout the day. Massage is contraindicated with the presence of GEPH. Pretreatment evaluations (see Chapter 3) are critical because they can help determine whether the client should receive bodywork.

Preeclampsia and other hypertensive disorders of pregnancy are responsible for at least 76,000 maternal and infant deaths each year.[16] Pregnancies complicated by preeclampsia or eclampsia have high maternal and perinatal death rates.[51] Acute kidney failure, pulmonary edema, and liver hematomas may result from untreated conditions.[52,53] Babies are often born prematurely, small for their gestational weight, and at risk for perinatal asphyxia.[54]

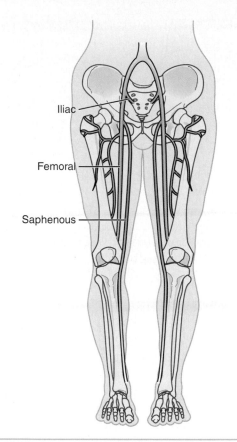

FIGURE 5-28 ■ Deep veins where blood clots might form are iliac, femoral, and saphenous veins.

Illness and death during pregnancy from venous thromboembolism occurs 1 in 1000 to 1 in 2000 pregnant and postpartum women.[45,46] During pregnancy, the clots most frequently begin in the veins of the calf muscles or in the iliofemoral portion of the deeper venous system. The left leg seems to be most susceptible.[47-49]

The symptoms of thrombi are localized heat, swelling, reddening, muscle contraction over the site of the clot(s), increased edema of the limb, sensitive dermatome above the clot, and very painful legs. Thrombi are also often asymptomatic, which is another reason all deep strokes are avoided on the legs during pregnancy (and up to 3 months postpartum).

Those clients who are most at risk of developing thromboembolism are sedentary women or those confined to bed rest, women over 30, overweight women, and those who suffer from autoimmune diseases such as lupus, and those having their fourth or more child.[50]

Changes and Adaptations to the Respiratory System

The **respiratory system** is responsible for breathing. Increased cardiac output and blood volume increases pulmonary blood flow.[55] Pregnant

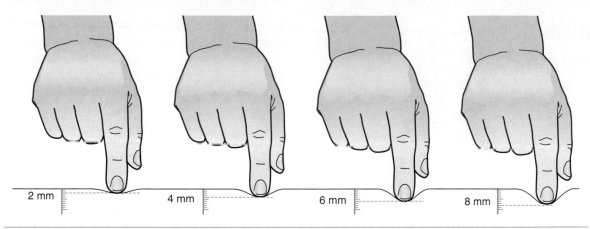

FIGURE 5-29 ■ To test for pitting edema, the practitioner should apply gentle pressure above her ankles and slowly count to 5. The impression should disappear between 10 and 30 seconds. If not, this could be a sign of preeclampsia and massage should be avoided.

BOX 5-9　*Preeclampsia*

Preeclampsia usually occurs after 20 weeks' gestation, although it can occur earlier or postpartum, and it affects both mother and fetus. Approximately 5% to 8% of all pregnancies are affected, and preeclampsia is a progressive condition with symptoms of high blood pressure, proteinuria, swelling, sudden weight gain, headaches, and vision changes. Eclampsia is a more serious and life-threatening condition than preeclampsia, although both can be very dangerous to mother and fetus. Signs of impending eclampsia are as follows:

A spike in blood pressure
Diminished urine output
Increase in proteinuria
Severe headache usually in the front of the head
Drowsiness or confusion
Visual impairment such as flashing lights or "floaters"
Stomachache denoting liver impairment
Vomiting or nausea

---

women are predisposed to nasal congestion, epistaxis (nose bleeds), and enlarged vocal cords, causing a deepened voice because increased blood volume and vasodilation create hyperemia and edema in the upper respiratory mucosa.[56] Almost 70% of healthy women develop pregnancy-induced dyspnea, or shortness of breath, in the first or second trimesters.[55] To compensate, some women hyperventilate and become dizzy.

As the uterus grows, the fundus indirectly compresses the respiratory diaphragm so that it is elevated from its normal position. The rib cage widens anterolaterally as much as 2 to 3 inches because of progesterone's influence on the ligaments to accommodate the gravid uterus. This often causes midthoracic discomfort. Inspiration becomes deeper, allowing for a 30% to 40% in tidal volume, which is the volume of air inspired or expired.[13] Oxygen use increases by 15% to 20% during pregnancy.[12,14]

By the third trimester, breathlessness is not uncommon. Some of the breathlessness is attributed to the extra weight the pregnant woman has to carry, her postural shifting, and an increase in basal metabolism (Box 5-10). As a result of the larger breasts and side-lying sleeping, shoulder medial rotation can create myofascial restrictions throughout the rib cage. Myofascial-releasing techniques and stretches are very helpful in relieving this congestion (Figure 5-30).

Changes and Adaptations to the Gastrointestinal System

One of the earliest signs of pregnancy is nausea, which is possibly caused by a reaction to hCG and experienced by almost 50% to 90% of pregnant women. This "morning sickness" can occur at any time during the day or night and at any trimester of the pregnancy. It generally abates by the second trimester as levels of a placental hormone, human placental lactogen (HPL), elevate, while hCG levels decline. An unfortunate 20% continually suffer from nausea throughout the entire pregnancy. For some women, nausea and vomiting can be extreme. This condition, known as *hyperemesis gravidarum*, can require

BOX 5-10	*Respiratory Changes during Pregnancy*
Minute volume	+40%
Oxygen consumption	+15%-20%
Cardiac output	+30%
Tidal volume	+30%-40%
Respiratory rate	Unchanged
Inspiratory reserve volume	Unchanged
Expiratory reserve volume	Reduces progressively
Residual volume	Reduces progressively
Total lung capacity	Unchanged
Vital capacity	Increased
Inspiratory capacity	Increased
Functional residual capacity	Reduces progressively
Residual volume	Unchanged
Physiological dead space	Increased
Alveolar ventilation	Increased

From Coad J: *Anatomy and physiology for midwives,* St. Louis, 2001, Mosby.

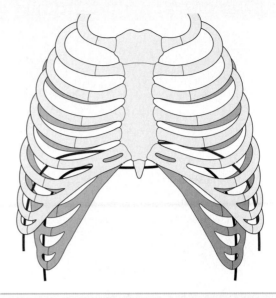

FIGURE 5-30 ■ The light rib cage represents the displaced rib cage of pregnancy. The dark rib cage is the nonpregnancy state. Note the raised diaphragm of pregnancy. (From Coad J: *Anatomy and physiology for midwives,* ed 2, 2005, London, Churchill Livingstone.)

medical intervention or hospitalization to treat the woman for dehydration.

As pregnancy continues, the growing uterus displaces the visceral organs by an increase in intraabdominal pressure (Figure 5-31). In addition, progesterone slows down the function of smooth muscle, affecting the gastrointestinal tract, uterus, ureters, and blood vessels.[31,57] These contribute to sluggish motility of the stomach contents into the intestines and peristaltic action of the intestines. The results are heartburn and constipation, two very common discomforts of pregnancy.

Heartburn is caused by the displacement of the stomach and slowed emptying time, with the resultant regurgitation of the stomach acid into the lower esophagus. This may become severe enough to cause esophageal ulcerations. It is best to massage these clients in a sitting position to minimize stomach acid reflux. Approximately 30% to 70% of women experience heartburn at some point in their pregnancies.[14] Progesterone lowers the tone of the esophageal sphincter, and regurgitation is likely. This usually occurs during the second trimester and gets worse as pregnancy continues.

Heartburn is increased with multiple pregnancies, obesity, and excessive bending over. Certain foods, such as alcohol, chocolate, and coffee, reduce esophageal muscle tone and exacerbate heartburn. Gastric acid secretions and pepsin levels abate during pregnancy as tone and motility decrease.

Constipation and intestinal gas may be caused by decreased gastric activity, pelvic congestion from the heavy uterus, iron supplements, and lax muscle tone. Exercise, postural considerations, and drinking at least 8 to 12 glasses of water a day are helpful.

Although intestinal tone and peristalsis are directly affected by progesterone, there is improved absorption of iron and calcium in late pregnancy. However, progesterone does inhibit transit of other nutrients such as the vitamin B group. Sodium and water absorption from the colon is increased, further adding to constipation. Recruiting the transverse abdominis muscle has been found to be helpful in relieving some of these symptoms by enhancing venous circulation to the bowel.[58]

Additional estrogen increases vascularity, sponginess, and softening to the gums. Even slight brushing can cause gums to bleed. Gingivitis and periodontal disease are not uncommon during the last trimester and are more pronounced in women who are older, had numerous pregnancies, and preexisting dental problems. Women who develop gum disease should discuss this with their

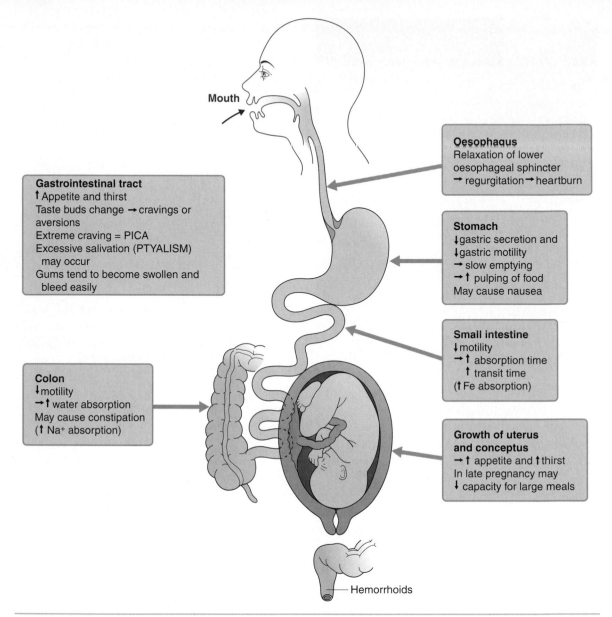

Oesophagus
Relaxation of lower
oesophageal sphincter
→ regurgitation → heartburn

Mouth

Gastrointestinal tract
↑ Appetite and thirst
Taste buds change → cravings or
aversions
Extreme craving = PICA
Excessive salivation (PTYALISM)
 may occur
Gums tend to become swollen and
 bleed easily

Stomach
↓ gastric secretion and
↓ gastric motility
→ slow emptying
→ ↑ pulping of food
May cause nausea

Small intestine
↓ motility
→ ↑ absorption time
 ↑ transit time
(↑ Fe absorption)

Colon
↓ motility
→ ↑ water absorption
May cause constipation
(↑ Na+ absorption)

**Growth of uterus
and conceptus**
→ ↑ appetite and ↑ thirst
In late pregnancy may
↓ capacity for large meals

Hemorrhoids

FIGURE 5-31 ■ Changes in the digestive system. (From Fraser D, Cooper M: *Myles' textbook for midwives*, ed 14, Edinburgh, 2003, Churchill Livingstone.)

obstetricians and dentists because preterm labor may be caused by gingivitis and severe periodontal disease. Teeth do not demineralize as a result of pregnancy because the fetus draws its calcium from maternal skeletal stores and not the teeth.[59] However, cavities do increase during pregnancy and the content of saliva changes to a more acidic pH.

Over 50% of women have an increase in appetite and an even higher rate of thirst, especially during the first trimester.[14,60] Estrogen has the tendency to suppress appetite, whereas progesterone is stimulating. Decreased plasma glucose and amino acid levels also stimulate the appetite.[14] Her eating habits might improve as she recognizes the need for carefully prepared, nutritious meals and snacks or she might have cravings or aversions. It is believed that the taste buds are somewhat dulled during pregnancy, so the spicier the food the better, whereas the sense of smell is heightened.[61]

Food cravings can become extreme, as in the case of pica, wherein women crave nonnutritious items such as coal, mothballs, ice, or toothpaste. African-American women in the south follow a tradition of eating laundry starch, chalk, and clay.[14]

Progesterone causes the gall bladder to become more flaccid, increasing bile volume storage and slower emptying time. In late pregnancy, some women complain of dry, itchy skin. It is believed that bile salts, which are retained in greater amount, are deposited in the skin, making it irritated.

The changes in the liver appear to be caused by organ displacement. Increased levels of glycogen and triacylglyceride are stored in the liver. The liver increases **fibrinogenic activity** (to produce clots) and there is an increase in cholesterol synthesis.

Changes and Adaptations to the Urinary (Renal) System

Urination (micturition) is very frequent during the first trimester because of the pressure of the uterus on the bladder. As the fundus rises out of the pelvis at about the fourth month, the urge to urinate lessens to some degree and reappears in the last trimester as the enlarged uterus compresses the bladder and squeezes it against the symphysis pubis. As the fetus grows, the bladder is displaced upward and flattened. Vascularity of the bladder increases, whereas muscle tone decreases. The walls of the bladder are edematous and hyperemic, lowering resistance to infection and trauma.[14]

Urinary tract infections are not uncommon in late pregnancy because the weight of the pelvis compromises circulatory and lymphatic drainage from the bladder. The pressure of the uterus can even block the ureters, particularly on the right side.[31] Stasis of urine in the bladder also increases the risk of bladder infections.[12]

Each kidney lengthens by 1 to 1.5 cm and the ureters also elongate, widen, and become more curved (Figure 5-32). The increase in progesterone level, the extra blood volume, and the growing uterus cause the smooth muscle of the ureters and renal pelvis to relax and dilate. There is up to 50% more glomerular filtration rate (GFR) from the kidneys during pregnancy, and the renal plasma flow increases 25% to 50%.[62] Increased GFR and impaired reabsorption increases glucose excretion (glycosuria) in about 50% of women.[36] This condition is often associated with gestational diabetes and increased infection rate and is usually carefully watched by doctors.[56]

Even though more waste is excreted, the volume of urine remains the same, making the **urinary system** more efficient during pregnancy. The kidney secretes an enzyme called *renin*, also stimulated by heightened levels of estrogen, that acts as a vasoconstrictor. Levels of this enzyme increase in the first trimester and continue to rise until the end of the pregnancy.

In the last trimester, the fetus needs more sodium, which results in maternal retention of

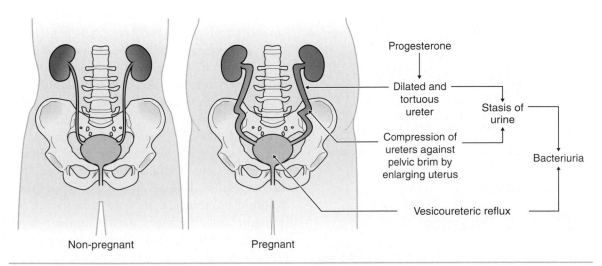

FIGURE 5-32 ■ Nonpregnant ureters *(left)* and pregnant ureters *(right)* showing enlargement, curving, and factors for urinary tract infection. (From Fraser D, Cooper, M: *Myles' textbook for midwives*, ed 14, Edinburgh, 2003, Churchill Livingstone.)

sodium and potassium and more swelling. Urinary release of calcium increases by calcium absorption to maintain maternal levels. The adaptations to the urinary system continue until approximately 6 weeks' postpartum, or the puerperium.

Changes and Adaptations to the Reproductive System

The **reproductive system** is involved in becoming pregnant and childbirth. The uterus undergoes dramatic changes during pregnancy. Before pregnancy, this 7.5 × 5 × 2.5 cm pear-shaped organ weighs only 2 oz (50 to 60 gm). At term, it becomes a thin-walled, muscular 30 × 22.5 × 20 cm housing for the fetus, placenta, amniotic sac, and amniotic fluid and weighs over 2 lbs (1000 gm).[12,36] The uterine lining, known as the endometrium, thickens into the decidua (a thickening and increased vascular lining). The layers of the myometrium become clearly delineated as new muscle fibers develop (Figure 5-33). The uterus grows as a direct result of estrogen and progesterone secretions, as well as the pressure of the fetus against the uterine walls, and can be explained by an increase in muscle cells (hypertrophy) and the creation of new cells (hyperplasia). The uterus is the major repository of the increased blood volume to nourish the fertilized egg as it implants and to support the growing fetus and placenta. Blood vessel diameter increases, and vascular resistance drops. These changes facilitate the increased blood flow to the placenta, which is balanced and maintained under conditions of low blood pressure.[14]

The uterus is actively contracting throughout the pregnancy. These contractions, called Braxton Hicks contractions, help circulate the blood through the placenta to the fetus and strengthen the uterus for labor. During the first trimester, these painless contractions are not noticeable. Women who have had previous pregnancies seem to be more aware of the Braxton Hicks contractions throughout the pregnancy.

In early pregnancy, the uterus stays pear-shaped. As the pregnancy progresses, the corpus and fundus become rounder. By the tenth week, the uterus is the size of an orange.[63] At the end of the first trimester, it grows to the size of a grapefruit and is no longer a pelvic organ but elevates and becomes upright, and the fundus can be palpated just above the pubic symphysis.[64] The uterus becomes spherical by week 16 as the isthmus and cervix develop into the lower uterine segments. This region of the uterus contains fewer muscle cells and blood vessels and is the site of the incision for most Cesarean sections (Figure 5-34).[55]

By the twentieth week, the uterus can be felt at the umbilicus and assumes an ovoid shape that it maintains to term.[65] As the uterus continues to rise into the abdominal cavity, the uterine tubes stretch vertically, creating more tension in the broad and round ligaments.[33] By week 30, the fundus can be felt between the umbilicus and xiphoid process. By the thirty-eighth week, the fundus reaches the xiphoid process. Upper uterine muscle contractions increase in frequency and strength, while the lower uterine segment develops faster and is stretched radially allowing the fetus to begin its descent into the pelvis. The upper uterine segment can contract 40 times higher than the distal cervix. For those women who have had

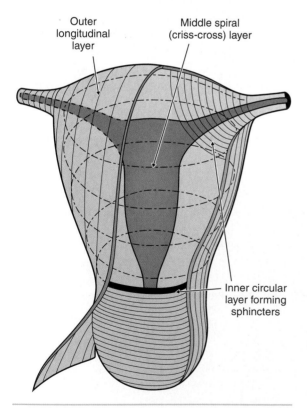

Outer longitudinal layer

Middle spiral (criss-cross) layer

Inner circular layer forming sphincters

FIGURE 5-33 ■ The three layers of uterine muscles during pregnancy. (From Fraser D, Cooper, M: *Myles' textbook for midwives,* ed 14, Edinburgh, 2003, Churchill Livingstone.)

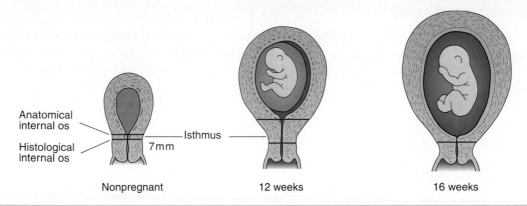

FIGURE 5-34 ■ Changes in the uterus from nonpregnant *(left)* to 12 weeks *(middle)* and at 16 weeks' gestation *(right)*. (From Fraser D, Cooper, M: *Myles' textbook for midwives*, ed 14, Edinburgh, 2003, Churchill Livingstone.)

previous pregnancies, the fetus might not engage until labor begins (Figure 5-35).

The cervix is made up of predominantly collagenous tissue, with only about 10% composed of muscle fibers. The cervix stays closed throughout the pregnancy and remains a constant 2.5-cm long.[66] Estrogen and progesterone cause the cervix to swell and soften. It is bluish in color because of increased vascularity. As the uterus starts contracting, the cervix gradually softens, or ripens, and the birth canal dilates. Effacement, or taking up of the cervix, generally occurs for the first-time mother about 2 weeks before labor. Effacement does not occur in the multigravida until labor begins.

Mucus fills the endocervical canal and a mucous plug, or operculum, is formed to protect against bacterial infections. The mucous plug is either expelled as effacement continues or during labor.[67]

Blood flow to the **vagina** (a musculomembranous tube that forms the passageway between the uterus and external opening) and vulva increases, making the vaginal tissue more distensible so it can stretch during birth. Venous engorgement creates more fluid in the vagina, and the additional cervical mucous production results in an increased white vaginal discharge during pregnancy called *leukorrhea*. Some clients might feel more comfortable or cleaner wearing a panty liner in her underwear during massage treatment because of the increased vaginal discharge. The pH of the vagina decreases, but acidic conditions prevent the growth of potentially harmful bacteria. The color of the vagina becomes a violet-blue because of increased vascularity.

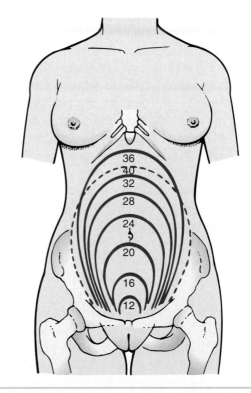

FIGURE 5-35 ■ The height of the fundus by weeks with a single fetus. The broken line represents uterine height after lightening. (From Lowdermilk DL, Perry, SE: *Maternity & women's health care*, ed 8, St. Louis, 2004, Mosby.)

The increased vascularity of the vagina and other pelvic viscera increases sensitivity. During the second trimester, sexual interest and arousal might peak. The vascularity might also increase congestion in the vulva, resulting in edema and varicosities that usually heal during postpartum.

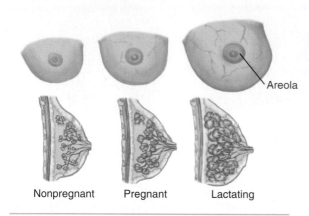

Areola

Nonpregnant   Pregnant   Lactating

FIGURE 5-36 ■ Breast changes of pregnancy. (From McKinney ES, James SR, Murray SS, et al: *Maternal-child nursing*, ed 2, St Louis, 2005, Saunders.)

During pregnancy, ovulation and menstruation cease. Estrogen and progesterone are still secreted by the ovaries until about the tenth to fourteenth week of gestation to support the pregnancy until the placenta can take over hormonal production. During pregnancy, the corpus luteum manufactures relaxin along with the placenta to relax the pelvic joints and ripen the cervix for labor.

One of the earliest signs of pregnancy is breast tenderness and a darkening of the nipples and areola. The breasts prepare for lactation through the interaction of several hormones: estrogen, progesterone, prolactin, and hPL. The breasts enlarge rapidly the first 2 months and thereafter progressively as a result of ductal growth.[12]

Women can secrete colostrum, which is baby's first food and a fatty, premilk fluid, as early as the tenth week and through the third day postpartum when it is replaced by milk. Lactation commences after the birth by dramatic drops of estrogen and progesterone levels and an increase in prolactin production (Figure 5-36).

Changes and Adaptations to the Endocrine System

The increase in hormones is vital to the progress and continuation of pregnancy. The corpus luteum of the ovaries initiates most of the hormonal production until the placenta takes over. The most dramatic adaptation to the **endocrine system** (the glandular system of the body responsible for the production and secretion of hormones) is the creation and growth of the placenta as an endocrine organ. The placenta synthesizes, elaborates, produces, and stores numerous hormones that regulate maternal and fetal development.[14]

Right after implantation, the fertilized ovum and the chorionic villi produce hCG until the placenta takes over. Progesterone, initially produced by the corpus luteum, relaxes smooth muscles, making the uterus less contractible and protecting against miscarriage. Progesterone and estrogen permit maternal fat stores to deposit over her abdomen, back, and upper thighs. This fat is necessary as a source of energy for pregnancy and lactation. Estrogen encourages enlargement of the genitals, uterus, and breasts and increases vascularity and vasodilation. Estrogen, with relaxin, relaxes the ligaments and joints.

Although serum prolactin is produced by the anterior pituitary gland, increased levels of steroid hormones progesterone and estrogen inhibit lactation until after the birth.[68] By the end of the pregnancy, progesterone has increased by 50% higher than luteal levels and threefold by term.[14] The primary estrogen of pregnancy is estriol that starts to rise during the ninth week. Estriol and estrone levels increase about 100 times and estradiol levels about 1000 times during the pregnancy (Figure 5-37).[69] The estrogens encourage growth of the endometrium, stimulate fluid retention, and increase the ability of connective tissue to retain water.

hCG, which is detected in home pregnancy kits, is produced very early in the pregnancy by the blastocyst. hCG stimulates the production of estrogen and progesterone until the placenta assumes this role. hCG levels peak between 60 to 90 days and then fall to a low level until term. In addition to steroid hormone production, this hormone stimulates fetal adrenal glands to increase its production of corticosteroids, may be a reason for morning sickness, stimulates maternal thyroid gland, increases appetite and fat deposits, suppresses maternal lymphocyte production, promotes myometrial growth, affects fetal nervous tissue and male sexual differentiation, and causes the fetal testes to produce testosterone.[14]

Relaxin is created in the ovaries and stored in the placenta. Relaxin softens the elastic ligaments

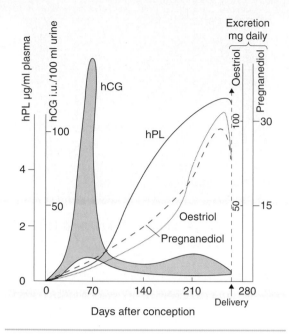

FIGURE 5-37 ■ Increasing levels of estrogen and progesterone during pregnancy. (From Coad J: *Anatomy and physiology for midwives,* St. Louis, 2001, Mosby.)

of the pelvis, allowing the bones to widen during birth. Clients often complain about lower back pain because of hypermobilization of the pelvis and stretching of the pelvic ligaments.

The adrenal and pituitary glands increase in size and hormonal production during pregnancy. Secretion of aldosterone is increased from the adrenal glands that help in the reabsorption of excess sodium. In addition, cortisol levels are increased.[40] The pituitary gland increases 135% in weight.[36] Prolactin is secreted by the pituitary gland and prepares the breasts for lactation. The number of prolactin-secreting cells increases from 10% to 50%, and prolactin levels increase throughout gestation to 20 times higher than prepregnant levels.[14] The pituitary gland also releases oxytocin, considered to be the hormone of love and maternal feelings. It also stimulates uterine contractions, is inhibited by progesterone during pregnancy (which explains why women do not go into labor after experiencing orgasms that release oxytocin), keeps the uterus contracted after the birth to encourage uterine involution, and stimulates the milk ejection reflex during breastfeeding.[12]

Pregnant women often remark that they tan more easily. They also notice darkened pigmenta-tion; irregular skin patches; chloasma, or melasma gravidarum ("the mask of pregnancy"); a linea nigra, or dark line up the middle of the abdomen; darkening of moles and freckles; and darkening of nipples and areolae. These changes are caused by an increase in melanocyte-stimulating hormone (MSH) production.

Elevated levels of thyroxine (T4) affect the size and activity of the thyroid gland. It increases basal **metabolism** (the sum of all physical and chemical changes) by 23%.[12] The rise in T4, like hCG, has also been associated with nausea and vomiting. The parathyroid hormone controls the metabolism of calcium and magnesium. There is a slight hyperparathyroidism during pregnancy that reflects the fetal need for calcium and vitamin D. This hormone peaks between weeks 15 and 35 when the fetus is growing its skeletal system.[13]

There is a delicate balance in maternal and fetal glucose levels. Since the fetus requires tremendous amounts of glucose to grow, it depletes maternal stores and decreases her ability to synthesize glucose by draining her amino acids. Therefore, maternal glucose levels drop. Maternal insulin does not cross the placenta so her body compensates by decreasing pancreatic production of insulin. Increased cortisol levels from the adrenal gland stimulates maternal insulin supplies but also derails her tissues' ability to use it. This is actually a protective mechanism to insure adequate amounts of glucose for the fetus and placenta. The maternal need for insulin increases at a steady rate and the beta cells of the islets of Langerhans in her pancreas satisfies this need.[13] It is interesting to note that a massage lowers glucose levels in everyone, so the pregnant client becomes more susceptible to diminished glucose levels. The client can avoid any problems by eating or drinking something light after the treatment to bring up her glucose levels.

Changes and Adaptations to the Neurological System

Functional changes to the **neurological system** (the system of the body made up of the brain, spinal cord, and nerves) during pregnancy have not been studied at any great length. The endocrine system influences hypothalamic-pituitary neurohormonal changes, but most of the neurological adaptations seem to result from structural or neuromuscular symptoms.

Sciatic nerve pain, numbness, or sensory changes in the lower extremities is mostly caused by the compression of the pelvic nerves and venous stasis by the enlarged uterus rather than nerve root damage. Altering positions and bringing the fetus off the sciatic region often eases the discomfort. Carpal tunnel syndrome or de Quervain's syndrome may result from a protracted cervical spine, swelling involving peripheral nerves, and flexor/extensor retinaculum softening from relaxin.[70] Pressure on the median nerve beneath the carpal ligament of the wrist from edema creates the numbness, pain, weakness and burning sensations in the hands or thenar region.

Poor posture is culpable in instances of acroesthesia, or tingling of the hands. The kyphotic stance and the exaggerated S curve of pregnancy inhibit neurological stimulation to the hand or hands resulting in numbness. This condition is associated with brachial plexus traction.

Neuromuscular conditions, such as leg and thigh cramping or tetany, may result from insufficient maternal calcium, magnesium, and potassium stores.

Changes and Adaptations to the Integumentary System

The pigmentation changes are often among the first signs of a confirmed pregnancy. As previously mentioned, the increase in MSH in pregnancy causes hyperpigmentation. The nipples and areolae darken very early, and skin darkening is observed from the third month on in 90% of pregnant women.[36] Most women develop a linea nigra, which is a darkened line running from the pubic bone to above the umbilicus (Figure 5-38). This line runs over the diastasis recti (Box 5-11). Itching, rashes, skin tags, hives, acne (improved or worsened), increased hair growth (including facial hirsutism), angiomas or vascular spiders (minute red elevations on the skin in the upper torso), and palmar erythema (reddening of the palms of the hands or soles of the feet) are not uncommon changes to the skin.

Other changes include chloasma, or "the mask of pregnancy," and stretch marks, or striae

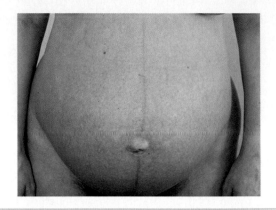

FIGURE 5-38 ■ Linea nigra. (From Lowdermilk DL, Perry, SE: *Maternity & women's health care*, ed 8, St. Louis, 2004, Mosby.)

BOX 5-11 *Linea Nigra*

The linea nigra is a darkened line (dark-skinned women have darker lines) that runs from the pubic bone to just above the umbilicus. One theory for its presence is that it is a response to the underlying diastasis, or separation of the linea alba.

Another theory is that the linea nigra serves as a road map for the newborn. When a newborn is placed on its mother's abdomen, it wiggles toward her darkened nipples to feed by following the darkened line.

---

gravidarum. Stretch marks occur in 50% to 90% of all pregnancies, usually in the second or third trimesters (Figure 5-39). They may be caused by the action of adrenocorticosteroids. They are separations along the underlying connective (collagen) tissue and occur at areas of maximum stretch such as the abdomen, breasts, and thighs. There is also a hereditary factor. Striae cannot be prevented or avoided, and no amount of expensive creams, oils, or lotions will stop them from developing. These lubricants can, however, minimize the itching and dryness that occur (Box 5-12).

Unique to pregnancy is pruritic urticated papules and plaques of pregnancy (PUPPP), which is an itchy, bumpy rash that often starts in the striae of the abdomen during the last trimester and disappears after birth.

Visceral Organ Adaptations

As previously mentioned, the heavy uterus compresses and displaces the organs of the gastrointestinal system and the hormone progesterone

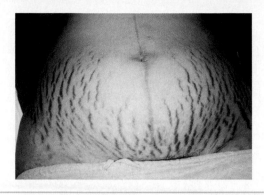

FIGURE 5-39 ■ Stretch marks, or striae gravidarum, on the abdomen. (From Lowdermilk DL, Perry SE: *Maternity & women's health care*, ed 8, St. Louis, 2004, Mosby.)

BOX 5-12   *Stretch Marks*

Stretch marks cannot be avoided, and no amount of oils or lotions can prevent them. Lubricants can, however, minimize the itching and dryness that occurs. A wonderful herbal recipe to speed up the healing of stretch marks is as follows:
 	
    20 drops of lavender and 5 drops of neroli (orange) mixed into 2 fluid oz. of wheat germ oil.
 	
    Cocoa butter or Shea butter are also effective when massaged on the abdomen.

From Stillerman E: *MotherMassage: massage during pregnancy professional manual*, New York, 1997.

slows down smooth muscle function and these result in constipation, heartburn, gas, and esophageal reflux. Visceral organs are also displaced during pregnancy (Figure 5-40). In addition, the gallbladder and liver change during pregnancy.

The gallbladder is often distended as a result of low muscle tone. It takes longer for the gallbladder to empty, and the bile thickens as a result of this longer retention. This may account for gallstones during pregnancy.

The liver is only mildly affected by the pregnancy. Occasional retention and accumulation of bile may occur in late pregnancy and may be somewhat responsible for itchy skin with or without jaundice. All of these changes reverse after birth.

Metabolic Adaptations

The pregnant woman experiences many metabolic changes that are needed to support her body, the developing fetus, and the placenta and to provide for the increase in basal metabolic rate and oxygen consumption. She needs an additional 200 kcal per day to maintain her energy level. Calcium, protein, and fat metabolism rates increase. In early pregnancy, bone reabsorption is increased and bone volume decreases. Placental calcium levels are higher than maternal supplies so that the fetus can be protected if maternal calcium stores decline. The maternal skeletal structure is conserved through maternal hormones. Even when a pregnant woman does not have enough calcium, she still maintains skeletal mass and bone density.[71]

Carbohydrate metabolism changes dramatically. The fetus needs glucose to grow and develop and gets its supplies from the mother's diet and enhanced secretion of insulin in response to glucose. Pregnancy has been referred to as having a diabetogenic effect, or causing diabetes, when in fact maternal energy metabolism shifts from carbohydrate to lipid oxidation.[36] During the first half of the pregnancy, the abdomen, breasts, and thighs add a layer of fat. This fat store is her primary energy source, with glucose used for the fetus. (It is the use of stored fat that protects the mother and fetus from prolonged starvation.)

Weight gain is slow in the first half of the pregnancy and rapidly increases in the second half. An average weight gain of 25 to 35 lbs for a single fetus is comprised of the fetus, placenta, amniotic fluid, hypertrophy of maternal tissues and organs, extra blood volume, extracellular fluid, increased breast tissue, and some maternal fat.

Adaptations of the Five Senses

The pregnant woman's nasal mucosa fills with extra blood and becomes congested, causing stuffiness and obstruction. This can dampen the sense of smell for some women and may clog the Eustachian tubes and affect her hearing. Other women experience a more sensitive sense of smell during pregnancy.

In the last trimester, mild cornea edema is common and the cornea becomes slightly thicker. Even her tears are affected and become greasier. Some women report feeling uncomfortable wearing contact lenses during pregnancy; because vision can change, it is best to wait until after the pregnancy before getting a new prescription. Women

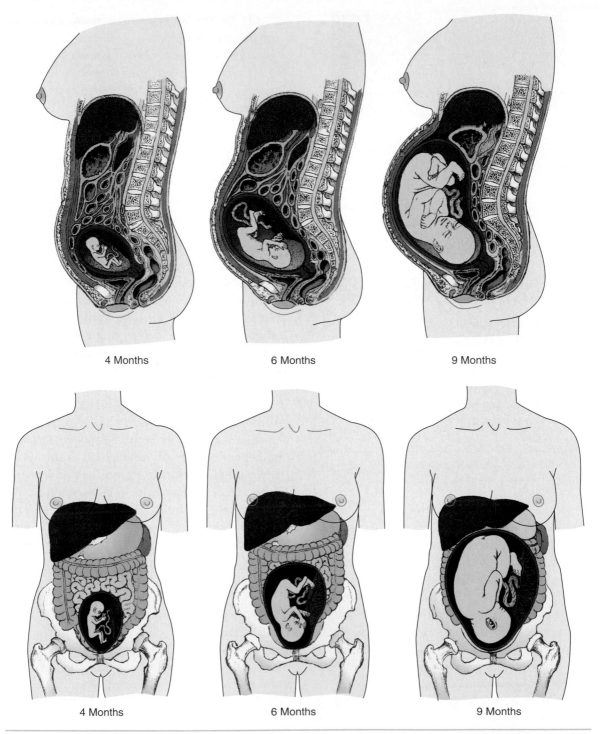

4 Months   6 Months   9 Months

4 Months   6 Months   9 Months

FIGURE 5-40 ■ Displacement of visceral organs and diaphragm at 4, 6, and 9 months. (From Lowdermilk DL, Perry SE: *Maternity & women's health care*, ed 8, St. Louis, 2004, Mosby.)

with preeclampsia, retinal edema, and diabetes are more vulnerable to vision problems.

Although her appetite increases in early pregnancy, her sense of taste becomes dulled and she may desire spicier foods.

In My Experience...

K was a colleague who studied with me and rented office space from me. One day, she called very distraught. During a massage, a pregnant client of hers had been insisting on deep leg work. K told her that it was inappropriate to work deeply on the legs of a pregnant woman because of the increased clotting factor and because lymphatic drainage is the best way to reduce swelling in the extremities. The client was adamant and told K when the massage was over, "I really shouldn't be paying you since you didn't do what I asked for." K told me that she kept hearing my voice in her head repeating, "I am emphatic about lymphatic!" but did not know how to deal with this client.

Two days later, K's client called me. I told her that K had done exactly what she should do during the pregnancy but perhaps could have told her before the massage what the leg massage was going to be—and why. The client responded with, "Well, I don't care what you *think*, I am going to find a massage practitioner who *will* work deeply on my legs." I told her if she did, she would be working with someone who either was not properly trained in prenatal massage or someone who is acting irresponsibly. The choice was hers.

Many pregnant women want to know the difference between prenatal massage and "regular" massage. Prenatal massage is regular massage, but it has been adapted to suit the pregnant woman's changing body. As such, when a technique is going to be different from what is generally expected—like prenatal and postpartum leg massage—it is advisable to let the client know before she gets on the massage table, so there are no surprises or disappointments. This communication can also assures the client that the practitioner knows what he or she is doing, and she can derive much comfort and satisfaction from that.

Summary

Dramatic changes occur in the anatomy and physiology of pregnant women to maintain optimal health and support the growing fetus. To effectively and appropriately treat a pregnant woman, it is essential to understand the physiological changes she undergoes. Almost all of the early adaptations are mediated by the increase of steroid hormones. In later pregnancy, these changes arise from structural and postural shifts. Her joints and connective tissue become lax and soft to allow her body to accommodate the growing uterus. Postural shifting results in muscle soreness, particularly at weight-bearing structures, and exaggerated curvature of the spine. Her cardiac output and blood volume increases. She has more clotting factor that must be recognized and addressed when massaging her legs.

Hyperventilation is normal, but her rib cage expansion might cause thoracic discomfort. Digestive disorders are common, and urinary incontinence can be an embarrassment. Reproductive organs adapt to support the growing fetus, and her nervous system might be affected by nerve compression. Changes in her skin and complexion are common in pregnancy but should be checked before massaging an affected area.

Women have many questions about how and why their bodies are changing. Practitioners should use their knowledge of physiology to assuage their concerns, calm their fears, explain these changes, and respect their magnificent bodies.

References

1. Sears W, Sears M: *The pregnancy book*, Boston, 1997, Little, Brown.
2. Ting RY, Brant H, Holt K: *The complete mothercare manual*, New York, 1987, Prentice Hall.
3. Bolane JE: *With child*, Waco, TX, 1999, Childbirth Graphics.
4. Goldsmith J: *Childbirth wisdom*, New York, 1984, Congdon & Weed.
5. Nei HT, Wen CS: *The yellow emperor's classic of internal medicine*, Vieth I, translator Berkeley, 1949, University of California Press.
6. Boaz F: *Kwakuitl ethnology*, Chicago, 1966, University of Chicago Press.

7. Lewis GC: *Astronomy of the ancients*, London, 1862, Parker, Son & Bourn.

8. Goodale JC: *Tiwi Wives—A study of the women of Melville Island, North Australia*, Seattle, 1971, University of Washington Press.

9. Roscoe J: *The Banyankole*, Cambridge, 1923, Cambridge University Press.

10. Roberts J: *Three Navaho households*, Paper of the Peabody Museum of American Archaeology and Ethnology Cambridge, MA, 1951, Harvard University.

11. Standlee MW: *The great pulse: Japanese midwifery and obstetrics through the ages*, North Clarendon, VT, 1959, Charles E. Tuttle.

12. Leifer G: *Maternity nursing: an introductory text*, ed 9, St. Louis, 2005, Saunders.

13. Lowdermilk DL, Perry SE: *Maternity & women's health care*, ed 8, St. Louis, 2004, Mosby.

14. Coad J: *Anatomy and physiology for midwives*, St. Louis, 2001, Mosby.

15. Hassid P: *Textbook for childbirth educators*, Philadelphia, 1978, Harper and Row.

16. Gray H: *Anatomy: descriptive and surgical*, ed 15, New York, 1977, Bounty Books, Crown Publishing.

17. Fraser D, Cooper M: *Myles' textbook for midwives*, ed 14, Edinburgh, 2003, Churchill Livingstone.

18. Blackburn ST, Loper DL: *Maternal, fetal and neonatal physiology*, Blackwell, 1992, Oxford.

19. Stillerman E: *MotherMassage: massage during pregnancy professional manual*, New York, 1997.

20. Kendall HO, Kendall FP, Wadsworth GE: *Muscles testing and function*, ed 2, Baltimore, 1971, Williams & Wilkins.

21. Walther DS: *Applied kinesiology*, vol 1, Pueblo, CO, 1981, Systems DC.

22. Tupler J: *Maternal fitness*, New York, 1996, Simon and Schuster.

23. Brill P: *The core program*, New York, 2001, Bantam Books.

24. Stillerman E: *MotherMassage: massage during pregnancy training manual*, 2004.

25. Sapsford RR, Hodges PW, Richardson CA, et al: Co-activation of the abdominal and pelvic floor muscles during voluntary exercises, *Neurol Urodynam* 20:31-42, 2001.

26. Hodges P, Richardson CA: Inefficient muscular stabilization of the lumbar spine associated with low back pain, *Spine* 21(22):2640-2650, 1996.

27. Richardson CA, Jull GA: Muscle control—pain control: what exercises would you prescribe? *Manual Ther* 1:2-10, 1995.

28. Ostgaard HC: Lumbar back and posterior pelvic pain in pregnancy. In Vleeming A, Mooney V, Dorman T, Sniders C, et al, eds: *Movement, stability and low back pain*, Edinburgh, 1997, Churchill Livingstone.

29. Noble E: *Essential exercises for the childbearing year*, ed 4, Harwich, MA, 1995, New Life Images.

30. Revelli A, Durando A, Massobrio M: Exercise and pregnancy: a review of maternal and fetal effects, *Obstet Gynaecol Surv* 47(6):355-367, 1992.

31. DeCherney P, Nathan L: *Current obstetric & gynecologic diagnosis & treatment*, ed 10, New York, 2003, McGraw Hill.

32. Gynecology and Obstetrics: Physiology of pregnancy. In Beers MH, Porter RS, Jones TV, eds: *The Merck manual of diagnosis*, ed 18, Whitehouse Station, NJ, 2006, Merck.

33. Cunningham FG, Gant NF, Leveno KJ, et al: *Williams obstetrics*, ed 21, New York, 2001, McGraw Hill.

34. Malone F, D'Alton M: Multiple gestation: Clinical characteristics and management. In Creasy R, Resnik R, eds: *Maternal-fetal medicine*, ed 4, Philadelphia, 1999, Saunders.

35. Monga M: Maternal cardiovascular and renal adaptation to pregnancy. In Creasy R, Resnik R, eds: *Maternal-fetal medicine*, ed 4, Philadelphia, 1999, Saunders.

36. Hermida R, Ayala D, Iglesias M: Predictable blood pressure variability in healthy and complicated pregnancies, *Hypertension* 38(3 Pt 2):736-744, 2001.

37. de Sweit M: The cardiovascular system. In Chamberlain G, Broughton-Pipkin F, eds: *Clinical physiology in obstetrics*, Oxford, 1998, Blackwell Science.

38. Dunlop W: Serial changes in renal haemodynamics during normal human pregnancy. *J Obstet Gynaecol* 88:1, 1980.

39. Girling JC: *Physiology of pregnancy, Obstetrics, anaesthesia and intensive care medicine*, Abingdon, England, 2001, Medicine Publishing Company.

40. Symonds E, Symonds I: *Essential obstetrics and gynaecology*, ed 3, Edinburgh, 1998, Churchill Livingstone.

41. Coustan D: Maternal physiology. In Coustan D, Haning R, Singer D, eds: *Human reproduction—growth and development*, London, 1995, Little Brown.

42. Letsky E: The haematological system. In Chamberlain G, Broughton-Pipkin F, eds: *Clinical physiology in obstetrics*, Oxford, 1998, Blackwell Science.

43. Alexander D: Deep vein thromboembolism and its management in pregnancy, *Massage Ther J* 32:58, 1993.

44. Toglia MR, Weg JG: Venous thromboembolism during pregnancy, *N Engl J Med* 335(2):108-113, 1996.

45. deSweit M, Fidler J, Howell R, et al: Thromboembolism in pregnancy. In Jewell D, ed: *Advanced medicine*, London, 1981, Pitman Medical.

46. Rutherford S, Montoro M, McGehee W, et al: Thromboembolic disease associated with pregnancy: an 11 year review, *Am J Obstet Gynecol* 164:286, 1991.

47. Bergqvist D, Hedner U: Pregnancy and venous thrombo-embolism, *Acta Obstet Gynecol Scand* 62:449-453, 1983.

48. Bergqvist A, Bergqvist D, Hallbook T: Deep vein thrombosis during pregnancy: a prospective study, *Acta Obstet Gynecol Scand* 62:443-448, 1983.

49. Hull RD, Raskob GE, Carter CJ: Serial impedance plethysmography in pregnant patients with clinically suspected deep-vein thrombosis: clinical validity of negative findings, *Ann Intern Med* 112:663-667, 1990.

50. Jeffries WS, Bochner F: Thromboembolism and its management in pregnancy, *Med J Australia* 155:253, 1991.

51. Rath W, Fardi A, Dudenhausen JW: HELLP syndrome, *J Perinat Med* 28(4): 249-260, 2000.

52. Lewis G, Drife J, eds: *Why mothers die 1997-1999. The confidential enquiries into maternal deaths in the United Kingdom*, London, 2001, RCOG Press.

53. Sibai BM: Hypertension in pregnancy. In Gabbe SG, Niebyl JR, Simpson JL, eds: *Obstetrics: normal and problem pregnancies*, ed 3, New York, 1996, Churchill Livingstone, 1996.

54. Harms K, Rath W, Herting E, et al: Maternal hemolysis, elevated liver enzymes, low platelet count, and neonatal outcome, *Am J Perinatology* 12(1):1-6, 1995.

55. Campbell S, Lees C, ed: *Obstetrics by 10 teachers*, New York, 2000, Oxford University Press.

56. Steinfeld J, Wax J: Maternal physiological adaptations to pregnancy. In Seifer D, Samuels P, Kniss D, eds: Philadelphia, 2001, Lippincott Williams & Wilkins.

57. Hellman LM, Pritchard JA: *Williams obstetrics*, ed 14, New York, 1971, Appleton-Century-Crofts.

58. Wiedenbach E: *Family centered maternity nursing*, ed 2, New York, 1967, Putnam's Sons.

59. Blackburn ST, Loper DL: *Maternal, fetal and neonatal physiology: a clinical perspective*, Philadelphia, 1992, Saunders.

60. Hytten F: The alimentary system. In Hytten F, Chamberlain G, eds: *Clinical physiology in obstetrics*, ed 2, Oxford, 1991, Blackwell.

61. Bowen DJ: Taste and food preference changes across the course of pregnancy, *Appetite* 19:233-242, 1992.

62. Sodre PM: Maternal physiology changes during pregnancy. *Obstetrics & gynecology*. http://www.medstudents.com.br/ginob/ginob5.htm

63. Lowdermilk D, Perry S, Bobak I: *Maternity nursing*, ed 5, St. Louis, 1999, Mosby.

64. Miller A, Hanretty K: *Obstetrics illustrated,* ed 5, Edinburgh, 1997, Churchill Livingstone.

65. Llewellyn-Jones D: *Fundamentals of obstetrics and gynaecology,* ed 7, London, 1999, Mosby.

66. Pollard I: *Guide to reproduction: special issues and human concerns,* Cambridge, 1994, Cambridge University Press

67. Calder A: Normal labor. In Edmonds K, ed: *Dewhurst's textbook of obstetrics and gynaecology for postgraduates,* ed 6, Oxford, 1999, Blackwell Science.

68. Guyton A, Hall J: *Human physiology and mechanism of disease,* ed 6, Philadelphia, 1997, Saunders.

69. Tulchinsky D, Hobel CJ: Plasma human chorionic gonadotrophin, estrone, estrdiol, progesterone, and 17-hydroxyprogesterone in human pregnancy. III. Early normal pregnancy, *Am J Obstet Gynecol* 117:884, 1973.

70. Padua L, et al: Symptoms and neurophysical picture of carpal tunnel syndrome in pregnancy, *Clin Neurophysiol* 112(10): 1946-1951, 2001.

71. Cross NA, Hillman LS, et al: Calcium homeostasis and bone metabolism during pregnancy, lactation, and postweaning: a longitudinal study, *Am J Clin Nutr* 61: 514-523, 1995.

REVIEW QUESTIONS

1 What are the early signs of pregnancy?

_____

_____

_____

_____

_____

_____

2 Describe the musculoskeletal adaptations of pregnancy and the massage practitioner's treatment goals.

_____

_____

_____

_____

_____

_____

3 What is relaxin? What is its influence on connective tissue?

_____

_____

_____

_____

_____

_____

4 What is the diastasis recti and how does it affect a pregnant woman's posture and contribute to lumbar instability?

_____

_____

_____

_____

_____

5 Which abdominal muscle is most important in minimizing the diastasis recti and supporting greater lumbar stability?

_____

_____

_____

_____

_____

_____

6 What can a pregnant woman do to encourage back stability during her pregnancy? How important are body mechanics in maintaining structural integrity during pregnancy?

_____

_____

_____

_____

_____

_____

7 What are the cardiovascular adaptations of pregnancy?

_____

_____

_____

_____

_____

_____

8 When does fibrinogenic activity begin during pregnancy and what is its purpose?

_____

_____

_____

_____

_____

9   How does supine (flat) positioning create a maternal hypotensive reaction and fetal hypoxia?

_____

_____

_____

_____

_____

_____

_____

10   What can be done to ease varicose veins and hemorrhoids?

_____

_____

_____

_____

_____

_____

_____

11   What is preeclampsia and what are some its signs? What is GEPH? Is massage recommended with either of these syndromes?

_____

_____

_____

_____

_____

_____

_____

12   Describe the respiratory changes of pregnancy.

_____

_____

_____

_____

_____

_____

13   How is the gastrointestinal system affected by pregnancy?

_____

_____

_____

_____

_____

_____

_____

14   Why is heartburn or esophageal reflux so common during pregnancy?

_____

_____

_____

_____

_____

_____

_____

15   What are the urinary changes during pregnancy?

_____

_____

_____

_____

_____

_____

_____

16   How has the pregnant woman's reproductive system adapted to the pregnancy?

_____

_____

_____

_____

_____

_____

17 What is the fundus?

_____

_____

_____

_____

_____

_____

18 What is the placenta and what are its many functions?

_____

_____

_____

_____

_____

_____

19 What is colostrum?

_____

_____

_____

_____

_____

_____

20 How does the endocrine system change to support the pregnancy? Name six hormones that support the pregnancy.

_____

_____

_____

_____

_____

_____

21 What are the neurological adaptations that might affect a pregnant woman?

_____

_____

_____

_____

_____

_____

22 How do the hormones of pregnancy affect the skin?

_____

_____

_____

_____

_____

_____

23 What is the linea nigra?

_____

_____

_____

_____

_____

_____

24 What are striae gravidarum? Can they be prevented?

_____

_____

_____

_____

_____

_____

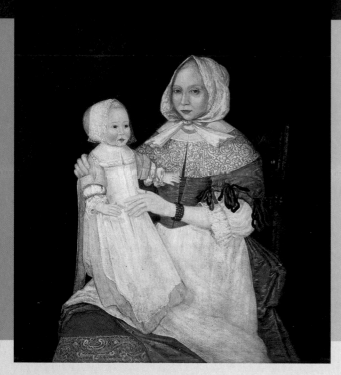

CHAPTER 6

Contraindications and Precautions of Prenatal Massage

Objectives

On completion of this chapter, the student will be able to do the following:

1   Understand the general contraindications and precautions of massage

2   Learn the specific pregnancy-related contraindications and precautions for massage

3   Identify the contraindicated acupuncture and reflex points

General contraindications	Local contraindications	Pretreatment evaluations
Keloid scar	Precautions	Regional contraindications

Within the first week of massage training, practitioners should be taught the basic guidelines to determine when a massage treatment is or is not indicated. When working with either the non-pregnant or pregnant population, certain rules still apply. Prenatal massage is absolutely not safe when any of the conditions, or **general contraindications,** listed in Box 6-1, are present. If a client has any of the symptoms or conditions in the category of general contraindications, it is best to have a doctor or midwife assess the client before proceeding with any bodywork. Once a massage is permitted, it is advisable to work with the health care provider to formulate a safe treatment plan.

Local, or **regional,** contraindications refer to specific areas of the body that have to be avoided until a diagnosis has been made by the client's health care provider or that require special care during massage (Box 6-2).

Prenatal Massage Contraindications

Practitioners should understand those pregnancy-related conditions, which are also included in the general contraindication category, in which massage must be avoided and the client must see **[DVD]** her health care provider. Massage is absolutely CONTRAINDICATED in cases of the following:

- Bleeding or staining
- Premature labor; labor between 20 to 37 weeks is considered preterm labor.
- Pitting edema, which could be symptomatic of more serious conditions such as preeclampsia (toxemia) or eclampsia
- A spike in blood pressure or a hypertensive condition
- Placenta previa
- Abruptio placentae

BOX 6-1 *General Contraindications to Prenatal Massage*

Do NOT massage the client if she presents with any of the following:
Fever
Nausea or diarrhea
Any acute vascular inflammatory condition such as Buerger's disease (an inflammatory disease of the blood vessels, primarily in the legs) or phlebitis (inflammation of a vein)
Acute stage pneumonia
Diabetes with complications such as gangrene, advanced coronary disease, or renal disease
High blood pressure
Bleeding or hemorrhaging
Severe hypertension
Shock
Metastatic cancers
Systemic contagious/infectious condition
Aneurysms

From Stillerman E: *MotherMassage: massage during pregnancy professional manual*, New York, 1997; Fritz S: *Mosby's fundamentals of therapeutic massage*, ed 3, St. Louis, 2004, Mosby.

BOX 6-2 *Local Precautions to Prenatal Massage*

Do NOT massage the following:
Over the site of a bruise, lesion, contusion, or undiagnosed dermatitis
Directly on top of keloid scars (Box 6-3)
Over varicose veins
On an inflamed nerve
Over cysts or tumors, including ovarian cysts or uterine fibroids
Acute flare-up of inflammatory arthritis wherever it occurs
Local contagious conditions anywhere on the body
Local skin irritability, lesions, warts, eczema, psoriasis
On an open wound, sore, herpetic lesion, recent burn, including sunburn
Undiagnosed lump or tumor

BOX 6-3 *Keloid Scars*

Scars are formed from connective tissue. When the body's repair reaction is excessive, it forms elongated, often irregularly shaped keloid scars. **Keloid scars** are fibrous, dimensional, raised and thick scars that contain more water and soluble collagen than regular scars. They can often be progressively enlarging due to the excessive amounts of collagen.

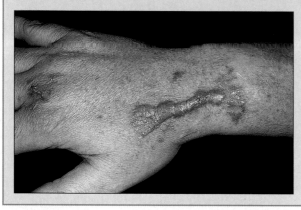

Keloid scar. (From Habif TP: *Skin disease: diagnosis and treatment*, ed 2, Philadelphia, 2005, Mosby.)

From Taber CW: *Taber's cyclopedia medical dictionary*, ed 8, Philadelphia, 1959, FA Davis; Wittlinger H and G: *Textbook of Dr. Vodder's manual lymph drainage*, ed 6, Heidelberg: 1998, Karl F. Haug Verlag.

- Fetal movement not felt for 8-10 hours
- Ectopic pregnancy
- Severe abdominal pain
- Throbbing or migraine headaches

Prenatal Massage Precautions

Local precautions in prenatal massage require that certain areas of the pregnant woman's body have to be avoided or treated in an appropriate manner. These precautions are as follows:

- Avoid using any electric heating pads, blankets, hot stones, or hydrocollators. If the client complains of being cold, warm the lotion in front of a space heater and cover her with an extra blanket.
- Avoid using any deep strokes on the legs at all times to prevent dislodging any clots and to maximize lymph drainage. Avoid the following strokes on the legs: Swedish massage strokes; percussion; vibration; cross-fiber friction; ischemic compression techniques, such as shiatsu, acupressure, Jin Shin Do, Jin Shin Jitsu, or trigger point therapy); and deep tissue bodywork or any technique that stimulates deep circulation. The lymphatic drainage massage that is

appropriate is superficial and about 10-30 gm of pressure.
- Wait 1 week after genetic testing (i.e., chorionic villi sampling (CVS) or amniocentesis) before giving a massage. These tests raise the chance of miscarriage.
- Make sure the client is not hungry before working with her. If she just had a large meal, wait at least 1 hour before treating her.
- Clients who are prescribed bed rest may be candidates for massage, depending on the reasons they are confined to bed. If they exhibit any of the contraindications as described, then a massage must be avoided. If, however, they are permitted a modest amount of movement and are generally in good health, a massage may be provided. With women confined to bed, the massage should not last longer than ½ hour. The client should stay on her left side during the treatment to facilitate circulation, and all leg and feet massage must be avoided because the incidence of blood clots increases appreciably.
- Abdominal massage should only be performed after the client has given her permission. At any trimester, the massage should be a light, open-handed, and gentle effleurage in a clockwise direction. The

myofascial releasing and stretching must also be done lightly, following the client's breathing pattern. These stretches never go beyond the superficial fascia.

- Breast massage must be performed only after the client has given her permission. Massage one breast at a time, keeping the other breast covered with a sheet. If need be, the massage can be performed under the sheet, or even above it. The pressure is always extremely light on this very sensitive area. Male practitioners should be particularly aware of avoiding any misconceptions about the work by asking permission and describing the technique before doing it.
- Make sure the client is comfortably positioned at all times (see Chapter 3) and is never in a supine (flat) position.
- Take care to avoid hyperextension of her joints. She is already hypermobile from the relaxin.
- Make sure that **pretreatment evaluations** are done before every treatment. These evaluate the arch of the foot and test for pitting edema and for the presence of blood clots in the leg. The Homan check, which is a test for blood clots specific to the calves, should also be done. (Chapter 3 includes additional information about pretreatment evaluations.)

Acupuncture Points

Traditional Chinese medicine (TCM) practitioners have been treating pregnant, laboring, and postpartum women for centuries with acupuncture or acupressure points. Each trimester has its own tsubo (acupuncture point) protocol to support the pregnancy. It has also been established that there are certain treatment points that should not be needled or pressed deeply during pregnancy because they might cause uterine contractions and possibly premature labor.

Deep, protracted pressure on these points should be avoided at all times during pregnancy; however, Chapter 17 includes a discussion of the use of acupuncture points to stimulate labor or speed up the progress of labor. Many of the contraindicated acupuncture points are located

Touch Points

The contraindicated points on the body described and detailed in this chapter are not exclusive to traditional Chinese medicine. Numerous bodywork techniques, such as Jin Shin Do, acupressure, shiatsu, and reflexology, also regard these same areas of the body as unsafe for deep, protracted stimulation during pregnancy. Practitioners do not have to be proficient in Oriental bodywork to learn where these points are located. The regions of the body to be aware of are the same regardless of what they are called or which bodywork technique is used.

on the legs and feet, which are places where swelling usually occurs. It is essential to treat pregnant clients for swelling and at the same time, avoid stimulating these points.

Lymphatic drainage is the principal technique of choice on a pregnant client's legs and feet. The 5 gm of light pressure employed will not penetrate to the level of these acupuncture points. Furthermore, lymphatic drainage is slow but is not static and the practitioner will not be pressing on any one area as long as the strokes are steady and constant.

There are definite areas on the pregnant woman's body that must be avoided with deep, sustained pressure (a count of 6 to 10, repeating 6 to 10 times, for example). On the legs is the massage practitioner should lightly move along the skin and superficial fascia lymphatically, without stopping to stimulate any specific points.

The same holds true in other areas of the body where prenatal contraindicated acupuncture points are found. As long as the massage pressure is light and constantly moving, specific stimulation to the area can be avoided. Therefore the massage techniques used are vitally important to which structures being affected.

Contraindicated Acupuncture and Reflex Points

In TCM, it has been said that "when Yin attacks and Yang separates,...a child has been conceived."[1] The following acupuncture and reflex points support pregnancy, and each point is bilateral. Chinese (Ch) and Japanese (J) names for the

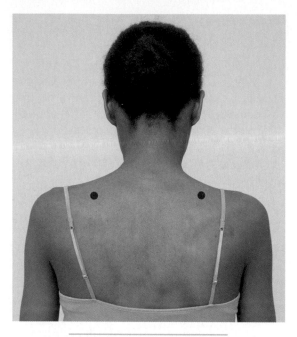

FIGURE 6-1 ■ Gall bladder 21.

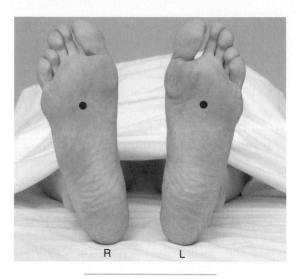

FIGURE 6-2 ■ Kidney 1.

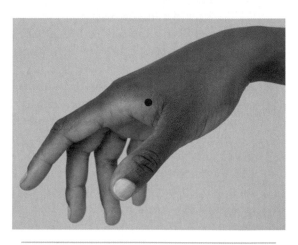

FIGURE 6-3 ■ Large intestine 4: the "great eliminator."

points are also given, as well as the English names. A "cun" (pronounced soon) is a Chinese measurement approximately a thumb's width.[2-5]

Gall Bladder 21

Gall bladder 21 (GB21), known as "well in the shoulder," is located on the highest point of the upper trapezius, slightly to the rear (Figure 6-1). This point is also known as Jianjing (Ch) and Ken Sei (J) and is fibrous to the touch. GB21 is also known as the nursing point and will stimulate milk let down. With the secretion of prolactin, oxytocin also gets released and that could initiate uterine contractions. GB 21 also stimulates uterine bleeding.

Kidney 1

Kidney 1, known as "gushing spring," is located on the soles of the feet (Figure 6-2), under the "red flesh" midway across the ball of the foot (following the vertical line from the middle toe). This point, also known as Yongquan (Ch) and Yu Sen (J), draws energy downward.

Large Intestine 4

Large intestine 4, known as "meeting mountains" or the "great eliminator," is located midway between the two bones of the thumb and index finger in the middle of the second metacarpal on the radial aspect (Figure 6-3). This point, also known as Hegu (Ch) and Go Koku (J), can stimulate uterine contractions and speed up the progress of labor.

Spleen 6

Spleen 6, known as "meeting point of the three Yin leg meridians," is located approximately 3 cun above the medial ankle posterior to the tibia (under the tibia) (Figure 6-4). This powerful point, also known as Sanyinjiao (Ch) and San Yin Ko (J), is the plexus of three Yin (personifying female energy) channels. Stimulation of this point will encourage uterine contractions and speed up a prolonged labor.

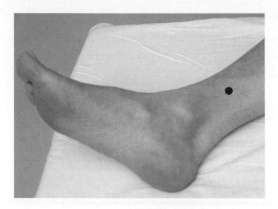

FIGURE 6–4 ■ Spleen 6.

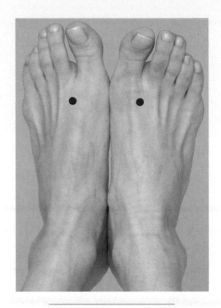

FIGURE 6–6 ■ Liver 3.

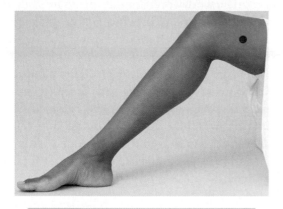

FIGURE 6–5 ■ Spleen 10: the "ocean of blood."

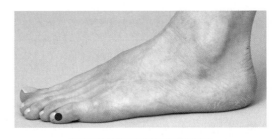

FIGURE 6–7 ■ Bladder 67.

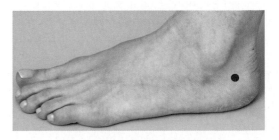

FIGURE 6–8 ■ Ovary reflex.

Spleen 10

Spleen 10, known as "ocean of blood" is located approximately 2 inches above the patellae at the middle of the belly of the vastus medialis (Figure 6-5). This point, also known as Xuehai (Ch) and Ketsu Kai (J), stimulates functional uterine bleeding and releases the contents of the uterus.

DVD

Liver 3

Liver 3 is located between the first and second toes, 2 cun proximal to the web (Figure 6-6). Liver 3, also known as Taichong (Ch) and Tai Chu (J), encourages uterine bleeding, has water influence, may also initiate the onset of labor, and may speed up a prolonged labor.

DVD

Bladder 67

Bladder 67 is located at the lateral side of the tips of the small toes, approximately 0.1 cun posterior to the corner of the nail (Figure 6-7). This point is also known as Zhiyin

DVD

(Ch) Shi Yin (J). Turns fetal presentation, is used to speed up a difficult labor. This point is considered to be extreme yin.

Ovary Reflex

Ovary reflex, known as bladder 61, is located midway between the lateral anklebone and heel where the tissue feels spongy (Figure 6-8). This point is also known as Pushen (Ch) and stimulates ovaries.

DVD

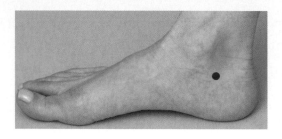

FIGURE 6-9 ■ Uterine reflex.

Uterine Reflex

Uterine reflex, known as kidney 5, is located **DVD** midway between the medial anklebone and heel where the tissue feels spongy (Figure 6-9). This point is also known as Shuiquan (Ch) and stimulates the uterus.

In My Experience...

F was a 41-year-old psychiatrist who had been trying to conceive for many years with no luck. Finally, after her third or fourth in vitro fertilization attempt, she became pregnant. She came to see me in her sixth month for regular massages as part of her prenatal care.

As I always do, I asked her to use the restroom before getting on the table so she could relax and be comfortable for the hour. Afterward, she got on the table and I started to cover her with the sheets when she said to me, "I don't know if I should say anything or not, but there was a little blood in the toilet." Without skipping a beat, I pulled back the sheets and told her to get dressed and call her doctor immediately.

She called 3 weeks later. She had been hospitalized with placenta previa for 2 of those weeks and finally had the time to call. Her doctor commented that if I had continued with the massage, she would have gone into preterm labor. She thanked me for being so insistent that she notify her doctor.

Summary

With any type of bodywork, practitioners have to determine whether treatment is indicated for their clients. In the presence of certain acute, contagious, or serious illness, massage is contraindicated. The physiology of pregnancy also requires additional knowledge so the practitioner can provide appropriate bodywork. During pregnancy, there are certain situations in which local or regional massages can be given, but care must be taken to avoid particular body areas.

There are specific areas on the body of a pregnant woman where sustained, deep pressure must be eschewed and replaced with superficial stroking. These ancient Chinese and reflex points can be massaged, but the touch must be light and constantly moving to prevent stimulating them.

References

1. Nei HT, Wen CS: *The yellow emperor's classic of internal medicine*, Vieth I, translator. Berkeley, 1949, University of California Press.
2. The Academy of Traditional Chinese Medicine. *An outline of Chinese acupuncture*, Peking, 1975, Foreign Languages Press.
3. Ohashi W: *Do-it-yourself shiatsu*, New York, 1976, Dutton.
4. Carter M: *Helping yourself with foot reflexology*, West Nyack, NY, 1969, Parker Publishing.
5. Ingham ED: *Stories the feet can tell*, Rochester, NY, Eunice Ingham, 1938.

REVIEW QUESTIONS

1 Describe the difference between local and general massage contraindications.

_____

_____

_____

_____

_____

_____

2 Name at least six general contraindications to prenatal massage.

_____

_____

_____

_____

_____

3 Name at least six local precautions during prenatal massage.

_____

_____

_____

_____

_____

_____

4 List at least six pregnancy-related contraindications to massage.

_____

_____

_____

_____

_____

_____

5 Describe the safest and most effective bodywork for the feet and legs of a pregnant woman. What physiological system is most enhanced by appropriate use of this technique and what does it protect against during pregnancy?

_____

_____

_____

_____

_____

_____

_____

6 Describe the massage given to a woman who is prescribed bed rest during a portion of her pregnancy.

_____

_____

_____

_____

_____

_____

_____

_____

7 What is a keloid scar? Is it ever safe to massage directly across the keloid? Why or why not?

_____

_____

_____

_____

_____

_____

_____

8 Describe the location of GB21. Why is it contra-indicated to deeply stimulate this point during pregnancy?

_____

_____

_____

_____

_____

9 Describe the location of kidney 1. Why is it contraindicated to deeply stimulate this point during pregnancy?

_____

_____

_____

_____

10 Describe the location of large intestine 4. Why is it contraindicated to deeply stimulate this point during pregnancy? Large intestine 4 is also known by what other name?

_____

_____

_____

_____

11 Describe the location of spleen 6. Why is deep pressure to spleen 6 contraindicated during pregnancy? How is this point expressive of female energy?

_____

_____

_____

_____

_____

12 Describe the location of spleen 10. Why is deep pressure to spleen 10 contraindicated during pregnancy? Spleen 10 is also known by what other name?

_____

_____

_____

_____

_____

13 Describe the location of liver 3. Why is deep pressure to liver 3 contraindicated during pregnancy?

_____

_____

_____

_____

14 Describe the location of bladder 67. Why is deep pressure to bladder 67 contraindicated during pregnancy?

_____

_____

_____

_____

_____

15 Describe the location of the ovary and uterus foot reflexes. Why is deep pressure to these reflexology points contraindicated during pregnancy?

_____

_____

_____

_____

_____

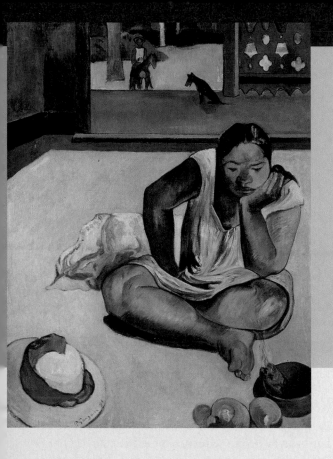

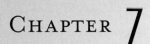

CHAPTER 7

Treating High-Risk Pregnancies and Clients Confined to Bed Rest

Objectives

On completion of this chapter, the student will be able to do the following:

1   Understand the medical definition of high-risk pregnancies
2   Recognize how low-, moderate-, and high-risk factors affect massage treatment
3   Know the dangers associated with smoking and alcohol and substance abuse as they pertain to maternal and fetal health
4   Recognize the issues involved with survivors of abuse
5   Learn the protocol of treating clients confined to bed rest

Key Terms

Abruptio placentae	Hydramnios	Pregnancy-induced hypertension
Anemia	Labor complications	Premature labor
Artificial reproductive technology	Morbidity	Premature rupture of membranes
Bed rest	Mortality	Preterm labor
Cephalopelvic disproportion	Oligohydramnios	Prolapse of umbilical cord
Cesarean section	Placenta previa	Risk factors
Dystocia	Polyhydramnios	Substance abuse
Gestational glucose intolerance	Postterm labor	Umbilical cord
High risk	Precipitate labor	Withdrawal

"According to early reporters, tribal childbirth—in addition to its ease—was distinguished by a dearth of complications," said Adriaen Van der Donck, who visited North America in 1641, of the natives. "They rarely are sick from childbirth, suffer no inconveniences from the same, nor do any of them die on such occasions."[1,2]

The Arikara of North Dakota were studied by Melvin Gilmore in the 1930s, and he reported "that among the tribe there was no extra-uterine pregnancy, no placenta previa, no septicemia nor eclampsia; and premature birth occurred only as a result of an accident. No phlebitis was seen among Arikara women 'until they started living like whites.'"[1,3]

In a massage practice, practitioners will be treating women whose pregancies are categorized as **high risk,** with an increased possibility of suffering harm, damage, injury, loss, or death to themselves or the fetus. Because there are no clear definitions of "risk," this assessment could be determined by a rigid, fixed medical or clinical definition that might be seen differently by another clinician or the women herself.[4] While the bodyworker has to take the **risk factors** (possible causes involved with miscarriage) seriously, massage often has little or no consequence on either maternal or fetal risk factors or the birth outcome.[5] The high-risk label puts additional stress on the mother, and the client needs to become better informed about her risk factors to control unnecessary worrying.

To understand the factors involved, it is important to recognize what exactly is at risk. The four risk categories that might cause serious trauma to or compromise the health of mother and/or fetus are as follows:

- The risk of miscarriage
- The risk of **premature** or **preterm labor** (between 20 and 37 weeks)
- The risk of **labor complications** (difficulties that may occur during labor)
- The risk of maternal or fetal **morbidity** (injury or disease) or **mortality** (death)

Touch Points

Practitioners should expect to massage many clients with high risk pregnancies. Because the term *high risk* can refer to a number of physical conditions, it is important that the right questions are asked to make sure the practitioner is providing them with safe, appropriate bodywork.

The client should be asked what the risk factors are and whether there are any reasons to modify or avoid massage. If more information is needed about their condition, the practitioner can ask to speak with the client's care provider or other health professionals about the risk factors. The Resources section can also provide a great deal of information about the condition before bodywork begins.

In most cases, massage will be safe. But the practitioner can make sure that all of the necessary research is done before massaging a client whose risk factors might increase the chances of losing the baby or having a preterm delivery.

Risk of Miscarriage

Miscarriages, or spontaneous abortions, occur in a high percentage of pregnancies (see Chapter 2). It is estimated that almost 40% to 50% of women will experience a natural termination of their pregnancies before 20 weeks' gestation, with 90% of them losing the pregnancy within the first 8 weeks.[6,7] Miscarriages are caused by fetal abnormalities or other maternal and environmental conditions.

Appropriate bodywork and massage will not cause a miscarriage, but if symptoms of miscarriage are present, the treatment is contraindicated.

Risk of Premature or Preterm Labor

Premature or preterm labor is the onset on active labor contractions and cervical dilation between 20 and 37 weeks' gestation. Nearly 8% of women go into labor before term, and although many of the babies survive, many will have serious health issues.[8] The signs of preterm labor include uterine or abdominal cramping with or without vomiting or diarrhea, vaginal bleeding, and a change in vaginal discharge. Women also experience vaginal or pelvic pressure, low back pain, and intermittent or persistent pain in the front of their thighs.[8] When any of these symptoms are present, bodywork is contraindicated.

Risk of Labor Complications

A prenatal massage will prepare the woman's body for labor but is not a factor in labor complications. Some of these complications are **premature rupture of membranes** (spontaneous rupture of the amniotic sac before 37 weeks' gestation), **dystocia** (abnormal or difficult labor), **postterm labor** and birth (a labor after 42 weeks' gestation), **precipitate labor** (a speedy labor completed in less than 3 hours), uterine rupture, **hydramnios** (excessive amniotic fluid), **oligohydramnios** (decreased amniotic fluid), **cephalopelvic disproportion** (fetus is too large to pass through the cervix or the maternal pelvis is too small), **prolapse of the umbilical cord** (the umbilical cord precedes the fetus), multifetal (multiples) pregnancy, and **Cesarean section**.[8]

Risk of Maternal and Fetal Morbidity or Mortality

Maternal and fetal morbidity or mortality is not influenced by a massage. Maternal death is described as "the death of a pregnant woman or death within 42 days of delivery, miscarriage, or termination of pregnancy related to or aggravated by the pregnancy or its management but from accidental or incidental causes."[9] The World Health Organization estimates that at least 600,000 women die annually from pregnancy-related causes, although the exact rate is difficult to obtain.[10,11] Around the globe, maternal death rate in developed countries is estimated to be 1 in 1800; in Africa the maternal death rate is 1 in 16; in Asia, 1 in 65; and in Latin America, 1 in 130.[12] In the United States, maternal mortality rates were static between 1980 and 1998 at 7% to 8% per 100,000. This number increased in 2000 to 9.8%, but this increases was attributed to the manner of reporting rather than an actual increase. The leading causes of maternal death differ around the world; however, three major health-related causes have persisted over the last 50 years: hypertensive disorders, infection, and hemorrhage.[6]

Statistics for stillborn death, perinatal death (within the first week of life), neonatal death, and infant death rates are hard to quantify. In the United States, infant mortality rates in 2000 were the lowest ever recorded at 6.9 per 1000 live births.[13] Other developed nations have much better rates than the United States.[14] Factors involved in perinatal death are low birthweight, intrauterine hypoxia, respiration depression at birth, intracranial injury, and congenital abnormalities, with the latter being the leading cause of neonatal death.[6,15]

Race is an indicator of certain risk factors. Nonwhite women are more than three times as likely as Caucasian women to die of pregnancy-related causes. African-American babies have the highest rates of prematurity and low birth weight. Infant mortality rates among African Americans are more than twice as high as Caucasians.[6]

For the massage practitioner, it is important to recognize that miscarriage, preterm labor, labor complications, and maternal and fetal morbidity or mortality can be caused by risk factors that vary in degrees of severity. These risk factors are classified here as low-, moderate-, or high-risk factors. The massage done for the low risk group follows typical prenatal protocol—there is no need to alter typical massage procedures. In the moderate-risk group, some techniques may have to be modified, the length of the treatment may be minimized, or certain areas may have to be avoided. In the high-risk group, the complications are usually so severe that massage treatment must be avoided until the condition reverses or improves.

In all instances, the practitioner should work in tandem with the client and her health care providers to promote the safest, most satisfying massage possible.

Low-Risk Factors

When treating a pregnant woman with low-risk factors, including maternal age, multifetal gestation, artificial reproductive techniques, previous pregnancy complications, multiple spontaneous miscarriages, or fetal genetic disorders, the practitioner's massage technique remains the same.

Maternal Age

If none of the risk factors associated with maternal age is present and the client is healthy, maternal age is a low risk factor. However, teenagers younger than 18 and women over 35 years of age are considered high risk. Teenage pregnancy is a major public health issue throughout the world. Among industrialized nations, the United States has one of the highest birth rates per 1000 teenagers age 15 to 19 years. In the mid1990s, the birth rate for this group was 54.4 births per 1000 women. In Japan, Australia, and Germany, the birth rates for teenagers age 15 to 19 years were 3.9, 19.8, and 12.5, respectively.[16] The District of Columbia had the highest rate in the country with 69.1 per 1000 births. Mississippi had the highest state rate (64.7 births) and New Hampshire the lowest (20.0). These rates are dropping, however. By 2002, there was a 5.30% drop in teen pregnancies.[16]

Pregnant teenagers generally do not eat nutritiously and are more likely to indulge in unhealthy habits such as drugs, smoking, and alcohol consumption. They are also more likely to have **anemia** (a condition caused by a decrease in red blood cells, hemoglobin, or both), **pregnancy-induced hypertension** (increased blood pressure during pregnancy), preterm delivery, babies with low birth weight, prolonged labors, babies with genetic disorders, and 60% higher infant and maternal mortality rates.[17,18] Girls under the age of 16 are 5 times more likely to die

TABLE 7-1	*Rates of Down Syndrome*	
Maternal Age (Years)	Probability of Positive Result	Detection Rate (%)
Under 25	1 in 45	35
25-29	1 in 30	40
30-34	1 in 15	55
35-39	1 in 5	75
40-44	1 in 2	95
45 and older	More than 1 in 2	More than 99
Average	1 in 20	60

From Kenard A, Goodburn S, Golightly S, et al: *Midwives* 108(1290):207-210, 1995.

during or right after the pregnancy than women 10 years older.[19]

Women over 35 years of age are also considered high risk, although the risks are very slight. Most older women can look forward to healthy, uncomplicated pregnancies and babies. However, older women do have more difficulties becoming pregnant because ova age as they do and chances of fetal genetic abnormalities, in particular Down syndrome, increase the older she gets (Table 7-1). Older women also have higher instances of gestational glucose intolerance, hypertension and pregnancy-induced hypertension, prolonged labor, Cesarean sections (in the United States, not in Europe or Asia), **placenta previa** (placental implantation that encroaches on the margin of the cervical os), **abruptio placentae** (premature separation of a normally implanted placenta from the uterine wall), varicose veins, and mortality.

Multiples or Multifetal Gestation

A multiple pregnancy is usually shorter than a pregnancy with one fetus. An average gestation for twins is 37 weeks, triplets 34 weeks, and quadruplets 33 weeks. As more women use artificial reproductive technology to become pregnant, the incidence of multiples increases. The woman carrying multiples presents greater symptoms of common aches and pains, she is more prone to anemia as the fetuses make tremendous demands on her iron reserves, and she may have **polyhydramnios** (more amniotic fluid) that adds to her discomfort. Her increased weight and size further impairs venous return from her legs, exacerbates edema of the lower limbs, and contributes to lower back pain, indigestion, constipation, and dyspnea. Many of these women prefer to remain on their left side during the treatment because turning can be rather awkward. Women with multiples need more attention paid to those body parts that are most compromised (Figure 7-1).

The Use of Artificial Reproductive Technology

Many women who have difficulty conceiving resort to **artificial reproductive technology** (ART) to become pregnant. They may undergo in vitro fertilization (IVF), intrauterine insemination, gamete intrafallopian transfer (GIFT), zygote intrafallopian transfer (ZIFT), or intracytoplasmic sperm injection (ICSI) or use an egg or sperm donor for any number of infertility reasons. Regardless of age or general health, women who conceive through these means are categorized as high-risk pregnancies. However, whether the pregnancy continues without complication, there is no reason for the practitioner to change his or her massage techniques.

Complications from Previous Pregnancies

Whether a previous pregnancy was considered a high-risk pregnancy, a woman's chances of having the same risk factor a second or third time are higher. Massage practitioners have to assess the woman's physical condition and treat her appropriately whether a problem exists. However, if this pregnancy is normal, there is no need to alter treatment.

Multiple Spontaneous Abortions or Miscarriages

Miscarriages occur as often as 40% to 50% of the time, but repeated miscarriages might indicate an unresolved physical problem. Women with this medical history often choose to wait until the second trimester before making a massage appointment. Although it is clear that massage does not cause a miscarriage, it is understandable that a woman may need to feel secure

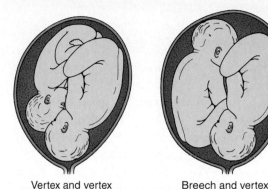

Vertex and vertex   Breech and vertex

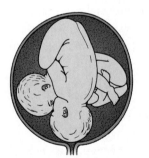

Breech and breech

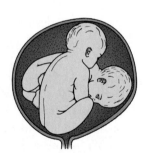

Vertex and transverse   Breech and transverse

FIGURE 7-1 ■ Presentation of twins in utero. (From Fraser D, Cooper M: *Myles' textbook for midwives,* ed 14, Edinburgh, 2003, Churchill Livingstone.)

and safe about her pregnancy before booking an appointment.

Fetal Genetic or Medical Disorders

It would be a wonderful thing whether a massage could change fetal genetic, hereditary, or medical abnormalities and complications, but it cannot. Although fetal genetic or medical disorders are medically serious risk factors, the massage treatment does not change.

Midlevel-Risk Factors

With symptoms and conditions of midlevel-risk factors, which include illnesses or preexisting conditions, drug exposure, surgery, trauma, obesity, low weight gain, smoking, Rh incompatibility, and physical or sexual abuse, the practitioner may have to minimize treatment time to see how the client tolerates the massage and then make certain adaptations to the treatment or avoid certain areas of her body.

Maternal Illnesses or Preexisting Conditions

Most maternal illnesses are not harmful to the fetus because the maternal immune system fights the illness. Certain conditions, such as rubella, cytomegalovirus, and toxoplasmosis, do affect the fetus, often with catastrophic results.[20] Some preexisting conditions require medical massage protocol in addition to the prenatal care. Because many old injuries resurface as a result of postural shifting, care must be paid to those weakened areas.

Gestational Glucose Intolerance

Gestational glucose intolerance (GGI) is glucose intolerance during pregnancy, affecting perhaps 5% of the population.[7] Symptoms include all the classic signs of a diabetic: excessive thirst, hunger, urination, and weakness.[8] Insulin resistance is common in pregnancy; some women have only slight glucose tolerance impairment, others may have a more serious reaction. The risk factors for the fetus, such as hydramnios, premature membrane rupture, and stillbirth, are increased, regardless of how mild the maternal reaction may be.

Although diet can control GGI during pregnancy, about 10% to 15% of women will require insulin to control glucose levels.[8] Many doctors want to manage the pregnancies carefully and will either induce labor at 38 weeks or schedule a Cesarean section to prevent the fetus from growing too large. The symptoms of GGI reverse a few weeks after the birth, but as many as 35% to 50% of these women demonstrate compromised

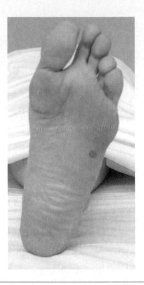

FIGURE 7-2 ■ The reflex point for the treatment of anemia is found on the left foot only. Press lightly and hold for a count of 6-10. Repeat 6-10 times.

carbohydrate metabolism over the next 15 years of life.[8]

A client with GGI is treated the same as a client who does not have the ailment. However, because glucose levels drop during a general massage, it is imperative that the client eats or drinks something before leaving the practitioner's office to elevate glucose levels. Clients may think that they are clear-headed, but their reaction times and ability to make decisions are impaired from the drop in glucose. Before the client gets behind the wheel of a car, the practitioner must insist that the client consume something. For that purpose, some kind of healthy snack food must be available for massage clients.

Anemia

Anemia is a decrease in the body's ability to bring oxygen to the cells. Symptoms are fatigue, immunological suppression, feeling chilly or cold, lackluster skin and hair, and brittle nails. Pregnant women with anemia are at increased risk for preterm labor and other complications.

Prenatal vitamins with additional iron can combat anemia, as well as eating a diet rich in iron and folic acid (see Box 5-8 for a list of iron-rich foods). A full body massage elevates red blood cell count and pressing the spleen reflex on the left foot helps the body produce more red blood cells to defeat anemia (Figure 7-2).

Heart Disease

Heart disease is a rare complication during gestation, affecting only about 1% of women.[8] The increase in cardiac output, heart rate, blood volume, and stroke volume can strain the cardiac functioning of a woman with preexisting heart disease. Massage treatment should minimize stress to the heart. A multidisciplinary approach is the most beneficial for the client. The practitioner must communicate with the primary care physician, cardiologist, obstetrician or midwife, and dietician to coordinate a treatment plan.

Depending on the severity of the heart problem, the practitioner should modify the work by limiting the initial visits to half-hour treatments to see how the client tolerates the work. The client should remain on her left side throughout the treatment, ensuring easier circulation and enhanced lymph drainage.

Urinary Tract Infections

Urinary tract infections (UTIs) are not uncommon during pregnancy, affecting from 5% to 20%.[8] The compression and loss of muscle tone in the urinary tract creates urinary stasis, making pregnant women vulnerable to UTIs. The pregnant client might urinate frequently and urgently with discomfort or pain (dysuria). She may notice blood in the urine (hematuria) and can develop a backache over the site of her kidneys.[8]

Increasing fluid intake will decrease the risk of chronic infections. She should also empty her bladder frequently and clean herself from front to back. Kegel exercises will promote strength to the pelvic floor and decrease frequency. When a client has to urgently urinate, relaxing on a massage table is very difficult, particularly if she is in pain. These infections are not contagious but are rather uncomfortable. A pregnant woman with a UTI should seek medical care and appropriate medication before receiving a massage treatment (Boxes 7-1 and 7-2).

Asthma

Along with other postural and respiratory compensations, pregnant women often hyperventilate and experience shortness of breath that can make flare-ups more common in women who suffer

---

BOX 7-1 Bladder Irritants to Avoid

The following list is known as the "C" list and contains foods and beverages that may irritate the bladder causing premature bladder contractions leading to urgency and incontinence or leaking.

Coffee and tea, even decaffeinated
Caffeine
Cold remedies
Chocolate
Carbonated beverages
Coke and colas
Citrus, fruit or beverage
C vitamin
Chardonnay (or Corona), alcohol in general
Crystal light or any artificially sweetened beverages
Candy and other sugars
Chili and other tomato-based foods
Chinese food, spicy or flavored with monosodium glutamate (MSG)
Cigarette smoking
Corn syrup

From Culligan P: *Challenges in women's healthcare*, Urogynecology for primary care providers seminar, New York, 2005.

BOX 7-2 Treatments for Bladder Control

Increase fluid intake to 4-6 glasses of water a day; 2-3 ounces every 20-30 minutes is the suggested way to drink the water.

Avoid reducing water intake that will cause urine concentration and further irritate the bladder.

Avoid caffeine and alcohol because caffeine will dehydrate the body and must be avoided in cases of UTIs; caffeine intake should be limited to 1-2 cups per day.

Drink grape, cherry, and apple juices and herbal teas.

Eat apricots, melons, homegrown tomatoes, bananas, prunes, and plums.

UTI, Urinary tract infections.
From Culligan P: *Challenges in women's healthcare*, Uregynecology for Primary Care Providers Seminar, New York, 2005.

---

from asthma. Medial rotation of her shoulders from sleeping positions and slouching can create myofascial restrictions and tightening in her chest. Massage treatment should include myofascial release to the rib cage and overhead stretches with her arms to decompress the pectoral girdle. If needed, inhaled steroid therapy used to treat asthma is safe during pregnancy and is not implicated in neonate low birth weight.[21]

Maternal Drug Exposure
Prescribed Medications

Some pregnant women have to take prescribed medications during their pregnancies to treat a preexisting condition. If they have to inject themselves, massage practitioners should take care to avoid the site of the injection. Some of these treatments can be very bruising, as in the case of heparin, where entire areas of the body can be covered with bruises in varying stages of healing.

Other women may take oral medications to treat an illness. It is advisable to discuss her reactions to the medication and whether any symptoms require special care. Cooperating with her health care team can help the practitioner devise the best treatment plan for her.

It is estimated that 1 in 1000 to 1500 pregnancies are complicated by malignancies.[22,23] Approximately 2% to 3% of women who are pregnant or lactating are diagnosed with breast cancer,[24] which is followed in frequency by cancers of the cervix (1 in 2000), melanomas, ovarian cancer, leukemia, lymphoma, Hodgkin's disease; colorectal, tubal, and thyroid have an incidence of 1 in 6000.[6,22,25]

Massage can mediate the side effects of chemotherapy and support the client emotionally, but the practitioner must work with her health care team to provide her with optimal care. Clients who undergo chemotherapy during pregnancy endure not only the physical reaction to the drugs but also extreme emotional duress. Most chemotherapy is avoided during the first trimester; however, if it must be administered, the placenta may be a powerful barrier against these toxic agents because most babies are born without significant abnormalities. Breastfeeding should be avoided, however.[24] Radiation seems to have dangerous side effects to the developing fetus.[25]

Diethylstilbestrol

From the late 1940s to early 1970s, approximately 2 to 6 million women were prescribed diethylstilbestrol (DES), a nonsteroidal synthetic estrogen, to prevent miscarriages and preterm deliveries (Figure 7-3). The theory was that by providing an estrogen

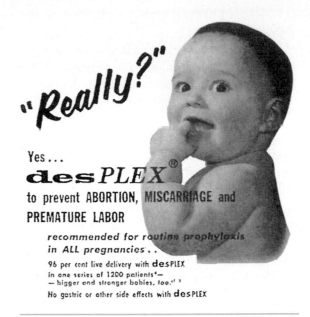

FIGURE 7-3 ■ This advertisement appeared in medical journals in 1957 encouraging doctors to prescribe DES to prevent miscarriages. (Reprinted by permission of the *New York Times*.)

substitute, miscarriages cold be avoided.[26] Doctors were advised that the prophylactic administration of DES could treat toxemia (preeclampsia), preterm deliveries, and stillbirths.[27]

In 1971, it was discovered that DES caused a rare vaginal cancer in young women who were exposed to DES in utero. Further studies linked the drug to anatomical abnormalities, menstrual dysfunction, infertility, miscarriages, premature births, stillbirths, vaginal adenosis (in 30% to 90% of DES daughters), cervical hypoplasia, tubal abnormalities, ectopic pregnancies, incompetent cervixes, and labor complications[28-30] (Figure 7-4). Men whose mothers were given DES also have an increased risk of reproductive anomalies such as epididymal cysts and testicular cancer.

Some doctors perform cerclage to prevent preterm deliveries on women who were exposed prenatally to DES. To stop the os, or mouth of the cervix, from dilating, sutures are placed within the cervix to keep it closed.

The massage practitioner must understand that many DES clients have had a difficult time conceiving and staying pregnant so the successful pregnancy is charged with anxiety, understandable concern, and possibly physical complications.

> **ARE YOU A DES DAUGHTER?**
>
> **Time may be running out on your claim for compensation**
>
> Recent studies report a significantly higher incidence of cancer, infertility, miscarriages, ectopic pregnancies and preterm delivery as a result of in utero exposure to DES *(Stilbestrol-Diethylstilbestrol)*, a synthetic hormone given to pregnant women in the 1950s and 1960s, subsequently banned as ineffective and dangerous. Even though many years have gone by, you may still have a claim for compensation if you act quickly. Medical records and the physicians and pharmacists involved are becoming difficult to locate. State statutes of limitations may bar a claim, if not pursued diligently. Our firm specializes in DES litigation and we have successfully represented hundreds of DES victims during the past 20 years. We can obtain your medical records, have our in-house medical professionals evaluate them and represent you on a contingent fee basis. No charge if no recovery.

FIGURE 7-4 ■ A law firm's advertisement for DES litigation. (Reprinted by permission of the *New York Times*.)

A practitioner can shorten the length of the massage treatment to under an hour to see how the client tolerates the bodywork and avoid direct contact with the client's abdomen until she feels comfortable with the massage. The time of the massage and depth of pressure can be increased with each ensuing treatment.

After Surgery, Trauma, or Injury

A pregnant client who undergoes a surgical procedure, trauma, or injury should wait until she feels strong enough to come for a treatment. The first time she sees the practitioner after the surgery, trauma, or injury, her care should be modified to suit her needs. The practitioner should take care to not overdo the work because she might still be feeling somewhat depleted or vulnerable. The massage treatment should be limited to 1 hour until her strength returns.

Obesity or Failure to Gain Weight

Excessive weight gain during (or before) pregnancy can lead to many complications including increased chances of macrosomia and fetopelvic disproportion, Cesarean section, postpartum hemorrhage, hypertensive disturbances, excessive swelling, thrombophlebitis, wounds, genital or urinary tract infection, birth trauma, and late fetal death.[14,31,32]

Failure to gain weight, or nutritional deprivation, may create a greater risk of anemia, preterm birth, low birth weight, and intrauterine growth restriction. A client with an eating disorder, such as bulimia, may be misdiagnosed as having hyperemesis gravidarum, or an anorexic pregnant woman may complicate her pregnancy with birth asphyxia and perinatal death.[15]

The average, healthy weight gain for a single pregnancy is 25-35 lbs; only about 5 lbs of this weight are maternal fat reserves.

Overeating or undereating may signal emotional problems, and practitioners are well-advised to suggest psychological counseling to their clients. Proper nutrition is essential to maintain maternal health and support fetal growth. A nutritionist or dietician can provide sound dietary solutions to keep the pregnancy healthy.

Smoking

Nicotine crosses the placenta and acts as a vasoconstrictor, causing fetal hypoxia. Cigarette smoke contains more than 4000 chemicals, including cyanide, lead, and numerous cancer-causing compounds.[33] In addition, the carbon monoxide in cigarettes inactivates hemoglobin also resulting in fetal hypoxia. Many fetuses have stunted growth, preterm birth, malformations and neurological defects from cigarettes. Infants demonstrate respiratory difficulties such as wheezing and asthma.[34] Smoking, drugs, alcohol and radiation have deleterious effects on cell division.[11,35] Smoking also increases maternal and fetal requirements for certain nutrients that can adversely affect fetal growth. In addition, a nursing woman should not smoke because nicotine crosses into breast milk.[36]

After 3 days without nicotine, a woman will begin to have **withdrawal** symptoms (painful, difficult reactions to the cessation of an addictive substance), and yet, these symptoms are still safer to her and the fetus than smoking. She may feel anxious, irritable, moody, or depressed. However, once she understands that she is giving up a very dangerous habit for the sake of the fetus, she has a better chance of succeeding.

Ideally, a client stopped smoking before her pregnancy, but it is never too late to stop smoking. Names of support groups should be given, and the client should discuss the best way to quit smoking with her health care provider (Box 7-3).

Rh Incompatibility

If the pregnant woman's blood is Rh negative, but her fetus is Rh positive, an incompatibility results. If fetal Rh positive blood leaks in to maternal circulation, her body may develop antibodies that will destroy fetal blood cells. The fetus will become anemic, develop heart failure, and die in utero. This can be avoided by injecting the woman with Rh-immune globulin (RhoGAM) at 28 weeks and within 72 hours after the birth.[11]

Physical or Sexual Abuse

Serious maternal and fetal consequences are the result when abuse is involved (see Chapter 4). Whether the client is a survivor of childhood abuse or a victim of spousal abuse while pregnant, she runs the risk of many prenatal and labor complications. The practitioner working with a survivor needs to be particularly sensitive to her emotional condition, as well as the physical sequelae. It is highly recommended that your client get psychological counseling in tandem with the bodywork so she can be more accepting of herself and embrace her pregnancy.

High-Level Risk Factors

High-level risk factors, which include drug or substance abuse, vaginal bleeding, hypertension, placenta previa, abruptio placentae, premature labor, pitting edema, and lack of fetal movement, are serious situations that require medical intervention before a massage is offered.

Drug or Substance Abuse

Drug or **substance abuse** can harm the mother and the fetus. No amount of alcohol is safe during pregnancy. Alcohol traverses the placenta and retards cell organization and growth resulting in neurological impairment, facial anomalies, mental deficiencies and hyperirritability (fetal alcohol syndrome). There is also an increased risk for miscarriage and abruptio placentae (Figure 7-5).

Cocaine or crack crosses the placenta and increases hypertension, irregular heart rhythms, vasoconstriction, preterm birth, and hyperglycemia in the mother. The fetus is at risk for preterm birth, irregular heart rhythms, hyperactivity, constricted intrauterine growth, poor feeding reflexes, irritability, and difficulty in soothing.

Heroin exposes the women to increased risk of human immunodeficiency virus (HIV) and other blood-borne infections and increases the chance of premature rupture of membranes, placentae abruptio, malnutrition, anemia, miscarriage, and the withdrawal from heroin causes fetal hypoxia. The newborn has the identifiable high-pitched cry coupled with hyperactivity, the continuous need for sucking, seizures, and disrupted sleep-wake cycles. These infants often recoil from cuddling or touch.

Speed, or crystal methamphetamine, causes maternal malnutrition, brain damage, paranoia, and powerful addiction. The fetus may suffer from heart problems, physical anomalies, and malformations and can be born undergoing withdrawal.

Sedatives or tranquilizers depresses the maternal central nervous system and are associated with other drugs and malnutrition. The fetus may experience seizures, delayed lung maturity, intrauterine growth restriction, and sensitivity to light.[11]

Vaginal Bleeding

Vaginal bleeding can be a symptom of more serious problems such as placenta previa or abruptio placentae. No massage should be provided until a medical diagnosis of the problem has been confirmed, the bleeding has stopped and her health care provider has given her permission to resume normal activity.

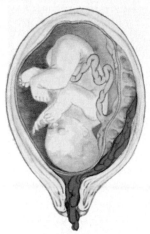

Marginal abruption
with external bleeding

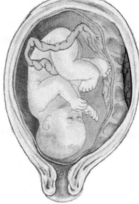

Partial abruption
with concealed bleeding

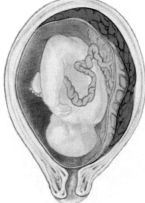

Complete abruption
with concealed bleeding

FIGURE 7-5 ■ Premature separation of the placenta is called abruptio placentae. (From Leifer G: *Maternity nursing: an introductory text*, ed 9, St. Louis, 2005, Saunders.)

BOX 7-4 Types of Pregnancy Hypertension

1. PIH or GH: Blood pressure elevates to over 140/90 mm Hg, after the twentieth week gestation, no proteinuria. Blood pressure usually stabilizes by the sixth week postpartum.
2. Preeclampsia: GH with proteinuria.
3. Eclampsia: Preeclampsia with seizures
4. Chronic hypertension: Elevated blood pressure before the pregnancy or before 20 weeks' gestation. Usually lasts about 1½ months' postpartum
5. Preeclampsia with superimposed chronic hypertension: Chronic hypertension with proteinuria, thrombocytopenia, and increased liver enzymes[37,38]
6. HELLP syndrome: A variant of chronic hypertension with superimposed eclampsia. The acronym stands for *H*, Hemolysis—anemia and jaundice; *EL*, Elevated liver enzymes—epigastric pain, nausea, and vomiting; *LP*, Low platelets—thrombocytopenia, abnormal bleeding and clotting time, bleeding gums.[11]

PIH, Pregnancy-induced hypertension; *GH*, gestational hypertension.

BOX 7-5 Symptoms of Hypertension

1. Vasospasm leading to increase in blood pressure and decrease flow to the uterus and placenta
2. Renal changes with decreased blood flow to kidneys and increase in proteinuria
3. Neurological changes leading to headaches and, cell damage, cerebral edema and visual disturbances
4. Liver enlargement causing abdominal pain preceding seizures
5. Possible stroke
6. Acute renal failure
7. Placentae abruptio
8. HELLP syndrome (10% of severe PIH)

HELLP, Hemolysis, elevated liver enzymes, low platelets; *PIH*, pregnancy-induced hypertension.

Pregnancy-Induced Hypertension or Gestational Hypertension

Pregnancy-induced hypertension (PIH), or gestational hypertension (GH), occurs if a pregnant woman's blood pressure exceeds 140/90 mm Hg, and a massage is contraindicated. A preexisting hypertensive condition can lead to abruptio placentae, renal failure, preeclampsia or eclampsia, and maternal or fetal death[37,38] (Box 7-4).

The origin of PIH may not be evident until halfway through the pregnancy. Hypertensive disease complicates 6% to 8% of all pregnancies.[39] Symptoms of HIP are vasospasm leading to an increase in blood pressure, renal changes lowering renal blood flow and filtration rate causing proteinuria, headaches and visual disturbances. Severe HIP can lead to strokes, acute renal failure, abruptio placentae, seizures and fetal and maternal death[15] (Box 7-5 and Table 7-2).

TABLE 7-2	Risk Factors for Pregnancy-Induced Hypertension (Gestational Hypertension)	
Factor		**Risk Ratio**
Nulliparity		3:1
Forty or older		3:1
African race		1.5:1
Family history of PIH		5:1
Chronic hypertension		10:1
Chronic renal disease		20:1
Diabetes mellitus		2:1
Twin gestation		4:1

PIH, Pregnancy-induced hypertension.
From Virtual Medical Library, Hypertension in pregnancy, Medical-Library.org.

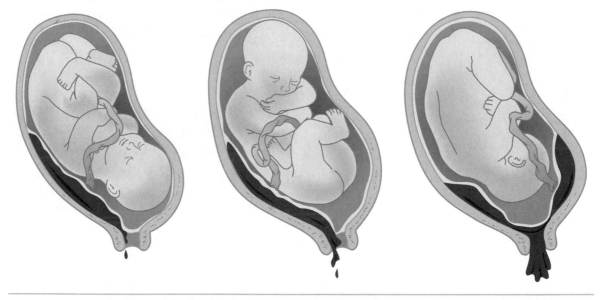

FIGURE 7-6 ■ The placenta *(dark red)* in three degrees of placenta previa. On the left, the placenta is low-lying and edges toward the cervical os. The middle picture shows the placenta partially covering the cervical os. On the right, the placenta completely covers the cervical os. (From Leifer G: *Maternity nursing: an introductory text,* ed 9, St. Louis, 2005, Saunders.)

Placenta Previa or Abruptio Placentae

In most pregnancies, the placenta attaches to the top, or fundus, of the uterus. When the placenta attaches abnormally near or directly over the cervix, placenta previa occurs (Figure 7-6). The amount of coverage over the os, or mouth, of the cervix determines the classification of the ailment. The two major threats are maternal hemorrhaging or fetal prematurity or death. Placenta previa occurs in 1 in 200 live births.[39]

Painless bleeding after 24 weeks' gestation may be a symptom of placenta previa. Women who develop placenta previa are carefully medically managed, and all bodywork must cease until the placenta migrates off the cervix and the medical team has established that she can resume normal activities.

Abruptio placentae is the premature separation of a normally implanted placenta from the uterine wall (see Figure 7-5).

Premature Labor

Any women experiencing labor contractions between 20 and 37 weeks' gestation is having preterm labor. It occurs in about 8% of the population and is responsible for most perinatal deaths not resulting from congenital abnormalities.[15] Infants born prematurely can have a lifetime of physical and cognitive difficulties. The signs of preterm labor are as follows:

- Menstrual-like uterine cramping
- Abdominal cramping with or without nausea, vomiting, diarrhea
- Vaginal bleeding
- Change in vaginal discharge

Those women experiencing preterm labor must receive medical attention to attempt to prolong the pregnancy and stop the contractions. Massage is absolutely contraindicated with preterm labor.

Pitting Edema

Before each treatment, it is essential for the practitioner to evaluate each client to make sure that she is a healthy candidate for bodywork. Pretreatment evaluations (see Chapter 3) include testing for the presence of blood clots. The practitioner lightly runs his or her hand down the back of the client's legs, dorsiflexing the client's feet with her knees slightly bent to check for the presence of clots in her calves. The last evaluation is a test for pitting edema. The practitioner lightly presses into the lowest part of the client's leg above the ankle; if the indentation does not fill in within a count of five, or if the ischemic coloration does not become red, the bodywork should not proceed and the client should seek medical attention immediately. Pitting edema may be symptomatic of renal disease or renal failure, preeclampsia, or any number of dangerous conditions.

Lack of Fetal Movement in 8 to 10 Hours

Fetuses have sleeping and waking cycles and some fetuses may be more active by nature than others. However, if a mother has not felt any activity from her fetus for a period of 8 to 10 hours, especially after eating, she should contact her health care provider.

Unfamiliar Conditions

If a client presents with a condition that the practitioner is not familiar with, it is advisable to book the appointment after researching the condition. The client's care provider or other resources may inform the practitioner that massage is not contraindicated or that certain modifications have to be made.

Treating Clients Confined to Bed Rest

There are many reasons why a woman may be confined to bed or be on restricted activity by her doctor or midwife. At least 20% of pregnant women are confined to **bed rest** for a week or more some time during gestation.[41] In the first half of the pregnancy, the conditions are bleeding, staining, or the threat of a miscarriage. During the second half, the threat of preterm labor is generally the reason for confinement.

Others conditions implicated in bed rest are preeclampsia, placenta previa, hypertension, incompetent cervix, premature rupture of the membranes, and chronic heart disease.[42] Bed rest decreases the pressure of the fetus on the cervix, reducing the likelihood of cervical stretching and contractions. A side-lying position increases blood flow to the placenta and can reduce high blood pressure.

On the other hand, bed rest increases the risk of thromboembolic disease, decreases cardiovascular conditioning, increases constipation and indigestion, bone demineralization and calcium loss, diuresis with accompanying fluid, electrolyte and weight loss, loss of muscle tone, sleep disturbances, fatigue, prolonged postpartum recovery and emotional guilt, depression, boredom, loneliness and psychological stress.[42,43] It is for these reasons that the idea of bed rest has become controversial.

With all of the previously mentioned complications, bodywork is contraindicated. If a client is prescribed bed rest for other reasons, such as impaired fetal growth and multiples, and she does not present any contraindicated symptoms, then a massage can be offered although all pregnancy considerations must be applied. Since the risk of thromboembolic disease is increased, all massage to the legs and feet must be avoided. In addition, the work is best performed with the client lying on her left side for enhanced placental profusion. Finally, considering all the other side effects of bed rest, limiting the treatment to under 1 hour will not deplete her of her energy reserve.

Bodyworks appropriate to bed rest include Swedish massage, lymphatic drainage, trigger point therapy, energy work, gentle myofascial release, craniosacral therapy, and passive and active exercises.

Coping With Bed Rest

A woman confined to bed, even for a short period of time, needs to find tools that can help eliminate the stress and concern that she feels. She also needs to make use of the time in a productive manner. The following are some suggestions to make the client on bed rest feel more comfortable, less achy, and proactive. Clients should be urged to do the following:

- Increase fluid intake to 8 glasses of water a day and add extra fiber and roughage to decrease constipation.
- Pass the time, including puzzles, reading, and crafts to reduce boredom.
- Maintain strength and muscle tone, such as isometric exercises, with gentle extension and flexion, circling arms, legs, and feet.
- Encourage the family to participate in the client's care and care of the house and older children.
- Combat the stress and anxiety of bed rest with relaxation activities, such as deep breathing exercises.
- Continue working from home on computer and phone.
- Use this opportunity to catch up on correspondences and projects
- Get help from others. A support group called *Sidelines* has a national hotline of volunteers to match the client with other expectant mothers on bed rest. Sidelines

toll free number is 1-888-447-4754 (HI-RISK4). E-mail address is Sidelines@sidelines.org and the Web site: www.sidelines.org.

- Spend some of the time bonding and communicating with the fetus.
- Learn a new skill, language, or craft.
- Enjoy the down time. This may be the last time you can rest so much.[41]
- Take it easy once bed rest orders have been removed.

In My Experience...

I often receive phone calls from clients who have been advised bed rest during their pregnancies asking whether I would come to their homes and give them a massage. The first question I always ask is, "Why has your care provider prescribed bed rest for you?" If the answer falls into the high-level risk category, I tell them that massage is not appropriate for them.

One day I received a phone call from a pregnant woman who was complaining how miserable she was feeling after so many weeks of bed rest. She was experiencing preterm labor contractions, and massage was out of the question. She pleaded with me to give her a massage and then she started sobbing. She felt miserable. Her body ached all over, and she confessed how guilty and depressed she was. All she wanted, she said, was to feel a little better.

While I commiserated with her and empathized with her situation, I made it clear that a massage was not in her or her baby's best interest. I offered her some coping suggestions and cautioned her to stop making any more calls for a massage. I told her that at some point, she would find someone who would go to her house. This person, I told her, would not have proper prenatal massage training or would be acting irresponsibly. In either case, the risk was too great.

She finally calmed down, thanked me, and promised not to make any more calls for a massage. She kept her word, except for a few weeks later when she called me to set-up an appointment at my office. Her doctor had given her a clean bill of health, and now she wanted to enjoy a well-deserved and much-needed massage.

Summary

Working with high risk pregnancies can be a challenge for the bodyworker. The conditions we are concerned with are those heightened risk factors that might increase the chances of a miscarriage, preterm labor, labor complications, and maternal or fetal morbidity or mortality.

Low-risk factors are those instances where the massage has no affect on outcome and the practitioner can proceed normally, within the safeguards of appropriate prenatal massage, without altering their techniques. Some of these factors are maternal age, multiples, the use of ART, complications from previous pregnancies, three or more spontaneous abortions, and fetal genetic or medical disorders.

With midlevel risk factors, the practitioner may have to adapt the techniques or modify them on some way that is appropriate to her condition. Treatment time may also be shortened if the condition requires. Some of the midlevel risk factors are maternal illness or preexisting condition, maternal drug exposure, expose to DES, after surgery, trauma or injury, obesity or low weight gain, smoking, Rh incompatibility, and physical or sexual abuse.

Those factors considered high-level risks require medical intervention and resolution before a treatment can be offered. These factors include maternal drug or substance abuse, PIH or GH, placenta previa, abruptio placentae, vaginal bleeding or staining, preterm labor, pitting edema, lack of fetal movement for 8 to 10 hours.

If practitioners are not certain about any specific condition, they should learn more about it before treating the client. With any high risk pregnancy, these conditions should be discussed with the client and her health care providers if necessary.

A woman confined to bed rest may or may not be a candidate for a massage. If she exhibits any of the high-level risk factors, massage should not be done until the condition heals and she has been given permission by her health care providers to resume normal activity. If she can receive a massage, then the time should be limited to suit her condition, she should remain on her left side, and all massage and bodywork to her legs and feet should be avoided because the blood is even more stagnant from her immobility.

References

1. Goldsmith J: *Childbirth wisdom*, New York, 1984, Congdon & Weed.
2. Van der Donck A: *A description of New Netherland*, Amsterdam, 1656.
3. Gilmore MR: Notes on gynecology and obstetrics of the Arikara tribe of Indians. Papers of the Michigan Academy of Sciences, Arts and Letters, vol XIV. Ann Arbor, 1930.
4. Hall P: Rethinking risk, *Can Fam Physician* 40:1239-1244, 1994.
5. Osborne-Sheets C: *Pre- and perinatal massage therapy*, San Diego, 1998, Body Therapy Associates.
6. Lowdermilk DL, Perry SE: *Maternity & women's health care*, ed 8, St. Louis, 2004, Mosby.
7. Gilbert ES, Harmon JS: *Manual of high risk pregnancy and delivery*, St. Louis, 1993, Mosby.
8. Leifer G: *Maternity nursing: an introductory text*, ed 9, St. Louis, 2005, Saunders.
9. Lewis G, Drife J, eds: *Why mothers die 1997-1999. The confidential enquiries into maternal deaths in the United Kingdom*, London, 2001, RCOG Press.
10. Clark PA: Maternal and neonatal morbidity and mortality: progress to date, *MIDIRS Midwifery Digest* 12(1):32-35, 2002.
11. Perinatal mortality: a listing of available information. Maternal health and safe motherhood programme, Geneva, 1996, WHO.
12. WHO World Health Day 1998 information kit, Geneva, 1998, WHO.
13. Minino A, Arias E, Kochanek KD, et al: Deaths: Final data for 2000, *Natl Vital Stat Rep* 50(15):1-119, 2002.
14. Hoyert D, Freedman MA, Strobino DM, et al: Annual summary of vital statistics, 2000, *Pediatrics* 108(6):1241-1255, 2001.
15. Fraser D, Cooper M: *Myles' textbook for midwives*, ed 14, Edinburgh, 2003, Churchill Livingstone.
16. Martin JA, Hamilton BE, Sutton PD: Births: final data for 2002, *Natl Vital Stat Rep* 52:10, 2003.

17. Albert B: *With one voice: American adults and teens sound off about teen pregnancy*, Washington, DC, 2003, National Campaign to Prevent Teen Pregnancy.

18. Singh S, Darroch J: Adolescent pregnancy: childbearing levels and trend in developed countries, *Fam Plan Persp* 32:1, 2000.

19. Black C, DeBlassie R: Adolescent pregnancy: contributing factors, consequences, treatment and plausible solutions, *Adolescence* 20:281-289, 1985.

20. Hassid P: *Textbook for childbirth educators*, Philadelphia, 1978, Harper and Row.

21. Namazy J, Schatz M, Long L: Use of inhaled steroids by pregnant asthmatic women does not reduce intrauterine growth, *J Allergy Clin Immunol* 113(3):427-432, 2004.

22. Munkarah AR, Morris R: Malignant disease in pregnancy. In James DK, Steer PJ, Weiner CP et al, eds: *High risk pregnancy options*, London, 1999, Saunders.

23. Berman M, DiSaia P, Brewster W: Pelvic malignancies, gestational trophoblastic neoplasia, and non-pelvic malignancies. In Creasy R, Resnik R, eds: *Maternal-fetal medicine*, ed 4, Philadelphia, 1999, Saunders.

24. Copeland L, Landon M: Malignant disease and pregnancy. In Gabbe S, Niebyl J, Simpson J, eds: *Obstetrics: normal and problem pregnancies*, ed 4, New York, 2002, Churchill Livingstone.

25. DiSaia P, Creasman W: *Clinical gynecologic oncology*, ed 6, St. Louis, 2002, Mosby.

26. Haney A: Fertility issues associated with pre-natal exposure to diethylstilbestrol, *The DES Research Symposium: looking back, looking ahead,* Oakland, CA, 1989, DES Action.

27. Stillman R: In utero exposure to diethylstilbestrol: adverse effects on the reproductive tract and reproductive performance in male and female offspring, *Am J Obstet Gynecol* 142(7):909-921, 1982.

28. Brody JE: *Prenatal exposure to DES can also hurt men, and they should be vigilant,* The New York Times, July 30, 1997.

29. Herbst A, Mishell D, Stenchever M, et al: *Comprehensive gynecology*, ed 2, St. Louis, 1992, Mosby.

30. Milhan D: DES exposure: implications for childbearing, *ICEA Review* 16:3, 1992.

31. Nucci LB, Schmidt ML, Duncan BB, et al: Nutritional status of pregnant women: prevalence and associated pregnancy outcomes, *Rev Saude Publilca* 35(6):502-507, 2001.

32. Sebire N, Jolly M, Harris JP, et al: Maternal obesity and pregnancy outcome: a study of 287, 213 pregnancies in London, *Int J Obes Relat Metab Disord* 25(8):1175-1192, 2001.

33. Woolston C: How smoking during pregnancy affects you and your baby, BabyCenter. Available at http://www.babycenter.com/refcap/pregnancy/pregquitsmoking/1405720.html, Accessed September, 2006.

34. Henderson AJ, Sherriff A, Northstone K, et al: Pre-and postnatal parental smoking and wheeze in infancy: cross cultural differences, *Eur Respir J* 18:323-329, 2001.

35. Coad J: *Anatomy and physiology for midwives*, St. Louis, 2001, Mosby.

36. Woodward A, Grgurinovich N, Ryan P: Breast feeding and smoking hygiene: major influences on nicotine in urine of smokers' infants, *J Epidemiol Community Health* 40(3):309-315, 1986.

37. Diagnosis and management of preeclampsia and eclampsia, *ACOG Practice Bulletin #33*, Washington, DC, 2002, American College of Obstetricians and Gynecologists.

38. National Institutes of Health: *National blood pressure workshop on blood pressure education*, Bethesda, MD, 2000, NIH.

39. Hypertension in pregnancy, Medical-Library.org.

40. Gabbe S, Niebyl J, Simpson J: *Obstetrics: normal and problem pregnancies*, ed 4, New York, 2002, Churchill Livingstone.

41. Sears W, Sears M: *The pregnancy book*, Boston, 1997, Little, Brown.

42. Enkin M, Keirse M, Neilson J, et al: *A guide to effective care in pregnancy and childbirth*, Oxford, 2000, Oxford University Press.

43. Maloni J: Home care of the high risk pregnant woman requiring bed rest, *J Obstet Gynecol Neonat Nurs* 23(8):696-706, 1994.

REVIEW QUESTIONS

1   What is meant by high risk pregnancy?

_____

_____

_____

_____

_____

2   What are the categories that might cause serious trauma or compromise the health of the mother or fetus?

_____

_____

_____

_____

_____

3   Are either maternal or fetal morbidity influenced by a massage?

_____

_____

_____

_____

_____

4   Describe and explain at least three low risk factors for massage during pregnancy.

_____

_____

_____

_____

_____

5   Describe and explain at least three midlevel risk factors for massage during pregnancy.

_____

_____

_____

_____

_____

6   Explain the importance of posttreatment observation for a client with gestational glucose intolerance.

_____

_____

_____

_____

7   List at least six foods or beverages that may cause further irritation to the bladder and lead to urgency and incontinence or leaking of urine.

_____

_____

_____

_____

8   What is DES, and what are some of the possible reproductive complications as a result to DES exposure?

_____

_____

_____

_____

_____

9 What suggestions can be made to help a pregnant woman stop smoking during her pregnancy?

_____

_____

_____

_____

_____

10 Describe and explain at least four high-level risk factors that would contraindicate massage during pregnancy.

_____

_____

_____

_____

_____

11 Describe various types of PIH.

_____

_____

_____

_____

_____

12 What are the symptoms of PIH?

_____

_____

_____

_____

_____

13 What is placenta previa? Abruptio placentae? Is massage indicated for these conditions?

_____

_____

_____

_____

_____

14 Describe situations where massage in not suitable for clients who have been prescribed bed rest during their pregnancy.

_____

_____

_____

_____

_____

15 Provide some helpful suggestions to help a client cope with bed rest during pregnancy.

_____

_____

_____

_____

_____

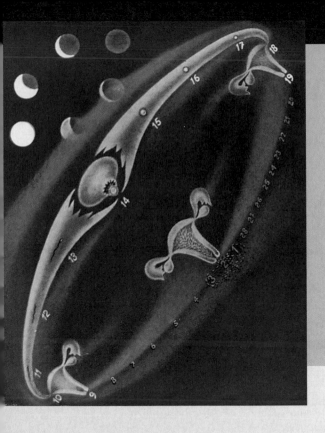

CHAPTER 8

Preconception Support

Objectives

On completion of this chapter, the student will be able to do the following:

1 Understand the causes of female and male infertility

2 Suggest a healthy lifestyle for the prospective parents

3 Learn how to do a kidney rub

4 Learn which muscles relate to the reproductive system and how to strengthen them

5 Understand the use of manual muscle testing

6 Learn effective massage protocol to treat neurolymphatic reflexes

7 Use a specific massage oil to increase clients' chances of conceiving

Preconception Support

In medical terms, **preconception** health care and screening help the medical team identify potential risk factors and lifestyle behaviors that can be managed, redirected, or changed before conception.[1] The medical information gathered includes a complete physical history and may also include psychological or psychosocial issues that might affect the birth outcome. The importance and potential impact of preconception care has only been recognized over the last 30 years. The purpose of this care is "to ensure that the woman and her partner are in an optimal state of physical and emotional health at the onset of pregnancy."[2] Preconception care may also give the prospective couple some options that would no longer be available to them once the pregnancy was confirmed.[3]

Preconception support provided by bodyworkers should enhance the client's general health and improve her chances of conceiving. These goals are achieved through specific bodywork techniques and client education. This chapter does not address issues related to infertility or the use of artificial reproductive technology (ART), although 1 in 7 couples will need medical intervention to get pregnant. However, (Boxes 8-1 and 8-2 include the causes of infertility in both females and males. For those clients, referral to a fertility specialist is suggested.

Referrals to other health care professionals are often appropriate and necessary. It is important to remember that the woman is only one-half of the couple, and if conception is going to be successful, both partners have to adopt healthy lifestyles and establish good habits. A few helpful suggestions for the couple are as follows:

- Eat well
- Include folic acid in the diet
- Maintain a healthy body weight
- Exercise
- Avoid first- or second-hand smoking

BOX 8-1 *Causes of Female Infertility*

Defective Ovulation

Endocrine disorders
- Dysfunction of hypothalamus, pituitary, adrenals, thyroid
- Systemic disease: diabetes mellitus, celiac disease, renal failure

Physical disorders
- Obesity
- Anorexia nervosa or strict dieting
- Excessive exercise

Ovarian disorders
- Hormonal
- Ovarian cysts or tumors
- Polycystic ovary disease
- Ovarian endometriosis

Defective Transport

Ovum
- Tubal obstruction
  - Infection (gonorrhea, peritonitis, pelvic inflammatory disease)
- Fimbrial adhesions
  - Previous surgery
  - Endometriosis

Sperm
- Vagina
  - Psychosexual problems (vaginismus)
  - Infection (causing dyspareunia)
  - Congenital anomaly
- Cervix
  - Cervical trauma or surgery (cone biopsy)
  - Infection
  - Hormonal (hostile mucus)
  - Antisperm antibodies

Defective Implantation
- Hormonal imbalance
- Congenital anomalies
- Fibroids
- Infection

From Fraser D, Cooper M: *Myles' textbook for midwives,* ed 14, Edinburgh, 2003, Churchill Livingstone.

<table>
<tr><td>

BOX 8-2 *Causes of Male Infertility*

Defective Spermatogenesis
Endocrine disorders
- Dysfunction of hypothalamus, pituitary, adrenals, thyroid
- Systemic disease: diabetes mellitus, celiac disease, renal failure

Testicular disorders
- Trauma
- Environmental (high temperature)
  - Congenital (hydrocele, undescended testes)
  - Occupational (furnace worker, long-distance truck driver)
  - Acquired (varicocele, tight clothing)
- Cancer treatment

Defective Transport
- Obstruction or absence of seminal ducts
  - Infection
  - Congenital anomalies
  - Trauma
- Impaired secretions from prostate or seminal vesicles
  - Infection
  - Metabolic disorders

Ineffective Delivery
- Psychosexual problems (impotence)
- Drug-induced (ejaculatory dysfunction)
- Physical disability
- Physical anomalies
  - Hypospadias
  - Epispadias
  - Retrograde ejaculation (into bladder)

</td></tr>
</table>

From Fraser D, Cooper M: *Myles' textbook for midwives,* ed 14, Edinburgh, 2003, Churchill Livingstone.

- Avoid excessive alcohol
- Address preexisting conditions
- Avoid environmental dangers

Diet

A nutritious diet and healthy maternal weight are essential elements to becoming pregnant. A woman's nutritional status before conception and during the first few weeks of pregnancy may actually be more important than what she eats once the pregnancy is confirmed.[4] This should not be interpreted as meaning that her prenatal diet is irrelevant. During pregnancy, it is vital that the woman maintain good eating habits to support and maintain her own well-being, as well as nourishing the developing fetus. Entering pregnancy in a less-than-healthy condition can lead to fetal damage and stunted growth.[5]

A preconception diet should be rich with a wide variety of wholesome foods such as lean meats, grains, legumes, and fresh fruits and vegetables. The diet should also consist of foods high in folate, which is found in dark green vegetables, fruit and fruit juices, beans, and yeast extract and can help protect the fetus against neural tube defects (NTDs).[6] Folic acid is the synthetic form of folate in vitamin supplements. An additional 800 mg of folate before conception and during the first trimester will help reduce the risk of NTDs.

Vitamin A is essential for the development, growth, and epithelial differentiation of the embryo, although excessive consumption of retinol, a form of vitamin A, is known to be teratogenic (causing birth defects). A diet with high levels of retinol consumed before the seventh week of pregnancy has caused birth defects such as cleft lip, ventricular septal defect, multiple heart defects, hydrocephaly, craniosynostosis, and transposition of the great vessels.[7] Since high levels of retinol are found in the livers of farm animals, women trying to conceive or who are recently pregnant should avoid eating, or consume only moderate amounts of, liver and liver products.

Overweight or underweight women often have difficulties trying to conceive. Overweight or obese women have higher risks of gestational diabetes and hypertensive disorders, higher instances of cesarean sections, and babies with low Apgar scores, fetal macrosomia, NTDs, and late fetal death.[8-10] Underweight women have delayed menses, secondary amenorrhea, and irregular periods, which create fertility problems.[11] Preconception support for these women includes helping them achieve a healthy body weight and educating them on healthy eating habits. Referrals to nutritionists, dieticians, or eating disorder clinicians, in addition to the bodywork, are recommended.

Caffeine consumption and birth defects do not seem to have any relationship.[12] However, caffeine is found in many food sources in addition to coffee, such as black and green teas, chocolate, colas, and certain medications, so the client may not

Touch Points

Talking to a client about changing her lifestyle—or her partner's lifestyle—to increase her chances of conceiving is not always easy. Some clients are more receptive to suggestions than others. The important thing to remember is to avoid making judgments about the way a person lives. The practitioner can offer evidence-based information about the effects of smoking, alcohol consumption, or drug use on conception and pregnancy. This information may make the client more aware of her dangerous behaviors and bad habits and more receptive to a practitioner's feedback instead of an accusing finger.

realize how much she is consuming. It is advisable to limit the amount of caffeine ingested.

Exercise

Moderate exercise is beneficial for a woman trying to become pregnant. It will strengthen and tone her body, improve her cardiovascular system, and ward off fatigue. Appropriate use of the abdominal muscles in exercises that recruit the transverse abdominis muscle will maintain and support the woman's core muscles and relieve and prevent back pain. These exercises will also enable her to use her abdominals more purposefully during labor.

Exercise can also address many emotional issues often associated with fertility by fighting depression and anxiety. The release of serotonin and beta-endorphins from exercising can reduce stress and potentially calm a woman's concerns.

Smoking

Part of a healthy lifestyle is staying away from or stopping smoking. Smoking can cut the chances of conception by almost 40%.[13] The evidence against smoking is well-established. Smoking can induce menstrual problems and early menopause in women; in men, smoking can cause changes in sperm morphology and motility. Smoking can increase the risk of spontaneous abortion, preterm labor, low birth weight, perinatal death, antepartum hemorrhage, and abruptio placentae (see Chapter 7). If a pregnant woman continues to smoke, the fetus often suffers from hypoxia and the harmful carcinogens that pass through the placenta.[14,15]

Nutritional habits are often less than ideal in smokers. Smokers may have diets high in total fat, saturated fat, cholesterol, and alcohol and have lower consumption of vitamins, antioxidants, and micronutrients.[16]

Alcohol Consumption

Consuming even small amounts of alcohol during pregnancy can have devastating results. During pregnancy, alcohol acts as a teratogen, which is an agent that can increase the risks of a congenital anomaly in the developing embryo or fetus. Fetal alcohol syndrome is generally associated with excessive prenatal drinking, but even social or moderate drinking can cause permanent damage to the fetus. The safest thing to do is avoid all alcohol consumption during pregnancy.

As a rule, social or moderate drinking does not carry the risk associated with high alcohol intake. Of course, this is an individual level. However, menstrual disorders and decreased fertility have been associated with heavy drinking—even among women who had five or fewer drinks a week.[17]

Preexisting Medical Conditions

A woman with a preexisting medical condition may have a difficult time conceiving. For example, a woman with diabetes mellitus suffers from the most common chronic medical disease in pregnancy. These women require medical supervision to regulate glucose levels. The safety of current oral hypoglycemic medications has not been adequately studied during pregnancy, and those women with type 2 diabetes should be switched to insulin therapy during preconception and for the duration of the pregnancy.[18]

A common neurological problem is epilepsy, and most drugs used to treat epilepsy are teratogenic. Newer medications have not been sufficiently studied for use during pregnancy.[19-21] The goal of preconception care for the woman with epilepsy is to control her seizures with the lowest dose of anticonvulsant medications.

If a client does have a seizure during massage treatment, practitioners should stop what they are doing and make sure the client does not fall off the table. The seizure should be allowed to run its course, and then the practitioner can help her off the table only when she is able to move. It is not uncommon for the seizure to be followed by a deep sleep. The client should not be awakened but should be observed closely until she awakens. She will rouse in a short time. Emergency medical help should be called if needed.

Environmental Factors

Environmental factors can have a tremendous effect on fertility. Certain solvents, ionizing radiation, and anesthetic gases are known toxins that can cause neurological defects, microcephaly, and increased risk of miscarriage.[22] Heavy metals, such as aluminum, cadmium, copper, lead, and mercury, are also toxic.[23] Other environmental factors that affect fertility are pesticides, defoliants, and industrial chemicals. Low levels of radiation from television sets, video display terminals, and microwaves may not be contributing factors in fertility or pregnancy complications.

Maintaining Support into the Bodywork

After all of the suggestions have been discussed with the client on how to improve the quality of her lifestyle, the support must continue into the bodywork. A full body massage is calming and relaxing and can minimize the stress factors often associated with trying to conceive. In addition, the enhanced circulation and increased red blood cell count can treat fatigue and make her feel more energized.

When a muscle is chronically weak, the effects are noticed with specific gland or organ dysfunction.[24] If a client is having difficulty conceiving, the muscles that correlate to the reproductive system will also be weak. According to the applied kinesiology technique, the muscles that correlate to the reproductive system are the **gluteus maximus**, **piriformis**, and **adductor muscles**.

Initially, the practitioner assesses a muscle's strength by testing it. **Manual muscle testing**

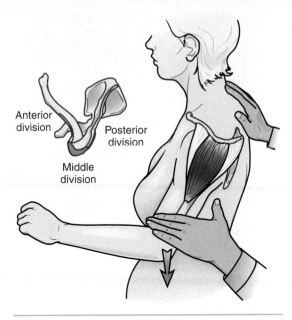

FIGURE 8-1 ■ Position for muscle testing the lateral deltoid.

requires the muscle being tested to contract against the examiner's applied but light pressure. The pressure should cause the isometric contraction to become an eccentric contraction, which means it produces force but lengthens against stronger opposing force. Manual muscle testing requires great skill and experience. The following is a simplified method of performing a manual muscle test.

The practitioner should have the client use a healthy muscle, such as the lateral deltoid, for muscle testing. The client should raise her arm laterally, parallel to the floor, and bend it at the elbow (Figure 8-1); this is the action of the lateral deltoid. The practitioner presses lightly at the client's elbow using downward pressure. A strong muscle will be able to hold the position, whereas as weak deltoid will fail. If this muscle proves to be strong, the practitioner can use it to assess the strength of the other muscles.

The client should assume the test position for the lateral deltoid and lightly touch the right and left gluteus maximus, piriformis, and adductor muscles. Her deltoid muscle can be tested each time she touches a muscle. Even though the lateral deltoid does not have the muscle/organ relationship to the reproductive system, it will fail if any of these muscles are weak.

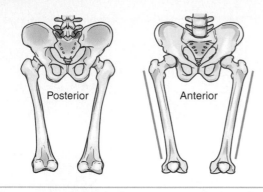

FIGURE 8-2 ■ If the gluteus maximus muscles test weak, treat the neurolymphatic reflexes located on the lateral aspect of both thighs and on the posterior aspect of the spine between L5 and S1.

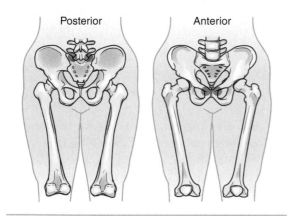

FIGURE 8-3 ■ Neurolymphatic reflexes for the piriformis muscles. The posterior points are found at L5 and S1, and the anterior points are located on either side of the symphysis pubis.

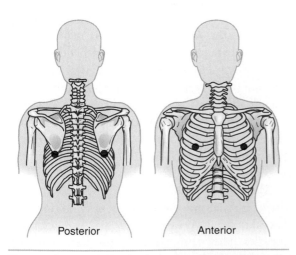

FIGURE 8-4 ■ Neurolymphatic reflexes for the adductors. The posterior points are located at the inferior angle of the scapulae, and the anterior points are found behind the areolae. This latter point may be too sensitive to treat.

Once the practitioner establishes which of the muscles are weak, they can be strengthened by stimulating their respective **neurolymphatic (NL) reflexes.** Dr. Frank Chapman developed a system of reflexes for improved lymphatic drainage in the 1930s. In 1965, Dr. George Goodheart, DC, noticed that weak muscles became dramatically stronger when certain reflexes were stimulated.[25] The NL reflexes are located on the anterior and posterior aspects of the body and are diagnostic and therapeutic. An active reflex is hypersensitive, generally more so on the anterior of the body.

A 15-second rotary massage with reasonable pressure, using the palmar surface of the fingertips, is the way to treat the NL reflexes (Figures 8-2 to 8-4). Once the reflexes have been treated, the lateral deltoid should be tested again as the client touches the muscle. The muscle should test stronger. The client should also be encouraged to eat foods rich in vitamin A (not retinol) and vitamin E that improve muscle functions.

Muscle testing takes a long time to understand and perform, but it can be a valuable assessment tool once learned correctly. Proper training is essential, and practice over time will give the practitioner the subtle touch needed for this technique.

In addition to muscle testing and treatment of related NL reflexes, other appropriate bodywork for preconception care consists of Swedish massage for relaxation, the kidney rub to stimulate "ancestral Qi" (Box 8-3), and stimulation of acupuncture points spleen 3 (Figure 8-5) for hormone balancing and conception vessel 3 (Figure 8-6) to tone the uterus. The woman's diet should also include drinking red raspberry leaf tea that contains fragine, a compound that tones the muscles of the uterus. She should drink 3 to 6 cups of this tea daily.

Massage Oil

A special massage oil can be used to help clients who are trying to conceive. The abdomen, back, inner thighs, and buttocks (gluteus maximus, piriformis, and adductors) can be massaged with 5 drops of rose oil and 15 drops of geranium oil added to 2 oz of any vegetable or carrier oil.

BOX 8-3 *The Kidney Rub*

In traditional Oriental medicine, the kidneys are the "hosts for the adrenal glands, which Oriental medicine says control the sexual function." The kidneys are regarded as the rulers of the sexual organs and the physical cause of most sexual problems. When the kidneys are healthy, sexual potency is high. The kidneys are called the "seat of life."*

Original Ki (Qi, Chi) (yuan-qi), also called prenatal Qi, is stored in the kidneys and is passed from parent to child at conception. It is believed that this Qi is partly responsible for a person's constitution.†

Another Oriental theory of yin and yang says, "When Yin (female) attacks and Yang (male) separates, it is said that a child has been conceived."‡

To stimulate original Qi (prenatal or ancestral Qi) and enhance the chances of conception, a kidney rub can be included in massage treatment. One way of doing a kidney rub is as follows:

1. Practitioners rub their hands together until they become hot and then place them on the client's kidneys.
2. Practitioners perform a broad, open-hand friction across the kidneys.
3. Kidneys are rubbed vigorously.
4. Then the client can rub her kidneys with her fists 100 times.

*Data from Muramoto N: *Healing ourselves,* New York, 1973, Avon.
†Data from Kaptchuk TJ: *The web that has no weaver,* New York, 1983, Congdon & Weed.
‡Data from Nei HT, Wen CS: *The yellow emperor's classic of internal medicine,* Vieth I, translator. Berkeley, 1949, University of California Press.

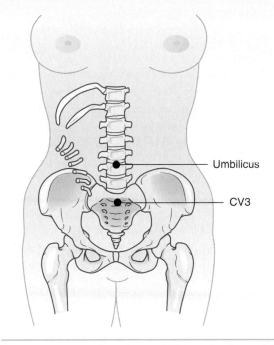

FIGURE 8-6 ■ Conception vessel 3 is located at the top of the uterus, 4 cun below the umbilicus. (Modified from Lowdermilk DL, Perry, SE: *Maternity & women's health care,* ed 8, St. Louis, 2004, Mosby)

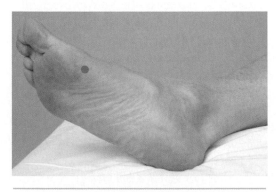

FIGURE 8-5 ■ Spleen 3 is used for hormone balancing.

In My Experience...

B and her husband were trying to conceive for about a year when I first met her. After a few massages, I decided to perform muscle testing on those muscles that relate to the reproductive system. Each muscle tested very weak.

I stimulated the NL reflexes, which were very sensitive to the touch, and noticed a modest improvement in muscle strength. I mentioned to B that I would continue including this during her massages until her muscles—and her reproductive system—became stronger.

I will never know for certain what did the trick: the massages that calmed her or the NL points that energized her reproductive system, but within 3 months, she became pregnant.

Summary

Couples planning to become pregnant can improve their chances by adopting a healthy lifestyle, maintaining good dietary habits and weight, giving up harmful habits such as smoking and drinking, and being cautious about environmental dangers.

The practitioner can help couples reach their goal by educating them about a healthy lifestyle and providing women supportive massage techniques that can relax them, promote greater health, and strengthen their bodies.

References

1. Leifer G: *Maternity nursing: an introductory text*, ed 9, St. Louis, 2005, Saunders.

2. The role of general practice in maternity care. Royal College of General Practitioners. Report of the RCGP Maternity Care Group, *Occas Pap R Coll Gen Pract* 3:1-14, 1995.

3. Chamberlain G: *Turnbull's obstetrics*, London, 1995, Churchill Livingstone.

4. Doyle W: Preconception care: who needs it? *Modern Midwife* 2:18-22, 1992.

5. Wynn M, Wynn A: The need for nutritional assessment in the treatment of the infertile couple, *J Nutr Med* 1:315-324, 1990.

6. Department of Health: *Folic acid and the prevention of neural tube defects: report form an expert advisory group*, London, 1992, DH Publications.

7. Rothman KJ, Moore LL, Singer MR, et al: Teratogenicity of high vitamin A intake, *N Engl J Med* 333(21):1369-1373, 1995.

8. Baeten JM, Bukusi EA, Lambe M: Pregnancy complications and outcomes among nulliparous women, *Am J Public Health* 91(3):436-440, 2001.

9. Cnattingius S, Bergstrom R, Lipworth L, et al: Prepregnancy weight and the risk of adverse pregnancy outcome, *N Engl J Med* 338(3):147-152, 1998.

10. Galtier-Dereure F, Boegner C, Bringer J: Obesity and pregnancy: complications and cost, *Am J Clin Nutr* 71:1242S-1248S, 2000.

11. Frische RE, Wyshak G, Vincent L: Delayed menarche and amenorrhea in ballet dancers, *N Engl J Med* 303(1):7-18, 1980.

12. Woolston C: How smoking during pregnancy affects you and your baby, BabyCenter. Available at http://www.babycenter.com/refcap/pregnancy/pregquitsmoking/1405720.html, Accessed September, 2006.

13. Sexton M: Smoking. In Chamberlain G, Lumley J, eds: *Prepregnancy care*, Chichester, England, 1986, John Wiley.

14. Department of Health: *Smoking kills— a white paper on tobacco*, London, 1998, DH Stationary Office.

15. Dallongville J, Marecaux N, Fruchart JC, et al: Cigarette smoking is associated with unhealthy patterns of nutrient intake: a meta-analysis, *J Nutr* 128:1450-1457, 1998.

16. Jensen TK, Hjollund NH, Henriksen TB, et al: Does moderate alcohol consumption affect fertility? Follow-up study among couples planning first pregnancy, *BMJ* 317(7157):505-510, 1998.

17. Cunningham FG, Gant NF, Leveno KJ, et al: *Williams obstetrics*, ed 21, New York, 2001, McGraw Hill.

18. American Diabetic Association: Clinical practice recommendations, *Diabetes Care* September 2001.

19. Crawford P: Epilepsy and pregnancy: good management reduces the risks, *Prof Care Mother Child* 7(1):17-18, 1997.

20. Holmes LB, Harvey EA, Coull BA, et al: The teratogenicity of anticonvulsant drugs, *N Engl J Med* 334(15):1132-1138, 2001.

21. Lloyd C, Hunter E: The care of pregnant women with epilepsy, *MIDIRS Midwifery Digest* 11(1):37-39, 2001.

22. Joffe M: Women's work and pregnancy. In Chamberlain G, Lumley J, eds: *Prepregnancy care*, Chichester, 1986, John Wiley.

23. Fraser D, Cooper M: *Myles' textbook for midwives*, ed 14, Edinburgh, 2003, Churchill Livingstone.

24. Walther DS: *Applied kinesiology*, vol 1, Pueblo, Colo, 1981, SDC Systems.

25. Goodheart GJ Jr: *Applied kinesiology*, ed 3, Detroit, 1965, ICAK.

REVIEW QUESTIONS

1 What is the purpose of preconception health care and screening?

_____
_____
_____
_____
_____
_____

2 What are practitioners' preconception treatment goals for their clients?

_____
_____
_____
_____
_____

3 What are some possible medical complications attributed to female infertility?

_____
_____
_____
_____
_____

4 What are some possible medical complications attributed to male infertility?

_____
_____
_____
_____
_____

5 Describe what is meant by adopting a healthy lifestyle to enhance fertility.

_____
_____
_____
_____
_____

6 Describe how environmental factors can affect fertility.

_____
_____
_____
_____
_____

7 Which nutrient is particularly important in reducing the risk of NTDs?

_____
_____
_____
_____

8 How much of this nutrient should a woman trying to conceive consume daily?

_____
_____
_____
_____
_____

9 What are some of the prenatal risks factors associated with being overweight?

_____

_____

_____

_____

_____

10 According to traditional Oriental medicine, which organs are considered to "control sexual function"?

_____

_____

_____

_____

_____

11 How does the "kidney rub" enhance fertility? How is it done?

_____

_____

_____

_____

_____

12 What is manual muscle testing? How does a "strong" muscle behave during muscle testing?

_____

_____

_____

_____

_____

13 Which muscles are related to the reproductive system?

_____

_____

_____

_____

_____

14 Where are the NL reflexes for these muscles located?

_____

_____

_____

_____

_____

15 How long should rotary pressure last on the NL points?

_____

_____

_____

_____

_____

16 Where on the body are the active NL reflexes generally more tender?

_____

_____

_____

_____

_____

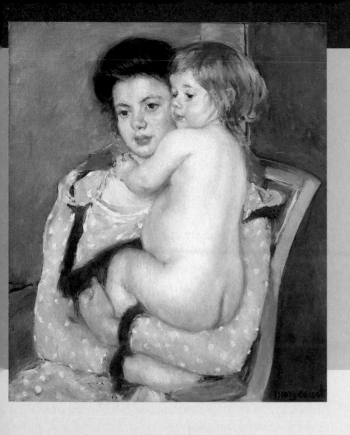

CHAPTER 9

The First Trimester

Objectives

On completion of this chapter, the student will be able to do the following:

1 Understand the basic facts of fertilization and how the embryo develops

2 Learn how the fetus develops during the first trimester of pregnancy

3 Understand the physical and emotional changes during the first trimester of pregnancy

4 Recognize the common discomforts associated with the first trimester

5 Learn massage considerations for the first trimester

Amniotic fluid	Dizziness	Human chorionic gonadotrophin
Amniotic sac	Fatigue	Hyperemesis gravidarum
Braxton Hicks contractions	Fertilization	Morula
Chorionic villi sampling	First trimester	Ovum

Pregnancy is characterized by three trimesters, each lasting approximately 3 months. The **first trimester**, known as the developmental period for the fetus, lasts from conception until 13 weeks.[1]

Fertilization and Embryonic Development

Within 30 minutes after **fertilization**, or the joining of the egg and sperm, the **ovum** (egg) divides from a single cell (called a zygote) to two cells, four cells, eight cells, sixteen cells, and so on[1] Figure 9-1). After 2 days, the group of rapidly dividing cells is called a **morula**, and after only 5 days, the conceptus, or morula, moves through the fallopian tube to the uterus where it implants. Implantation generally occurs in the upper part of the uterus, called the *fundus;* the conceptus is now called a *blastocyst* (Figures 9-2 to 9-4). A fertilized ovum that implants outside of the uterus

usually in the fallopian tubes is an ectopic pregnancy and requires prompt medical care (Box 9-1).

As the blastocyst continues to grow, a watertight sac forms around it that gradually fills with fluid. This **amniotic sac** contains **amniotic fluid,** which is produced by the amniotic membrane. The amniotic fluid protects and cushions the growing embryo, keeps the embryo at a steady temperature, allows fetal movement, and prevents fetal body parts from adhering to each other. Amniotic fluid is also important in the development of the fetal respiratory system and has bacteriostatic properties.

By week 3, the blastocyst is made up of about 100 cells. The outer cells will become the placenta, and the inner layer will become the embryo. At the end of 4 weeks, the fetus is 0.014 to 0.04 inches in length and is made up of 150 cells. Its cells are already specialized according to function. The outer layer will mature into the nervous system, skin, and hair. The inner layer will become organs

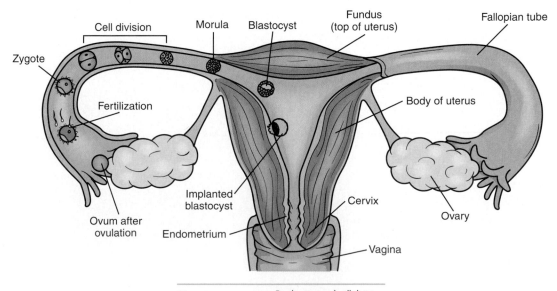

FIGURE 9-1 ■ Fertilization and cell division.

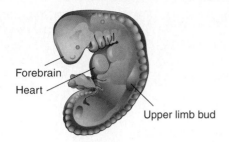

FIGURE 9-2 ■ Pregnancy at 1 month. (From Leifer G: *Maternity nursing*, ed 9, St Louis, 2005, Saunders).

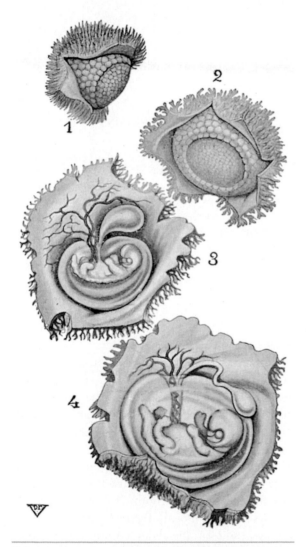

FIGURE 9-3 ■ "Evolution a few days after fecundation and embryos in the first months of pregnancy." (Reprinted from Willy A, Vander L, Fisher O: *The illustrated encyclopedia of sex*, New York, 1950, Cadillac Publishing.)

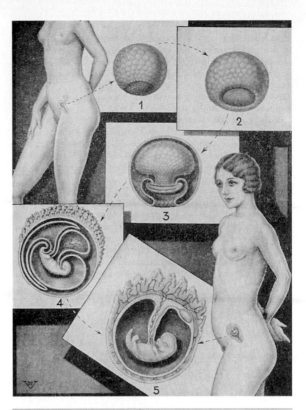

FIGURE 9-4 ■ Evolution of the fetus. (Reprinted from Willy A, Vander L, Fisher O: *The illustrated encyclopedia of sex*, New York, 1950, Cadillac Publishing.)

BOX 9-1 *Ectopic Pregnancy*

A fertilized ovum that implants outside the uterus is called an ectopic ("out of place"), or tubal pregnancy because 95% of these pregnancies occur within the fallopian tubes.* These pregnancies always result in miscarriage or surgical resolution. Symptoms include abdominal pain, bleeding, nausea, vomiting, dizziness, tenderness over the tubes, and severe pain on pelvic examination. Damage to the fallopian tubes may result in future fertility difficulties or hemorrhaging.† Prompt, appropriate medical care is essential for this potentially life-threatening emergency.

*Data from Sears W, Sears M: *The pregnancy book*, Boston, 1997, Little, Brown.
†Data from Coad J: *Anatomy and physiology for midwives*, St. Louis, 2001, Mosby.

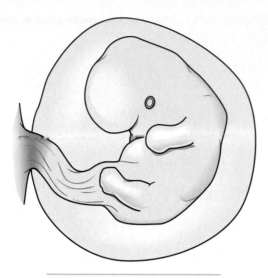

FIGURE 9-5 ■ Embryo at 5 weeks.

of respiration and digestion. The middle layer will grow into the skeletal and circulatory systems, muscles, kidneys, and sex organs.[2]

By the end of the second month, or weeks 5 to 8, the embryo is about 0.05 inches long. Its heart, brain, spinal cord, muscles, and bones are forming.[2] Facial features continue to form, and the ears are little folds of skin at the side of the head. Tiny buds that will become the arms and legs are forming, and the fingers, toes, and eyes are developing. The embryo's neural tube (brain, spinal cord, and other neural tissue of the central nervous system) is well-delineated, and the digestive tract and sensory organs begin to form (Figures 9-5 and 9-6).

The embryo takes on a tadpole shape and is about 0.08 to 0.16 inches long. The eyes and limbs are forming, and a heartbeat can be detected with an ultrasound. The embryo is floating inside the fluid-filled amniotic sac, and its spine is clearly visible.[2,3] (Figure 9-7).

Seven weeks marks a large growth spurt for the embryo. It is now ¾ of an inch long, and it can move its hands on which there are clearly delineated fingers. Eye lenses form, and its internal organs are visible.[3] The heart and lungs are becoming more developed, and the brain and spinal cord are forming from the neural tube[2] (Figure 9-8).

In the next week, the embryo will grow about 1½ inches more and weigh ½ oz and is complete. The heart has divided into four chambers. Hands, feet, and fingers are complete with fingerprints. Toes are

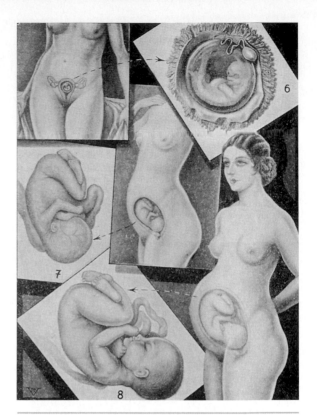

FIGURE 9-6 ■ "(6) After approximately five weeks, the head, limbs, eyes and mouth already distinguishable; (7) In fourth month the foetus in every way resembles a human being; (8) After eight months, a few days before delivery, the breasts are now fully prepared for lactation." (Reprinted from Willy A, Vander L, Fisher O: *The illustrated encyclopedia of sex,* New York, 1950, Cadillac Publishing.)

fully formed. Major joints are developing, and the mouth, tongue, gums and teeth buds, and nose and nostrils are more mature. Earlobes are visible, and all of the structures of the eyes are present. Gender, which was determined at conception, cannot be determined by looking, although external genitalia may become evident. The genital tubercle, a slit with a bump of tissue, is seen between the developing leg buds. If the embryo is a male, the Y chromosome stimulates these rudimentary sex glands to produce male hormones that bring the two sides of the slit together, forming the scrotum. The genital tubercle will develop into a penis. Before birth, the testicles will descend from the abdomen into the scrotum. If the embryo is female, hormones cause the slit to develop into the vulva and the genital tubercle to become the clitoris. Her ovaries are also formed.[1]

The embryo's primitive brain is sending neural impulses that coordinate the function of many of its organs. Between days 46 and 48, permanent

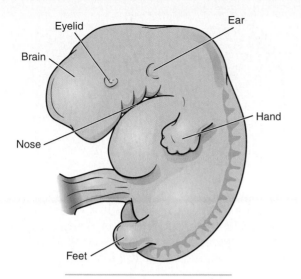

FIGURE 9-7 ■ Fetus at 6 weeks.

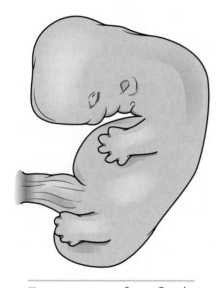

FIGURE 9-8 ■ Fetus at 7 weeks.

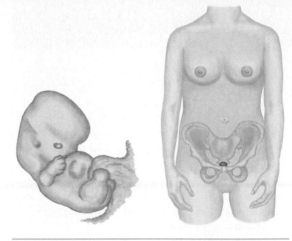

FIGURE 9-9 ■ Fetus at 8 weeks. Crown-rump length is 13 mm. Embryonic stage, with heart developed, beginning to pump; arm and leg buds present; head is large, with facial features beginning to form. (From Sears W, Sears M: *The pregnancy book*, Boston, 1997, Little, Brown.)

At 10 weeks, the fetus is 1.25 to 1.68 inches long. Its eyes are covered by skin that will split to form eyelids. The fetus is now the size of a medium shrimp. At 11 weeks, the fetus is the size of a large lime and measures 1.75 to 2.5 inches in length. Fingernails and external genitalia are clearly visible, and the fetus can swallow and kick.

By the end of the twelfth week, the fetus is 2½ to 3 inches long and chances of miscarriages drop appreciably (Figure 9-10). By the end of the first trimester, week 13, the fully-formed fetus measures 2.6 to 3.1 inches in length and is the size of a peach. The head is still larger than its body, but physical growth is rapid. The fetal face is looking more like a baby, and its fingers and toes are separate. It has functioning wrists and ankles, and its intestines are moving into place.[1]

Physiological Changes in the Pregnant Woman

When conception occurs, hormonal orchestration begins to prepare the woman for pregnancy. **Human chorionic gonadotrophin** (hCG), detected in home pregnancy tests, is produced by the developing placenta, which stimulates the ovaries to produce estrogen and progesterone until the mature placenta can take over this function.

bone cells replace the cartilage in the skeletal system. Embryologists have suggested that when these first bone cells appear in the upper arm, the embryonic period is over and the growing baby is a fetus (Figure 9-9).[1,4]

Fetal Growth

The fetus at 9 weeks can now move its body and limbs, although the mother cannot feel the movement. Its head is more erect, and its neck is more developed. If the mother is going to have a **chorionic villi sampling** (CVS) genetic test, it will be scheduled during weeks 10 to 12 (Box 9-2).

BOX 9-2   *Chorionic Villi Sampling*

Chorionic villi sampling (CVS) is a prenatal test used to detect genetic defects such as Down syndrome, fragile X syndrome, Tay-Sachs disease, sickle cell anemia, and most types of cystic fibrosis. CVS is performed between 10 and 12 weeks' gestation and is an invasive test. Small amounts of developing placental (chorionic villi) cells are extracted transvaginally and are grown in a culture to produce enough cells for testing. The results of the CVS can be determined in a matter of days.

From Leifer G: *Maternity nursing: an introductory text,* ed 9, St. Louis, 2005, Saunders.

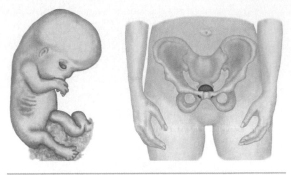

FIGURE 9-10 ■ Fetus at 12 weeks. Crown-rump length is 6 to 7 cm (2.4 to 2.8 inches). Fetal stage begins at 10 weeks after last menstrual period. Extremities are developed, fingers and toes differentiated, external genitalia show signs of male or female sex. Weight is 14 gm (0.5 oz). (From Sears W, Sears M: *The pregnancy book,* Boston, 1997, Little, Brown.)

Nausea and vomiting, often associated with elevated levels of hCG, disappear after the first trimester, when levels of hCG decline between 60 and 90 days after conception.

Estrogen enhances the growth of reproductive tissue by increasing the size of the uterine musculature, encouraging the growth of the endometrium (uterine lining) and blood supply, increasing vaginal mucus production, and stimulating the duct system and blood supply of the breasts. Water retention, subcutaneous adipose tissue build-up, and changes in skin pigmentation are all influenced by estrogen.[1]

Progesterone relaxes smooth muscle contraction, thereby preventing the uterus from excessive contractions. This hormone also relaxes the walls of blood vessels to maintain low blood pressure and slows functioning of the gastrointestinal system to enhance absorption of nutrients. The secretion of relaxin, which softens the connective tissue, is also promoted by progesterone.[1]

Although the newly pregnant woman does not have the pregnant contour, her body starts to make subtle changes that she may identify with being pregnant. Her breasts may feel tender, and she may notice a darkening of her nipples and areolae. She has missed her period, yet some women still feel cramping in the lower abdomen. These cramps are the **Braxton Hicks contractions** that strengthen the uterus and enhance uterine circulation. Her waist starts to feel thicker, and she may experience shortness of breath and feel very tired. Nausea or morning sickness affects about two-thirds of all pregnant women

and usually occurs during the first trimester.[5] No one has definitively explained the cause of morning sickness, but it is thought to result from a combination of hormonal changes, psychological adjustments, and neurological factors.[7] About 0.3% to 2% of pregnant woman develop a serious condition known as **hyperemesis gravidarum**, or excessive vomiting during pregnancy, which may require hospitalization if dehydration is threatened.[7] Practitioners can make the following suggestions for treating morning sickness:

- Eat protein at the last meal of the night because protein takes longest to digest
- Eat dry, unsalted crackers in the morning
- Eat small but frequent meals throughout the day to maintain blood sugar levels
- Drink ginger tea or ginger ale
- Avoid foods or smells that make nausea worse
- Stimulate acupuncture point pericardium 6 (Figure 9-11), a stomach-soothing point, manually or with electrical stimulation
- Drink red raspberry leaf tea
- Eat one umeboshi plum (found in Oriental or health food stores) and suck on the pit for several hours
- Stimulate acupuncture point spleen 3 (Figure 9-12) for hormonal balancing
- Avoid massage if experiencing nausea or vomiting[2,8,9]

The pregnant woman will experience frequent urination and notice increased vaginal secretions.

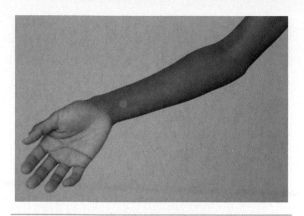

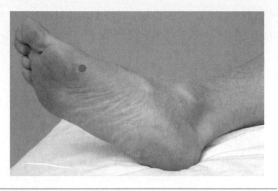

FIGURE 9-11 ■ Each point should be held for a count of 6 to 10 and repeat 6 to 10 times. Pericardium 6 has been found to be effective in minimizing or eliminating nausea.

FIGURE 9-12 ■ Both feet should be treated for a count of 6 to 10 and repeat 6 to 10 times. Spleen 3 can mediate the effects of nausea by helping to balance hormones.

Mood swings and erratic emotions may affect some women during this trying first trimester.

During the first month of pregnancy, the pregnant woman's uterus and cervix become softer and by the end of the first month, tiny finger-like projections called *chorionic villi* surround the ball of cells and help it attach to the lining of the uterus.[10]

By week 6, the client may have gained a bit of weight around her legs and breasts (unless the nausea and vomiting has caused her to lose weight). Her clothes are getting tighter around her waistline. A pelvic examination performed by a medical practitioner will reveal uterine changes. Dry and itchy skin is usually part of later pregnancy, although some women will experience this symptom as early as the second month.[5] Other physical discomforts of the second month might include mouth watering and taste changes, additional thirst, difficulty sleeping, constipation, flatulence, abdominal bloating, and heartburn.[5]

By the eighth week, the mother's uterus is the size of a grapefruit and some cramping may occur. The uterus tightens and contracts throughout the entire pregnancy. Unless the cramping is accompanied by bleeding, the pregnant woman should not be concerned.

At 9 weeks, maternal weight gain is still small, although she may be experiencing certain food aversions or cravings, heartburn, indigestion, nausea, and bloating. Her moods are unstable and she may feel weepy sometimes. At 11 weeks, the mother's uterus just about fills the pelvis and can be palpated in the lower abdomen.

By the end of the first trimester, morning sickness may start to subside, but occasional headaches and **dizziness**, or lightheadedness and vertigo, may bother the mother. Second-time mothers might start to show at this early point. The mother's uterus can be felt into the abdomen.

First Trimester Massage Considerations

During the first trimester, the most common discomforts the pregnant client will experience are the following:

- Nausea and vomiting (massage is contraindicated while she is feeling queasy or vomiting)
- **Fatigue** (or lack of energy)
- Heartburn, flatulence, abdominal bloating, constipation
- Minor uterine cramping
- Tender and sore breasts
- Frequent urination
- Food aversions and cravings
- Increased vaginal secretions
- Shortness of breath
- Hormonal adjustments
- Possible emotional lability and psychological adjustments

Treatments for the common discomforts of pregnancy are described in detail in Chapter 14.

Touch Points

During the first trimester, the practitioner can set the stage for a healthy, comfortable, and exciting pregnancy by addressing an expectant mother's physical needs and emotional concerns in a nonjudgmental, supportive environment. This is a very special time in a woman's life, and the practitioner must assure her that the bodywork is safe and designed to support her changing body.

Many practitioners want to know how to address the issue of miscarriage with their first-trimester clients. This is an understandable concern when so many pregnancies end in early miscarriage. Practitioners can give clients a pamphlet published by the ICEA called *Facts About Miscarriage** that explains the possible causes of miscarriage and demonstrates that miscarriages are rarely caused by something the expectant mother did or did not do. Practitioners must reassure their clients that they are not going to do any type of technique or bodywork that would jeopardize the pregnancy. It is important for the practitioner to talk with their clients and explain that proper prenatal massage training has taught them the kinds of techniques that will support their changing bodies and provide numerous benefits to them and their babies.

*Feldman P, Covington SN: *Facts about miscarriage and the grief it causes*, ICEA, Minneapolis, Minn, 1994.

The first trimester does not affect her structural integrity nor alter her center of gravity to any great degree. The woman's enlarging breasts may cause some medial rotation of her shoulders and tightened muscles of the pectoral girdle. She may also compensate for her enlarged chest by adapting a kyphotic, hunched stance. To address these issues, the practitioner should encourage her to recruit her transverse abdominis muscle for enhanced postural alignment and support. The massage should include stretches and myofascial release to prevent further muscle restrictions.

The bodyworker should also encourage her to strengthen her pelvic floor musculature by providing information about Kegel exercises that maintain structural integrity and function (Box 9-3).

Although fibrinogenic activity and increased interstitial fluid are not characteristic of the first trimester, it is advisable to massage her legs and feet using lymphatic drainage technique, which is light pressure moving toward her heart. Light pressure is also necessary on her abdomen. The rest of her body can be massaged with as much pressure as she prefers.

BOX 9-3   *How To Do Kegel Exercises*

Kegel exercise or pelvic floor muscle exercise is a technique used to strengthen the muscles that make up and support the pelvic floor. The exercise involves voluntarily contracting (tightening) and releasing the muscles that support the bladder and urethra. If a woman cannot identify which muscles are involved, she should be advised to pretend to stop the flow of urine or the passage of intestinal gas. Each contraction should be as strong as possible without recruiting the abdomen, thighs, or buttocks. The woman should feel the muscles pulling up so that the contractions reach the highest level of the pelvis, as she does the following:

- Hold each contraction for 10 seconds, if possible
- Rest for 10 seconds between each contraction
- Spend 15 minutes each day, up to 30 to 80 contractions daily

From Lowdermilk DL, Perry SE: *Maternity & women's health care*, ed 8, St. Louis, 2004, Mosby.

Positioning in the First Trimester

Most women can comfortably lie face down on the treatment table, although cushions with either breast recesses or cutouts are preferred. The practitioner can also alleviate pressure on the breasts by placing a towel across her chest and under both shoulders. Other positions for the first trimester can include supine, side-lying, sitting, and semi-recumbent. Pillows and wedges should be placed under her ankles (and chest) when she is prone and under her neck, knees, and feet when she is supine. For side-lying, a pillow should be placed under her neck and between her knees and legs to make sure her hips, knees, and ankles are on the same horizontal plane.

In My Experience...

L was in her first trimester and experiencing serious morning sickness (hyperemesis gravidarum). She had to be hospitalized in her second month and was intravenously hydrated because she was vomiting so much.

When she called for an appointment, I told her that massage was contraindicated when a person was experiencing nausea but suggested that she purchase "sea bands" and wear them on her forearms at pericardium 6 (P6). I explained the procedure and offered other suggestions to alleviate some of her symptoms.

One week later, she called to say that the morning sickness had mostly disappeared. No doubt her hormone levels were adjusting, but the stimulation of P6 had made a tremendous impact on how she felt.

Years later, I was massaging a nurse who worked on the pediatric floor at Sloan Kettering Memorial Hospital in New York City. Her young patients were receiving bone marrow transplants and were very sick from the chemotherapy. I suggested she offer the sea bands to the children to see whether that would help relieve some of the nausea. The next time I saw her, she was ecstatic. The children were wearing the sea bands on P6 and were now drinking and tolerating food. The doctors could not believe this worked, but the proof was right before their eyes.

Summary

The first trimester of pregnancy lasts for 3 months. Within 5 days of fertilization, the conceptus, or blastocyst, implants into the uterus. The cells of the blastocyst are specialized according to function, and eventually form an embryo. By weeks 5 to 8, the heart, brain, spinal cord, muscles, and digestive and respiratory organs begin to form. Eyes, hands, feet, fingers, toes, genitals, earlobes, and facial features are developing. The skeletal system begins to change from cartilage into permanent bone cells and the embryo becomes a fetus. During weeks 9 to 12, fetal growth is rapid.

During the first trimester, the pregnant woman is adjusting to the physical changes of early pregnancy and trying to accept and adjust to the fact the she is going to be a mother. She has emotional highs and lows, which can be mollified by loving, supportive massage. During the first trimester, most women experience fatigue, morning sickness, shortness of breath, frequent urination, heartburn, flatulence, constipation, tender breasts, and headaches. A pregnant woman also may develop compensatory posture because of the increased size of her breasts, resulting in shoulder medial rotation and tightened pectoral muscles. With appropriate bodywork, the practitioner can minimize these common discomforts and prepare the pregnant woman for a healthier, stronger pregnancy.

Many women feel the need to talk during the massage to address the reasonable fears and concerns most first-time mothers share. The practitioner should actively listen and be supportive by creating a nonjudgmental therapeutic environment where women are free to speak their minds and hearts. Educating them about their bodies and choices and offering appropriate referrals can often resolve many of their concerns. This is a very exciting yet stressful time in her life. Massage practitioners have the ability to make this journey a smooth and enjoyable one through loving, nurturing touch.

References

1. Simkin P, Whalley J, Keppler A: *Pregnancy childbirth and the newborn*, New York, 1991, Meadowbrook Press.
2. Grayson C, ed: Your pregnancy week by week: weeks 1-4, Available at http://www.webmd.com/content/article/64/72360.htm. Accessed on 2003.
3. NOVA: *The miracle of life*, Boston, 1983, WGBH Educational Foundation.
4. Sears W, Sears M: *The pregnancy book*, Boston, 1997, Little, Brown.
5. Snell LH, Haughey BP, Buck G, et al: Metabolic crisis: hyperemesis gravidarum, *J Perinat Neonat Nurs* 12(2):26-37, 1998.
6. Nagendran T, Nagendran S: Mechanism and treatment of nausea and vomiting, *Ala Med* 60:12-16, 1990.
7. Eliakim R, Abulafia O, Sherer DM: Hyperemesis gravidarum: a current view, *Am J Perinatol* 17(4):207-218, 2000.
8. Evans AT, Samuels SN, Marshall C, et al: Suppression of pregnancy-induced nausea and vomiting with sensory afferent stimulation, *J Reprod Med* 38:603-606, 1993.
9. Stillerman E: *MotherMassage: massage during pregnancy professional manual*, New York, 1997.
10. Bolane JE: *With child*, Waco, TX, 1999, Childbirth Graphics.

REVIEW QUESTIONS

1   How many weeks does the first trimester last?

_____

_____

_____

_____

2   How soon after fertilization does the conceptus undergo changes?

_____

_____

_____

_____

3   What is an "ectopic" pregnancy?

_____

_____

_____

_____

_____

4   When does the placenta start to develop?

_____

_____

_____

_____

_____

5   How big is the fetus at by the end of the first trimester?

_____

_____

_____

_____

6   Which hormone is detected in pregnancy tests and is often associated with first trimester nausea and vomiting?

_____

_____

_____

_____

_____

_____

7   How does estrogen support the reproductive system during pregnancy?

_____

_____

_____

_____

_____

_____

8   What effect does progesterone have on smooth muscle? How does this action prevent excessive uterine contractions?

_____

_____

_____

_____

_____

9   What are some of the changes a pregnant woman may experience in her first trimester?

_____

_____

_____

_____

_____

10 How common is morning sickness and what suggestions can practitioners offer their clients to help treat nausea?

_____

_____

_____

_____

_____

11 By the end of the first trimester, how large has the mother's uterus grown and where can it be felt?

_____

_____

_____

_____

_____

12 Describe the common discomforts some women experience during their first trimester.

_____

_____

_____

_____

13 How are first-trimester clients positioned on the massage table?

_____

_____

_____

_____

14 Is light leg pressure advisable during the first trimester even though fibrinogenic activity and increased interstitial fluid retention are not characteristic of the first trimester?

_____

_____

_____

_____

15 What is the purpose of Kegel exercises? How are they done?

_____

_____

_____

_____

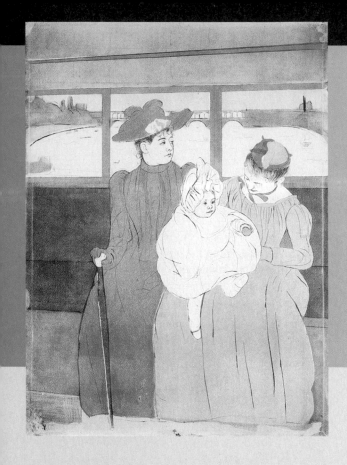

CHAPTER **10**

*The Second
Trimester*

Objectives

*On completion of this chapter, the student will be able to do
the following:*

1 Understand the physical and emotional changes during the
   second trimester of pregnancy

2 Recognize the common discomforts associated with the
   second trimester

3 Learn how the fetus develops during the second trimester
   of pregnancy

4 Learn massage consideration for the second trimester

Key Terms

Alpha fetoprotein
Amniocentesis
Blood volume
Broad uterine ligament
Chloasma
Constructive rest position
Down syndrome
Femoral vein

Glucose tolerance screening
Iliac vein
Iliopsoas (iliacus and psoas) muscles
Lanugo
Linea nigra
Plasma fibrinogen
Quickening
Round uterine ligaments

Saphenous vein
Second trimester
Stretch marks
Striae gravidarum
Triple screen
Ultrasound
Vernix caseosa

"For psychic and emotional states that have no small part in determining marital fertility. The thorough exploration of this theme and formulation of any guiding principles would need along and special monograph. But its most important constituent is Love—Love which indescribably alters and influences the natures of men and women, making them desire complete self-abandonment, union and communion, through the fibres of their bodies and all the faculties of their minds and souls."[1]

Physiological Changes in the Woman

Many of the first trimester's discomforts are relieved in the **second trimester,** or weeks 14 to 26 of pregnancy. Levels of human chorionic gonadotrophin (hCG) start to decline between 60 to 90 days, and the pregnant woman's morning sickness and fatigue usually abate or disappear. She is now starting to feel energetic and is emotionally more secure, having resolved many of her earlier conflicts about the pregnancy.[2] She is also relieved that the sensitive first trimester is behind her and the chance of miscarriage is small (Figure 10-1). The pregnancy is now a confirmed reality as she starts to look pregnant and feels the fetus moving for the first time between weeks 18 to 22 (for a first-time mother) and earlier for a second-time mother. For many women, this is the most exciting and comfortable time of their pregnancy.

As her uterus grows into her abdomen, the pregnant woman's need to urinate as frequently diminishes, but she begins to experience postural shifting. It is essential that she is offered information about appropriate abdominal exercises, such as those that employ the transverse abdominis muscle, to maintain relative postural alignment and minimize musculoskeletal discomforts (see Chapter 5).

Elevated levels of relaxin are making the woman's connective tissue relax and soften to accommodate the growing uterus, but these effects of relaxin also makes the weight-bearing joints unstable. The effects of relaxin can be felt as early as 10 weeks. As her abdomen swells and heightens, the anterior musculature and myofascia stretch and weaken, while her posterior musculature compensates by shortening.

Blood volume, the amount of blood within the circulatory system, is starting to increase during the second trimester and peaks between weeks 16 and 28.[3] This increase causes many pregnant women to feel warm. The client should be encouraged to drink extra water and fluids and wear comfortable loose clothing made of natural fibers. The increase in blood volume might contribute to sensitive, swollen, and bleeding gums or pregnancy gingivitis, as well as varicose veins (Box 10-1).

During the second trimester, the woman's white blood cell count increases and peaks during the final trimester.[3] Between weeks 14 and 20, her resting pulse increases about 10 to 15 beats per minute and maintains that level until the end of the pregnancy. She might notice palpitations and arrhythmias as a result, most of which are not dangerous.[4] Her blood pressure starts to decrease by week 20 but then increases and should stay the same as early pregnancy.[5,6]

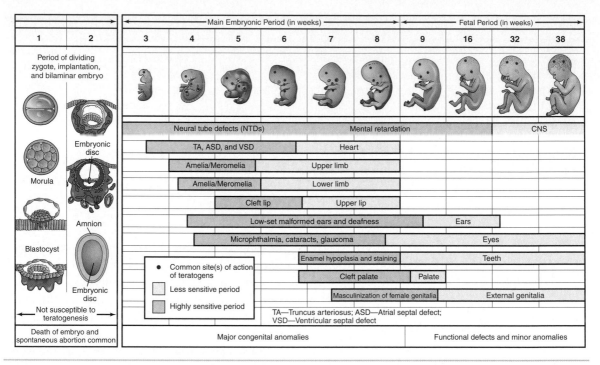

FIGURE 10-1 ■ Critical periods in fetal development. Purple bars denote highly sensitive periods, and green bars indicate stages that are less sensitive to teratogens. (From Lowdermilk DL, Perry SE: *Maternity & women's health care,* ed 8, St. Louis, 2004, Mosby.)

BOX 10-1   *How to Treat Bleeding Gums*

- Eat more fruits and vegetables that are rich in vitamin C.
- Rinse with a mild antiseptic mouthwash after each meal and throughout the day.
- Brush gently after each meal and snack using a soft bristle toothbrush or an ultrasonic toothbrush to effectively remove more plaque.
- Floss gently after each meal and snack.
- Avoid sticky foods and candies that could collect under the gums.*
- If gum disease develops, contact a dentist and obstetrician or midwife. Preterm labor may occur in cases of severe gum disease.

*Data from Sears W, Sears M: *The pregnancy book,* Boston, 1997, Little, Brown.

During the second trimester, there is an increase in the synthesis of **plasma fibrinogen** (clot-making enzyme) to protect the mother from hemorrhaging during labor that continues throughout the first few months of postpartum recovery. When massaging a pregnant woman during the second trimester, it is necessary to massage her legs with lymphatic drainage massage, using only 10-30 gm of pressure to prevent dislodging any clots that may be harboring within the deeper **femoral, saphenous,** and **iliac veins** of the legs.[4,7-9]

In preparation for a smooth passage of the fetus, a woman's vaginal discharge increases.[10] However, there are times when a vaginal discharge may be symptomatic of a yeast infection. Signs and symptoms of yeast infections are included in Box 10-2, as well as tips to help reduce the frequency and intensity of the infections.

The increase in progesterone may cause a pregnant woman's mucous membranes to swell, creating an annoying postnasal drip. The client can flush her sinuses with a facial steam bath or Neti pot, which is an Indian ceramic designed to cleanse the sinuses. Women with asthma, allergies, and hay fever often complain of exaggerated symptoms during the second trimester.

Changes to her skin and complexion may develop during the second trimester. The **linea nigra** appears from her navel to pubis. This shows the embryonic folding and fusion line of the abdomen.[11] Some practitioners theorize that this darkened pigmentation is a road map for the newborn to locate the breast. A neonate who is placed

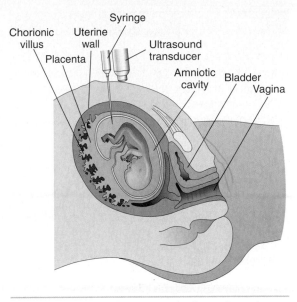

FIGURE 10-2 ■ Amniocentesis. The ultrasound scans the woman's abdomen to locate the fetus and placenta. A needle is inserted into the uterine wall and amniotic fluid is withdrawn. (From Leifer G: *Maternity nursing: an introductory text,* ed 9, St. Louis, 2005, Saunders.)

on the mother's abdomen follows the line up to the darkened nipple and areola where it latches on to the breast to nurse.

The pregnant woman also develop a mottled pigmentation around her eyes and forehead, called the *mask of pregnancy,* or **chloasma.** Freckles and recent scars may darken, and she may grow neck tags, notice changes in moles, and develop rashes. Acne may clear up in some pregnant women. As her abdomen grows, **stretch marks,** or **striae gravidarum,** may appear. Her abdomen can be massaged with Shea butter, cocoa butter, olive oil, or vitamin E oil to ease the itching and speed up healing. A massage oil for stretch marks is 20 drops of lavender plus 5 drops neroli (orange) oil in 2 fluid oz of wheat germ oil.

Fetal Growth and Physical Changes in the Mother

By week 14, the fetus measures about 3.2 to 4.1 inches and its ears are moving from the neck to the sides of the head. The fetus can bring its hands together and suck its thumb.[12,13] At this time, the pregnant woman might be experiencing constipation because progesterone relaxes the bowel.

At week 15 of the pregnancy, the fetus is 13 weeks old (pregnancy is determined from the day of the last menstruation and not the day of conception, so there is a discrepancy of about 2 weeks) and is 4.1 to 4.5 inches long. Its sensory organs are almost completely developed. Its body is covered by a protective layer of ultrafine hair, or **lanugo,** that falls off by birth or within days after birth. Eyebrows and the hair on its head start to grow, and bones mineralize and harden.

At this time, the woman can palpate her uterus about 3 to 4 inches below the navel. Within the next 5 weeks, she may have a **triple screen** maternal serum screening test. This genetic evaluation tests a fetal antigen, **alpha-fetoprotein** (AFP), hCG, and placental estrogen levels to determine the presence of any fetal genetic defects. Another genetic test, **amniocentesis,** extracts a sample amniotic fluid transabdominally to test for **Down syndrome** (mental impairment caused by an abnormal chromosome) and other genetic defects (Figure 10-2). This test is suggested for those women 35 years and older because the risk of fetal genetic disorders increases in older women[12] (Box 10-3).

AFP, Alpha fetoprotein.

At this time, the expectant mother also may find side-lying a more comfortable position in which to sleep because it keeps pressure off her abdomen and breasts. The practitioner should make appropriate adjustments in positioning her on the massage table.

Week 16 brings a growth spurt to the fetus that now measures 4.3 to 4.6 inches. The fetal nervous system is functioning and muscles are reacting to stimulation from its brain. The heartbeat is audible with ultrasound equipment. At 16 weeks, the uterus weighs almost 9 oz.

The structure of the placenta was complete by the end of the first trimester or at 12 weeks. It continues to grow wider until 20 weeks, when it covers almost half of the uterine surface. Throughout the pregnancy, the placenta grows thicker, and the villi still develop within the placenta, increasing the functional surface area.[4] If there is a multiple pregnancy, there may be more than one placenta. Most identical twins share one placenta, whereas fraternal twins have separate placentas.

At week 17, the fetus is almost 4.8 inches long and fat is beginning to form. The lungs are exhaling amniotic fluid and its circulatory and urinary systems are functioning. Hair on its eyebrows, head and eyelashes is getting thicker. The expectant mother looks pregnant now, and she may have gained 5 to 10 lbs as her appetite increases.

At week 18, the fetus measures 5 to 5.6 inches and weighs about 5.25 oz. Growth is slowing a bit, but its reflexes are quickly developing. It can yawn, stretch, and grimace. Taste buds are developed enough to differentiate between sweet and bitter flavors. If its lips are stroked, the fetus will suck and it can swallow. The retinas of its eyes are light sensitive, and a fetus will move away from a light shined on the abdomen.

The expectant mother's uterus is the size of a cantaloupe and is felt just inferior to the navel. The first-time mother may feel the first signs of movement, which is called **quickening**. Initially, it feels like a bubble of gas or gentle "butterfly wing" fluttering. It eventually gets stronger and is readily identified as fetal movement.[12]

Some doctors perform a midpregnancy **ultrasound**, which is a prenatal examination that uses high-frequency waves directed through a transducer on a woman's abdomen, between weeks 18 and 22 to assess the growth and development of the fetus. An ultrasound may also help the doctor estimate the due date and gender of the fetus. The maternal heart is now working 40% to 50% harder to support the pregnancy.[12]

At the nineteenth week after conception, the fetus is 5.2 to 6 inches and weighs almost 7 oz. Skin is transparent, and blood vessels can be seen through it. A protective coating called the **vernix caseosa** starts to cover the skin.

The pregnant woman's center of gravity has shifted to the anterior, and good alignment with proper posture can ease many of the muscle stiffness and soreness (Figure 10-3). She needs to pay attention to her abdominal muscles and remember to bring them in toward her spine (recruiting the transverse abdominis muscle). These muscles will encourage a posterior pelvic tilt to elongate her lumbar spine. In this more appropriate posture, her back and **iliopsoas** muscles (iliacus and psoas) should stretch passively and her rectus femoris muscle should remain relaxed. The latter will permit the distal ends of the femurs to move anteriorly, causing the hyperextended knees to relax. With proper alignment, the curvature of her spine is minimized.[2] By using her muscles correctly earlier in the pregnancy, they will strengthen and help support her in better postural alignment as the uterus continues to grow.

At 20 weeks, the fetus is 5.6 to 6.4 inches long and weighs about 9 oz. It can hear sounds and will cover its ears if a loud sound is made near the

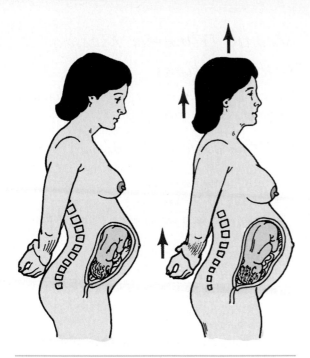

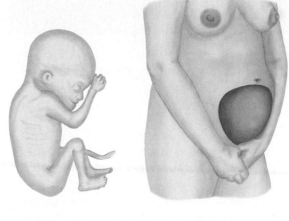

FIGURE 10-4 ■ Fetus at 5 to 6 months. (From McKinney ES, James SR, Murray SS, et al: *Maternal-child nursing,* ed 2, St. Louis, 2005, Mosby.)

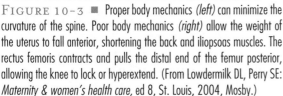

FIGURE 10-3 ■ Proper body mechanics *(left)* can minimize the curvature of the spine. Poor body mechanics *(right)* allow the weight of the uterus to fall anterior, shortening the back and iliopsoas muscles. The rectus femoris contracts and pulls the distal end of the femur posterior, allowing the knee to lock or hyperextend. (From Lowdermilk DL, Perry SE: *Maternity & women's health care,* ed 8, St. Louis, 2004, Mosby.)

mother. The fetus is very active now. The expectant mother's uterus is now at navel level, and her waistline has spread out. Bladder infections may increase because of progesterone's relaxing effects on the smooth muscles of the urinary tract. Her breathing might deepen, and she may perspire more from a more active thyroid gland[12] (Figure 10-4).

By week 21, the fetus is 7.2 inches long and weighs 10.5 oz. It is developing fat to keep warm, and buds for permanent teeth start to form. The expectant mother's uterus is now extending above the navel, and she has gained approximately 10 to 14 pounds for a single pregnancy.

By week 22, the fetus measures 7.6 inches and weighs 12.3 oz. Its movements and stretches strengthen its muscles, and eyelids and eyebrows are developed. As the uterus expands, postural shifting may occur, along with increased swelling of her legs and feet. Lymphatic drainage massage is essential to relieve the lymphatic congestion, and when the woman can, she should elevate her legs. Leg and foot cramps may start to plague her as the fetus

absorbs calcium, magnesium, and potassium for its muscle and bone growth. She should consume a wide variety of calcium and potassium-rich foods and stretch her legs to prevent painful cramping.

During week 23, the fetus is almost 8 inches long and finally reaches 1 lb. Its physical proportions look more like a baby, but its skin will remain wrinkled until it adds on more fat. The expectant mother's skin may begin to itch from the growing uterus. Any emollient lotion can ease the itching, although there is no cream, lotion, or unction that can prevent stretch marks, or striae gravidarum, from occurring.

At week 24, the fetus is 8.4 inches long and weighs just over 1 lb. Hiccups are not uncommon, and its circulatory system is starting to produce white blood cells to help it fight infections and disease.[12] The expectant mother's uterus is 1.5 to 2 inches above her navel, and she should expect to gain a pound a week until the end of the pregnancy. At any time between weeks 24 and 28 weeks, a medical doctor might suggest a **glucose tolerance screening** to test for gestational glucose intolerance (gestational diabetes) (Box 10-4).

By the end of the second trimester, the fetus measures about 8.8 inches and weighs 1½ lbs. Its skin takes on an opaque quality replacing transparency, and its heartbeat is strong enough to be heard through a traditional stethoscope or by placing an ear against the woman's abdomen.

BOX 10-4   *Glucose Tolerance Screening*

It is normal for pregnant women to excrete additional sugar into their urine on occasion because the hormones of pregnancy suppress insulin release. This gives the developing fetus more glucose from which to grow. Small but frequent meals throughout the day provide this much-needed supply of glucose to the fetus. In about 2% to 10% of pregnant women, the blood sugar is higher than average. This condition, which is temporary, is called **gestational glucose intolerance** (formerly referred to as gestational diabetes mellitus).

This condition is based on the belief that protracted exposure to high blood sugar can cause exaggerated fetal growth, fetal macrosomia, and lead to birth complications. The extended exposure to high blood sugar may cause the fetus to manufacture too much of its own insulin, causing the baby's blood sugar to drop precipitously immediately after birth.

These theories have their detractors. In 1973, an attempt was made to link prediabetic women to perinatal outcome. This association is believed to be weak, but it gave rise to the idea of gestational glucose intolerance as a disease and glucose tolerance tests were devised to screen for the condition.*

Careful attention to diet can control blood sugar levels. Gestational glucose intolerance is more prevalent in women who are overweight or older, those with a family history of diabetes, or women who have previously given birth to a baby weighing in excess of 9 lbs.

At the doctor's office, the pregnant woman drinks a glass of very sweet liquid called Glucola on an empty stomach. Her blood sugar levels are tested an hour later. If this screening is positive for excessive blood sugar, she will take another test, which is the more reliable 3-hour test. Only 15% of those who test positive for the 1-hour test also test positive for the 3-hour test.

The test itself is under debate because the 50 gm of sugar reacts differently on women of various sizes.†

*Data from Enkin M, Keirse M, Nellson J, et al: *A guide to effective care in pregnancy and childbirth,* Oxford, 2000, Oxford University Press.
†Data from Sears W, Sears M: *The pregnancy book,* Boston, 1997, Little, Brown.

During the last weeks of the second trimester, the pressure of the growing uterus may cause lower gastrointestinal complaints, such as hemorrhoids, constipation, and indigestion, in the woman. The expectant mother may also notice a change in vision. Increased fluid retention can alter the shape of her eyeballs and consequently her vision. These changes are temporary and will reverse during postpartum recovery.

Second Trimester Massage Considerations

During the second trimester, the most common discomforts the pregnant client experiences are as follows:

- Postural shifting with compressed lumbar spine and anterior pelvic tilting
- Round ligament pain
- Breast tenderness
- Sore and tired legs and feet from swelling
- Leg cramps
- Varicose veins or spider veins
- Constipation, flatulence, indigestion, hemorrhoids
- Postnasal drip and sinus stuffiness
- Skin dryness and itchiness
- Feeling hot as blood volume increases, bleeding gums, nosebleeds
- Body image issues as her shape takes on the distinctive pregnancy silhouette

Treatments for the common discomforts of pregnancy are detailed in Chapter 14.

Postural Shifting

During the second trimester, the bodyworker should introduce massage techniques that address postural alignment to support her shifting center of gravity and prevent further postural discomforts as the pregnancy continues. It is also necessary to make positioning changes to accommodate the growing uterus.

The importance of an integrated abdominal core to maintain postural alignment and lumbar stability as pregnancy progresses is understood, but it is important to recognize and work with other muscles that also function to support her changing contour. Special attention should be paid to releasing tension in the core iliopsoas muscles to make room for the growing fetus. Because the psoas is the only muscle that attaches the spine to the leg, releasing tightness in this muscle transfers the support from the muscle to the skeletal system. This relieves some of the hip and pelvic pain she maybe experiencing and increases blood circulation through her legs and feet.[14] Palpation or deep massage of this intrinsic muscle is contraindicated during pregnancy and in general because it may be implicated in bruising, intestinal hernias, rupture of major arteries, and retraumatization of this sensitive muscle.[14] Thus it is necessary to employ nonmanipulative techniques to release this muscle.

The iliacus and the psoas muscle are often referred to as one muscle, the iliopsoas, because they share a common action: thigh flexion and minimal lateral rotation and abduction (psoas) of the thigh.[15] The psoas originates at the anterior surface of the transverse processes, lateral border of the vertebral bodies, and intervertebral discs T12 through L5. It inserts at the lesser trochanter of the femur with the iliacus[15] (Figure 10-5).

The iliacus originates at the upper two-thirds of the iliac fossa, internal border of the iliac crest, anterior sacroiliac, and the lumbosacral and iliolumbar ligaments. It inserts at the lesser trochanter of the femur with the psoas major.[16] The origin of the iliopsoas is in the lower lumbar spinal segment and moves the lower back anterior, or in the supine position, raises the back up as it raises the legs, creating more of an anterior pelvic tilt. If the abdominal muscles are also weakened, as in the case of pregnancy and the presence of the diastasis, the client may experience lower back problems when walking or lifting her legs because this function is primarily a hip flexion not an abdominal action. Intact abdominal muscles, or strong abdominal muscles, prevent lower back pain by pulling up on the front of the pelvis (where they attach at the pubic bone) and flatten, or elongate, the lower back.[16,17]

Although iliacus massage is inappropriate during pregnancy, posterior pelvic tilting can be effective in elongating the lumbar spine, relaxing the iliopsoas, and shortening the abdominal muscles. The client can perform this exercise while standing, leaning over a support, or on her hands and knees (the client should be advised to keep her wrists and ankles in neutral positions when she is leaning on them). With her abdominals pulled in, she slowly brings rounds her lower back and brings her sacrum forward. Breathing normally, she relaxes to a neutral spine and repeats the same movement 10 more times. The practitioner can affect the same release by doing a pelvic tilt on the client (Box 10-5).

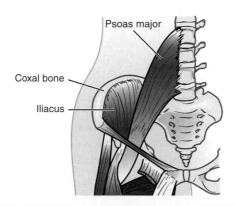

FIGURE 10-5 ■ **The psoas muscle:** Origin: anterior surface of transverse processes, lateral border of vertebral bodies, and corresponding intervertebral discs from T12 to L5. Insertion: lesser trochanter of the femur with the iliacus. The psoas muscle is the only muscle to connect the spine to the leg. **The iliacus muscle:** Origin: upper two-thirds of the iliac fossa, internal bodies of the iliac crest, anterior sacroiliac, and the lumbosacral and iliolumbar ligaments. Insertion: lesser trochanter of the femur with the psoas.

BOX 10-5	*Pelvic Tilt*

DVD Pelvic tilt is one of the most powerful and muscle tension—relieving techniques a practitioner can offer a pregnant or laboring woman. This gentle stretch elongates the lumbar spine and releases compressed muscles.

With the client in a side-lying position, the practitioner stands behind her and places his or her right hand on the woman's sacrum, with the heel of the practitioner's hand at S1. (If the heel of the hand is on the lumbar spine, it is too high). The practitioner's hand should be relaxed and fingers should be lifted slightly off the woman's body. (Practitioners with long fingers need to pay attention to finger placement and avoid her gluteal cleft.) The opposite hand or fleshy portion of the forearm is placed on the top ASIS. The practitioner should avoid grabbing the lymph area by pointing his or her fingers toward the woman's feet.

Practitioner posture and body mechanics are important. The practitioner's knees are bent and he or she is in a lunge position facing the woman's feet. For additional support and lower back relief, the practitoner can lean against the massage table. The arm on the woman's sacrum is bent into the practitioner's body for additional strength. The practitioner leans horizontally on his or her forward leg toward the client's feet and pushes the woman's sacrum anterior (elongating the lumbar spine) and pull up on her ASIS. The movement is gentle. The practitioner holds (and breathes) for a count of 10. The practitioner releases slowly and repeats 5 more times.

ASIS, Anterior superior iliac spines.

BOX 10-6   *Positional Release of the Iliopsoas*

Positional release, also known as *origin-insertion technique,* is a neuromuscular and educational technique that places a muscle in a shortened position to trick the proprioceptors into releasing.*

The client should be placed in a semisitting or recumbent position, propped with pillows, on the table or the floor. Her knees are bent and her feet are parallel to each other and a hip-width apart. The heels of her feet should be placed about 12 to 16 inches away from her buttocks. Her spine should be neutral by maintaining its natural curves. Her arms can rest comfortably at her sides or over her abdomen.

This **constructive rest position** (a recumbent position with legs bent, feet wider than the shoulders and placed 12 to 15 inches away from the hips to relax and shorten the overstretched psoas muscles) should be maintained for 10 to 20 minutes. She should get off the table or the floor by rolling to her side and recruiting her transverse abdominis.†

Rocking in a rocking chair can also provide release of the iliopsoas muscle and other core abdominal muscles.†

*Data from Stillerman E: *The encyclopedia of bodywork,* New York, 1996, Facts On File.
†Data from Koch L: *Midwifery Today Int Midwife* 74:26-29, 2005.

BOX 10-7   *Myofascial Release*

Myofascial release is a mild and gentle form of stretching that evaluates and treats the fascial system. This work addresses the fascia, a tough connective tissue, that spreads throughout the body in a three-dimensional network. Fascia is made up of two types of fibers: collagenous fibers, whose main component is collagen, that provide support with little elasticity; and elastic fibers, whose main component is elastin, that are stretchable. Fascia is divided into three layers: the superficial layer that lies directly below the skin and contains fat, nerve endings, and blood vessels; the second layer, known as *potential space,* may increase in size with extra tissue fluid or edema; and the third, or deep, layer.* During pregnancy, practitioners work predominantly with the superficial layer of fascia.

Any malfunctions, restrictions, or tightness in this pervasive network can create abnormal pressure in all structures it covers, causing pain or dysfunction. During the release, elastic fibers release, followed by collagenous fibers. The practitioner should follow the motion of the tissue, barrier after barrier, until release is felt. Tissue release can have many forms: a change in client's breathing pattern, muscle twitching, digestive noises, or the sensation of heat emanating from the tissue.

Hand placement should be comfortable for the practitioner and client. The hands, fingers, thumbs, or pisiform bones (see Box 10-10) should be placed proximal to the attachments of the muscle being stretched. The pressure is strong enough to stretch the superficial skin, fascia, and underlying muscle in the direction of the fibers. The traction is held until tissue release is felt. The stretch is repeated, taking up additional slack produced by the release. This process is repeated until the muscle and related soft tissue are fully elongated and relaxed.†

*Data from Koch L: *Midwifery Today Int Midwife* 74:26-29, 2005.
†Data from Stillerman E: *The encyclopedia of bodywork,* New York, 1996, Facts On File.

Positional release is a powerful yet gentle noninvasive technique to relax the iliopsoas and other core abdominal muscles (Box 10-6).

As her growing uterus shifts her center of gravity anterior, trigger points may develop in her hips, gluteals, along her erector spinae, vertebral borders of the scapulae, and abdominal attachments. Myofascial release (Box 10-7) and trigger point therapy (Box 10-8) are effective techniques to release tension areas. Medial compression along the hips and down toward her greater trochanters addresses the widening of her hips, can help reduce sciatic pain, and realigns the sacroiliac and lumbosacral joints softened by relaxin.

She might notice abdominal weakness as the separation of the linea alba, the diastasis, begins to develop. This separation will affect lower back stability and create lower back pain. It is important to remind her to avoid conventional sit-ups and crunches and replace them with the pregnancy-friendly transverse abdominal exercises that can help minimize the diastasis and maintain lumbar spine integrity.

Ligament Pain

Pain in the **round uterine ligaments,** which are the ligaments that attach to the sides of the uterus, usually starts in the second trimester as the uterus grows and these ligaments must stretch. Relaxin allows the collagenous connective tissue to relax, but sudden movements or stretching with normal activity can cause sharp pains on one or both the sides of the uterus. These pains are not harmful to the fetus, but they can be painful for the expectant mother. The pain is usually the sharpest between 14 to 20 weeks when the uterus is large and heavy enough to pull the ligaments but not big enough to place some of its weight on the pelvic bones.[10]

To minimize the pain, a standing leg lift can help The woman should stand barefoot, supporting herself with one hand against a table, countertop, or chair. Recruiting her transverse abdominis muscle, she should lift the foot on the side of the pain just 2 inches off the floor. Hold the lift for 10 seconds and repeat 10 times. Then she should reverse legs.[10] The expectant woman should use her abdominals correctly with all movements and activities to avoid or minimize round ligament pain. She should also avoid sudden movements and changes of position, particularly standing from a sitting position. Side-lying may also relax the round ligaments. As pregnancy progresses into the third trimester, this pain usually abates as the ligaments adapt to uterine growth.

Pain in the round or **broad uterine ligaments** (the broad uterine ligaments attach to the uterine wall and sacrum) may cause referred pain in other areas of her body. Round ligament pain can be felt in her abdomen, groin, and anterior thigh, whereas lumbar and gluteal discomforts are a result of the stretching broad ligament. A strong abdominal core will help support these ligaments, and avoiding sudden movements is also helpful. A hands and knees position (wrists and feet in neutral positions) or side-lying positioning can help relieve the pain caused by these ligaments stretching.

As the uterus grows, it may cause sudden shooting pains down the client's lower back, buttocks, or legs that can be alarming. Weight displacement during this trimester has shifted her pelvis anterior, compressing the lumbar spine and the sciatic region and she is feeling sciatic pain. Her femoral nerve, which runs along the outer thighs, stretches and this causes pain along its pathway. In addition, relaxin has made the lumbar spine and pelvic girdle unstable and prone to subluxations, creating more referred pain. Sudden movements can also make the uterine ligaments stretch, creating a referred pain pattern.

The client should be taught proper body mechanics (i.e., how to lift using her transverse abdominis and legs instead of her back, how to bend over by bending her knees and not her waist), and proper alignment can reduce the pains she may be feeling.

Gentle myofascial abdominal stretching during the second trimester helps avoid future restrictions caused by the growing uterus (Box 10-9).

DVD *Leg and Foot Soreness*

The client's legs and feet are now assuming much of the pressure of the heavier uterus and increased blood volume and interstitial fluid. Each massage must begin with the pretreatment evaluations (test for pitting edema, full leg palpation, and Homan check for blood clots; see Chapter 3) before commencing with any bodywork. Appropriate leg and foot massage is lymphatic drainage: light, slow pressure pushing in the direction of the heart. Lymphatic drainage strokes consist of light strokes that stretch the skin (using 10-30 gm of pressure and affecting the precollector lymph vessels just under the skin) repeated several times starting from the knee to the thigh. These strokes are followed with circular pétrissage around the knee. Lymphatic compression on the thigh is the last stroke. There are 6 compressions on the thigh, and each is held for 10 seconds. The pressure and steady rhythm never changes, although the stroke does.

The practitioner should follow this with an effleurage from the ankle to the hip, repeating several times. If hyperemia is visible, it means the massage is being done too deeply. If practitioners are not comfortable such light work, they must concentrate to make sure that their pressure does not get deep. (Practitioners will also be amazed at how powerful this light work can be. A client can feel tremendous relief from her sore and tired legs, and

BOX 10-8   *Trigger Point Therapy*

A trigger point is a hypersensitive nodule or area in the muscle, its tendon, or in fascia that can be palpated as a fibrous point. Digital pressure over the trigger point will elicit pain in a specific, referred area.* Finger pressure can also be effective in relieving trigger points. From 5 to 7 seconds of direct pressure usually sedates the point and reduces the pain in the referred area. Once the point is calmed, a general massage can be applied to remove the waste products and restore circulation to the area.† Practitioners can use an open hand, fingertips, thumbs, or pisiform bones to treat trigger points (see Box 10-9).

Trigger points in the second half of the pregnancy often manifest in the client's hips, gluteals, erector spinae, scapulae, and abdomen. To treat the clients hips and gluteals, the practitioner should gently press along the sacrum to the gluteus maximus attachments at the posterior gluteal line of the ilium where she feels these sensitive points. The pressure should be firm enough to elicit a pleasure/pain response. The practitioner holds each point 5 to 7 seconds, works into deeper layers of the gluteal muscles, and then continues pressing laterally to the posterior superior iliac spine and down to the greater trochanters. The practitioner presses into the ischial tuberosities and works laterally to the greater trochanters. Care should be taken to avoid direct pressure on the sciatic nerve. The practitioner presses along the piriformis to its insertion at the superior border of the greater trochanter and continues to press all around the greater trochanters.

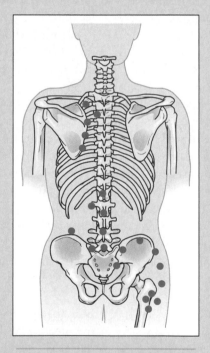

Trigger points of the back, shoulders, and hips.

The paravertebral erector spinae muscles can hold trigger points at any area. The practitioner presses bilaterally along the spine (if the woman is in a prone position, unilaterally if in a side-lying position) to locate tender areas and treats all trigger points bilaterally. The sacroiliac joints, lumbar segments of the spine, and quadratus lumborum attachments are vulnerable to trigger points, particularly as the pregnancy progresses. The practitioner palpates along the longissimus thoracis (extends the thoracic spine), iliocostalis thoracis (maintains erect posture of the spine), and the iliocostalis lumborum (extends the lumbar spine).

The trigger points of the scapulae are usually found along the vertebral border. The practitioner cups the head of the humerus with one hand and brings the scapula posterior to expose the trigger points for more effective treatment. The practitioner presses into the rhomboids, levator scapulae, iliocostalis cervicis (extends neck), and longissimus cervicis (extends neck) feeling for tender nodules.‡

*Data from Walther DS: *Applied kinesiology,* vol 1, Pueblo, CO, 1981, Systems DC.
†Data from Stillerman E: *The encyclopedia of bodywork,* New York, 1996, Facts On File.
‡Data from Tortora GJ, Anagnostakos NP: *Principles of anatomy and physiology,* ed 3, New York, 1981, Harper & Row.

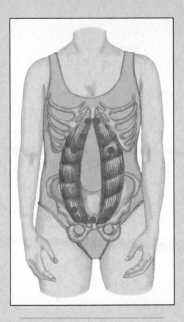

Trigger point release on the abdomen.

The abdominal trigger points become active as the pregnancy progresses and are particularly sensitive if the woman has a large diastasis that results in a weakened abdominal core. The practitioner can press along the muscles' origins at the xiphoid process and lower ribs and the insertions at the pubic bone and anterior iliac crests.

this work is.) This should be followed with circular pétrissage a few times around her ankle and effleurage once again up to her hip. Six lymphatic compressions from her ankle to her knee are done, each held for 10 seconds, then followed by another 6 compressions from her knee to her hip. (This routine is 1½ minutes of just compressions.) The practitioner should use gentle effleurage on the client's foot, making sure that the direction of the stroke is toward her heart. The bodyworker can twist her foot, massage the sole, rotate and circumduct each toe, and end the leg massage with a final few effleurages from her foot to her hip. This gentle, slow, and very specific technique will treat her sore, tired, and swollen legs; ease leg cramps; and reduce the pressure from varicose and spider veins.

At this time of pregnancy, fibrinogenic activity begins to prevent hemorrhaging at birth. It is essential that all leg and feet massages follow lymphatic drainage sequence, pressure, and direction of strokes. All deep pressure to the limb must be avoided to prevent dislodging a blood clot.

Common discomforts of the second trimester also include leg cramps brought on by the fetal need for calcium, a potential maternal electrolyte imbalance, decreased leg circulation and pressure of the growing uterus impeding blood flow, and hand tingling or carpal tunnel weakness. Carpal tunnel weakness affects almost 25% of the pregnant population and is brought on by swelling, neck protraction, and relaxin softening the extensor and flexor retinaculum at the wrist.[10]

Breast Tenderness

Breast soreness is often accompanied by engorgement, breast growth, and a compensatory thoracic stiffness. Larger breasts may create pectoral shortening, medial shoulder rotation, and a kyphotic

BOX 10-9 *Abdominal Myofascial Release*

To prevent myofascial restrictions in the abdominal region, gentle myofascial stretching may be provided with the client's permission. Starting this work in the second trimester helps maintain pelvic and fascial fluidity and suppleness for the months that follow. This work can be offered in a semisitting or recumbent position, as well as in a side-lying position. Care must be taken to keep the direction of the stretch horizontal—head to toe—and not vertical or down into her body. Practitioners also have to make sure that their hands are placed on either side of the woman's uterus but never directly on it.

DVD In a side-lying position, the practitioner places the heel of one hand (the "mother hand") on the woman's top iliac crest and the opposite open hand (the "wanderer") on her lower ribs. The practitioner gently stretches the fascia in opposite directions and returns slowly to the neutral position. The practitioner should repeat 3 more times. The practitioner should keep the "mother" hand on the client's iliac crest and move the "wanderer" higher on her rib cage. Practitioners should stretch gently and allow the woman to breathe normally and perhaps deeply. The "mother" hand should remain stationary, pushing toward her feet, as the practitioner brings the client's arm over her head to maximize the stretch. Then she is returned to a neutral position.

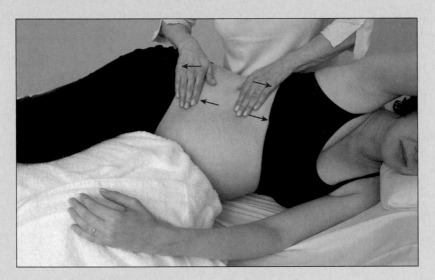

DVD To stretch the underlying side, the client should be in a side-lying position tilted forward slightly to enable the practitioner to place his or her hands under the client's side. After the client shifts back, the practitioner places the "mother" hand at the client's iliac crest and the "wanderer" at her lower ribs. The practitioner should lift slightly while stretching the fascia. The practitioner's "mother" hand stays at the same spot as the "wanderer" hand moves further up the client's rib cage. The practitioner stretches and takes the "wanderer" hand as far as possible, stretching in opposite directions with each new position. The client leans forward as the practitioner removes his or her hands. If the client can turn over, the practitioner can effectively stretch the opposite side once she turns.

DVD The next myofascial stretch is more anterior on the client's abdomen but lateral to the uterus. The practitioner places one hand on the lateral side of her uterus just under the rib cage and the other hand lateral to the bottom of her uterus. The practitioner gently stretches and releases slowly and repeats a few more times. The practitioner can lean over the massage table and lift the client's abdomen to reach under her belly. Lateral to the uterus, the practitioner's hands are placed in the same positions and gently stretches, releases slowly, and repeats a few more times.

spine when she sits or lies down. Sleeping in a side-lying position also shortens the pectorals. Breast massage is addressed in Chapter 14, but myofascial stretching of the pectorals is very helpful in elongating this restricted musculature. Practitioners with large fingers should pay careful attention to hand placement and should follow the same directions as the rib cage myofascial release.

Miscellaneous Discomforts

The second trimester brings major changes to the pregnant woman's silhouette and contour. During this trimester, she not only starts to look pregnant but also feels the fetus move and kick for the first time. Her partner can also become more accepting of the pregnancy as the pregnancy becomes more visible.

BOX 10-9 *Abdominal Myofascial Release—cont'd*

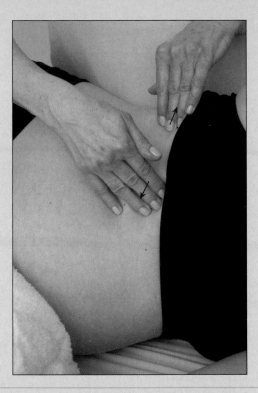

Abdominal fascial stretch on the ribs. Pressure should be light, and stretch should be horizontal.

DVD Myofascial stretching of the rib cage can relieve some of the congestion caused by the displacement of the ribs by the growing uterus and ease the restrictions created by shortness of breath. The practitioner should remember that the stretch is horizontal. The fingertips of the "mother" hand are placed on the costal edge of the ribs, with the "wanderer" touching just behind the "mother" hand. "Mother" pulls toward the midline of the body as the "wanderer" pulls three "steps" in the opposite direction. The traction should be held. "Mother" catches up to the "wanderer," and once again, the "wanderer" pulls away three "steps." Each time, the "mother" catches up. The practitioner should stretch as far as possible on one side, then lean over the table and stretch the underlying ribs.

DVD The abdominal myofascial stretching should be followed by gentle abdominal and rib massage. The rib massage pulls laterally from the midline, following the anterolateral expansion of the ribs. If the client is recumbent or sitting, the same stretches can be provided equally to both sides.

Some women find they have the need to slow down a bit by the end of the second trimester. They will feel particularly tired, often exhausted, if their day was stressful and overly busy. It is important to remind them to respect what their bodies are telling them: slow down. There is a delicate balance between work and rest to get through the day and grow a child.

Women should be advised to drink 8 to 12 glasses of water daily to combat dehydration, which is a major cause of preterm labor, and to cool down. Drinking water will also facilitate elimination, minimize skin dryness and itchiness, ease nasal congestion, and help fight swelling.

Hemorrhoids and incontinence may plague and embarrass her during the second trimester as a heavy uterus compresses the pelvic structures and can cause veins in the rectal wall to enlarge and swell. They may or may not bleed, which is not harmful but can be very irritating and uncomfortable (see Chapter 14). All rectal bleeding, however, should be brought to the attention of the care provider.

BOX 10-10   *The Pisiform Bones*

The pisiform bones are the most medial bones in the proximal row of carpals (see Box 10-7). They are shaped like hooks and can be used in lieu of the thumbs or fingertips as a hand-saving technique. Practitioners with any wrist problems are cautioned against using this technique.

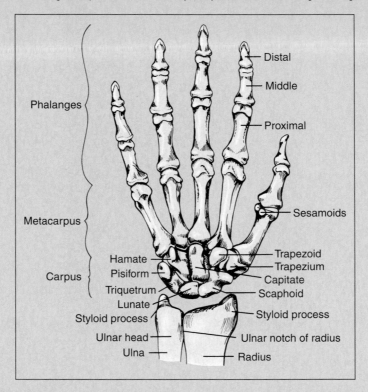

With wrists relaxed, the practitioner flexes them slightly to expose the pisiform "hook" and leans into the trigger point. Pisiform myofascial stretching is also extremely effective and hand saving. The practitioner bring his or her hands together with all five fingertips and the heels of both palms touching, presses into the fascia, and pronates the hands slightly, keeping the fingertips together while maintaining pressure on the pisiform bones. The movement is very small but can be used instead of the thumbs.

Positioning in the Second Trimester

Breasts and abdominal swelling make it uncomfortable for most women to lie prone on the massage table during the second trimester without the use of contoured cushions such as the bodyCushion system. When used correctly, these cushions safely support the growing uterus without raising intrauterine pressure or straining the lumbar spine. Prone positioning on conventional tables without these cushions, however, is neither comfortable nor recommended. Other positioning options are side-lying, sitting, or semisitting (recumbent). Flat supine positioning is not recommended and can cause a decrease in maternal blood pressure (supine hypotension), nausea, hyperventilation, and fetal hypoxia. When the client is on her back, her upper torso should be raised with a bolster or several pillows (from her hips to her head) to an angle between 45 to 70 degrees, her legs should be elevated above her heart, and she should be tilted slightly to the left to get the growing uterus off the vena cava. The client will provide the best feedback about what feels most comfortable.

In My Experience...

S was 6 months pregnant and complaining about hip and pelvic pain and instability. She also walked with an awkward gait. I addressed two things with her. First, I showed her how to use her transversus abdominis muscles to ensure greater lumbar stability. Then I placed her on the massage table in a semisitting position with the heels of her feet 12 to 16 inches away from her buttocks. She stayed in this **constructive rest position** for about 15 minutes after the massage was over.

When she got up (using her transversus abdominis), she walked more upright and with more stability. She also said that her entire pelvis felt stronger and the pain was gone.

Summary

The second trimester is a time of exciting growth and change. The fetus grows from 3 to 4 inches and weighing a few ounces to more than doubling its length and weighing over a pound. During this trimester, the expectant woman feels the fetus move for the first time and her body starts to look pregnant.

Many changes and adaptations are occurring in her body. Postural shifting begins with associated muscle and ligament aches and pains. There are noticeable differences in her skin, slowing down of bodily functions, and increased heat output as her blood volume increases. Massage techniques that address and strengthen her structural variances make the second trimester more comfortable and help her avoid more extreme discomforts during the last trimester.

A woman learns more about her pregnancy during this trimester. Prenatal genetic tests can provide her with information about the gender and genetic health. Many women become more accepting of the pregnancy now because the fetus moves and there is physical proof in the new shape of her body. This exciting process can be thrilling for the expectant mother, as well as the bodyworker.

References

1. Van De Velde TH: *Fertility and sterility in marriage: their voluntary promotion and limitation*, New York, 1929, Random House.
2. Hassid P: *Textbook for childbirth educators*, Philadelphia, 1978, Harper and Row.
3. DeCherney P, Nathan L: *Current obstetric & gynecologic diagnosis & treatment*, ed 10, New York, 2003, McGraw Hill.
4. Lowdermilk DL, Perry SE: *Maternity & women's health care*, ed 8, St. Louis, 2004, Mosby.
5. Cunningham FG, Gant NF, Leveno KJ, et al: *Williams obstetrics*, ed 21, New York, 2001, McGraw Hill.
6. Hermida R, Ayala D, Iglesias M: Predictable blood pressure variability in healthy and complicated pregnancies, *Hypertension* 38(3 Pt 2):736-744, 2001.
7. Girling JC: *Physiology of pregnancy, Obstetrics, anaesthesia and intensive care medicine*, Abingdon, England, 2001, Medicine Publishing Company.
8. Symonds E, Symonds I: *Essential obstetrics and gynaecology*, ed 3, Edinburgh, 1998, Churchill Livingstone.
9. Coustan D: Maternal physiology. In Coustan D, Haning R, Singer D, eds: *Human reproduction—growth and development*, London, 1995, Little Brown.
10. Sears W, Sears M: *The pregnancy book*, Boston, 1997, Little, Brown.
11. Coad J: *Anatomy and physiology for midwives*, St. Louis, 2001, Mosby.
12. Grayson C, ed: Your pregnancy week by week: weeks 1-4, Available at http://www.webmd.com/content/article/64/72360.htm. Accessed 2003.
13. NOVA: *The miracle of life*, Boston, 1983, WGBH Educational Foundation.
14. Koch L: Birthing fear: the iliopsoas muscle, *Midwifery Today Int Midwife* 74:26-29, 2005.
15. Walther DS: *Applied kinesiology*, vol 1, Pueblo, Colo, 1981, Systems DC.
16. Fritz S, Grosenbach J: *Essential sciences for therapeutic massage*, ed 2, St. Louis, 2004, Mosby.
17. Stillerman E: *MotherMassage: massage during pregnancy training manual*, New York, 2004.

REVIEW QUESTIONS

1   Explain how the second trimester brings relief from many of the first trimester's discomforts and concerns.

_____
_____
_____
_____
_____

2   When does a first-time mother usually feel the fetus move?

_____
_____
_____
_____

3   How are elevated levels of relaxin affecting her connective tissue? When does she start feeling the effects of relaxin?

_____
_____
_____
_____

4   When does blood volume peak? What can she do about the increased warmth she feels?

_____
_____
_____
_____

5   Within which deeper veins do potential blood clots lodge? Where are they located?

_____
_____
_____
_____
_____

6   What is an amniocentesis? When and why is it performed?

_____
_____
_____
_____

7   At what point in the pregnancy does her center of gravity start to shift anterior? How does her body compensate for this postural shift?

_____
_____
_____
_____
_____

8   What is glucose tolerance screening and what does it test for?

_____
_____
_____
_____

9   Describe the uterine ligaments and how they are changing during the second trimester.

_____

_____

_____

_____

_____

10   List at least six massage considerations for the second trimester.

_____

_____

_____

_____

_____

11   How is the iliopsoas muscle affected by the shift in center of gravity? What can be done to treat it during the second trimester of pregnancy?

_____

_____

_____

_____

_____

12   What are some of the advantages of the pelvic tilt?

_____

_____

_____

_____

_____

13   Where do trigger points develop during pregnancy? Describe the technique to help ease trigger point discomfort.

_____

_____

_____

_____

_____

14   What are some of the benefits of abdominal myofascial release?

_____

_____

_____

_____

_____

15   Describe safe and comfortable positioning for the second trimester.

_____

_____

_____

_____

_____

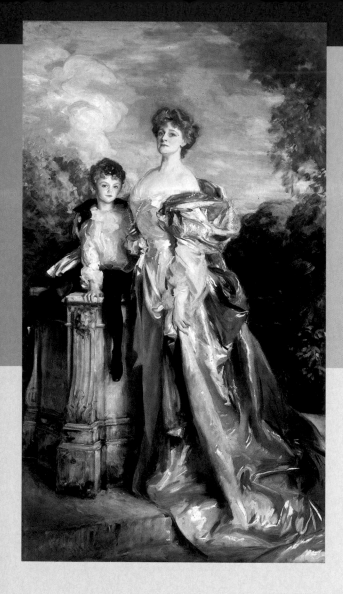

CHAPTER 11

The Third Trimester

Objectives

On completion of this chapter, the student will be able to do the following:

1 Understand the physical and emotional changes that take place during the third trimester of pregnancy

2 Recognize the common discomforts associated with the third trimester of pregnancy

3 Learn how the fetus develops during the third trimester of pregnancy

4 Learn massage considerations for the third trimester of pregnancy

Arrhythmias
Breech
Colostrum
Due date
Interstitial fluid

Labor
Manual version
Moxibustion
Occiput anterior
Occiput posterior

Pelvic station
Position
Presentation
Third trimester

"...All our mothers and grand-mothers used in due course of time to become with-child, or, as Shakespeare has it, round-wombed...but it is very well known, that no female, above the degree of a chamber-maid or laundress, has been with-child these ten years past: every decent married woman now becomes pregnant; nor is she ever brought-to-bed, or delivered, but merely, at the end of nine months, has an accouchement; antecedent to which, she always informs her friends that at a certain time she shall be confined."[1]

Physiological Changes in the Woman

The **third trimester** is defined as weeks 27 through 40 of a woman's pregnancy. The adaptations her body made during the first two trimesters are now exaggerated as the uterus continues to grow and her body prepares for **labor** (the process by which the fetus, membranes, and placenta are expelled) and childbirth.

Some women are cognizant of uterine tightness during the second trimester, but many more become aware of Braxton Hicks contractions during the third trimester (Box 11-1). By the beginning of the seventh month, an expectant mother may find that simple activities and movements, such as bending over to tie her shoes, are becoming awkward. She may gain a pound per week during this trimester, and her uterus will expand to just below her rib cage, compressing her respiratory diaphragm and resulting in shortness of breath. Also compressed are the organs of her upper gastrointestinal tract, resulting in indigestion and heartburn.

Recognizing that the pregnancy is almost over can prove emotionally exhilarating, as well as challenging. The pride and stature of pregnancy can make a woman feel special yet fragile, and

---

BOX 11-1 *Braxton Hicks Contractions*

In 1872, an English doctor, Dr. John Braxton Hicks, explained the prelabor, "practice" uterine contractions that many women confused with true labor. These are often referred to as "false labor" contractions. These contractions can start during the second trimester but are most common with the third trimester. Uterine muscles tighten anywhere from 30 seconds to 2 minutes, and the contractions serve to strengthen the uterine muscle in preparation for labor and increase placental blood profusion. These contractions are described as follows:

- Irregular and not increasing in intensity
- Infrequent and not increasing in frequency
- Unpredictable
- Without rhythm or pattern
- Feeling more like uncomfortable menstrual cramps rather than painful
- Tapering on and off
- Not involved with cervical dilation

Braxton Hicks contractions are stimulated by the following:

- Maternal or fetal activity
- Touching the pregnant abdomen
- A full bladder
- Sexual activity
- Dehydration

Clients can ease these contractions by doing the following:

- Changing positions or walking around
- Taking a warm bath for less than half an hour
- Drinking water to combat dehydration
- Eating a snack or drinking tea or milk

From Braxton Hicks Contractions, American Pregnancy Association. Available at http://www.americanpregnancy.org/labornbirth/braxtonhicks.html.

---

preoccupation with the birth may make her forgetful and anxious.[2] As the pregnancy nears an end, most women are looking forward to relief from pregnancy's physical discomforts but are deeply concerned, and even frightened, about the prospects of labor, birth, and motherhood.[3]

Touch Points

Massage during the third trimester offers relief from somatic discomforts and prepares a woman for labor physically and emotionally. It is not at all uncommon for a woman, especially the first-time mom, to articulate her concerns and fears about labor. The third trimester is the time for the practitioner to be patient, compassionate, and nurturing.

One of the biggest reasons women fear labor is because they do not understand what it is or how their bodies function. So much of the concern could be eliminated and so many more women could be empowered, if they understood more about the process and the numerous techniques available to them to control pain. A supportive practitioner can really help. Clients can be empowered when they are provided information, resources, and options. They (and their babies) will thank the practitioner for the support.

By the third trimester, her blood volume has increased by 30% to 50%. To circulate the additional blood, her heart rate increases by an additional 10 beats per minute and her heart pumps about 30% more blood with each beat.[2] Occasional pounding, irregular heartbeats, and **arrhythmias** (irregular heart actions) are noticeable during this last trimester.

During pregnancy, a woman's hands, legs, **DVD** and feet may swell because increased **interstitial fluid** (fluid within the tissues) is needed to nourish the pregnancy, continuously supply amniotic fluid, and provide for the fetus' fluid needs. By the end of the pregnancy, the pregnant woman is carrying an extra 10 quarts or 20 lbs of fluid.[2] The swelling she experiences will contribute to muscle and joint soreness and stiffness but is considered normal. The practitioner must remember to test for pitting edema before each treatment to ensure that the swelling is not associated with preeclampsia or eclampsia (Box 11-2). If a client tests positive for pitting edema or if the practitioner is unsure, refrain from massage and have the client see her health care provider.

Backaches, particularly in the lower back, are common during the last trimester (Box 11-3). During pregnancy, a woman's abdomen displaces her weight anteriorly, creating an anterior pelvic tilt that compresses her lumbar spine. Her diastasis, the separation of the rectus abdominis along the linea alba, and overstretched abdominal

BOX 11-2   *Edema in the Third Trimester*

To test for pitting edema, the practitioner presses his or her **DVD** finger into the client's leg, above her ankle for a count of 5. If the indentation in her leg fills in and the color returns to normal, pitting edema is not present and the treatment can proceed. If the indentation still remains or if the impression is still blanched (ischemic), the massage should not be performed and she should advise her health care provider.

The quantity of swelling is not as important as the quality of the swelling. Swelling is normal with the following:

- Swelling shifts with gravity, which is known as *gravity swelling,* and at different times of the day. The swelling should reduce after an hour of elevating the affected limbs.
- Weight gain is slow and steady, rather than sudden.
- Blood pressure remains normal.
- Diet is balanced and nutritious.
- No protein shows in the urine during a routine medical check-up.

Swelling is not normal with the following:

- Swelling is excessive, and light finger pressure leaves an indentation on the limb.
- Elevation for an hour does not relieve the swelling.
- There is a sudden weight gain.
- Blood pressure becomes high or suddenly spikes.
- Diet is not balanced or adequate.
- Urine checks reveal excessive protein in the urine.
- The fetus is not growing normally.
- Client does not feel well in general (her skin may feel clammy and damp to the touch).

Normal swelling should be treated with the following:

- Follow the lymphatic drainage sequence and **DVD** protocol. Light touch (about 10-30 gm of pressure) on the skin and superficial fascia, in the direction of the heart, will help rid the body of excess fluid (see Chapter 14).
- Avoid standing or sitting for extended periods of time
- Elevate swollen feet or hands for at least one hour
- Engage in a cardiovascular activity such as swimming, walking, or riding a stationary bicycle.
- Lie on the left side for 15 minutes at least 3 to 4 times per day
- Sleep on the left side
- Drink plenty of water and fluids
- Perform isometric contractions on the legs and feet to encourage muscle contractions which stimulate lymph circulation
- Avoid tight waistbands or socks that may restrict circulation

BOX 11-3 *Preventing and Treating Backaches*

Backache is one of the most common reasons a pregnant client seeks a massage. Practitioners can teach their clients prevention techniques that will make pregnancy more comfortable as the uterus continues to grow.

Pregnant clients can be taught the following to prevent backaches:

- Use the transverse abdominis muscle while exercising and throughout the day to encourage lumbar stability and core muscle integrity. (This will have a tremendous impact on aligning her posture and minimizing back weakness.)
- Do a pelvic tilt to elongate the lumbar spine and shorten her overstretched abdominal muscles
- Use proper body mechanics when standing from a sitting position, sitting from a lying position, turning on the bed or treatment table, bending and lifting.
- Wear shoes with a medium heel (no higher than 2 inches) for work or dress, and wear comfortable walking shoes for everyday wear.
- Go swimming, which is the preferred cardiovascular activity. Also, walking on natural surfaces such as grass, earth, or sand is kinder and less jarring to the spine.
- Avoid twisting the spine or awkward reaching motions.
- Elevate the legs when sitting and sleep in a side-lying position, changing sides as necessary.

To treat backaches, the practitioner can elongate compressed areas and shorten overstretched muscle groups by performing the following:

- With the client in a side-lying position, the bodyworker begins with a gentle myofascial pelvic tilt. In a prone position (on supportive cushions), the client's lumbar spine can be stretched by placing the heel of the practitioner's hand on the client's sacrum and the other hand at L3 or L4 and then releasing. Then the practitioner keeps one hand on the sacrum and move the other hand higher on her lumbar spine to L1 and gently stretches. Practitioners use their fingers, thumbs, or pisiform bones to stretch paravertebrally next to **[DVD]** each transverse process from C7 to the woman's sacrum. Each traction is held for a slow count of 5. The pressure is outward (horizontal) rather than downward (vertical).
- Gently stretch the cervical spine. Massage along the occipital ridge to release the neck and upper back muscles.
- Massage her back, pelvis, and hips using effleurage strokes. The pressure should start lightly and gradually become deeper **[DVD]** to client's comfort level.
- Palpate and treat any trigger points along her spine, hips, and scapulae.
- Finish with several more effleurage strokes from her sacrum over her shoulders.

muscles coupled with the hormone relaxin contribute to ligament, hip, pelvic, and lumbar instability. The "waddle" of late pregnancy is attributed to hip and pelvic instability. Thoracic spine pain may be brought on by the weight of her enlarged breasts.

Other common discomforts associated with the third trimester are clumsiness, forgetfulness, sore hips, frequent urination, increased breast growth and changes, additional thirst, lightheadedness, increased vaginal discharge, heartburn, constipation, and vaginal, pelvic, and groin pain.[2]

Fetal Growth and Corresponding Changes to the Mother

At the start of the third trimester, the fetus measures 9.2 inches and weighs almost 2 lbs. It can hear and react to all noises and has a definite sleep-wake cycle. Fetal movement, especially kicking in the rib cage, is rather constant. The fetal lungs still need more time to mature.

At week 27, the fetus now measures 9.6 inches from crown to rump and weighs over 2 lbs. The fetus can suck its thumb and cry. Maternal weight gain for a single baby is 16 to 22 lbs by the beginning of the third trimester. Stretch marks, striae distensae or striae gravidarum, may start to appear.[4] The development of stretch marks during pregnancy has been ascribed to the rise in adrenal cortical hyperfunction and not to the size of the abdomen.[5] In a study conducted in 1959, it was concluded that there may be a biochemical "stretch factor" that influences the skin to stretch. In addition, women with a 25% weight gain were more likely to develop stretch marks and light-skinned women develop more stretch marks than dark-skinned women.[5] Marks found on the breasts, which do not stretch as the abdomen does in later pregnancy, also demonstrate a relation to increased adrenal cortical activity.

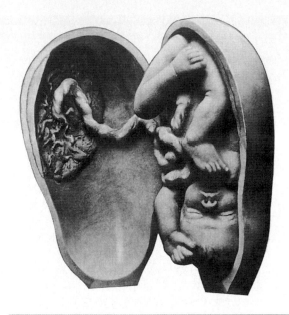

FIGURE 11-2 ■ Fetus at 30 weeks. (From Offen JA: *Adventure to motherhood,* New York, 1964, Simon and Schuster.)

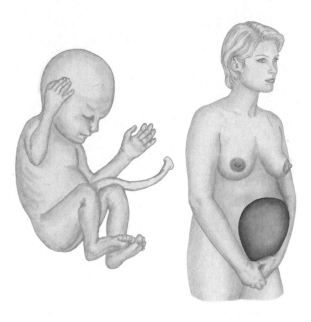

FIGURE 11-1 ■ Fetus at 25 to 28 weeks. Crown rump length 25cm (9.8 in). Weight 1000 g (2 lb, 3 oz). Eyes partially open; eyelashes present. Skin covered with vernix. Respiratory system immature, but fetus may survive if born. (From McKinney ES, James SR, Murray SS, et al: Maternal-child nursing, ed 2, St. Louis, 2005, Mosby.)

Acne or skin eruptions during pregnancy can be caused by an increased production of ketosteroids, a possible striae factor. Research demonstrates that when facial acne occurs, breast stretch marks also appear. Women who do not breakout during pregnancy are less likely to develop striae.[6] Box 11-4 contains a recipe for a stretch mark massage oil.

By week 28, the fetus is 10 inches long from crown to rump or 15.75 inches from head to toe and weighs 2.4 lbs (Figure 11-1).[4] The uterus is above the navel, just under the ribs, and pushes all of the organs up, creating pressure in the lungs and stomach.[7] The pregnant woman may experience pain in the rib cage from this pressure. Urination is becoming very frequent.

By week 29, the fetus measures 16.7 inches from head to toe and weighs over 2½ lbs. Braxton Hicks contractions are becoming very apparent, although not painful.

The fetus can start controlling its own temperature by week 30 (Figure 11-2). Eyebrows and eyelashes are completely formed, and the hair on its head is getting thicker. Its body is now in the proportion of a newborn, and its hands are completely developed, with growing fingernails. The maternal uterus is about 4 inches above the navel, and the rib cage continues to expand and cause discomfort.

At week 31, the fetus weighs 3½ lbs and measures 18 inches long from head to toe. In 1 week, the fetus grows another 0.9 inches and weighs close to 4 lbs. It can still do somersaults within the uterus and is developing a layer of fat under its thin skin. Eyes are opening and closing, and it is practicing its breathing. Backaches and leg cramps continue to bother the mother. She also might notice a yellowish discharge coming from

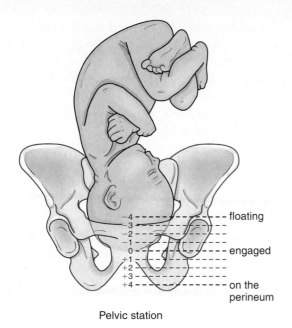

FIGURE 11-3 ■ Pelvic station. When the fetal head is in the false pelvis, it considered to be "floating" at -4 through 1l. At 0, the fetus is engaged within the true pelvis and the numbers ascend to +4 when the fetus is at the perineum.

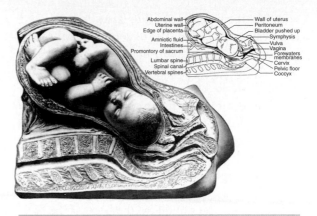

FIGURE 11-4 ■ Fetus at 40 weeks ready to be born. (From Offen JA: *Adventure to motherhood,* New York, 1964, Simon and Schuster.)

her breasts. This discharge is **colostrum**, which is the baby's first sustenance, preceding milk production.

By week 33, there is a noticeable lessening of fetal movement because there is little room for it to move in the uterus. The fetus measures 19.4 inches and weighs 4.4 lbs. Over the next 7 weeks, it will gain more than half its birth weight.[4] The maternal uterus is 5.2 inches above the navel and half of the weight the mother is gaining is going to the fetus.

At week 34, the fetus measures 19.8 inches and weighs 5 lbs. It is settling in to its head-down, or vertex, position in preparation for birth, although it may still change position several more times.

By week 35, the fetus is 20.25 inches long and weighs 5½ pounds. Its lungs are almost completely developed, but it still does not have enough subcutaneous fat to keep warm outside of the womb and would need to be incubated if it was born now. The maternal uterus is about 6 inches above the woman's navel.

The final month of pregnancy features increased fetal growth. At 36 weeks, the fetus is about 20.7 inches long and weighs about 6 lbs. The fetus may now settle into a vertex **presentation** (the part of the fetus that first enters the pelvis). The maternal uterus is under the ribs, and the pregnant woman may be experiencing increased backaches, abdominal pressure, constipation, heartburn, and pain in her groin, buttocks, and pelvis. Anxiety about labor and birth may cause insomnia, anxiety, and increased moodiness.

At week 37, the fetus is about 21 inches long and weighs almost 6½ pounds. Fat continues to fill out its skin. During this week, the uterus stays the same size and the woman's weight gain should peak. At week 38, the fetus is 21 inches long and weighs 6.8 lbs. The lanugo and vernix caseosa is disappearing. Antibodies are passing through the placenta to the fetus to protect the newborn from infections and illnesses. Maternal discomforts are high at this point and many women feel a combination of restlessness, anxiety, fatigue, and excitement.

At week 39, the fetus is 21.5 inches long and weighs 7 lbs. The fetal muscles are strong and its lungs are practicing breathing movements. At this point, the first-time mother may notice that the baby has dropped or engaged into the **pelvic station,** or the pelvic brim (Figure 11-3). This brings the woman relief from upper respiratory and digestive complaints; however, she exchanges this relief for increased lower back instability and pain, sciatica, increased leg and feet swelling, abdominal pressure, and hemorrhoids or vaginal varicosities. Her gait is rather wobbly, and she is clumsier than usual.

Week 40 marks the end of gestation for most women (Figure 11-4). Only 5% of babies are born on their estimated **due dates** (which used to be called estimated date of confinement) so the expectant mother should not worry about being late. Approximately 95% of babies are born within 2 weeks of their due dates.[4] The practitioner should mention this to the client in order to avert any additional fears and concerns about a late delivery.

By week 40, the fetus is about 21.5 inches long and weighs about 7.5 lbs. Most of the lanugo has fallen out, although some may still remain after birth on the shoulders, the back of the ears, and in the folds of skin. This will wear away after a few days postpartum. The baby's reflexes are coordinated so he or she can respond to stimuli such as light, sounds, and touch.

The mother's uterus repositions from a posterior to anterior placement as the fetal head aligns itself with the birth canal. She is certainly eager to end the pregnancy but still may be harboring concerns about labor, birth, and parenthood. The more supportive, responsive, and sensitive the practitioner is to her needs, the better prepared and more in control she will feel.

Group B Streptococcus

Group B streptococcus (GBS) is a gram-positive bacterium that colonizes primarily in the gastrointestinal tract, although it can be present in the vagina in up to 25% of women.[8] The risks associated with GBS in the vagina during pregnancy are preterm labor, prolonged rupture of the membranes, maternal pyrexia (fever) during labor, and infiltration of GBS into the amniotic cavity, leading to infection of the fetal lungs.[9]

The expectant mother will be tested for GBS bacteria between weeks 36 and 37. GBS is the most common cause of sepsis in newborns. The respiratory infection progresses rapidly to sepsis, shock and finally death.[10]

Presentation

Breech Presentation

Breech presentation is considered to be any fetal position that is buttocks first and not vertex, or head-down (Figure 11-5). Before week 27, almost 40% of all pregnancies are not vertex. That number drops to 17% between weeks 28 and 38. By weeks 38 and 40 that number drops further to only 3% to 5% of pregnancies.[11] It is important to explain these statistics to clients who worry after being told that the fetus is "breech." Most fetuses spontaneously convert to a head-down presentation before birth.[12]

In this country, 95% of breech presentations are delivered by cesarean section so turning the fetus into vertex noninvasively is desirable.[13]

Week 37 and before the fetus drops deeper into the pelvis is the recommended time to try the following procedures for conversion to head-down presentation. As the client performs these maneuvers, she should use active visualization, imagining that the fetus is turning.

- Crawl on all hands and knees. This allows gravity to bring the head of the fetus down. It also provides more room for a fetus in an occiput posterior position to turn.
- Climb stairs. This can also help turn a fetus in an occiput posterior position by widening the pelvic outlet.
- Rock the pelvis. This movement is even more effective when used in conjunction with crawling. The client should be on her hands and knees, with wrists and feet in neutral positions, and should pull the belly toward the spine and arch the back. She then returns to a neutral spine position and repeats 9 more times. This should be done 3 times a day.
- Gentle lateral lunges. Lunges widen the pelvic outlet and help a fetus in an occiput posterior presentation to turn.
- Breech tilt. With the client positioned supine on a firm surface, she should raise her hips about a foot so pillows can be tucked under her hips. She should concentrate on relaxing the abdominal muscles. Do this 3 times a day for 15 minutes on an empty stomach.
- Ironing board tilt. An ironing board or wide slanted plank should be placed on a secure surface at a 45-degree angle. The client should lie on the board, head down, with her knees bent. The breech tilt and ironing board tilt are based on the same principle: when the mother's head is lower

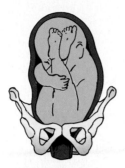

A

Frank breech

Lie: Longitudinal or vertical
Presentation: Breech (incomplete)
Presenting part: Sacrum
Attitude: Flexion, except for legs at knees

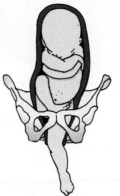

B

Single footling breech

Lie: Longitudinal or vertical
Presentation: Breech (incomplete)
Presenting part: Sacrum
Attitude: Flexion, except for one leg extended
at hip and knee

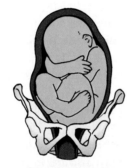

C

Complete breech

Lie: Longitudinal or vertical
Presentation: Breech (sacrum and feet presenting)
Presenting part: Sacrum (with feet)
Attitude: General flexion

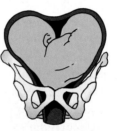

D

Shoulder presentation

Lie: Transverse or horizontal
Presentation: Shoulder
Presenting part: Scapula
Attitude: Flexion

FIGURE 11-5 ■ Breech presentation. **A-C,** Breech (sacral) presentation. **D,** Shoulder or transverse presentation. (From Lowdermilk DL, Perry SE: *Maternity & women's health care,* ed 8, St. Louis, 2004, Mosby.)

than her hips, gravity encourages the fetus to move toward the fundus, flex its chin, and turn under. The fetus slowly rotates, first into the transverse presentation, and then into vertex (Figure 11-6).

■ Heat and cold compresses. A cold or ice pack can be placed on the fundus and a warm pack at the bottom of the uterus. The fetus will seek out the warmth.

■ Singing and talking. A tape of the mother's voice talking, reciting nursery rhymes, or singing can be played through earphones placed near the pubic bone. Because the fetus can hear, it will move toward its mother's voice.

■ **Moxibustion.** A heated herb (mugwort) is used to treat acupuncture point Bladder 67 (B67). B67 is found on the outside edge of each little toenail. (Do **not** stimulate this point before 37 weeks and only stimulate it if the fetus is still in a breech presentation.) Moxa, from the Japanese word *mogusa,* is a common weed known as Artemisia or mugwort. Moxibustion is the traditional Chinese medicine method of employing heat from burning herbs to

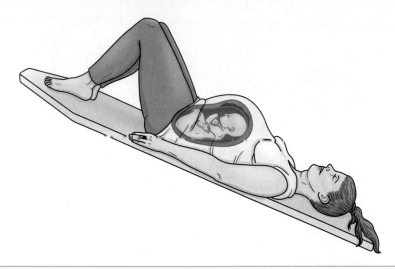

FIGURE 11-6 ■ Ironing board tilt to turn breech presentation to vertex should be done for 15 minutes, 3 times a day.

stimulate a specific acupuncture point such as B67. The theory is that radiating heat on this point stimulates the Yang energy of the body and increases fetal movement. The treatment is suggested twice a day for 5 days, although most fetuses will turn before 5 days. The British Medical Acupuncture Society reports a success rate of 84.6% after 34 weeks.[14] Reports out of China, where moxibustion is routinely used, cite a success rate of 90%. Moxibustion should only be used by a licensed acupuncturist and is not suitable for women with high blood pressure, multiple births, and other medical conditions.[14,15]

■ Bodywork, such as myofascial release, craniosacral therapy, sacral-occipital blocking, and other modalities, can help remove the myofascial restrictions in the pelvis that prevent the fetus from turning.

If all of these techniques fail to turn the fetus into a cephalic presentation, the client can have the doctor or midwife try **manual version,** also called external cephalic version. Before manual version, an ultrasound is performed to confirm the breech presentation and to locate the site of placental attachment. A nonstress test may also be performed to make sure the fetus is in good heath. A tocolytic drug is then administered to slow or prevent the onset of labor, and the doctor or midwife presses and pushes the fetus in an attempt to turn it into the vertex position. This can be very uncomfortable, even painful, for some women. Success rates are about 70%.[16-20] In some instances, the fetus will turn to an anterior position during labor.

Vertex Presentation

The fetus may also be in a vertex presentation, but with its **occiput posterior** rather than the preferred **occiput anterior**, or face down. Approximately 1 of 4 vertex presentations are in the occiput posterior position. **Position** refers to the direction the fetus lies within the uterus (i.e., front, back, or transverse). In this position, the back of the fetus' head presses against the mother's sacrum, stretching the sacroiliac ligaments (Figure 11-7) and causing back labor. Attempts should be made to turn the fetus to occiput anterior to prevent this painful labor. Back labor often slows the progress of labor. The preferred position for labor is the fetus in a vertex presentation and an occiput anterior position.

Third Trimester Massage Considerations

The pregnant woman's exaggerated posture places enormous stress on her weight-bearing joints and musculature. Extra interstitial fluid, increased

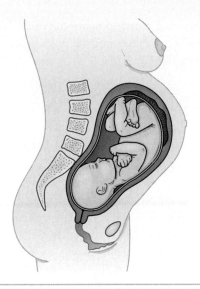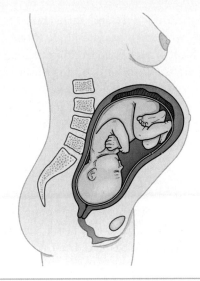

FIGURE 11-7 ■ Occiput anterior *(left)* is the preferred position for the fetus. In an occiput posterior position *(right)*, the fetal head presses against the mother's sacrum, causing painful back labor and possibly slowing the progress of labor.

blood volume, and weight gain contribute to stiffness and soreness throughout her body. The bodyworker should pay special attention to lower back, rib cage, pectoral girdle, hips, pelvis, legs, and feet.

During this trimester, the practitioner should concentrate on elongating the compressed areas of the client's body and shortening the overstretched regions. Exercises should be suggested that recruit the transverse abdominis muscle to minimize the diastasis and help maintain postural integrity. Trigger point release on the sacrum, lower back, hips, pelvis, abdomen, and rib cage can bring welcome relief to the pregnant client. Pelvic tilts and sacral lifts are helpful for relief of lower back pain, abdominal pressure, and hemorrhoids. They can also enhance lymphatic drainage.

Manual lymphatic drainage is the only bodywork technique appropriate on the woman's sore and tired legs and feet. Aside from bodywork, elevation of her legs and Epsom salt soaks (see Chapter 14) can help reduce swelling. Calf cramps or "nervous" legs often result from her hyperextended knees and an imbalance in or insufficient amounts of calcium, magnesium, potassium, and phosphorus. The client can be referred to a nutritionist to help prevent or treat these painful muscle spasms.

Carpal tunnel syndrome or de Quervain's syndrome can also plague a pregnant woman during the third trimester. These conditions are caused by increased swelling, loose extensor and flexor retinaculum, and neck protraction. Appropriate body mechanics can help alleviate symptoms. Massage techniques should include lymphatic drainage, myofascial stretching of the forearm, and use of acupuncture points. Acupuncture points to use are large intestine 11 coupled with small intestine 3 (see Chapter 14). Both points should be held for a count of 6 to 10 and repeated 6 to 10 times.

During the third trimester, clumsiness, falling, incorrect exercises, or the simple fact that relaxin is doing its job, may create a condition known as symphysis pubis separation. With this condition, the symphysis joint of the pubis becomes lax and the pubic bones separate and shear. This is very painful for the pregnant woman and getting in and out of bed, moving on and off the massage table, sitting, going to the bathroom, or standing can be excruciating for some women. At this stage of pregnancy, all types of hip and pelvic tractions must be avoided. Only techniques such as medial compression to realign the pubic bones and gentle positional release are appropriate. The client can be referred to a professional who can reposition her bones and balance her legs by using sacral-occipital blocking techniques.

Positioning during this and each trimester is based on the woman's comfort level. Prone on the bodyCushion system is appropriate as long as the cushions are used correctly, and she feels supported and comfortable. Side-lying, with or without the cushions, is always appropriate. Sitting or semireclining massage is also appropriate during the third trimester.

In My Experience...

M was 7 months pregnant with twins and complaining of lower back pain. She had a large diastasis, and her pelvis was displaced to the anterior with an exaggerated lordotic curve.

After teaching her transverse abdominis exercises and how to use her deep abdominal muscles throughout the day to enhance lumbar stability, I showed M how to do the pelvic tilt in standing and leaning positions to avoid having to get on the floor. I also carefully instructed her on the importance of proper body mechanics to protect her back.

After about a month, she reported less discomfort in her lower back even though the twins continued to grow. She also kept her diastasis from getting any larger and was able to complete her pregnancy without any further back pain. Of course, the swelling in her legs was another matter....

Summary

The last trimester brings exaggerated physical discomforts and emotional highs and lows. Eager to be finished with the pregnancy, many women are fearful of labor, birth, and impending motherhood. The expectant mother may experience backaches, swelling, headaches, frequent urination, and additional thirst. Most women become more aware of Braxton Hicks contractions during this time. Possible breech presentation is also a concern during her third trimester.

During the last trimester, the fetus grows to 21 inches and weighs more than 7 lbs. The fetus can hear and has a definite sleep-wake cycle. Fetal movement is constant in the early part of the final trimester but slows as its size increases.

The role of the practitioner during this final trimester is to provide the client relief from her aches and pains, prepare her for labor, and reassure her that her body knows exactly what to do during labor.

References

1. The Gentlemen's Magazine, December 1791. In Smith L: *The mother book: a compendium of trivia and grandeur concerning mothers, motherhood & maternity*, Garden City, NJ, 1978, Doubleday.
2. Sears W, Sears M: *The pregnancy book*, Boston, 1997, Little, Brown.
3. *Emotions during pregnancy*, Department of Nursing: Children's and Women's Services/OB-GYN Patient Education Committee, Iowa City, IA, 1997, The University of Iowa.
4. Grayson C, ed: Your pregnancy week by week: weeks 1-4, Available at http://www.webmd.com/content/article/64/72360.htm. Accessed 2003.
5. Poidevin LO: Striae gravidarum. Their relation to adrenal cortical hyperfunction, *Lancet* 436-439, 1959.
6. Stillerman E: Stretch marks: what can be done about them? *Natural Physique* 30: April 1987.
7. Bolane JE: *With child*, Waco, TX, 1999, Childbirth Graphics.
8. Feldman RG: Group B streptococcus prevention of infection in the newborn, *Practising Midwife* 4:16-18, 2001.
9. Fraser D, Cooper M: *Myles' textbook for midwives*, ed 14, Edinburgh, 2003, Churchill Livingstone.
10. Blumberg RM, Feldman RG: Neonatal group B streptococcal infection, *Curr Paediatr* 6:34-37, 1996.
11. Bilodeau R, Marier R: Breech presentation at term, *Am J Obstet Gynecol* 130:555, 1978.
12. Cox JP: Delivery alternatives in the term breech pregnancy, *ICEA Review* 12:4, 1988.
13. Gaskin IM: The undervalued art of vaginal breech birth, *Mothering* 125:52-58, July-August, 2004.
14. Ayman E, Olah K: Moxibustion in breech version: a descriptive review, *Acupuncture Med* 20(1):26-29, 2002.

15. Saunders: Moxa–what? *Mothering,* 125:63, 2004.

16. Stillerman E: Head over heels: what you can do when your baby's breech, *Mothering* 125:59-61, 2004.

17. Ferguson JM, et al. Maternal and fetal factors affecting success of antepartum external cephalic version, *Obstet Gynecol* 70(5):722-725, 1987.

18. Simkin P: Turning breech to vertex, ICEA tear sheet. In Weston MB: *Maternal Health News* 8:3, 1983.

19. Savona-Ventura C: The role of external cephalic version in modern obstetrics, *Obstet Gynecol Surv* 41(7): 393-400, 1986.

20. Stine LE: Update on external cephalic version performed at term, *Obstet Gynecol* 65(5):642-646, 1985.

REVIEW QUESTIONS

1   What are prelabor or labor preparation contractions called? What purpose do they serve?

_____

_____

_____

_____

_____

2   During the third trimester, how much has the woman's blood volume increased?

_____

_____

_____

_____

_____

3   Explain some of the common discomforts of pregnancy during the third trimester.

_____

_____

_____

_____

_____

4   Describe the swelling of the extremities during the third trimester. What is considered normal edema and what is considered abnormal?

_____

_____

_____

_____

_____

5   How does the massage practitioner treat normal swelling of the legs?

_____

_____

_____

_____

_____

6   What can massage practitioners do to help their clients prevent or treat backaches during the third trimester?

_____

_____

_____

_____

_____

7   Can stretch marks be prevented? Describe striae gravidarum.

_____

_____

_____

_____

_____

8   At what point does the fetus settle into a vertex presentation?

_____

_____

_____

_____

_____

9 How high in the mother's abdomen does the fetus reach in the last few weeks of pregnancy? What common discomforts can she experience from this fetal position?

_____
_____
_____
_____
_____
_____

10 What is meant by breech presentation? How common is it? What can massage practitioners suggest their clients do to help turn the breech presentation naturally?

_____
_____
_____
_____
_____

11 What is meant by occiput posterior and how can this position affect labor? What is the preferred position for the fetus to promote a faster labor?

_____
_____
_____
_____
_____

12 How does the position of the maternal uterus shift in preparation for labor?

_____
_____
_____
_____
_____

13 What types of bodywork are most efficient to treat the common discomforts accompanying the third trimester? On what areas of the body are they most effective?

_____
_____
_____
_____
_____

14 What are the possible contributing factors contributing to carpal tunnel syndrome or de Quervain's syndrome during the third trimester?

_____
_____
_____
_____
_____

15 Describe positioning options for the client during her third trimester.

_____
_____
_____
_____
_____

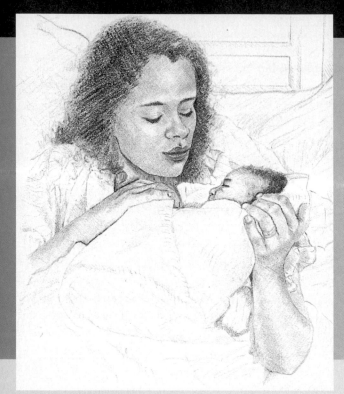

CHAPTER 12

Massage for Labor Preparation

Objectives

On completion of this chapter, the student will be able to do the following:

1   Identify prelabor maternal physical changes

2   Recognize and explain the importance of perineal massage and Kegel exercises

3   Understand and treat the common discomforts associated with prelabor

4   Provide an appropriate prelabor massage

Key Terms

Bloody show	Episiotomy	Operculum
Dilation	Kegel exercises	Perineal massage
Effacement	Lightening	Perineum
Engagement	Mucous plug	Prelabor
Engorgement	Nesting instinct	

Prelabor Physiology

A number of discernible maternal physical and emotional changes occur in the last few weeks of pregnancy that herald the onset of labor. In Malaysia, the midwife touches the expectant woman's feet as she gets closer to labor. When the big toes feel cold, they believe it means that the pregnant woman's body heat has shifted to her uterus in preparation for labor. Once her ankles become cold, labor will soon follow.[1] In traditional societies, birth lore is rife with symbolism and rituals. Undoing knots, for example, is thought to prevent knots in the umbilical cord, so African women undo their braided hair and Navaho women do not wring their hands while washing them.[1] Other traditions believe slippery treatment helped the baby slide out easily. Cherokee women bathe in a ritual bath filled with slippery bark, and Yemeni women are fed milk and oil.[1]

A pregnant woman's body undergoes dramatic changes as preparation for labor. Some of these physical changes are external and easy to recognize, whereas others occur internally. Most of these changes occur during the last few weeks of pregnancy with first-time mothers because their bodies need to make these adaptations. The body of a woman who has given birth before has already made some of these changes and may not present some of these signs.

Mood swings and emotional lability are common as the expectant woman is eager for the discomforts of pregnancy to be over but anxious about labor, birth, and impending motherhood. She may have vivid dreams or premonitions about the birth as she waits impatiently and nervously for signs of labor. Some women become easily distractible, especially during Braxton Hicks contractions, and may feel confused as to whether these **prelabor** (before labor begins) contractions are actually labor contractions.[2]

She may experience a surge of energy, which is known as the **nesting instinct**, and she may clean and prepare her home and the baby's room for its arrival.

Approximately 2 or 3 weeks before labor, the lower segments of the uterus expand to permit the fetal head to sink lower into the pelvis and perhaps engage in the pelvic brim. This **lightening** is noticeable in first-time mothers. When this occurs, the fundus of the uterus descends and the expectant woman experiences a relief from respiratory and upper gastrointestinal discomforts (Figure 12-1).

When **engagement** occurs, the fetus drops, or engages, into the pelvis and the uterus tilts from a posterior position to an anterior position. Her abdomen looks pointier and even larger, although it is only the change in uterine position not any change in size (see Figure 12-1). The symphysis pubis widens in reaction to hormonal secretions, and the pelvic floor softens and relaxes, permitting the uterus to descend further into the pelvis (Figure 12-2).

The respiratory and upper gastrointestinal relief that the woman experiences when the fetus drops is exchanged with an increased pressure in the pelvis as the fetus' head causes venous congestion of the pelvis. Her legs and feet swell, vaginal secretions increase to ease passage through the birth canal, and there is an increase in frequency and urgency of urination and possibly some incontinence.

The cervix dilates, or opens, and becomes softer. The practitioner can palpate spleen 6 to see if **dilation** of the cervix has begun. If the pregnant woman's cervix has softened or dilated, spleen 6 will feel softer and watery. It will be very sensitive to the touch (Figure 12-3). An internal examination by

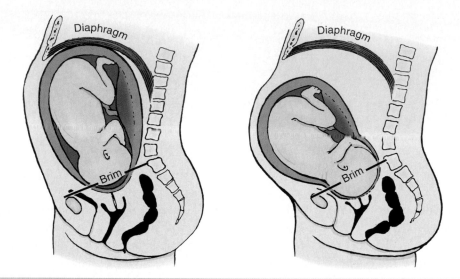

FIGURE 12-1 ■ The fundus compresses the diaphragm *(left), and* the lower uterine segment has not stretched to allow the fetal head to descend. After lightening *(right),* the fundus drops away from the diaphragm, easing respiratory systems, and the lower uterine segment softens and widens to accommodate the fetal head. Notice the anterior tilt of the uterus as the fetal head engages into the pelvic brim. (From Fraser D, Cooper M: *Myles' textbook for midwives,* ed 14, Edinburgh, 2003, Churchill Livingstone.)

her doctor or midwife may also reveal that her cervix has started to efface, or thin out. **Effacement** is measured from 0% to 100% (Figure 12-4).

She might experience more backaches, often characterized as restless backaches, which are caused by the fetus now lower in the uterus, stretching the uterine and pelvic ligaments, as well as pelvic joints. She notices stronger and more frequent Braxton Hicks contractions that are helping the uterus efface. These contractions get stronger before labor but abate with ambulation.

In late pregnancy, the expectant mother takes on the "pregnancy waddle" because of the hypermobility of the symphysis pubis and sacroiliac joints. This hypermobility often causes lower back pain and may give rise to symphysis pubis dysfunction or separation.[3]

The woman experiences a weight loss of a pound or so. Birth hormones are causing intestinal cramps and loose, frequent bowel movements. This diarrhea empties the intestines to make more room for passage through the birth canal. It also allows the laboring woman's uterus to utilize the essential blood supply rather than rerouting it for elimination.

The **mucous plug,** or **operculum,** which once sealed the cervix and acted as an additional barrier against infection, loosens. The combination of the fetal head dropping into the pelvic cavity and the prelabor contractions thinning out the cervix causes this plug, or **bloody show,** to release. The consistency of the mucus varies from women to women from stringy to thick and sticky.

For some women, the mucous plugs passes one time. Other women notice increased blood-tinged vaginal discharge. Tiny blood vessels rupture as the cervix thins, so pink-stained or brown-stained discharge is very common. Clients should be made aware that if the discharge shows more blood than mucus, such as a menstrual period, this must be brought to the attention of the health care provider. Loss of the mucous plug can mean that labor will start within a few days or up to a week or so.

Only about 10% to 12% of women have their membranes rupture during prelabor. This usually does not occur until labor is well established. The labor may start anywhere from a few minutes to within 24 hours of the membranes rupturing. Perineal massage (vaginal massage), baths, and sexual intercourse should be avoided once the membranes have ruptured because there is no longer any protection for the fetus against infection.[4,5,6]

A network of prominent blood vessels may be seen across the pregnant woman's chest and breasts

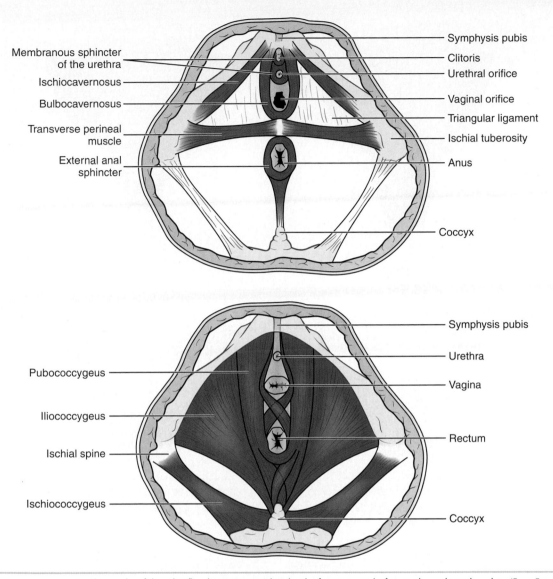

FIGURE 12-2 ■ The muscles of the pelvic floor become more relaxed and softer to permit the fetus to descend into the pelvis. (From Fraser D, Cooper M: *Myles' textbook for midwives*, ed 14, Edinburgh, 2003, Churchill Livingstone.)

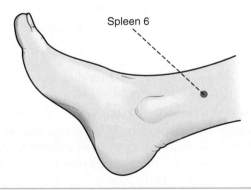

FIGURE 12-3 ■ When spleen 6 on both legs feels soft and watery, it means the cervix is softening and the uterus may be dilated. (From Lowdermilk DL, Perry SE: *Maternity & women's health care*, ed 8, St. Louis, 2004, Mosby.)

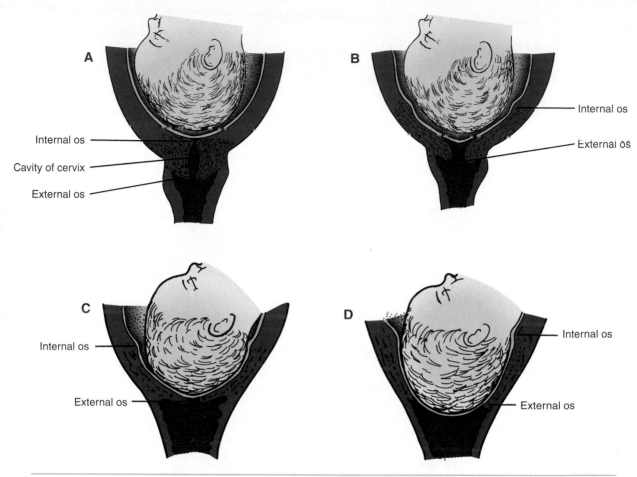

FIGURE 12-4 ■ Cervical dilation increases from 0 cm to 10 cm at birth. The cervix can be dilated as much as 3 centimeters for a number of weeks before labor begins. **A,** Before labor begins; **B,** early effacement; **C,** 100% effacement; **D,** complete dilation at 10 cm. (From Lowdermilk DL, Perry SE: *Maternity & women's health care,* ed 8, St. Louis, 2004, Mosby.)

as her body is preparing for lactation. Some women may already be lactating, whereas others start secreting colostrum (Box 12-1). The breasts may be sore, heavy, and swollen. This **engorgement** of the breasts may also contribute to midback pain.

Perineal Massage

In preparation for labor, women at 34 weeks' gestation should begin **perineal massage.** Many care providers will perform this massage during the second stage of labor to smooth out the tissues of the perineum as the baby's head crowns and stretches the tissue. The technique is called *ironing.*[6] Some care providers will support the **perineum,** the area between the vagina and anus, with a warm compress as the baby's head crowns.

Perineal massage is not done if any of the following are present:

- Active genital herpes lesion
- Vaginal varicosity
- Ruptured amniotic membranes
- Urinary tract infection, or any other bacterial or viral vaginal infection, including venereal disease

Perineal massage is not done on any region other than the vagina, nor is it done by the bodyworker or massage practitioner. The woman, her partner, her doctor, or midwife are the only people who can massage the perineum.

Bodyworkers should advise their clients of the numerous benefits perineal massage offers, which are as follows:

- During labor, levels of relaxin permit the vaginal opening to stretch wide enough to

BOX 12-1 *Colostrum*

During pregnancy, levels of estrogen and progesterone stimulate breast alveolar and ductal growth along with the secretion of co-lostrum. Although colostrum is present from week 16 of pregnancy, lactation is repressed until after birth when placental hormone levels fall. Colostrum is produced for the first 3 to 4 postpartum days and contains high levels of antibodies (immunoglobin to protect the immature newborn gastrointestinal tract from infections), protein, minerals, and fat-soluble vitamins. Colostrum has twice the amount of vitamin A, which gives colostrum its yellowish color, present in mature human milk. Colostrum is high in protein, low in sugar and fat, and easy for the newborn to digest. Colostrum's antibodies help establish the baby's normal intestinal flora, and its laxative effect eases the passage of meconium, which is the viscid waste of new-borns that contains mucus, bile, and epithelial shreds.

From Fraser D, Cooper M: *Myles' textbook for midwives*, ed 14, Edinburgh, 2003, Churchill Livingstone; Butt A: *The Nilotes of the Sudan and Uganda*, London, 1952, International African Institute.

BOX 12-2 *Cultural Care of the Perineum*

In most traditional societies the perineum was relaxed by steaming, bathing, or lubricating the area with oil just before the onset of labor.* The Buganda women of Uganda sit in a shallow bath infused with herbs during the final few weeks of pregnancy.† In Sudan, women steamed the perineum by squatting over a pot of herbs.‡

In Japan, India, and Thailand, oil was used as a lubricant to prevent tears, and women of Botswana used fat to keep the skin loose and to prevent lacerations.*

*From Goldsmith J: Childbirth wisdom from the world's oldest societies, New York, 1984, Congdon & Weed.
†From Butt A: The Nilotes of the Sudan and Uganda, London, 1952, International African Institute.
‡From Evans-Pritchard EE: Man and woman among the Azande, London, 1974, Faber and Faber.

accommodate the baby's head. The perineal massage performed by the client on herself cannot approximate this same tissue elasticity before labor, however, the technique does provide a modest amount of tissue elasticity and muscle memory to prepare the perineum for birth in the hopes of preventing an episiotomy, which is a surgical incision to widen the vaginal opening.

- Massaging the perineum will help prevent lacerations and tears (Box 12-2). Those women who do not massage their perineum are almost three times more apt to tear than women who do the technique.[8] The technique enables the client to identify the pelvic floor muscles she has to release with each contraction.

- If she performs the perineal massage correctly, it should burn when the tissue is maximally stretched. This sensation, known as the *rim of fire*, is the same sensation she will feel as the baby's head crowns. If she becomes inured to this sensation by repeating the massage often, she will not fight or contract against the burning when she experiences it during labor. On the contrary, she knows it means that her baby is being born.

- In addition, she learns that her body responds to pain by rushing endorphins to the area and putting out the "fire." This is the same response her body has during labor. The pressure of the baby's head on the perineum acts as a natural anesthetic and reduces perineal pain.

The client should empty her bladder and bowels, if necessary, before performing perineal massage. Her hands should be washed and fingernails trimmed. She may want to prepare the area by applying a warm, moist washcloth, although this is not necessary. The steps for perineal massage are as follows:

1. Thumbs or fingers should be inserted into the vagina about 1 to 1½ inches. The perineum should be stretched downward toward the rectum until maximum stretch, and she feels a stinging or burning sensation. She should breath normally and maintain the stretch until the sensation subsides, in about 1 or 2 minutes. The stretch should be released slowly and repeated five more times.

2. The perineum should be stretched down toward the anus until maximum stretch and the stretch should be maintained until the burning subsides. The same pressure should be maintained while gliding and stretching the tissue from the midline to either side of the vaginal opening.

This massage should be performed every day or several times a week, beginning at 34 weeks.

Episiotomy

No discussion of perineal massage is complete without addressing the episiotomy. This surgical incision is performed at the lower end of the vaginal opening, usually with a pair of surgical scissors, just before the baby's head crowns. It is the second most common surgical procedure performed in the United States (cutting the umbilical cord is the most common procedure).[9] Medical literature establishes the need for episiotomy with the following reasons:

- To prevent a tear
- To widen the vaginal opening to reduce pressure on the baby's head, particularly if the woman is not laboring in a gravity-friendly position
- To reduce trauma and damage to the muscles surrounding the vaginal opening
- To speed up the second stage of labor

Most research indicates that routine episiotomy actually does more damage to the pelvic floor than the vaginal birth.[10] Clinical trials suggest that routine episiotomies result in severe perineal lacerations (which is what it was supposed to prevent), pain, fecal and urinary incontinence, impaired sexual function, and damage to the pelvic floor muscles.[11]

Some physicians perform an episiotomy when the baby's shoulder blocks the birth canal to prevent fetal injuries. A study performed at the Johns Hopkins School of Medicine in 2004 analyzed 127 cases of shoulder dystocia, which is injury to the fetus' shoulder when it catches on the maternal pelvic bone. When attending physicians manually manipulated the fetus, only 35% of the babies suffered injuries, compared with 60% of the babies delivered after episiotomies. The study also established more anal tearing in the group who received the episiotomies.[12]

One study found that perineal postpartum pain and subsequent bruising and swelling and the need for pain medication was the highest for women who had episiotomies.[13] The study also proved that there was no evidence that babies benefited by routine episiotomies and questioned the wisdom of this practice.[13-16]

Touch Points

When clients start to exhibit prelabor changes, a certain amount of anticipation, anxiety, and fear may go hand-in-hand with the excitement and relief they often feel. This is the time to continue nurturing, supportive bodywork and help her stay calm and focused. First-time mothers in particular often articulate that they are scared and nervous about labor. Talking with them and explaining the process can often assuage many concerns. By keeping clients relaxed, bodyworkers are encouraging and promoting a natural transition into the next phase—labor—with calmness and preparedness being the primary factors.

Kegel Exercises

Kegel exercises are the voluntary tightening and relaxing of the pelvic floor muscles or the pubococcygeal muscles, to strengthen the vagina and perineum and control urinary incontinence. They were developed in 1948 by Dr. Arnold Kegel as a way for women to control incontinence after childbirth, although they are effective in controlling incontinence during pregnancy as well. These same exercises are now recommended to women with urinary stress incontinence. These exercises should strengthen the muscles of the pelvic floor to improve urethral and rectal sphincter function and structural integrity. Kegel exercises are performed as follows:

1. Begin by emptying the bladder. (Some women learn to identify these muscles by stopping the flow of urine midstream.)
2. Tighten the muscles of the pelvic floor and hold for a count of 10.
3. Relax completely for a count of 10.
4. Perform this 10 times, 3 times a day.[17]

Prelabor Discomforts

Once the fetus has lightened and is engaged within the pelvis, the expectant woman experiences a relief from respiratory and upper gastrointestinal disturbances but exchanges these discomforts with increased lower back pain, pelvic and hip instability, sciatica, lower abdominal pressure, pelvic floor pressure that may aggravate preexisting hemorrhoids or vaginal varicosities, and increased leg swelling and soreness.

BOX 12-3 *Hypnosis for Childbirth*

Hypnotherapy can provide deep relaxation to a laboring woman and thereby reduce fear, tension, and subsequently pain. Hypnotherapy addresses the fear-tension-pain cycle. Women are taught relaxation techniques and cues to bring them into complete relaxation while being very much aware of their environment and all that is going on around them without the fear and pain.

From Weiss RE: Hypnosis for labor. Your guide to pregnancy/birth, About: Pregnancy and Childbirth. Available at http://pregnancy.about.com/cs/naturalchild-birth/a/aa082501a.htm.

She is also emotionally unstable during these last few weeks of pregnancy as labor gets closer and more real to her. Her anxiety levels might escalate, especially for a first-time mother. She should be allowed to express her fears, hopes, and concerns in a nonjudgmental environment and taught relaxation techniques such as the tension-releasing scan (see Chapter 19), deep breathing exercises, and positive visualization (Box 12-3).

DVD *Prelabor Bodywork*

The practitioner can assuage a pregnant woman's fears by making her more comfortable physically and preparing her body for labor. The practitioner should concentrate on increasing flexibility to the woman's hips, pelvis, and legs, so she can labor comfortably in several positions without joint stiffness or muscle soreness. The bodywork should address all postural changes that have recently occurred, with an emphasis on her body mechanics and the use of the transverse abdominis muscle for better alignment.

The massage for her legs must continue to follow manual lymphatic drainage procedure. At this time in the pregnancy, because the engaged fetus has created more swelling in her lower extremities, more of the hour may be spent reducing the swelling in her legs and elongating her exaggerated lordotic curve.

Trigger point therapy and myofascial stretching to release tension in her hips, pelvis, and abdomen are effective and particularly important for the muscles of her lower back, lumbodorsal fascia, hip rotators, and pectoral girdle. This work

will also help the client be more comfortable in a variety of birthing positions. Pain in the symphysis pubis and sacroiliac and lumbosacral joints can be relieved through general massage techniques, transverse friction at the joints, medial joint compressions, pelvic tilting, and sacral lifts.

In My Experience...

D was 39 weeks' pregnant with her first baby. When she came for her massage, she exclaimed "Look how big I got! How is this baby going to get *out*?" I explained to her that the baby really had not grown that much bigger. Instead, her uterus had tilted anterior to help the baby's head align with the birth canal and that made her look bigger. I also asked her if her breasts were more sensitive, if she noticed more swelling in her legs, or if she had a change in her energy levels. Her answers were "Yes, yes, and yes."

"Well," I told her, "it only means that you are soon going to have a baby!" She looked at me and said, in wide-eyed innocence, "Isn't this *amazing*?!"

Summary

The final few weeks of pregnancy are defined by many physiological changes in a women's body in preparation for labor. Some of these adaptations are visible, whereas others are occurring internally. The fetus descends into the pelvic station, and the pregnant woman can breathe deeply once again but now feels more discomfort in her legs, sciatic region, lower back, hips, pelvis, pelvic floor, and lower abdomen. The pregnant woman is also actively involved in labor preparation by doing perineal massage and Kegel exercises daily. These important activities can help her avoid tearing during labor and hasten recovery.

In preparation for labor, the bodyworker should release tensions in these regions with appropriate massage techniques. The amount of time spent in any particular area is predicated by her needs. Because the pregnancy is coming to an end and labor is quickly approaching, providing her with exercises and methods to relax during labor will help eliminate fear and minimize pain.

References

1. Jackson D: *With child: wisdom and traditions for pregnancy, birth and motherhood,* San Francisco, 1999, Chronicle Books.

2. Simkin P, Whalley J, Keppler A: *Pregnancy, birth and the newborn,* New York, 1991, Meadowbrook Press.

3. Fraser D, Cooper M: *Myles' textbook for midwives,* ed 14, Edinburgh, 2003, Churchill Livingstone.

4. Siemens R: Signs of labour (labor), Pregnancy Health Information Organization. Available at http://pregnancy.health-info.org/labour-signs.html.

5. Lowdermilk DL, Perry SE: *Maternity & women's health care,* ed 8, St. Louis, 2004, Mosby.

6. Sears W, Sears M: *The pregnancy book,* Boston, 1997, Little, Brown.

7. Leifer G: *Maternity nursing: an introductory text,* ed 9, St. Louis, 2005, Saunders.

8. Mynaugh PA: *The effectiveness of prenatal health practices and two instructional educational methods on labor and delivery: a case study of perineal massage.* Dissertation Abstracts International, Ann Arbor, MI, 1988, University Microfilms.

9. Banta D, Thacker SB: The risks and benefits of episiotomy, *Birth* 9(1):25-30, 1982.

10. Livingston C: *Just the facts about episiotomy,* Minneapolis, 1996, ICEA.

11. Hartmann K, Viswanathan M, Palmieri R, et al: Outcomes of routine episiotomy, *JAMA* 293:2141-2148, 2005.

12. *Clearing the way for baby, safely,* The New York Times, October 5, 2004.

13. Harrison RF, Brennan M, North PM, et al: Is routine episiotomy necessary? *BMJ* 288:1971-1975, 1984.

14. Homsi R, Daikoku NH, Littlejohn J, et al: Episiotomy: risks of dehiscence and rectovaginal fistula, *Obstet Gynecol Surv* 49:803-808, 1994.

15. Lede R, Belizan JM, Carroli G: Is routine use of episiotomy justified? *Am J Obstet Gynecol* 174:1399-1402, 1996.

16. Shiono P, Klebanoff MA, Carey JC: Midline episiotomies: more harm than good, *Obstet Gynecol* 75:765-770, 1990.

17. Gaudier FL: *Kegel exercises,* Jacksonville, FL, 2005, Maternal Fetal Medicine.

REVIEW QUESTIONS

1   Describe at least 10 of the prelabor physiological and emotional changes many women experience.

_____
_____
_____
_____
_____
_____

2   As the baby descends deeper into the pelvis, what set of symptoms are relieved and which take their place?

_____
_____
_____
_____
_____
_____

3   What is lightening?

_____
_____
_____
_____
_____

4   What is the significance of the widening of the symphysis pubis?

_____
_____
_____
_____
_____

5   How do the muscles of the pelvic floor change in preparation for childbirth?

_____
_____
_____
_____
_____
_____

6   What is cervical dilation? What acupuncture point can you press after 38 weeks to see if the cervix is starting to soften?

_____
_____
_____
_____
_____
_____

7   What causes a "restless backache"?

_____
_____
_____
_____
_____
_____

8   How common is it for the amniotic membranes to rupture before labor? When does it often occur?

_____
_____
_____
_____
_____

9   What are the contributing factors in the "pregnancy waddle" that some women exhibit before labor begins?

_____

_____

_____

_____

_____

10   What is the significance of the network of blood vessels that appear across the chest and on the breasts of some women?

_____

_____

_____

_____

_____

11   What is colostrum and what is it composed of ?

_____

_____

_____

_____

_____

12   Explain the importance of perineal massage and when the client should start doing it.

_____

_____

_____

_____

_____

_____

13   When should be perineal massage not be done?

_____

_____

_____

_____

_____

_____

14   Describe some of the physical discomforts a woman may experience as her body prepares for labor.

_____

_____

_____

_____

_____

15   What are some of the bodywork techniques practitioners can use to help prepare a woman's body for labor?

_____

_____

_____

_____

_____

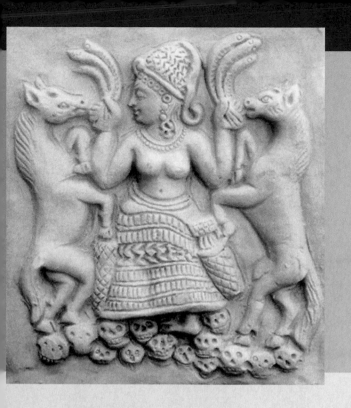

CHAPTER 13

Sitting Massage

Objectives

On completion of this chapter, the student will be able to do the following:

1 Comfortably position the client for the sitting massage
2 Identify the conditions that warrant a sitting massage
3 Employ proper body mechanics while performing a sitting massage
4 Recognize appropriate bodywork techniques for this massage

Key Terms

Esophageal reflux	Pelvic squeeze	Sitting massage
Nasal and sinus congestion	Sacral lift	Symphysis pubis separation

A **sitting massage** is a massage given with the client sitting on a stool or regular chair that does not make use of the standard massage chair. Standard massage chairs are not designed to accommodate or support the pregnant woman's uterus, ligaments, and breasts. The standard massage chair also positions a person's extremities in a way that increases swelling rather than offering lymphatic drainage through elevation.

Client Positioning

A wooden stool without wheels or a regular chair is used and placed against the massage table or any high surface. The client is supported with a pillow on the stool or chair, and another pillow is placed against her abdomen as she leans over another pile of pillows. The woman's neck should be comfortably supported to minimize neck flexion (Figure 13-1). Face cradles can be used to support her head (Figure 13-2). A footstool can also be used to elevate her feet and provide a slight posterior pelvic tilt.

The client may feel more comfortable wearing underpants, but she is draped with a sheet wrapped around her and secured at the back. The sheet can be pulled through her legs and secured at the back to provide a more modest draping (Figure 13-3).

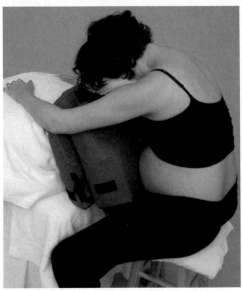

FIGURE 13-2 ■ The use of a face cradle makes a sitting massage more comfortable for the client.

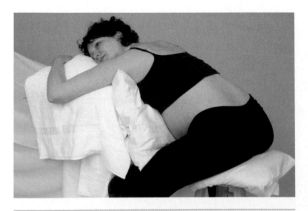

FIGURE 13-1 ■ A pillow should be placed on the wooden stool and another in front of her abdomen for support. Pillows should be added to the table so she can comfortably lean over them without excessive neck flexion.

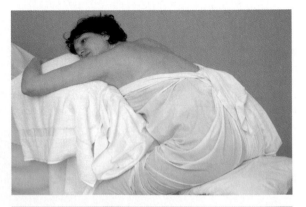

FIGURE 13-3 ■ The client should be draped by wrapping the sheet around her body and securing it in the back. The sheet can be pulled through her legs for additional coverage.

Conditions that Warrant a Sitting Massage

In some instances, a pregnant client may be unable to get on the massage table or another pregnant client may find it more comfortable sitting upright. Some physical conditions during pregnancy warrant a sitting massage. These conditions include the following:

- **Esophageal reflux,** or heartburn. This condition can be minimized by an upright position. Some women suffering from esophageal reflux have to sleep in a semisitting or recumbent position and are more comfortable having a sitting massage.
- **Nasal or sinus congestion** (stuffed nose and sinuses). It is easier for the sinus membranes to drain in an upright position
- **Symphysis pubis separation,** a separation and shearing of the symphysis pubis. A footstool might make it easier to get on the table for some, but other women may find raising their legs to get on the table quite painful. Sitting permits them to move their legs and find a comfortable position.
- **Sciatica.** Lying on the affected side might be too painful for some women. Although side-lying on the opposite side may offer some relief, a number of women prefer the sitting position.
- With multiples, particularly in late pregnancy, getting on and off the massage table might be too difficult.

- In early labor.
- After a cesarean section. Many women feel more comfortable and less vulnerable in a sitting position with a pillow compressing against the incision.
- After any type of surgery, infirmity, or in a hospital setting. Sitting massage is warranted when treating a client in a bed is awkward or uncomfortable.

In addition, when the practitioner's massage table is not available, a sitting massage can be a useful and effective positioning alternative.[1]

Practitioner Body Mechanics

The practitioner seats the client on a cushioned wooden stool at the foot or head of the massage table, with a pillow at her abdomen, leaning comfortably over a pile of pillows. Her arms should be placed on the pillows to enhance lymphatic drainage. The practitioner stands behind the client, with knees bent slightly and one leg behind, in a lunge position (Figure 13-4). The practitioner gets strength from his or her legs and by leaning into the client. The practitioner should remember to keep his or her shoulders and arms relaxed. In this position, the practitioner can massage the woman's back and neck. To massage the woman's neck in a neutral position, she should cup her hands and place her forehead in them. The practitioner

Touch Points

Learning how to massage a client sitting on a stool without wheels or a chair has numerous applications. The client may have esophageal reflux or congested sinuses that requires a sitting position, or she may have a difficult time getting on and off the massage table. Practitioners may also find that there is limited time to do a massage and it is more expedient sitting, or perhaps you do not have a treatment table available.

Whatever the reason, learning to do a massage with a client in a sitting position will provide a practitioner with enhanced massage skills and tools to make your clients comfortable and provide them with wonderful, therapeutic care.

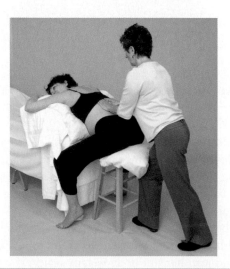

FIGURE 13-4 ■ The practitioner's knees should be slightly flexed in a lunge position with one leg behind. Her weight shifts forward to attain more pressure.

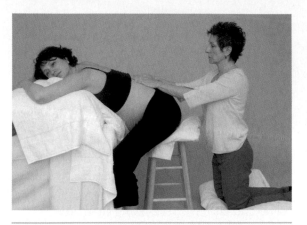

FIGURE 13-5 ■ Leaning on pillows allows the practitioner to use his or her body more effectively and comfortably.

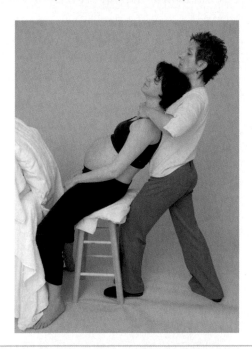

FIGURE 13-6 ■ With the client leaning on the practitioner, the practitioner firmly anchors his or her back leg to support the client's body weight.

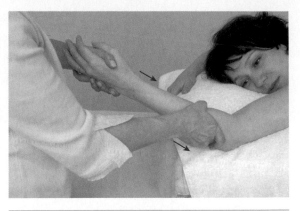

FIGURE 13-7 ■ The practitioner stands on either side of the massage table to massage the client's arms. Lifting the client's arm enhances lymphatic drainage. Her wrists should be kept in a supported, neutral position and care should be taken to avoid squeezing the contraindicated acupuncture point large intestine 4.

woman's face, scalp, and chest. The client should be returned to the original position leaning over the pillows, with the practitioner moving to either side of the table to massage her arms (Figure 13-7).

To massage her legs, the client can turn and face outward or lean over the pillows sideways, whichever position feels most comfortable. The practitioner sits down next to her and lifts one of her legs, supporting the leg behind the knee and at the ankle. The practitioner places the client's leg on his or her leg (a towel over the practitioner's lap will protect the practitioner's clothing), knee to knee, so the practitioner can massage her leg using lymphatic drainage procedure and light pressure. Excess lubrication should be wiped from her feet, and her foot should be replaced on the floor by supporting her leg under the knee and ankle (Figure 13-8). The practitioner then massages her other leg. As she faces outward, a towel should be placed across her breasts and her abdomen should be massaged with gentle, clockwise effleurage strokes (Figure 13-9). The sheet should be replaced, and she should be repositioned in a comfortable position as she rests a few moments after the treatment.

Appropriate Bodywork

The pressure of the strokes should be based on the client's comfort level. Some women enjoy deep work, whereas others, feeling more fragile, prefer a lighter touch. Swedish massage, myofascial

should kneel down or lean on a pillow to access her lower back and hips (Figure 13-5). In this position, the practitioner can offer a **pelvic squeeze** (hip squeeze) or **sacral lift** (lifting of the sacrum and attached pelvic floor muscles).

The practitioner stands up and repositions in the lunge position with one leg behind. The client should lean her full body weight against the practitioner's body as the practitioner firmly anchors on his or her slightly flexed back leg (Figure 13-6). In this position the practitioner can massage the

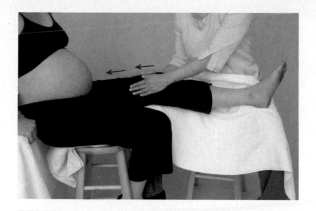

FIGURE 13-8 ■ When lifting the client's leg, the practitioner supports it under the knee and ankle.

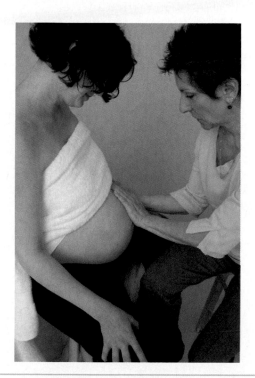

FIGURE 13-9 ■ A towel should be placed over the client's breasts for abdominal massage in a sitting position.

release, trigger point release, strain-counterstrain, shiatsu and lymphatic drainage on her extremities are all appropriate techniques the practitioner can use with the client in a sitting position.

In My Experience...

R had a cesarean section about 3 weeks before her appointment and felt very uneasy about getting on the massage table and lying down either prone or on her side. When I suggested a sitting massage, she was eager to do it.

I placed numerous pillows on the end of the table so R could lean over comfortably. Another pillow was positioned in front of her abdomen that she leaned against for more support and to compress the incision. She said she felt very secure like this. As the massage proceeded, R had to shift her weight to accommodate the massage, but this did not pose any problem for her. By the time I asked her to turn around so I could massage her legs, she had fallen asleep.

Summary

Certain physiological or practical reasons warrant a full body massage in a sitting position. A sitting massage can be a pleasant and therapeutic hour for the client who is either unable to get on the massage table or finds it more comfortable to be sitting. Sitting massage is also required for clients with some conditions, such as esophageal reflux, sinus congestion, symphysis pubis separation, sciatica, and others, and can increase the client's comfort level.

Reference

1. Stillerman E: MotherMassage: massage during pregnancy professional manual, New York, 2004.

REVIEW QUESTIONS

1   How would you comfortably position a client for a sitting massage?

_____

_____

_____

_____

_____

_____

2   Describe at least six reasons to offer a client a sitting massage.

_____

_____

_____

_____

_____

_____

3   Describe how the sitting position can ease those discomforts.

_____

_____

_____

_____

_____

_____

4   What are the proper body mechanics for the practitioner who is performing a sitting massage?

_____

_____

_____

_____

_____

_____

5   What are some of the appropriate bodywork techniques a practitioner can use for a sitting massage?

_____

_____

_____

_____

_____

_____

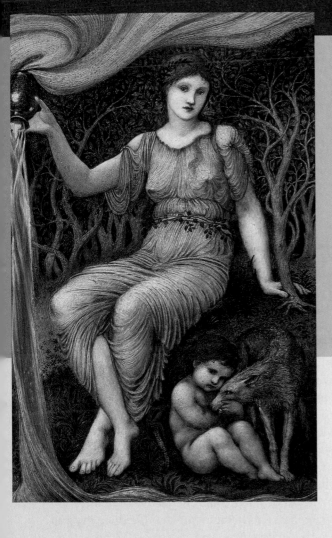

 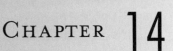
Massage for Common Discomforts of Pregnancy

Objectives

On completion of this chapter, the student will be able to do the following:

Understand the causes of the common discomforts of pregnancy

- Apply appropriate bodywork techniques to treat the aches and pains of pregnancy such as backaches, breast soreness, headaches, leg cramps, sciatica, and symphysis pubis separation
- Apply appropriate bodywork techniques to treat common complaints of pregnancy such as abdominal pressure, constipation, esophageal reflux, fatigue, heartburn, hemorrhoids, insomnia, morning sickness, and varicose veins
- Apply appropriate bodywork techniques to treat medical conditions during pregnancy such as anemia, carpal tunnel syndrome, de Quervain's syndrome, edema, gestational glucose intolerance, nasal and sinus congestion, and shortness of breath

Key Terms

Abdominal pressure	De Quervain's syndrome	Insomnia
Anemia	Edema	Leg cramps
Backaches	Fatigue	Sciatica
Breast soreness	Gastrointestinal disturbances	Shortness of breath
Carpal tunnel syndrome	Headaches	Varicose veins
Charley horses	Heartburn	
Constipation	Hemorrhoids	

Massage instructions for prenatal (labor and post-partum) massage and techniques for treating specific discomforts of pregnancy are best learned in a hands-on classroom setting such as the *Mother-Massage: massage during pregnancy* course. Professional demonstration and on-site supervision reinforces the concepts behind the techniques used to treat the common discomforts of pregnancy.

Common Pregnancy-Related Discomforts

Abdominal Pressure

The dramatic changes in the pregnant woman's body and the postural adaptations she has to make just to stand upright can cause a respectable amount of stiffness, soreness, and discomfort. As pregnancy progresses, her shifting posture creates joint, myofascial, and muscular stresses throughout her body. One of the bodyworker's many goals is to minimize these strains and improve her alignment.

Because postural shifting is one of the major contributing factors and causes of her aches and pains, offering the expectant mother ways to minimize this maladaptive posture is essential. The importance of recruiting her abdominal muscles correctly when she sits, stands, lifts, and exercises to help support her posture has been stressed in earlier chapters. In particular, the transverse abdominis muscle, which acts as a girdle around the midsection, provides lumbar stability, protects articulating structures, and assists in skeletal stress absorption.[1,2] When the pregnant woman draws in her abdominal wall, especially the lower segment, she contracts the transverse abdominis muscle.[3]

Other factors that contribute to **abdominal pressure** in pregnancy are the diastasis (separation of the abdominal muscles),

weakened and overstretched abdominal muscles, multiple pregnancy, stretching of uterine ligaments (particularly the round ligaments), anterior pelvic tilt, weight of the uterus, and fetal engagement into the pelvis in late pregnancy, which places more pressure on the lower abdomen. Rib soreness and bruising may be attributed to fetal kicking. Care must be taken to avoid further irritating a bruised area.

Groin pain may happen when the client moves too quickly or when she sneezes, laughs, or coughs when her hips are in extension—lying down or standing. The sudden stretching of one or both of the round ligaments causes the pain. Moving slowly often avoids the pain and if she anticipates a sneeze or cough, she should flex her hips and draw in her abdominal muscles to reduce the pull on the ligaments.

Treating abdominal pressure includes the following massage techniques that support the abdomen and pelvic floor and positions that relieve abdominal compression:

- The client's bladder and intestines should be emptied when necessary to prevent additional congestion in the lower abdomen.
- The client should be taught the importance of engaging her transverse abdominis muscle during any activity to stabilize her lumbar spine, support the uterus, shorten the abdominal muscles, and minimize the diastasis.[4]
- Pelvic tilting during the massage elongates the compressed lower spine and shortens the overstretched abdominal muscles. The client can also perform these movements several times throughout the day in a variety of positions: standing, leaning over a secure surface, on her hands and knees (she

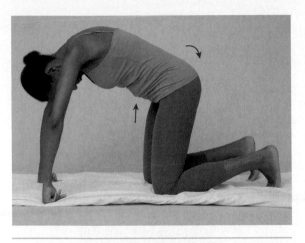

FIGURE 14-1 ■ A four-point pelvic tilt eases abdominal pressure and relieves lower back pain. The client's wrists and ankles should be in neutral positions. Those clients with hand or wrist pain can lean on their elbows. The abdominal muscles should be pulled in while holding this position.

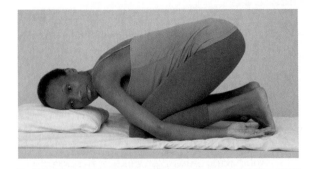

FIGURE 14-2 ■ The knee-chest rest eases abdominal pressure. Ankles in a neutral position.

should keep her wrists and feet in a neutral position to avoid wrist pain or calf cramps), or on her elbows and knees. She should draw her abdominal muscles in as she holds these positions, breathing normally (Figures 14-1 and 14-2) Using the bodyCushion system with the client in a prone position approximates the pelvic tilt by bringing the fetus forward and decompressing and elongating the lumbar spine.

■ The sacral lift should not be done on anyone

   DVD with coccygeal pain or dislocation, but it provides tremendous relief from a bulging pelvic floor. With the client in a side-lying position, the practitioner scoops one hand down the pregnant woman's lumbar spine to approximate a pelvic (posterior) tilt and brings it to rest on the woman's lower sacral segments near her coccyx. The practitioner should bend his or her elbow and lean into it. This will allow the practitioner to perform the lift by simply leaning into the arm. The practitioner's other hand rests softly on the client's hip. In a lunge position at the side of the massage table, the practitioner leans into the arm that is resting on the client's sacrum and pushes at a 45-degree angle toward the client's umbilicus (Figure 14-3). Another way to perform the sacral lift that spares the practitioner's wrists is to use an outstretched arm and the flat surface of the practitioner's fist at the client's sacrum, avoiding bone-on-bone contact. This is also a stronger lift for the client. The sacral lift can also be performed while the client is sitting on a chair or stool. While kneeling behind her, the practitioner places one hand under her sacrum and the other hand on top for added strength and lifts toward her navel at about a 45-degree angle. The practitioner can also employ his or her fist in this position.[5]

■ With the client in a side-lying position,

   DVD the practitioner stands behind the client and reaches over the client's abdomen. Both open palms are placed under the lowest part of the client's abdomen. The practitioner gently lifts the pregnant woman's abdomen (the fetus is well protected within the amniotic sac) and performs effleurage hand over hand.

Anemia

Anemia is the reduced ability of the blood to carry oxygen to the cells of the body.[6] Symptoms of anemia are fatigue, pallor, dizziness, reduced immune function, loss of appetite, susceptibility to infection, and feeling chilled. During pregnancy, anemia often occurs because of the fetal need to build hemoglobin; the frequent use of antacids to treat **heartburn**, or gastric indigestion, which decreases dietary iron absorption; and the slowness with which red blood cells reproduce as blood volume increases.

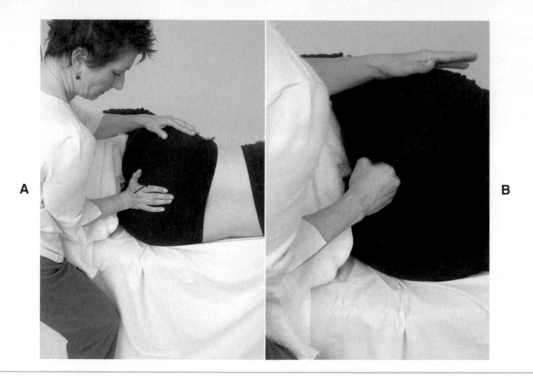

FIGURE 14-3 ■ **A**, The sacral lift reduces abdominal pressure and eases the pain of hemorrhoids and vaginal varicosities. **B**, The practitioner uses either the palm of the hand or the fist and pushes up at a 45° angle.

Anemia increases the risk of pregnancy complications such as early labor. The client should first establish with her physician which form of anemia she has. The practitioner may want to refer the client to a nutritionist to help with her dietary adjustments to combat anemia. The four kinds of anemia are as follows:

■ Iron deficiency anemia is defined as a serum iron concentration of less than 60 mg/dl with less than 16 transferrin saturation.[7] Fetal iron demands coupled with overuse of antacids predisposes a woman to iron deficiency anemia. Dietary changes are prescribed to treat this type of anemia. Foods rich in iron, such as meat, chicken, and dark, leafy green vegetables, are suggested. Iron supplements, along with vitamin C and zinc to enhance absorption, are recommended. These supplements, however, can cause constipation, nausea and vomiting, and abdominal discomfort.

■ Folic acid deficiency anemia is associated with neural tube defects such as anencephaly, spina bifida, and encephalocele. The United States Public Health Services recommend that all women of childbearing age take 0.4 mg of folic acid daily. Leafy green vegetables, citrus fruits, beans, yeast, and fortified breakfast cereals are high in folic acid. During pregnancy, the need for folic acid increases, but anemia may result form insufficient quantities, poor absorption, or drug interactions.

■ Sickle cell anemia is an inherited disease caused by the presence of abnormal hemoglobin in the shape of a sickle. The cells group together and block blood vessels and lead to infarcts in organs. Approximately 1 out of 11 African Americans carries the trait, although less than 1% will develop the disease.[6] Sickle cell anemia increases the likelihood of miscarriage and stillbirth. Women are treated with oxygen, intravenous fluids, or antibiotics, as medically determined.

■ Thalassemia is a genetic defect resulting in anemia and hemolysis. In this instance, too much iron creates an overload situation that may lead to either a reduction in red blood cell production or destruction of these cells.[6]

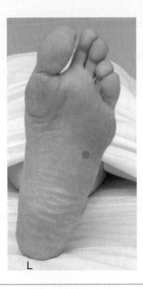

FIGURE 14-4 ■ The spleen reflex point is found on the left foot. To help treat anemia, this reflex point should be pressed for a count of 6 to 10, repeating a total of 6 to 10 times.

Massage considerations in a patient with anemia are as follows:

- A full body massage reintroduces lazy red blood cells back into the client's blood stream, thus elevating her erythrocyte count. The reflex point for the spleen, found on the left foot, can be pressed for a count of 10, repeating 10 times (Figure 14-4). The spleen recycles and plays an important role in the manufacture of hemoglobin.
- The shiatsu points found between L3 and L4 and L5 and S1 stimulate the spleen. Bladder 25 and bladder 27 should each be pressed on both sides of the spine for a count of 6 to 10, repeating 6 to 10 times.[5]

Backaches

Backaches are a major reason clients seek therapeutic massages, and poor posture is the most frequent cause of back pain.[8] In early pregnancy, elevated levels of relaxin loosen the pelvic and lumbosacral joints, creating an unstable and hypermobile pelvis. As pregnancy progresses, the anterior shift in the woman's center of gravity and postural displacement cause stress on her muscles, joints, and myofascia. Her pelvis tilts anteriorly, and her lumbar spine and its musculature are compressed. Her neck protracts, creating headaches, neck soreness, and arm weakness.

Abdominal muscle weakness and the presence of the diastasis contribute to her maladaptive posture and lumbar instability. These core muscles have to be strengthened to support her in an upright position and to minimize these postural compensations. A multiple pregnancy, constipation, and obesity are other factors contributing to backaches during pregnancy.

The practitioner should explain to the client the importance of using her transverse abdominis muscle throughout the day. Her posture will improve once she gets used to drawing her abdominal muscles in on a regular basis. In good alignment, a large portion of the weight of the uterus rests in the pelvic basin and the client's buttocks are tucked under, in a mild posterior pelvic tilt. Her abdominal muscles should be strong enough to support the fundus. Her weight is carried slightly anterior to her instep, and her head sits neutrally on her neck. Her shoulders are slightly laterally rotated to make room for her expanding ribcage.[8]

The client should be advised about proper body mechanics during daily activities. She should be reminded of the correct way to get on and off the massage table (or out of bed) by drawing her abdominal muscles in, turning to the side, and using her arms. She should never "jackknife" when getting in or out of bed.

She should also wear comfortable shoes to minimize back pain. As pregnancy progresses, the heels of her shoes should become shorter and broader. Soft and flexible shoes absorb more of the impact of walking than firm shoes.[9] Hip and shoulder soreness from sleeping on one side can be reduced by changing positions while she sleeps. Round ligament stretching may cause referred pain to the front of the thighs, and the sacrouterine and broad ligaments refer pain down the buttocks and to the lower back. Recruiting the transverse abdominis helps support and lift the uterus, thereby easing the stretching of the ligaments.

The back pain a woman experiences during pregnancy is rarely nerve root damage, such as a herniated disc, but is mainly caused by postural shifting and poor alignment. Appropriate bodywork techniques include myofascial release, Swedish massage, trigger point release, strain-counterstrain, postural release, lomilomi, craniosacral technique, sacral-occipital technique, and shiatsu or acupressure. An effective approach to treating back pain is to begin by releasing the superficial tissues first and gradually addressing the deeper musculature. One technique for back massage is as follows:

- With the client in either a side-lying or prone position, the practitioner starts with a gentle pelvic tilt (lumbosacral stretch). Hold for a count of 6-10 and release the traction slowly. Repeat several more times.
- The pelvic tilt is followed with a sacral lift.
- Myofascial stretching of the muscles of the cervical spine can also help ease lower back congestion due to the dural attachments at C1 to C3 and L3 to the periosteum of the coccyx. With the client in a prone position, the practitioner stretches laterally and diagonally on either side of the spine all the way down the client's erector spinae muscles.
- The practitioner then moves on to more traditional massage strokes all over her back, including effleurage, pétrissage, and friction strokes. The pressure should start out light and gradually progress deeper to the client's comfort level and tissue resistance.
- Trigger point release along the lower back, hips, pelvis, and scapulae is effective in addressing referred pain and local muscular congestion.
- The practitioner can release her sacroiliac joint by placing one finger into the joint at the posterior iliac spine and the other hand posterior to her anterior superior iliac spine (ASIS). The finger at the sacroiliac joint remains stable while the practitioner tractions and gently pulsates from the ASIS, decompressing and stretching the joint.
- The client's neck and the occipital ridge should be massaged.
- The practitioner can perform a medial compression behind the ASIS. In a side-lying position, the client leans forward slightly so the practitioner can position his or her fist behind the underlying ASIS. Practitioners should find a comfortable hand position. The client's hips should be squeezed together. Many women

experience relief from abdominal pressure and back pain with this hip squeeze.

- Deep friction around the greater trochanters reaches some of the attachments of the lateral leg rotators. The practitioner can use the fingers, thumbs, knuckles, pisiforms, or elbows for deepest pressure. The practitioner should take care to start out lightly before working deep into the acetabulum. Because many women sleep on their sides, some women are extremely sore and sensitive in this area.
- The back massage is completed with several more effleurage strokes.

When the client is in a side-lying position, using both hands to do the massage does not give the practitioner enough resistance to work deeply and makes the client feel as if she has to hold on to something or else she will be pushed off the table. To avoid this, it is helpful if the practitioner holds the woman's shoulder or hip (wherever the practitioner is working) with one hand and learns how to give a massage with the other. This is especially useful for long, flowing strokes, such as effleurage, and not nearly as important in more local treatment.

Breast Soreness

In the early weeks of pregnancy, **breast soreness** is caused by heightened levels of estrogen and progesterone. The increase in these hormones causes a fullness, tingling, or increased sensitivity to the breasts. The nipples and areolae darken, secondary pinkish areolae extending beyond the primary areolae develop, and the nipples become more erectile. Montgomery's tubercles, the sebaceous glands in the breasts, appear to have a protective role in keeping the nipples lubricated for breastfeeding and are visible around the nipples.[10]

The blood vessels beneath the skin dilate from increased blood volume, and these vessels become prominent, often appearing bluish. Venous congestion is more prevalent in the breasts of primigravidas.[10] Stretch marks may appear on the side of the breasts.

During the second and third trimesters, the breasts enlarge from an increase in the growth of mammary glands. Glandular tissue replaces connective tissues so the breasts feel looser and softer.

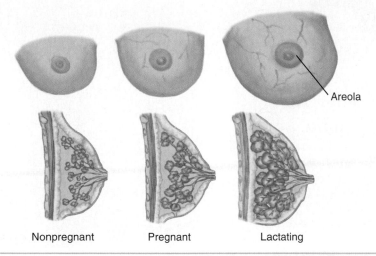

Nonpregnant   Pregnant   Lactating

FIGURE 14-5 ■ Breast tissue changes. (From McKinney ES, James SR, Murray SS, et al: *Maternal-child nursing,* ed 2, St. Louis, 2005, Mosby.)

BOX 14-1	*Creation of the Milky Way*

According to ancient Greek legend, Heracles was the son of the god Zeus and a mortal named Alcmene. When Heracles ascended to heaven, he had to be "reborn" by a goddess to achieve immortality.

In a mock labor, Hera, the goddess of marriage and maternity, gave birth to Heracles. Zeus placed his son in Hera's bed to nurse her divine milk. Heracles sucked so powerfully (he was, after all, fully grown), that Hera's milk spilled out across the night sky and created the Milky Way.

From Jackson D: *With child: wisdom and traditions for pregnancy, birth and motherhood,* San Francisco, 1999, Chronicle Books.

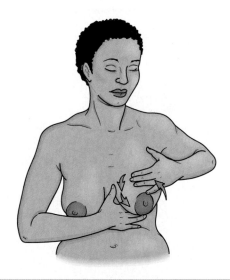

FIGURE 14-6 ■ Gentle effleurage with the fingertips around the breast 6 times relieves congestion.

Lactation does not occur until after birth when there is a decline in estrogen. A precolostrum can be found within the breast tissue by the third month of gestation, and colostrum can be expressed by week 16[11] (Figure 14-5 and Box 14-1).

In early pregnancy, prone positioning on the massage table might be uncomfortable for women with sensitive breasts. The practitioner can place a rolled towel across the woman's shoulders to elevate her upper chest. It is advisable to ask permission before massaging the client's breasts. If she declines, the practitioner can demonstrate the massage over the clothing so she can do this lymphatic drainage technique on her own. Breast massage should also include myofascial stretching across her chest, intercostals, and thoracic spine (when she is turned to a supine position). The practitioner avoids all contact to her nipples and areolae. Breast massage is as follows:

- First, the practitioner performs light lymphatic effleurage around the base of her breasts 6 times (Figure 14-6).
- Then, the practitioner does light circular pétrissage around the base of her breasts 6 times.

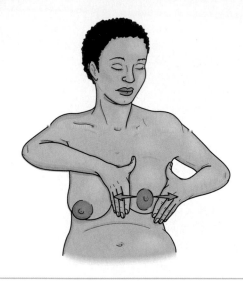

FIGURE 14-7 ■ Gliding effleurage helps reduce swelling of the breasts. Contact with the areolae should be avoided.

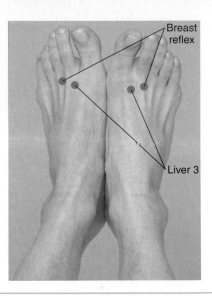

FIGURE 14-9 ■ Liver 3, found between the big and second toes, is a contraindicated point during pregnancy. However, light stimulation—one count of 6-10—can help reduce breast swelling and engorgement. Lateral to liver 3 on both feet is the breast reflex point that can safely be held to a count of 6 to 10, repeating 6 to 10 times.

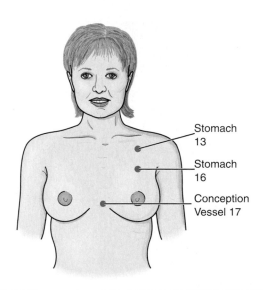

FIGURE 14-8 ■ Each of these acupuncture points (stomach 13, stomach 16, and conception vessel 17) can be pressed for a count of 6 to 10 for 6 to 10 repetitions.

■ Next, the practitioner performs a light effleurage glide outward from the outside of her areola (on the face of a clock, this would be 9 to 3), followed with light effleurage glide superior and inferior (12 to 6). Each glide is performed 6 times (Figure 14-7).

■ Acupuncture point stomach 13 (St13) is found under the middle of the clavicle, and stomach 16 (St16) is found 3 inches below St13 at the beginning of the breast.

Conception vessel 17 (CV17) is located midsternum and can be stimulated to treat breast soreness. Each point should be pressed for a count of 6 to 10, repeating 6 to 10 times in total. Special attention should be paid to the sensitivity of the sternum; CV17 should be pressed softly at first, with pressure gradually getting deeper (Figure 14-8).

■ The foot reflex to the breasts should be pressed for a count of 6 to 10, repeating a total of 6 to 10 times. Medial to the breast reflex is liver 3, which is a contraindicated acupuncture point. However, in prenatal discomforts associated with excess water, liver 3 can be lightly stimulated to encourage the body to absorb the fluid. Liver 3 can be pressed for a count of 6 to 10 only one time (Figure 14-9).

Relief for Breast Engorgement

Bodyworkers can remind a client to stand in the shower and let warm water cascade over her shoulders to ease breast engorgement. A warm ginger compress placed on the breasts dilates the blood vessels and reduces engorgement. The recipe for a warm ginger compress is as follows:

- Grate one cup of raw ginger root (peeled) and tie it up in cheesecloth.
- Place the ginger in 1 quart of water that is taken up to the boiling point. (It is important not to let the water boil which will destroy ginger's value.)
- Let the ginger steep until the water turns a pale yellow color, about one-half hour. Squeeze the ginger out.
- When the water temperature is warm but comfortable, take two washcloths and place them in the ginger water.
- Wring them out (make sure the water temperature is not too hot) and place them over the breasts. Keep the water warm and use the compress for 15 minutes, replacing as it cools.[12,13]

Carpal Tunnel Syndrome and de Quervain's Syndrome

Carpal tunnel syndrome is entrapment of the median nerve at the wrist, affecting one or both hands. During pregnancy, carpal tunnel syndrome is caused by fluid retention and swelling of the hands, protracted neck compressing the lower cervical vertebrae, or relaxin's effect on softening the flexor and extensor retinaculum that can no longer support the carpals. Repetitive stress and poor postural habits may also be culpable. Symptoms include numbness, tingling, and pain in the arms, hands, or fingers and seem to be worse at night.[14,15]

The best way to treat carpal tunnel syndrome is to avoid positions that hyperextend the wrist and put additional pressure on the median nerve. Antiinflammatory creams, cortisone injections, splinting, and joint immobilization are also used to treat carpal tunnel syndrome. It can become so painful that surgery to remove fibrous bands compressing the nerve may be the final resort for some women.

De Quervain's syndrome, also called washerwoman's sprain, is swelling and inflammation of the tendons or the tendon sheaths that abduct the thumb. It is caused by repetitive use of the wrist, swelling of pregnancy, protracted neck, and the effects of relaxin on the retinaculum. Symptoms include pain and weakness on the side of the thumb and at the base of the thumb that worsens with movement. Rest, warm soaks, splinting, and immobilizing the wrist and nonsteroidal antiinflammatory medications help in a small percentage of cases. Injections of corticosteroids into the tendon sheath help nearly 80% to 90% of sufferers. Surgery may be an option for some.[16]

Some women avoid hand complications during pregnancy but develop them during the postpartum period. Maintaining proper body mechanics and keeping the wrists as neutral as possible will help a pregnant or postpartum woman prevent these painful and sometimes debilitating syndromes (Figure 14-10).[17] Swelling of the hands can be relieved with lymphatic drainage massage on the arms. Postural considerations must include retracting the cervical spine and encouraging better alignment by recruiting the abdominal muscles correctly. Massage treatment for these common discomforts is as follows:

- To help drain the arm of excess fluid, the practitioner starts the treatment with lymphatic drainage massage. The practitioner can lightly effleurage the client's arm from the elbow to the shoulders 5 to 7 times. The pressure should be light, approximately 10 gm, on the arms.
- The practitioner follows with circular pétrissage around the elbow and shoulder. To help the valves of the lymphatic system close more efficiently, lymphatic compression should be performed (using the same light pressure) from the elbow to the shoulder. Each compression should be held for a count of 10, with 4 compressions on each arm.
- A few more effleurage strokes should be done on the arms before moving to the forearm.

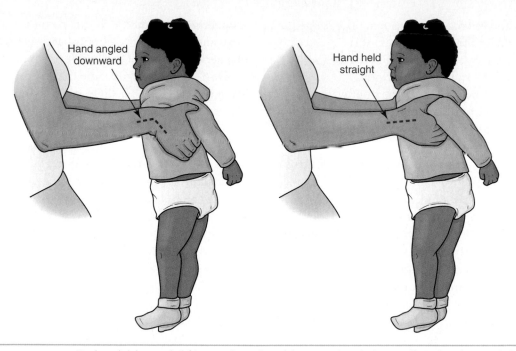

FIGURE 14-10 ■ Hands angled downward *(left)* strains the tendons of the wrist and can lead to carpal tunnel syndrome or de Quervain's syndrome. Neutral wrists *(right)* minimize the strain on the tendons.

- The same routine is followed on the forearm but the strokes should be taken all the way to the shoulder.
- The woman's hands should be massaged, taking care to keep her wrist in a neutral position. To stretch the palmar fascia, her hand should be turned palm down, with the practitioner's fingertips placed next to each other in the center of her palm. The practitioner should not massage or pull her fingers outward. Instead, the stroking should be done in the direction of her heart.
- Excess lubrication should be wiped from the practitioner's hands. To perform a muscle-stripping, or myofascial stretching, from the client's wrist to elbow on each side, the practitioner uses his or her thumb, fingertips, or ulnar surface of the hand. Myofascial or muscular congestion on the palmar surface of the forearm near the elbow is often palpable. This tissue should be stretched longitudinally, laterally, and diagonally to ease the stress pattern.
- Acupuncture point large intestine 11 is on the belly of the brachioradialis, and small

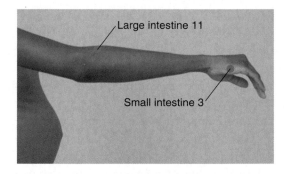

FIGURE 14-11 ■ After lymphatic drainage on the arm is performed and muscle stripping has been done, the practitioner presses both acupuncture points, large intestine 11 and small intestine 3, simultaneously to treat carpal tunnel syndrome or de Quervain's syndrome. These points should be held for a 6 to 10 count, repeating 6 to 10 times.

intestine 3 is midway between the first knuckle and ulnar head under the metacarpal. These points treat hand pain. Both points should be held at the same time for a count of 6 to 10, repeating 6 to 10 times (Figure 14-11).
- The massage is finished with range of motion movements at the neck, shoulder, elbow, and wrists—all along the course of the median nerve.

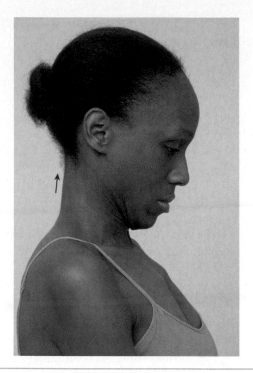

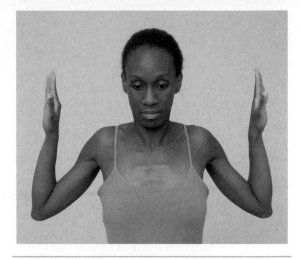

FIGURE 14-13 ■ The "chicken" helps to realign the cervical and thoracic spine.

FIGURE 14-12 ■ Neck retraction elongates and decompresses the lower cervical spine.

Physical therapy exercises are important in preventing and treating hand discomforts. The practitioner can instruct the pregnant client on the following exercises:

- Neck retraction helps to realign the cervical vertebrae that are compressed and protracted during pregnancy. The client tucks the chin in, elongating the cervical spine and holding for a count of 10 (Figure 14-12).[18]
- The "chicken" stretches tightened pectorals, strengthens upper back muscles, and decompresses the lower segments of the cervical spine. The client tucks the chin in, elongating the cervical spine, then pushes the chest out and lifts it, pinching the shoulder blades together. The client bends the arms and pulls the hands back toward the shoulders, elbows close to the body with palms facing outward. She should hold for a count of 10 and release (Figure 14-13). A variation is the "dead chicken," in which the head is extended back, with her face parallel to the ceiling. The client holds for a count of 10 and releases (Figure 14-14).[18]

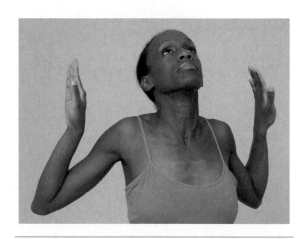

FIGURE 14-14 ■ The "dead chicken" provides additional neck stretching.

- The rapid movements of the median nerve exercise glide the median nerve through its sheath and soft tissues. The client raises both arms to shoulder level with palms facing forward. The hands are flexed backward as far as possible and released. This should be done 10 times in rapid succession (Figure 14-15).[18]
- The radial nerve glide is performed by raising both arms to shoulder level with the palms facing backward. The client grasps the fingers around both thumbs and forms a fist, flexing the wrists rapidly back and forth 10 times (Figure 14-16).[18]

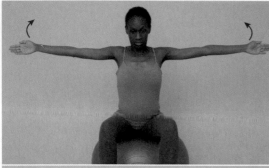

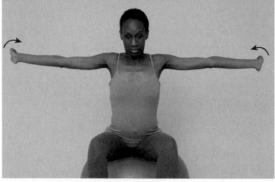

FIGURE 14-15   ■   The median nerve glide.

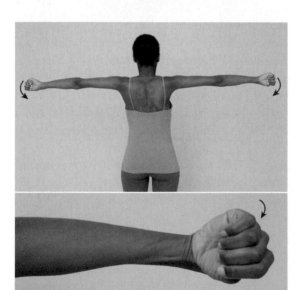

FIGURE 14-16   ■   The radial nerve glide.

■ The ulnar nerve glide relieves pressure on the ulnar nerve. The client makes the "okay" sign with the thumbs and index fingers of both hands and then turns the fingers toward the face and place the "circles" over the eyes. The other fingers rest

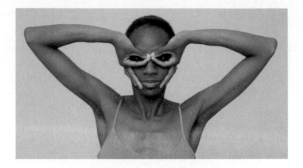

FIGURE 14-17   ■   The ulnar nerve glide.

on the cheeks, and the elbows are pushed back as far as possible. This position should be held for a count of ten (Figure 14-17).[18]

■ Fist extension exercises allow the tendons in the wrist to glide freely during movement (Figure 14-18).[15]

■ Stimulating acupuncture point liver 3 for a single count of 6 to 10 can help absorb excess fluid (see Figure 14-9).

All massage practitioners and bodyworkers can benefit from doing the neck and hand exercises in Figures 14-11 through 14-18 at least once a day. These exercises will promote hand health and help the practitioner achieve career longevity.

Edema

Edema, or swelling, is normal during pregnancy. By the end of the third trimester, most women have a 40% increase in interstitial fluid in their bodies, particularly in the legs and feet. Edema is aggravated by myofascial restrictions, compression of the heavy uterus on the iliac and femoral veins, the effects of progesterone on smooth muscles slowing the efficiency of lymph vessels, prolonged standing, hot weather, restrictive clothing, poor diet, excessive sodium in the diet, lack of exercise, and poor posture. Edema during pregnancy is defined as an accumulation of fluid (water) in the interstitial tissues. The lymph system is intact and healthy but overworked and affected by progesterone and excessive fluid. Lymphedema, however, is an accumulation of fluid and protein in the tissues brought about by mechanical insufficiency as the transport capacity of the lymph system cannot remove the water or protein from the interstitial spaces. This pathological condition is caused by surgery, radiation, inflammation, or trauma but not pregnancy.[19]

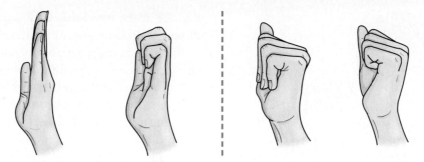

FIGURE 14-18 ■ Fist extension exercises. Start with the fingers in a straight position *(left)*, then moves the fingers into a hook fist position *(second from left)*, continues flexing the fingers *(right)*, and ends with a full fist *(far right)*. This exercise should held for 5 seconds and repeat 5 more times.

Practitioners should be concerned about the quality of the pregnant woman's swelling. Before each treatment, it is essential to test for pitting edema by pressing above the ankle at the site of swelling for a slow count to 5. The depression should fill in, and the skin's normal color should return in 10 to 30 seconds. If the depression remains, the massage should not be done. the woman's doctor or midwife should be called immediately. Massage should also be avoided if her upper body and face swell during early pregnancy. The pitting may be symptomatic of preeclampsia, a serious and life-threatening condition, that affects almost 25% of all pregnancies (Box 14-2). Lymphatic drainage massage must always accompany prenatal massage (and postpartum care for 8 to 10 weeks postpartum) of the legs whether or not edema is present. Two major factors are involved: increased interstitial fluid and fibrinogenic activity.

The bodyworker can instruct clients to do the following to reduce swelling:

- Treat liver 3 lightly for one count of 6 to 10.
- Increase water intake to 8 to 12 glasses daily.
- Elevate the legs or hands above heart level.
- Lie on the left side 2 to 3 times daily for 15 minutes to increase lymph absorption.
- Soak in a tub, hand, or foot bath with Epsom salts. Dissolve 1 part salts in 2 parts boiling water, and add this solution to the tub.
- Increase cardiovascular activity to encourage speedier lymph absorption.

BOX 14-2 *Preeclampsia and Eclampsia*

Preeclampsia is a pregnancy specific hypertensive syndrome that develops after the 20 weeks' gestation. It is a multisystem, vaso-spastic disease of reduced organ perfusion and increased hypertension and proteinuria.* One of the first signs of preeclampsia is a rise in blood pressure, or a systolic reading greater than 140 mm HG or diastolic pressure greater than 90 mm HG.* It is unique to human pregnancy, and certain high risk factors involved in preeclampsia are first-time pregnancy, multifetal pregnancy, maternal age under 19 or over 40, diabetes, Rh incompatibility, chronic renal disease, chronic hypertension, obesity, or a family history of preeclampsia.*

Eclampsia is the onset of seizure activity or coma in a preeclamptic woman who never had seizures before pregnancy.*†

Massage is contraindicated with the presence of preeclampsia or eclampsia. The client must see her health care provider at once.

*From Diagnosis and management of preeclampsia and eclampsia, *ACOG Practice Bulletin #33,* Washington, DC, 2002, American College of Obstetricians and Gynecologists.
†From Roberts J: Pregnancy-related hypertension. In Creasy R, Resnik R, eds: *Maternal-fetal medicine,* ed 4, Philadelphia, 1999, Saunders.

- Do pelvic tilts to reduce the weight of the uterus on the blood vessels in the pelvis and abdomen. Rocking movements promote blood circulation.
- Soak in a large tub or pool to reduce swelling for up to 48 hours because the hydrostatic pressure of the water reduces edema and increases diuresis.
- Wear supportive hosiery.

Deep abdominal breathing enhances lymphatic drainage of the thoracic, abdominal, and pelvic

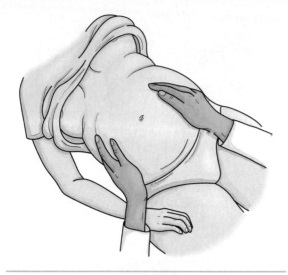

FIGURE 14-19 ■ During pregnancy, contact breathing is used to help affect lumbar lymph trunks for enhanced lymph absorption.

organs and extremities by influencing intraabdominal and intrathoracic pressure. During pregnancy, deep abdominal lymphatic drainage treatment is contraindicated but is substituted with contact breathing to affect the lumbar lymph trunks with a stretch and pull stimulation (Figure 14-19).[12,20] The massage routine described is this text is sufficient to address normal swelling during pregnancy but should not be construed as the complex manual lymphatic drainage technique, such as the Vodder technique. The massage here follows similar principles but is not meant to treat lymphedema or other lymphatic pathologies.

Lymphatic Massage for Edema of the Extremities

DVD

The light pressure of lymphatic massage is surprising to many bodyworkers who use deep pressure techniques. It is important to recognize that the system and tissues practitioners are working with are superficial, and pressure beyond these structures bypasses the system massage during pregnancy addresses and may actually do more harm than good. The arm receives this treatment when swelling is problematic or with the presence of carpal tunnel syndrome or de Quervain's syndrome. Unlike the legs, the hand and arm massage can be firm when edematous conditions are not present, but it is suggested that the practitioner begin the

massage at the proximal portion of the limb and direct the pressure toward the heart.

The basic manual lymphatic drainage principles characteristic to this technique are as follows:

- The proximal area is always treated before the distal area. In the leg, this means starting at the knee and working up to the hip. In the arm, the practitioner begins at the elbow and works toward the shoulder.
- Pressure must be limited to 30 to 40 mm Hg (between 5 to 10 gm).
- The direction of pressure in the limbs is toward the heart.
- The techniques and variations are repeated rhythmically about 5 to 7 times.
- The pressure phase of a circle lasts longer than the relaxation phase.
- There should be no visible reddening, or hyperemia, of the skin.
- There should not be any pain from this gentle technique.
- Circles are made with the skin and not on the skin.
- The skin contact areas should not be too smooth, rough or moist. Only a few drops of lubrication should be used. This equalizes the moisture of the skin. Traditional Swedish massage lubrication that permits gliding over the skin is excessive for lymphatic drainage.[21]

Most classic massage strokes are too aggressive for this technique. Swedish (classic) massage and manual lymph drainage are two distinct bodywork systems that should not be interchanged or confused with each other. Swedish massage encourages an increase in arterial blood flow accompanied by blood capillary pressure and subsequent increase in ultrafiltration of water in the area of the blood capillaries. This causes more fluid to accumulate in the interstitial spaces, counterproductive to the massage practitioner's goals with pregnant women.

In addition, the superficial lymph vessels are vulnerable to external pressure and damage to lymphatic anchoring filaments and endothelial lining can result from deep pressure.[22,23] The following massage is slow and rhythmic. The practitioner performs the following:

- Light effleurage from the knee (elbow) to the hip (shoulder), repeat only 5 to 7 times.

- Light circular pétrissage at the knee (elbow) 5 to 7 times.
- Light effleurage from knee (elbow) to hip (shoulder).
- Light lymphatic compression from knee to hip, 6 compressions per limb, and each compression is held for a count of 10 (4 compressions at the arm, each compression is held for a count of 10).
- Light effleurage from knee to hip (elbow to shoulder).
- Light effleurage from ankle to hip (wrist to shoulder), 5 to 7 times.
- Light circular pétrissage at the ankle (wrist).
- Light effleurage from ankle (wrist) to hip (shoulder)
- Light lymphatic compression from ankle to hip with 6 compressions each at the leg and thigh (a total of 12 on the leg), 4 compressions are the forearm and arm (with a total of 8 on the arm)
- Light effleurage on the entire leg (ankle to hip) or arm (wrist to shoulder).
- Light effleurage of the foot to hip, 5 to 7 times (fingers to shoulder), effleurage the muscles between toes and fingers.
- Range of motion on the foot and toes or hands and fingers. The Achilles tendon is stretched, the plantar fascia is stretched, and the foot is lightly twisted.
- Final light effleurage of the entire limb, from foot to hip, fingers to shoulder.

Fatigue and Insomnia

Newly pregnant women feel tired and in need of more sleep and rest. The demands of pregnancy, the change in metabolism, hormonal adjustments, and emotional highs and lows all contribute to fatigue and weariness.[20] As pregnancy progresses, the additional weight she carries, her postural shifting, and accompanying muscle aches and pains, coupled with the difficulty of finding a comfortable position at night, all add to her **fatigue.** Fatigue can also be symptomatic of more serious conditions such as anemia, nutritional deficiencies, or dehydration. **Insomnia** usually occurs in the latter part of pregnancy when labor and birth are near and the gravida cannot sleep, or does not get enough

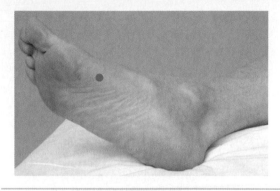

FIGURE 14-20 ■ Spleen 3 can help ward off fatigue in the early months of pregnancy.

restful sleep, because her mind is active with concerns about labor and delivery. The following can help the pregnant woman relax and get more rest:

- A light, general massage to oxygenate the blood will help energize her. The practitioner should take care not to work too deeply, which may further exhaust her.
- The practitioner should massage spleen 3, especially in early pregnancy, to help balance her hormones (Figure 14-20).
- Acupuncture point governing vessel 20 (at the crown of the head to draw the energy upward) (Figure 14-21), pericardium 8 (the "Palace of Anxiety" in the center of both palms—in hand reflexology, this is the solar plexus), pericardium 6 (1½ inches below the wrist—the morning sickness point), and heart 7 (at the head of the ulna) can all be stimulated for a count of 6 to 10, repeated 6 to 10 times (Figure 14-22).
- Light foot massage can also be stimulating.
- The pregnant woman should drink at least 8 to 12 glasses of water daily to maintain adequate hydration.
- The client should eat a wide variety of wholesome foods to ensure adequate nutrition. Iron-rich foods should also be included in her daily diet. Eating small but frequent meals throughout the day is easier on her gastrointestinal system.
- For insomnia, in addition to the above-mentioned treatments, it may be necessary to refer her to a psychologist or counselor to help her deal with her fears and concerns.

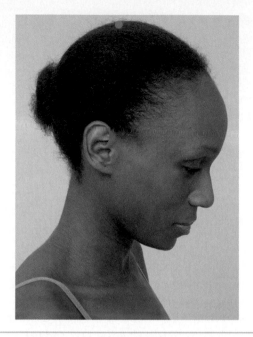

FIGURE 14-21 ■ Governing vessel 20, at the crown of the head, draws energy upward to help fight fatigue and general weakness.

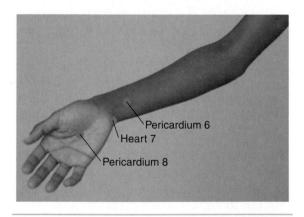

FIGURE 14-22 ■ Pericardium 8, in the center of the palm, pericardium 6 on the forearm, and heart 7 on the ulnar aspect of the wrist can help ward off fatigue.

Gastrointestinal Disturbances

Gastrointestinal disturbances (constipation, esophageal reflux, gas, and heartburn) plague many women during pregnancy. These conditions can be very uncomfortable, and some women find them embarrassing to discuss, but gentle coaxing can provide the practitioner with the information needed to help them.

High levels of progesterone slow the emptying of food through the intestines, creating a situation known as *decreased gastrointestinal motility* or *hypoperistalsis.*[9] The slower movement allows the body to absorb more water but that results in harder stools. **Constipation** (difficulty or inability to have a bowel movement) may also result from poor diet and food choices, lack of fluids, iron supplementation, decreased activity, abdominal distention by the uterus, and displacement and compression of the intestines.[10] Increasing water consumption raises the amount of water in the intestines, resulting in faster bowel evacuation. In the later stages of pregnancy, the weight and pressure of the uterus compressing the intestines adds to the sluggishness of the bowel.

Intestinal gas and bloating often accompany constipation. This discomfort may increase as pregnancy progresses as the uterus and bloated intestines try to fill the same limited space in the abdominal cavity.

Progesterone, causing decreased tone and movement of the stomach, is also involved in heartburn, or pyrosis. When foods and acids travel back into the lower esophagus as the stomach contracts, esophageal reflux, or acid reflux disorder, results. As the uterus grows and pushes against these digestive organs, symptoms of heartburn and esophageal reflux exacerbate. Practitioners can help clients alleviate some of the gastrointestinal discomforts with the following suggestions:

- Clients should be encouraged to drink at least 8 to 12 glasses of water daily and eat small but frequent meals slowly throughout the day.
- Clients should be encouraged to eat foods rich in natural digestive enzymes and natural fiber, such as papaya, mango, and grapefruit, or foods with live lactobacillus culture, such as yogurt.
- Clients should be encouraged to avoid foods that may produce gas such as cabbage, cauliflower, peppers, and carbonated beverages. Fried and greasy foods are difficult to digest and should also be avoided.
- Clients should increase their physical activity and exercise level to encourage improved peristaltic activity.
- Clients should be encouraged to use postures for abdominal pressure (see Figures 14-1 and 14-2) to relieve the compression

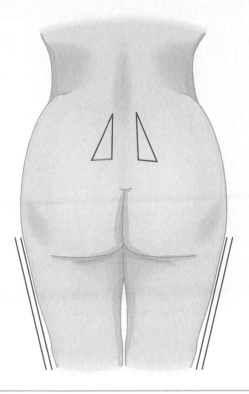

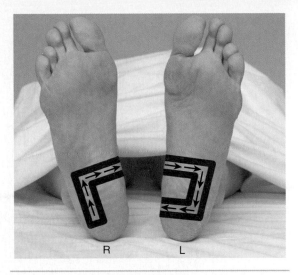

FIGURE 14-24 ■ To stimulate the intestinal foot reflexes, the practitioner massages up the right foot (the ascending colon) and across the foot (transverse colon). At the same point on the left foot, massage is done across the foot (transverse colon), down and across (descending colon). The flexures might feel tender if the pregnant woman is constipated or has intestinal gas.

FIGURE 14-23 ■ Massaging the neurolymphatic reflexes for the tensor fascia lata and colon may help stimulate normal intestinal peristaltic activity.

of the uterus on the intestines and support improved peristalsis.

- Clients who suffer from heartburn should be encouraged to lie on the right side to allow gravity to empty the stomach faster. The hands and knees position relieves gas by using gravity to pull the uterus away from the stomach, allowing the contents to pass more easily into the intestines rather than refluxing into the esophagus. Some women find relief by eating or drinking dairy products before a meal to coat their stomachs.
- Chamomile or mint teas can be soothing to the digestive tract.

Some women with serious heartburn or esophageal reflux feel more comfortable receiving their massages in a sitting position. Myofascial stretching of the lower back and massage to the tensor fascia lata will ease lumbar congestion and encourage normal intestinal function by stimulating the neurolymphatic reflex (Figure 14-23). Massage should include stimulation of the foot intestinal reflexes to stimulate peristalsis (Figure 14-24). Massage treatment for heartburn or esophageal reflux is as follows:

- A light abdominal massage can loosen myofascial restrictions, encouraging normal peristaltic activity.
- In a prone position, kenbiki of the lower segment of the erector spinae may encourage peristaltic activity (Figure 14-25). This gentle, wave-like rocking stroke can be performed two ways: heel of hand and fingertips or with the fingertips. Hands should be soft and relaxed.
- Practitioners place the heels of their hands on one side of the lower erector spinae muscle and push the muscle toward the spine. With the fingertips on the opposite side of the spine, the erector spinae should be pulled in toward the spine. The stroke should be light and rhythmic. When doing this stroke, the fingertips push and pull on the same side of the spine.

Gestational Glucose Intolerance

Gestational glucose intolerance (GGI) is not a contraindication for massage, although risk factors for the mother and fetus are increased. Fetal

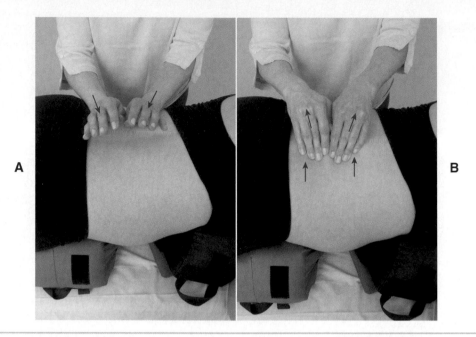

FIGURE 14-25 ■ Kenbiki is a Japanese massage applied to the lower back muscles to stimulate peristaltic activity of the intestines and can only be administered on a client in a prone position.

risk factors include hydramnios, elevated fetal weight gain, newborn hypoglycemia, and premature membrane rupture and stillbirth, regardless of how mild the maternal reaction may be. Maternal complications may include induced labor, elevated chances of cesarean section, and compromised carbohydrate metabolism in 35% to 50% of women with GGI over the next 15 years.[6] This condition of pregnancy affects about 5% of the population.[24] The symptoms are similar to adult-onset diabetes: excessive thirst, hunger, and frequent urination. Because glucose levels drop after a massage, the practitioner must be vigilant after each treatment to make sure that the client's glucose level is not too low. Although the client may appear levelheaded and unimpaired, a drop in glucose level can be very dangerous. To avoid an injury or serious accident from impaired reactions and decisions, practitioners should provide clients with a nourishing snack or fruit juice before they leave the office.

Headaches

Headaches are another common complaint of pregnancy. Most of them occur during the first two trimesters and generally subside or disappear as she starts the third trimester.[9] They can be mild or more intense like a migraine. Some migraine sufferers often find their headaches are more frequent and severe during pregnancy, whereas others actually experience relief from these symptoms. Over-the-counter products used to treat migraines are not safe during pregnancy. Any medications containing ergot or ibuprofen (Advil, Motrin) should be avoided.

Hormonal fluctuations and the intense emotional and physical changes of pregnancy can cause headaches. Other factors include stress; musculoskeletal tensions and trigger points, especially in the neck and upper back areas; temporomandibular joint (TMJ) subluxations; fatigue; insomnia; eye strain; constipation; and nasal and sinus congestion.

The practitioner must be vigilant about prenatal headaches because they can be symptomatic of pregnancy-induced hypertension. If the following measures fail to reduce the severity or frequency and the headache persists, the client should notify her health care provider.

■ A general massage with special attention to the neck, especially the occipital ridge, head, face, and scalp, is soothing. The trigger points in the neck, scapulae, and upper back should be treated.

Corrective posture will minimize the typical neck protraction of pregnancy and ease neck and upper back strain.[25]

- Craniosacral therapy can be used to address headache symptoms.
- The jaw should be treated for TMJ problems. The masseter muscles should be massaged, and any trigger points can be released.
- The foot reflexes (see Figure 14-24) should be treated for constipation to relieve intestinal congestion that might cause a headache. The client should be instructed to do the pelvic tilt to bring the fetus off the intestines and encourage improved peristaltic activity.
- Sinus points on the face (Figure 14-26) and reflexes on the tips of the fingers and toes should be treated to help drain the sinuses. Vascular engorgement, increased mucus production, constipation, and slower mucus drainage all contribute to sinus congestion. If sinus congestion is suspected as a cause of headaches, the client should increase her fluid intake to 8 to 12 glasses of water daily, avoid excessive dairy products, do a sinus flush, or use a facial steamer for 20 minutes to encourage sinus drainage.
- The client should be referred to an acupuncturist who can assist her with headache relief.[26]
- Relaxation exercises can help control tension headaches.

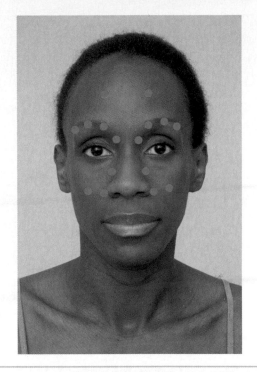

FIGURE 14-26 ■ Each point on the face can be held for a count of 6 to 10, repeating 6 to 10 times to treat nasal and sinus congestion.

Hemorrhoids

In late pregnancy, uterine compression of the iliac veins and inferior vena cava results in increased venous pressure and reduced blood flow to the legs (except when a woman is side-lying). These adaptations contribute to leg and foot swelling, varicose veins (swollen, distended and twisted veins) in the legs and vulva, and **hemorrhoids** (varicosities of the anus).[10] Lightening also establishes pressure-related symptoms such as dependent edema and hemorrhoids.[8] Other factors that contribute are constipation or straining during a bowel movement, a multifetal pregnancy, and abdominal pressure. Hemorrhoids are extremely common in postpartum recovery as a result of hard pushing during labor. Practitioners can relieve this common discomfort of pregnancy through the following:

- Lymphatic drainage on the legs eases lymph congestion and increases lymph reabsorption.
- The sacral lift takes the pressure off the pelvic floor muscles and is particularly helpful in treating hemorrhoids. Care must be taken to avoid pressing directly on the hemorrhoids while performing this lift.
- Reflex points on the feet can be pressed for a 6 to 10 count, repeating 6 to 10 times (Figure 14-27).
- Acupuncture point, governing vessel 20, can be stimulated (see Figure 14-21 for the crown of the head). This point is pressed for a count of 6 to 10, repeating 6 to 10 times.
- The tensor fascia lata is the muscle relating to the intestines (see Figure 14-23). The iliotibial band above the patellae can be

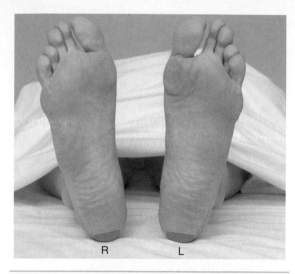

FIGURE 14-27 ■ The reflex point for the treatment of hemorrhoids is found on the heels of both feet. This is also the sciatic nerve reflex. Each point can be held for a 6-10 count, repeating 6 to 10 times.

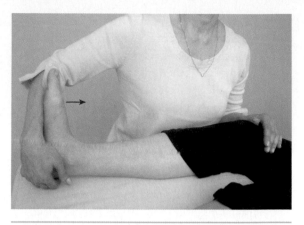

FIGURE 14-28 ■ Gently stretching the gastrocnemius and Achilles tendon treats a calf cramp.

Leg Cramps

Leg cramps, as well as thigh, foot, and toe cramps, and **charley horses** usually occur in latter pregnancy, often during periods of rest or sleep.[20] These cramps are caused by musculoskeletal strain, fatigue in the calf muscles created by the hyperextension of the knees, compromised leg circulation, or electrolyte imbalance and can be very painful and alarming, especially when they rouse the client from sleep. Restless leg syndrome affects about 10% of the pregnant population within 10 to 20 minutes of getting into bed. The cause is unknown but anemia is suspected.[27] Practitioners can offer clients the following to relieve these common discomforts of pregnancy:

- The lymphatic leg massage should include
  [DVD] gentle stretching of the Achilles tendon to relieve the cramp and stretch the gastrocnemius and soleus muscles (Figure 14-28). A gentle rolling of the legs muscles also loosens the painful cramp (Figure 14-29). Foot and toe cramps can be relieved by stretching the toes and plantar fascia.
- Musculoskeletal imbalance can be addressed by encouraging the client to recruit her transverse abdominis muscle to minimize postural shifting and support better alignment. The client can practice posterior pelvic tilting to lengthen the rectus femoris and release the posterior pull of the femur that allows the knees to lock.

> **BOX 14-3   *Hemorrhoid Treatment***
>
> Macrobiotic medicine suggests an albi plaster to reduce hemorrhoids. Taro, yucca, or white potatoes can be substituted. The plaster is a combination of 50% grated albi (or taro, yucca, or white potato), 45% white flour, and 5% grated ginger. Mix all the ingredients into a cheese or cotton cloth and wear the plaster for at least 4 hours, changing to a fresh plaster after 2 hours.[13]
>
> Another effective treatment is to peel a white potato and shape it like a suppository. The pregnant woman places the raw potato suppository into the anus and wears it overnight. The potato will disintegrate, soften the stool, and shrink the hemorrhoids. This is not advised in postpartum care until perineal swelling has subsided.

rubbed vigorously to stimulate the reflex for hemorrhoids.
- Witch hazel, lemon juice, vitamin E, Bach Flower "Rescue Remedy" (a floral remedy), calendula (a homeopathic remedy), or over-the-counter astringents can be applied directly on the hemorrhoids to ease pain, swelling, and itching.
- 15 drops of geranium and 5 drops of cypress diluted in 2 tablespoons of base (vegetable) oil can be topically applied to the hemorrhoids (Box 14-3).

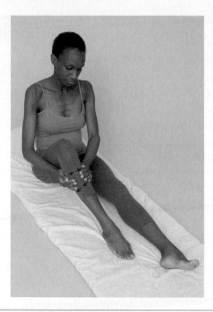

FIGURE 14-29 ■ A gentle calf roll will help relieve a calf cramp.

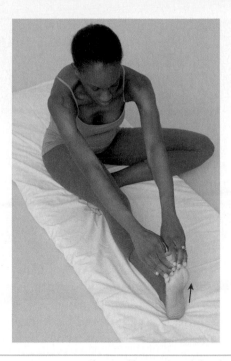

FIGURE 14-31 ■ The seated leg stretch can help reduce painful leg cramps.

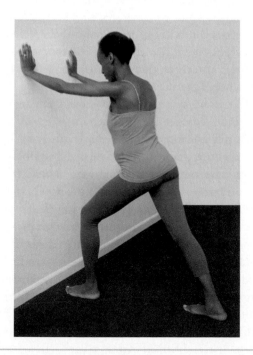

FIGURE 14-30 ■ Stretching the calves can reduce the frequency and severity of leg cramps.

- Posterior pelvic tilting, prone positioning on the bodySupport cushions, and postures for abdominal pressure move the uterus off the iliac and femoral veins, which helps restore circulation to the legs.
- Imbalances of calcium, phosphorus, magnesium, and potassium are often the cause of these painful cramps or nervous legs. The client should be encouraged to eat a wide variety of foods rich in these essential nutrients and avoid carbonated drinks that may interfere with assimilation of these electrolytes. Raised phosphate levels are implicated in cases of leg cramps and reducing dairy is helpful.[28]
- Comfortable shoes that promote good posture are recommended.
- Clients should avoid excessive plantarflexion of the foot that may cause a cramp to occur. Exercises that elongate the legs muscles, such as wall push-ups and leg stretches, are suggested before bed (Figures 14-30 and 14-31).
- Support stockings during the day may be helpful for some women.[9,12,20]

Morning Sickness

Almost 70% of pregnant women are afflicted with nausea or vomiting, or morning sickness, primarily during the first trimester of pregnancy.[29] Although it can occur at any time throughout gestation, these symptoms can start as early as 4 to 6 weeks' gestation and get worse as the weeks progress. For

BOX 14-4   *Risks Factors Contributing to Nausea and Vomiting*

- Multiple pregnancies
- History of nausea and vomiting in a previous pregnancy
- Nausea or vomiting as a side effect of birth control pills
- History of motion sickness
- Genetic predisposition to nausea and vomiting during pregnancy
- Migraine headaches

BOX 14-5   *Signs of Dehydration*

- Vomiting does not ease.
- Frequency of urination is less and the urine is darker in color.
- Mouth, eyes, and skin are dry.
- Fatigue and weakness increase.
- Mental acuity lowers.
- Feeling faint.
- Cannot keep food or fluid down for 24 hours.

From Hassid P: *Textbook for childbirth educators,* Philadelphia, 1978, Harper and Row.

half of the women who suffer from nausea and vomiting, the symptoms abate and disappear by the end of the first trimester or the beginning of the second. The remainder of women might feel nauseous for another month or longer. For still other women, nausea and vomiting comes and goes throughout their pregnancies.[30] The severity of morning sickness varies from mild queasiness to severe vomiting. The fetus is usually unaffected, but expectant mothers are miserable.

Some studies have indicated that those women affected with nausea and vomiting are less likely to miscarry or have preterm labor or intrauterine growth restriction.[31,32] One theory was that nausea evolved to protect mother and fetus from toxins, which naturally exist in certain foods, that may cause birth defects. These foods are meat, which leads the list of prenatal food aversions,[32] poultry, fish, eggs, fruits, vegetables, and spices.

Other theories suggest the elevated levels of human chorionic gonadotrophin (hCG) during early pregnancy may contribute to nausea and vomiting. Nausea seems to peak at the same time hCG levels are highest and starts to decline as these hormonal levels decrease. Estrogen may also be a factor in nausea or vomiting in pregnancy.

Heightened sense of smell and the sensitivity to odors may also be a cause of nausea. Gastric changes and an association between *Helicobacter pylori,* a gastrointestinal bacteria that can cause ulcers, and severe nausea have also been suggested[30] (Box 14-4).

When vomiting continues and causes serious dehydration, starvation, debilitation, and excessive

weight loss before 20 weeks' gestation, the condition is called *hyperemesis gravidarum,* and in the United States, it affects about 0.3% to 2% or 5 per 1000 pregnancies. It seems to be more common in westernized countries than rural regions.[33] The dehydration may result in a maternal electrolyte imbalance and she may require hospitalization and intravenous infusion to control the dehydration and prevent preterm labor. All foods and oral intake of fluids is stopped until the women can retain small amounts of fluid.

The causes of hyperemesis gravidarum are controversial. Before 1940, hyperemesis gravidarum was a major cause of maternal death. Some doctors theorize that there may be a psychological component for those women who cannot accept the pregnancy, have personality disorders, relationship problems, major depression and psychiatric illnesses. Some women with hyperemesis gravidarum have clinical hyperthyroidism. Estradiol levels may be implicated, as well as gastric and hepatic functions.[33] Other risk factors are previous pregnancies with hyperemesis gravidarum, obesity, multiple pregnancy, trophoblastic disease and nulliparity. The risk of hyperemesis gravidarum decreases with advanced maternal age[33] (Box 14-5).

Massage is contraindicated when a client is feeling nauseous or is vomiting. Practitioners can offer clients the following to relieve the nausea and vomiting of pregnancy:

- If the client has specific times when she is not nauseous, massage can be done during the time the queasiness has passed. Pericardium 6 (P6) and spleen 3 (Sp3) acupuncture points should be included in massage treatment. P6 is a stomach point, and Sp3

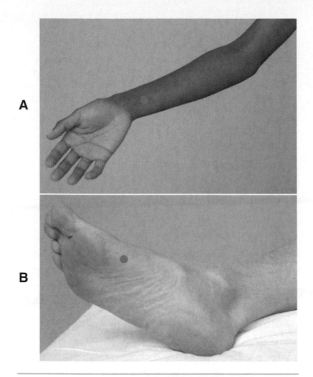

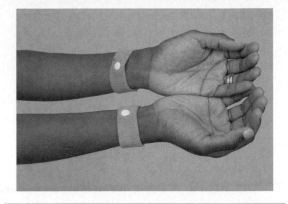

FIGURE 14-33 ■ "Sea bands" can be worn on pericardium 6 to treat morning sickness and nausea. They can be purchased at any drug store.

FIGURE 14-32 ■ **A,** Pericardium 6 on both forearms is a stomach point used to treat nausea and vomiting. **B,** Spleen 3 helps balance hormones.

is a hormone balancer. Each point should be held for a count of 6 to 10, repeating for 6 to 10 times (Figure 14-32).

■ The client can purchase "sea bands," which are motion sickness elastic bands, and wear them all night with the plastic button pressing on P6 (Figure 14-33). The client should remove the bands in the morning and keep them off for at least 2 hours before wearing them again for an hour. She can continue this pattern throughout the day. Another form of this bracelet uses a mild pulsating electric current at P6 to ease nausea and vomiting.

■ The last meal at night should be protein-rich. Protein takes longest to digest, and the pregnant woman will not wake up with an empty stomach.

■ The client should snack throughout the day. Unsalted crackers on waking can stave off that empty stomach in the morning.

■ The client should eat small but frequent meals.

■ The client should avoid fatty, rich, and acidic foods.

■ Vitamin B6 has helped some women treat morning sickness. It is safe during pregnancy, and a therapeutic dose is 10 to 25 mg 3 times a day.[12,30]

■ The client can cut up a lemon, place the pieces in a plastic bag, and then inhale the citrus fragrance whenever nausea starts.

■ Red raspberry leaf tea seems to help some women. Other women get relief from ginger tea, ginger drinks, ginger root, or ginger candies.

Nasal and Sinus Congestion

Increased blood volume and vasodilation of pregnancy causes hyperemia and edema in the upper respiratory mucosa. This usually occurs during the second trimester and results in nasal and sinus congestion, sinusitis, epistaxis, snoring, and vocal changes.[28,34] Progesterone slows smooth muscle function, which then slows sinus drainage. If a client's diet includes excessive amounts of dairy products, she may have increased mucus production. Constipation also creates congestion in the nasal and sinus cavities.

Women who suffer from allergies, hay fever, or rhinitis usually find these symptoms worsen during pregnancy, although there are some women for whom pregnancy is curative. Swollen nasal membranes trap the secretions in the sinuses, which results in sinus infections, nasal discharge, or chronic rhinitis. Practitioners can offer clients the following to relieve these common discomforts of pregnancy:

■ A general massage that focuses on the face, sinuses and occipital ridge will encourage nasal drainage (see Figure 14-26).

- The sinus reflex points found on the tips of the fingers and toes can be treated.
- Reflexes for the intestines should be massaged (see Figure 14-24).
- The client should drink at least 8 to 12 glasses of water daily.
- Inhaling steam with a facial steamer or placing warm, moist compresses over the sinus region can relieve sinus congestion.
- The client should avoid excessive dairy products
- Exposure to allergens and pollutants, such as dust, animal dander, smog, and cigarette smoke, should be avoided.
- The client should flush the sinuses with a saline solution (¼ teaspoon salt to 1 cup of water) or a Neti pot
- Nasal or oral decongestants with the following ingredients are possibly harmful to the fetus and must be avoided during pregnancy: ephedrine, phenylpropanolamine, neo-synephrine, and phenylephrine. These ingredients can constrict the vessels in the maternal airway passages and may also constrict the placental blood vessels. Any other sprays, decongestants, antihistamines, or nasal steroids should be discussed with a medical health care provider before the client uses them.[9]

Sciatica

Sciatica, or inflammation of the sciatic nerve, is rarely nerve root damage or injury during pregnancy but rather a manifestation of poor posture, muscular restrictions and tightness, hormonal influences, the stretching of uterine ligaments, uterine pressure on the sciatic region, and prelabor physiology.

Massage during an acute flare-up of sciatica, regardless of its genesis, is contraindicated. During this acute phase, the sciatic notch should be iced and the sciatic reflexes on the feet treated but direct contact with the affected leg should be avoided (see Figure 14-27).

When the pain is intermittent or chronic, appropriate sciatic (lymphatic) leg massage can be very helpful in reducing the sciatic pain. Practitioners can offer clients the following to relieve sciatic pain:

- **DVD** Manual lymphatic massage technique, including the gluteal region.
- Light (5 to 10 gm pressure) transverse friction across the path of the sciatic nerve.
- Light (5 to 10 gm pressure) sciatic beat along the path of the nerve.
- Reflex point stimulation.
- Ice applied to the sciatic notch. Before the client goes to bed, she should be encouraged to ice the region again.
- Sciatic nerve glide: lift the affected leg 4 inches off the floor, keeping the knee extended and point and flex the foot.[12]

In early pregnancy, about weeks 11 to 14 before there is any substantial weight gain, some women complain about a burning sensation or a dull, aching pain in the area of the sacroiliac joint and buttocks. This pain often stays local, although it can refer down the back of the leg. This lower back discomfort is caused by the hormone relaxin that has loosened the connective tissue between the sacrum and ilium, creating a hypermobility to the joints and pressure on the sciatic nerve. Treatment for early sciatic pain includes the previously mentioned massage, medial compression behind the ASIS, and ice, as well as the following exercises to help stabilize the pelvis:

- Strengthening the gluteals to restore medial placement will ease the lower back and leg discomfort. While standing, the client squeezes her buttocks and holds for a count of 10 and repeats for a total count of 10.
- In a standing position, the client leans to the affected side and squeezes those gluteal muscles for a count of 10, repeating for a total count of 10.

Most of the sciatic pain a woman experiences in later pregnancy is caused by the pressure of the uterus on the sciatic region, weakened abdominal core muscles, postural misalignment, and stretching uterine ligaments. The treatment for sciatica in these instances includes the previously mentioned massage and pelvic tilting to bring the fetus off the sciatic region. Prone positioning on the bodySupport systems is especially helpful in repositioning the fetus and reducing sciatic involvement. Postural adjustments, such as recruiting the abdominal core muscles, can also effectively reduce sciatica by elongating the lumbar spine and supporting the uterine ligaments more efficiently.

Another cause of sciatica is a taut piriformis muscle pressing directly on the sciatic nerve. The

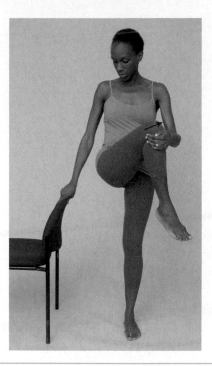

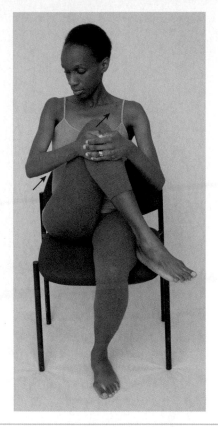

FIGURE 14-34 ■ The standing piriformis stretch releases the pressure of the muscle directly on the sciatic nerve. *1,* Legs are shoulder width apart with the affected leg next to the chair. *2,* The client holds the back of the chair and flexes the affected leg as shown. *3,* With the opposite hand, the client pulls the bent knee across her body, feeling the stretch. *4,* The client holds the position for a count of 10.

FIGURE 14-35 ■ The seated piriformis stretch is a variation of the standing stretch. *1,* The client sits up straight and draws in the abdominal muscles. *2,* She then crosses the affected leg over the opposite leg. *3,* With both hands, she pulls the affected knee upward toward the opposite shoulder. *4,* The client holds the position for a count of 10.

piriformis originates on the anterior surface of the sacrum and lateral to the anterior sacral foramen, sacroiliac joint, greater sciatic foramen, and sacrotuberous ligament. It inserts at the superior border of the greater trochanter. This muscle is a lateral hip rotator and slight abductor when the hip is flexed.[35] It is superficial to the sciatic nerve. If a client medially rotates her hip, which should stretch the muscle, and this movement elicits pain, chances are reasonable that the piriformis is implicated in her sciatica.

In additional to the massage technique, the bodyworker should include positional or gravitational release to stretch the tightened piriformis or strain-counterstrain to relax the muscle's tension. In a side-lying position, the affected leg should be flexed to the discomfort level and left in that position until the pain subsides. The leg should be flexed again to the next position that causes pain and left until the pain subsides. This will stretch the muscle and release it from pressing on the sciatic nerve. Using strain-counterstrain technique,

the leg is brought to a position that releases the discomfort and held for 90 seconds.

Trigger point release for the piriformis is helpful in freeing the pressure on the sciatic nerve. In a side-lying position, the gluteal region can be palpated until tension spots are located. Pressure should be maintained on these nodules. The affected leg can be gently rocked as the practitioner presses into the trigger points. In a prone position, the gluteals are palpated until tension areas are located. The client's leg is bent as the practitioner exerts a constant pressure on the trigger point as her hip is rotated medially and laterally.

The standing piriformis stretch stretches the piriformis and releases tension in the buttocks (Figure 14-34). The seated piriformis stretch is a variation of the standing stretch that releases the pressure on the sciatic nerve (Figure 14-35).[18]

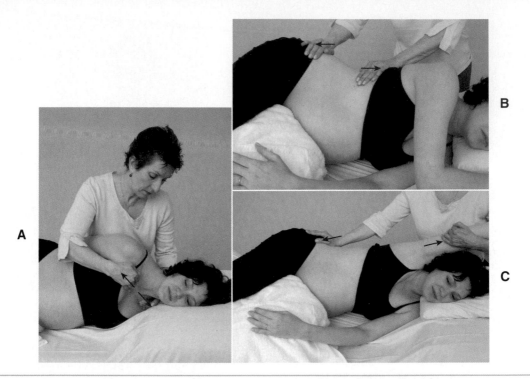

FIGURE 14-36 ■ Stretching the myofascia of the chest and upper ribcage can improve breathing. **A,** The client's arms are behind her back for the lateral stretch of the myofascia. **B,** One hand is on her hip, the other one on her true ribs. The stretch is horizontal. **C,** Lateral position for maximum stretch of the myofascia.

In the last few weeks of pregnancy, fetal lightening often causes sciatic pain. Once the fetus has settled deep within the pelvic station, there is little room for the fetus to move off of the sciatic region. In this instance, ice packs, the sciatic glide, and general massage may be helpful, but birth will be curative.

Shortness of Breath

Even with a 15% increase in oxygen consumption, minimal activity can cause **shortness of breath,** or dyspnea, in some women, particularly in early pregnancy.[6] It is important to remind the client that her breathing is actually more efficient during pregnancy, so she should not be concerned about not having enough oxygen for the fetus. She is feeling the inability to have expansive breathing, but the breathing is deeper. Consequently, myofascial restrictions of the rib cage may develop.

During the third trimester, uterine compression of the respiratory diaphragm limits lung expansion and the pregnant woman compensates by breathing more rapidly. These symptoms subside once the fetus has engaged into pelvic station.

Practitioners can offer clients the following to relieve breathlessness:

- Massage should include myofascial release of the rib cage and pectoral girdle. Some women may find a sitting position easier for breathing purposes.
- In a side-lying position, the client's underlying arm is brought behind her back (she will have to lift herself up slightly to slid the arm behind her) and the top arm behind her back to stretch the pectorals. In this position, the practitioner glides one hand under her neck and the other hand over her body and with fingertips positioned at the sternal-clavicular articulations. Using her body weight as she slightly leans forward, the practitioner stretches from the joints outward to the lateral lip of the head of the humerus (pectoralis attachment) (Figure 14-36). This stretch helps open the upper chest and encourages deeper breathing.
- A similar stretch can be accomplished with the client in a semisitting or sitting

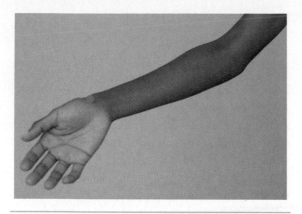

FIGURE 14-37 ■ Lung 9 points can be pressed for a count of 6 to 10, repeating for 6 to 10 times.

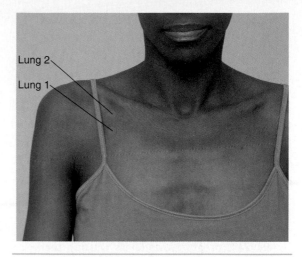

FIGURE 14-38 ■ Lung 1 and lung 2 can be stimulated for a count of 6 to 10, repeating 6 to 10 times to treat shortness of breath.

position. The practitioner presses the head of each humerus to stretch the pectoralis muscles.

- The practitioner should press acupuncture point lung 9, located inside the wrist crease near the radial head (Figure 14-37); lung 1, located between the first and second ribs, about 6 cun from the sternum; and lung 2, which is 1 inch above lung 1 (Figure 14-38).
- The client should exercise regularly and carefully, including aerobic activity that improves function of her respiratory and cardiovascular systems.
- When she feels short of breath, she should change positions and slow down her activity. (This is not contradictory to exercising. The more she exercises, the less fatigue and breathlessness she will feel.)
- The client should practice yoga or labor breathing exercises.

Symphysis Pubis Separation

Symphysis pubis separation, or symphysis pubis dysfunction, is brought about by abnormal relaxation of the ligaments of the symphysis joint because of relaxin. The increased mobility of the joint, often accompanied by painful shearing of the joint, places additional strain on the sacroiliac joints as well. The pain initially starts at the site of the separation, but after 28 weeks' gestation, backaches and sciatic pain may also arise. There may be pain in the abdominal muscles as muscular activity tries to stabilize the joint. In some cases, it is very difficult to stand, sit, or walk or even find a comfortable position lying down. It can be debilitating to some women. An injury, fall, aggressive exercising, or labor positions can cause this separation, or diastasis, of the pubic bone. After the birth, the ligaments slowly heal, although pain and discomfort may plague the woman for quite a while.[10] Practitioners can offer clients the following to relieve symphysis separation:

- During the massage, it is best to keep the client on one side and avoid turning her. Bolsters, pillows, or wedges that support her abdomen and prevent further stretching of the uterine ligaments are helpful. All pelvic, hip, and leg traction should be avoided.
- Medial compression behind the ASIS should be included to restore alignment and offer a gentle massage to the affected muscles.
- Sacral-occipital technique, performed by a chiropractor or osteopath, gently realigns the pelvis by positioning the client on strategically placed wedges.
- The client should avoid nonessential weight-bearing exercises and straddle activities. Proper body mechanics is very important, and the client should be reminded to use her abdominal core muscles with any activity.[36]

- Some women find it beneficial to wear a belt around the greater trochanters to promote medial compression.[5]

Varicose Veins

Increased uterine pressure on the blood vessels of the lower limbs slows down the flow of blood to the legs.[37] Sluggish venous return and increased pressure in the legs increases the distensibility and pressure in the veins of the lower extremities, vulva, rectum, and pelvis. This in turn can lead to dependent edema, varicose veins, and hemorrhoids.[38] Peripheral blood vessels are also affected by elevated progesterone levels causing the veins to enlarge and burst, creating spider veins or spider nevi.

The practitioner should recognize that varicosities are a predisposing cause of deep vein thrombosis and should take particular care in assessing the legs during their pretreatment evaluations for clients with varicosities. Areas that appear white or ischemic may be caused by deep vein thrombosis. The client should be asked to describe if there is any localized pain or tenderness in her legs or calves. If she indicates that there is localized pain, massage should not be done and she should be referred to her health care provider.[39]

Varicose veins may also be caused by hereditary predisposition, progesterone relaxing the muscle walls of the blood vessels encouraging engorgement, gravity, and straining during a bowel movement. The following techniques can relieve the pain and discomfort of varicose veins:

- Lymphatic leg massage should avoid all direct contact with these weakened vessels.

  DVD

- The client should elevate her legs above the level of her heart for 15 minutes, 3 times a day. Sleeping on the left side enhances blood circulation.
- The client should avoid standing for long periods of time and avoid crossing her legs when sitting.
- Loose fitting clothes and comfortable shoes should be worn. Some women find support hose a great relief.
- A bath containing 6 drops of cypress oil, 3 drops myrtle, 2 drops frankincense, and 3 drops German chamomile in 1 oz of

either St. John's Wort or oil base poured into a tub is a very soothing soak.[9,10,12]

In My Experience...

J was 8 months pregnant and suffering from painful sciatica. She limped as she walked down the hallway to my office. Sensing that her sciatic pain was a result of how the baby was positioned within her pelvis, I placed her in a prone position on the cushions I use. It took her a few minutes to relax into them, but when she did, she felt very supported and comfortable.

I continued my massage as usual then carefully had her turn over into a semisitting position so I could massage the front of her body. All the while, she was safely situated on the cushions and commented how comfortable and pain-free she felt.

When the massage ended and she stood up, the sciatic pain was gone. The prone positioning had allowed her baby to move off the sciatic region, thereby relieving her discomfort. She went home and told her husband, a physician, about the massage and how terrific she felt. The doctor was so pleased, he wrote the foreword to my first book, *MotherMassage*.

Summary

Most of the common discomforts, or typical physical aches and pains, of pregnancy can be easily treated with appropriate massage techniques. The hands-on therapies are very effective in easing common aches and pains of pregnancy and are best learned in a classroom setting. Many of these discomforts are symptomatic of the client's poor posture and can be remedied, even eliminated, with proper kinesthetic awareness, postural adjustments, and corrective massage. It is important that practitioners understand the etiology of these problems so the fears and concerns of the clients can be relieved by explaining how and why they are experiencing them.

References

1. Baratta R, Solomonow M, Zhou BH, et al: The role of the antagonist musculature in maintaining knee stability, *Am J Sports Med* 16(2):113-122, 1988.

2. Cresswell AG, Grundstrom A, Thorstensson A: Observations on intra-abdominal pressure and patterns of abdominal musculature activity in man, *Acta Physiol Scand* 144: 409-418, 1992.

3. Lacote M, Chevalier AM, Miranda A, et al: *Clinical evaluation of muscle function*, Edinburgh, 1987, Churchill Livingstone.

4. Tupler J: *Maternal fitness*, New York, 1996, Simon & Schuster.

5. Stillerman E: *MotherMassage: massage during pregnancy training manual*, New York, 2004, Dell.

6. Leifer G: *Maternity nursing: an introductory text*, St. Louis, 2005, Saunders.

7. Gabbe S, Niebyl J, Simpson J: *Obstetrics: normal and problem pregnancies*, ed 4, New York, 2002, Churchill Livingstone.

8. Hassid P: *Textbook for childbirth educators*, Philadelphia, 1978, Harper and Row.

9. Sears W, Sears M: *The pregnancy book*, Boston, 1997, Little, Brown.

10. Lowdermilk DL, Perry SE: *Maternity & women's health care*, ed 8, St. Louis, 2004, Mosby.

11. Lawrence R: *Breastfeeding: a guide for the medical profession*, ed 5, St. Louis, 1999, Mosby.

12. Stillerman E: *MotherMassage: a handbook for relieving the discomforts of pregnancy*, New York, 1992, Dell.

13. Muramoto N: *Healing ourselves*, New York, 1973, Avon Books.

14. American Society for Surgery of the Hand: *Carpal tunnel syndrome*, Rosemont, IL, 1998, the Society.

15. American Physical Therapy Association: *What you need to know about carpal tunnel syndrome*, Alexandria, VA, 2005, The Association.

16. de Quervain's syndrome. Available at http://www.merck.com/mmpe/sec04/ch042/ch042g.html?qt=de%20Quervain's%20syndrome&alt=sh, Accessed March, 2005.

17. Miller L: *When mothering is a pain in the wrist*, The New York Times, June 6, 2004.

18. Brill P: *Instant relief: tell me where it hurts and I'll tell you what to do*, New York, 2003, Bantam.

19. Zuther J: Traditional massage: manual lymph drainage in the treatment of lymphedema, *AMTA Florida J* 18:22-25, 2001.

20. Simkin P, Whalley J, Keppler A: *Pregnancy, childbirth and the newborn*, Minnetonka, MN, 1991, Meadowbrook Press.

21. Wittlinger G, Wittlinger H: *Textbook of Dr. Vodder's manual lymph drainage: volume I: basic course*, ed 6, Heidelberg, 1998, Karl F. Haug Verlag.

22. Zuther J: Traditional massage therapy in the treatment and management of lymphedema, *Massage Today* 2:6, 2002.

23. Eliska O, Eliska M: Are peripheral lymphatics damaged by high-pressure manual massage? *Lymphology* 28:21-30, 1995.

24. Gilbert ES, Harmon JS: *Manual of high risk pregnancy and delivery*, St. Louis, 1993, Mosby.

25. Wylie KR: Relaxation and massage often helpful, *JTCM* 17(2):130-139, 1997.

26. Melchart D, Streng A, Hoppe A, et al: Acupuncture in patients with tension-type headache: randomised controlled trial, *BMJ* 331:376-382, 2005.

27. Blackburn ST, Loper DL: *Maternal, fetal, and neonatal physiology: a clinical perspective*, Philadelphia, 1992, Saunders.

28. Coad J: *Anatomy and physiology for midwives*, St. Louis, 2001, Mosby.

29. Gordon M: Maternal physiology in pregnancy. In Gabbe S, Niebyl J, Simpson J, eds: *Obstetrics: normal and problem pregnancies*, ed 4, New York, 2002, Churchill Livingstone.

30. Morning sickness: causes, concerns, treatments, BabyCenter. Available at www.babycenter.com/refcap/254.html. Accessed June, 2006.

31. Furneaux E, Langley-Evans A, Langley-Evans S: Nausea and vomiting of pregnancy: endocrine basis and contribution to pregnancy outcome, *Obstet Gynecol Surv* 56(12):775-782, 2001.

32. Brody JE: *What could be good about morning sickness? Plenty*, The New York Times, p F7, June 6, 2000.

33. Ogunyemi DA, Michelini GA: Hyperemesis gravidarum. Available at http://www.emedicine.com/med/topic1075.htm.

34. Steinfeld J, Wax J: Maternal physiologic adaptations to pregnancy. In Seifer D, Samuels P, Kniss D, eds: *The physiologic basis of gynecology and obstetrics*, Philadelphia, 2001, Lippincott Williams & Wilkins.

35. Walther DS: *Applied kinesiology*, vol 1, Pueblo, Colo, 1981, Systems DC.

36. Fry D, Hay-Smith J, Hough J, et al: National Clinical Guideline for the care of women with symphysis pubis dysfunction, *Midwives* 110(1314):172-173, 1997.

37. de Sweit M: The cardiovascular system. In Chamberlain G, Broughton-Pipkin F, eds: *Clinical physiology in obstetrics*, Oxford, 1998, Blackwell Science.

38. Cunningham FG, Gant NF, Leveno KJ, et al. *Williams obstetrics*, ed 21, New York, 2001, McGraw Hill.

39. Fraser D, Cooper M: *Myles' textbook for midwives*, ed 14, Edinburgh, 2003, Churchill Livingstone.

REVIEW QUESTIONS

1   What are some of the factors that contribute to abdominal pressure? When does a pregnant woman generally experience this discomfort? What can the massage practitioner do to help ease this discomfort?

_____
_____
_____
_____
_____

2   The sacral lift has to be avoided on women with what condition?

_____
_____
_____
_____
_____

3   What causes iron deficiency anemia and folic acid deficiency during pregnancy? What can the massage practitioner suggest to help ameliorate this condition once a physician has diagnosed it?

_____
_____
_____
_____
_____

4   Backaches are one of the most common complaints during pregnancy. Explain what causes this discomfort and what massage practitioners can do to make their more comfortable.

_____
_____
_____
_____

5   How are the breasts affected by the pregnancy? What is the treatment for sore, tender breasts? What are the acupuncture points that effectively treat breast soreness?

_____
_____
_____
_____
_____

6   Describe the massage for carpal tunnel syndrome and de Quervain's syndrome.

_____
_____
_____
_____
_____

7   Why and how is the gastrointestinal system affected by the pregnancy and what remedies can massage practitioners offer?

_____
_____
_____
_____

8   How much additional interstitial fluid do pregnant women have by the end of their third trimester? What is the difference between pitting edema and general swelling? Is it safe to massage a client with pitting edema?

_____
_____
_____
_____

9   Describe preeclampsia and eclampsia.

_____

_____

_____

_____

_____

10 Describe appropriate leg massage for the reduction of edema.

_____

_____

_____

_____

_____

11 Why are fatigue and insomnia common during pregnancy and how can massage practitioners help alleviate these problems?

_____

_____

_____

_____

12 Describe gestational glucose intolerance and its implication in pregnancy.

_____

_____

_____

_____

_____

13 What are some of the causes of prenatal headaches? How can they be treated?

_____

_____

_____

_____

_____

14 What are hemorrhoids and how can they be relieved

_____

_____

_____

_____

_____

15 What are some of the causes of leg cramps? What massage techniques can help reduce their frequency and severity?

_____

_____

_____

_____

_____

16 How common is morning sickness? What is hyperemesis gravidarum?

_____

_____

_____

_____

17 What suggestions can practitioners offer their clients to ease the severity of nausea and vomiting during pregnancy?

_____

_____

_____

_____

_____

18   What risk factors contribute to nausea and vomiting of pregnancy?

_____

_____

_____

_____

_____

19   What are some of the signs of dehydration during pregnancy?

_____

_____

_____

_____

_____

20   Why do many pregnant women suffer from nasal and sinus congestion? What can be done to relieve these symptoms?

_____

_____

_____

_____

_____

21   What are some of the causes of pregnancy-related sciatica? How can they be treated?

_____

_____

_____

_____

_____

22   In early pregnancy, between weeks 11 and 14, what is the cause of sciatica? How it is it treated?

_____

_____

_____

_____

_____

23   Why is shortness of breath so common in pregnancy? At what point in the pregnancy do some women experience this symptom?

_____

_____

_____

_____

_____

24   What is a symphysis pubis separation? How is it treated?

_____

_____

_____

_____

_____

25   What are the reasons for varicose veins during pregnancy? Describe appropriate massage techniques for the treatment of varicose veins.

_____

_____

_____

_____

_____

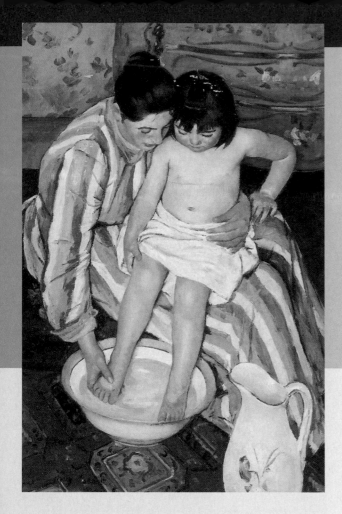

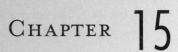

Chapter 15

Multiples

Objectives

On completion of this chapter, the student will be able to do the following:

1 Understand the physiology of a multiples pregnancy

2 Recognize the physiological effects and risk factors of a multiples pregnancy

Key Terms

Binovular	In vitro fertilization	Twins
Dizygotic	Monozygotic	Uniovular
Gestation	Multiples	
Infertility	Triplets	

"I always say, 'You show me a woman with fifteen children, and I'll show you an overbearing woman.'"—Phyllis Diller.[1]

As more women use artificial reproductive technology (ART) to help them conceive, the number of multiple births increases. In the United States in 1998, 39% of pregnancies conceived with the assistance of **infertility** (reproductive difficulties) treatments were **multiples** (more than one fetus).[2] In 2000 in the United Kingdom, 14.67 out of 1000 births were multiples. This percentage is up from 11.3 out of 1000 in 1989.[3-5] The rise in the birth of multiples is almost entirely the result of treatments involving ovulation induction[6] (Box 15-1).

A history of fraternal **twins** (two fetuses) in the female lineage will also increase the chances of twins.[7] Incidences of multiple pregnancies in other parts of the world are different. The highest rate of multiple pregnancies comes from West Africa, and the lowest rate is reported in Japan.[6]

Twins are classified as either **monozygotic** (MA) or **dizygotic** (DZ). Monozygotic, or **uniovular,** twins are identical twins developed from one egg and sperm that split into two. Dizygotic,

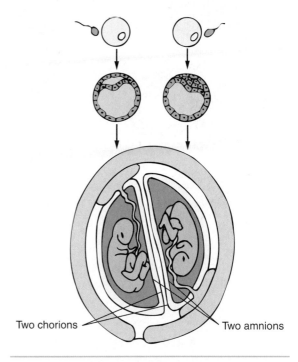

FIGURE 15-1 ■ Dizygotic twins. Note the two implantations, two placentas, two chorions and two amnions. (From Lowdermilk DL, Perry SE: *Maternity & women's health care,* ed 8, St. Louis, 2004, Mosby.)

Labels in figure: Two chorions — Two amnions

or **binovular,** twins grow from two separate ova fertilized by two different sperm. One half of the dizygotic twins will be boy-girl, a quarter will be boy-boy, and a quarter will be girl-girl (Figures 15-1 and 15-2).[6] The **gestation** period (duration of the pregnancy) for a multiple pregnancy is shorter than a single pregnancy. For twins, the average gestation lasts 37 weeks, 34 weeks for **triplets** (three fetuses), and 33 weeks for quadruplets.[6]

Physiological Changes to the Woman

The effects of a multiples pregnancy on the expectant woman exacerbate the common complaints of pregnancy. She may experience more nausea and

---

BOX 15-1 Multiple World Records

The most number of fetuses recorded by the *Guinness Book of World Records* was a woman with 15 fetuses in 1971 in Rome, Italy. A fertility drug was responsible for the 10 girls and 5 boys, although none survived.

The most number of babies who survived was a set of septuplets born in Iowa in 1997 conceived through **in vitro fertilization** (the ovum is fertilized in a glass dish and then implanted into the woman's uterus), and another set of septuplets was born in Saudi Arabia in 1998 from an unplanned pregnancy that was the result of a fertility drug used to regulate the mother's menstrual cycle.

From *The Guinness Book of World Records.* Available at http://www.guinnessworldrecords.com. Accessed 2005.

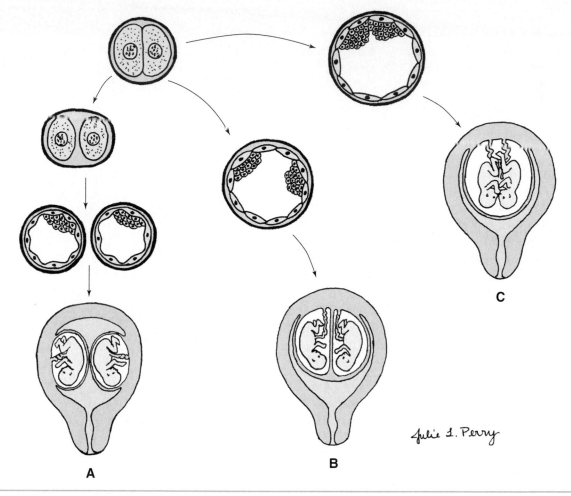

FIGURE 15-2 ■ Monozygotic twins. **A,** One fertilization with two implantations, two placentas, and two sets of membranes. **B,** One fused placenta, one chorion, and separate amnions. **C,** An incomplete separation of cell mass results in conjoined twins. (From Lowdermilk DL, Perry, SE: *Maternity & women's health care,* ed 8, St. Louis, 2004, Mosby.)

vomiting because of higher hormone levels. She may also experience gastrointestinal discomforts, such as constipation, gas, and heartburn, which may be worse as a result of the heavier uterus.

Swelling, leg and feet soreness, varicosities, hemorrhoids, and backaches are more troublesome because of the additional uterine pressure. An increased strain on the pregnant woman's cardiovascular system can also occur. Nutritionally, these women are commonly afflicted with iron and folic acid deficiency leading to anemia, especially after the week 28.[6] They also need to consume more calories and nutrients. Shortness of breath is also common as the larger uterus compresses the respiratory diaphragm. Nasal congestion can worsen, leading to rhinitis or sinus infections.

Abdominal distension is greater, and her diastasis will be larger.

Polyhydramnios is often associated with identical twins. It can lead to a miscarriage or premature labor if the condition becomes acute. Other concerns of a multiple pregnancy are increased risk of miscarriage, ectopic pregnancy, preeclampsia, more vaginal bleeding and placenta previa, malpresentation, longer postpartum recovery, and preterm labor and the sequelae of prematurity.[8,9] The perinatal morbidity rate for twins is four times the rate with singletons and 12 times higher with triplets.[3,10]

Women carrying triplets are even more at risk, are more likely to spend some of their pregnancy on bed rest, and are mostly likely going to have

Touch Points

When a woman is carrying twins or triplets, she most probably experiences more of the physical discomforts associated with pregnancy. Lower backaches, enlarged diastasis, swelling of the extremities, increased weight gain, additional muscle soreness and stiffness, sinus congestion, and fatigue are some of the discomforts she may have. Although multiple pregnancies are medically considered to be high-risk pregnancies, practitioners should make the woman feel more comfortable, treat discomforts with appropriate massage techniques, and teach proper body mechanics.

Equally important is to teach her about strengthening and utilizing her core abdominal muscles correctly. This will help stabilize her lumbar spine and pelvis and provide greater support for her enlarged uterus.

BOX 15-2 *Cultural Views of Multiples*

In Southeast Africa, along the arid coastline of Delagoa Bay, twins and their mothers are believed to have the power to bring much needed rain. The mother is called the "Sky" and her children are known as "Children of the Sky." Fresh water is poured over the mother and once the "Sky" is wet, the rains will come.

The Navajos of the United States looked down on multiple births and compared them to the litter of lower animals.

In other parts of the world, twins are said to bring magic. The Ga people of Africa have an annual celebration in honor of the pair.

From Jackson D: *With child: wisdom and traditions for pregnancy, birth and motherhood,* San Francisco, 1999, Chronicle Books.

a cesarean delivery. Perinatal mortality rates are higher for triplets than they are for twins, and neonate cerebral palsy rates are increased.[11] If a woman is confined to bed rest, lateral or side-lying positioning promotes an increase in placental profusion and reduces lower back strain.

There may be an emotional toll in multiple pregnancies, particularly if the pregnancy was unexpected, as well as the additional financial burden, limited living space, excessive workload, and coping difficulties for the family. The emotional stresses of any pregnancy can compound with multiples and seem overwhelming to the expectant mother and father. The practitioner should be sensitive and supportive of the clients' concerns and work to make them feel as comfortable as possible by addressing their physical and emotional needs.

Side-lying without turning the client, sitting, or prone on the bodySupport system with additional bolsters are the best positions for treating the client with a multiple pregnancy. In a side-lying position, the woman should be offered additional pillows and wedges for her abdomen and lower back, with the pillows between her knees and legs kept parallel. The bodySupport system should only be used if the client feels comfortable on them and if additional bolsters are used to elevate her abdomen. Lower back decompression should be achieved by placing her hips correctly on the pelvic cushion, so that her breasts are not compressed and her enlarged uterus is not pressing against the table (Box 15-2).

In My Experience...

P was pregnant with twins and suffering from severe edema in her legs. Her lower back was very sore and she commented that "her bras were bigger than some of her mini skirts." I had her prone on the cushions early in her pregnancy, and side-lying as the pregnancy advanced.

When it came to allocating the hour's massage, I had to concentrate on those areas that bothered her the most, which were usually her lower back and legs. The pelvic tilts and myofascial stretches I did on her lower back were usually greeted with sighs of relief. The lymphatic drainage, which often took half the hour, helped relieve her legs from the congestion caused by the pressure of her large uterus on the lymph vessels.

P received a massage just hours before she went into labor. She said she felt ready and eager to meet her babies—a boy and a girl.

Summary

The number of multiple pregnancy clients is increasing as more women become pregnant through the use of fertility drugs and treatments. The practitioner must recognize that the pregnant woman's complaints and discomforts will be exaggerated and care must be taken to find a comfortable position that supports her body.

References

1. Smith L: *The mother book: a compendium of trivia and grandeur concerning mothers, motherhood & maternity*, Garden City, NJ, 1978, Doubleday.
2. National Summary and Fertility Clinic Reports: *Artificial reproductive technology success rates*, Atlanta, 1998, Centers For Disease Control and Prevention.
3. Office of National Statistics: London, 2000, ONS.
4. General Register Office (Northern Ireland): Belfast, GRO, 2000.
5. General Register Office (Scotland): Edinburgh, GROS, 2000.
6. Fraser D, Cooper M: *Myles' textbook for midwives*, ed 14, Edinburgh, 2003, Churchill Livingstone.
7. Lowdermilk DL, Perry SE: *Maternity & women's health care*, ed 8, St. Louis, 2004, Mosby.
8. Edwards RG, Brody SA: *Principles and practice of assisted human reproduction*, Philadelphia, 1995, Saunders.
9. Addor V, Santos-Eggimann B, Fawer CI, et al: Impact of fertility treatments on the health of newborns, *Fertil Steril* 69(2): 210-215, 1998.
10. Cunningham FG, Gant NF, Leveno KJ, et al: *Williams obstetrics*, ed 21, New York, 2001, McGraw Hill.
11. Patterson B, Stanley F, Henderson D: Cerebral palsy in multiple births in Western Australia, *Am J Med Genet* 37:346-351, 1990.

REVIEW QUESTIONS

1   What is artificial reproductive technology? How does it influence the birth of multiples?

_____

_____

_____

_____

_____

_____

2   What is the difference between a monozygotic twin and a dizygotic twin?

_____

_____

_____

_____

_____

3   How long is the gestation period for multiples?

_____

_____

_____

_____

_____

4   What are some of the physical discomforts you would expect a woman carrying multiples to experience?

_____

_____

_____

_____

_____

5   What are some of the risk factors often associated with carrying multiples?

_____

_____

_____

_____

_____

6   If a woman is confined to bed rest, what is the most efficient position to promote increased placental profusion and ease back strain?

_____

_____

_____

_____

_____

_____

7   What ways can you safely and comfortably position your multiple pregnancy client for her massage?

_____

_____

_____

_____

_____

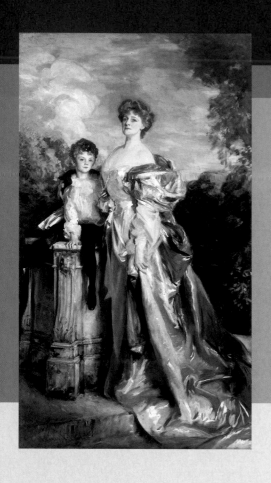

PART TWO

Labor Massage

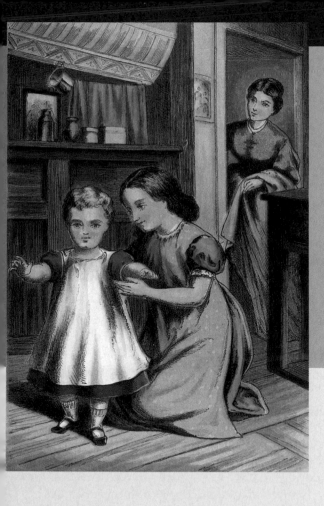

CHAPTER 16

The Physiology of Labor

Objectives

On completion of this chapter, the student will be able to do the following:

1 Explain the physiological and emotional stages of labor
2 Discuss the effects of epidural anesthesia with clients
3 Understand the hormonal influences that start labor
4 Understand the factors involved in a cesarean section and be able to describe the procedure
5 Explain vaginal birth after cesarean (VBAC)

A 2002 study conducted by Harris Interactive for Childbirth Connection (formerly Maternity Center Association) in New York City reported that only one-third (36%) of expectant mothers took childbirth education classes. Seventy percent of the women were first-time mothers, and almost 88% of these classes were held at a hospital site, doctor's office, or midwife's office.[1] This indicates that most women get their information about labor from friends, books, magazine articles, or television and go into labor without any class preparation.

Massage practitioners have a unique opportunity to educate pregnant clients about labor and delivery and offer a supportive, respectful, and dignified explanation of this astounding process. Most childbirth education classes are held at medical facilities, and these classes tend to provide few details on the anatomy and physiology of labor and instead concentrate more on hospital procedures. Childbirth educators who are independent of a medical facility seem to offer classes geared more to understanding the physiology of labor and teach a variety of coping skills.

The Physiology of Labor

Labor is a complex and interrelated physiological process that involves harmonious signaling and communication between the fetus, the placenta, and the mother's body. Interwoven stimulatory and inhibitory mechanisms are actively orchestrated to encourage uterine contractility, fetal membrane integrity, and cervical maturation.

Normal labor can occur any time between 37 and 42 weeks' gestation, although unlike other mammals, human gestation is not an exact science.[2] Gestation lasts about 280 days, with a margin of 10 days on either side. The World Health Organization (WHO) defines normal labor as "low risk throughout, spontaneous in onset with the fetus presenting by the vertex, culminating in the mother and infant in good condition following birth."[3,4] By the end of pregnancy, the uterus is the largest and strongest muscle in the female body.

No one knows exactly what precipitates the onset of labor, but five factors affect the process of labor and birth. These factors, known as the *five Ps*, are detailed in Box 16-1.[5]

Other factors that may be involved in the labor process are the woman's previous labor experience(s), her cultural approach to labor, and her preparedness, as well as the place of the labor and birth, the type of provider, and the procedures she receives.[5,6]

Labor consists of four **stages,** or divisions. Stage one consists of dilation and **descent** and is further subdivided into three **phases.** These phases are the **latent phase** (phase one), the **active phase** (phase two), and **transition** (phase three) phase. Stage two, descent and birth, is also subdivided into the same three phases. Stage three is the expulsion of the placenta, and stage four is recovery.

Stage One

The first stage of labor lasts from the beginning of regular uterine contractions and ends with full cervical dilation at 10 cm. This stage is longer than the second and third stages combined.[5] For the first-time mother, or nullipara, stage one can last up to 20 hours. General variations may occur because of specific maternal and fetal risk factors, clinical management of the labor and birth process, parity, birth interval, psychological state, fetal presentation and position, maternal pelvic shape, maternal mobility, and the size and strength of the uterine contractions.[7,8] A parous woman usually has a shorter first stage (Figure 16-1).

Uterine Contractions

Each uterine contraction starts in a corner (cornua) of the uterus and spreads across and downward. The uterine contraction lasts the longest and is the most intense in the **fundus,** the upper portion of the uterus, but the contraction peak recedes at the same time throughout the organ. This rhythm allows the cervix to dilate, and the upper segment, or fundus, to expel the fetus and placenta. The fundus is thick and muscular, and

the lower segment, the isthmus and cervix, is designed for distension and dilation.

Polarity describes the neuromuscular connection between the two poles of segments of the uterus. The upper pole contracts and retracts strongly to expel the fetus, whereas the lower pole contracts slightly and dilates to allow expulsion to occur.

The uterine muscle has unique capabilities. Instead of completely relaxing and lengthening after each contraction, the uterus retains some of the shortening called *retraction* (Figure 16-2). This function assists in the expulsion of the fetus as the upper segment becomes gradually shorter and thicker, and its cavity gets smaller. By the end of the first stage of labor, uterine contractions occur at 2 to 3 minute intervals, which last for about 1 minute and are very powerful.

Cervical effacement occurs when muscle fibers surrounding the internal os are drawn upward by the retracted upper segment and the cervix merges into the lower uterine segment. The cervical canal of the internal os widens, but the external os remains unchanged (Figures 16-3 and 16-4).[4,9,10]

Dilation, or the opening of the cervix (os uteri) from 0 to 10 cm to allow passage of the fetus, occurs because of uterine contractions and counterpressure of either the intact bag of waters or the presenting fetal part, or both. When pressure is applied evenly to the cervix, it makes the fundus contract and retract (Figures 16-5 and 16-6).[11,12]

Uterine contractions depend on the amount of intracellular calcium that activates the myosin-actin contractile unit. Oxytocin stimulates uterine contractions by increasing intracellular calcium.[13]

Stage One: Latent Phase

During the latent phase, there is more progress in uterine effacement than fetal descent.[5] When labor has been established, the contractions progress and the cervix dilates. This is called the latent phase of stage one. It is impossible to predict how long this phase will last. In early labor, the contractions sometime feel like a dull backache or menstrual cramps.[14] The contractions themselves are short and mild and will last for about 30 to 40 seconds. The rest interval between the contractions can be as long as 15 to 20 minutes. During the latent phase, the cervix dilates to 3, 4, sometimes 5 cm.[14]

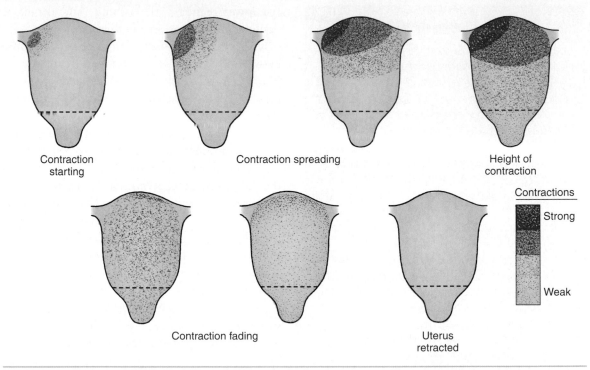

Contraction starting

Contraction spreading

Height of contraction

Contraction fading

Uterus retracted

Contractions
Strong
Weak

FIGURE 16-1 ■ The contractions begin at either cornua of the fundus and spread evenly throughout the uterus. Dark red indicates the strongest contracting uterine segment. (From Fraser D, Cooper M: *Myles' textbook for midwives,* ed 14, Edinburgh, 2003, Churchill Livingstone.)

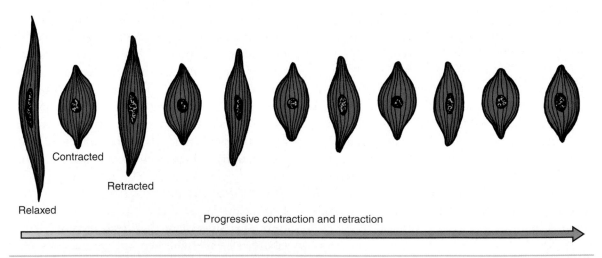

Contracted

Retracted

Relaxed

Progressive contraction and retraction

FIGURE 16-2 ■ The progress of uterine contraction during labor. (From Fraser D, Cooper M: *Myles' textbook for midwives,* ed 14, Edinburgh, 2003, Churchill Livingstone.)

The laboring woman may feel excited or a little nervous, but for the most part she can continue doing whatever activity she feels comfortable doing. This is not the time to be alone and become preoccupied with labor. The focus should be on relaxation and an activity that complements relaxing such as a massage, taking a bath or shower, reading, listening to music, or going for a walk. Small amounts of nutritious food and liquid should be consumed to help the expectant woman maintain her strength and keep her glucose levels balanced. Being ambulatory can speed up the process of labor (Figure 16-7).

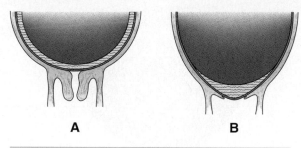

FIGURE 16-3 ■ A, Cervix before effacement: 0%. B, Fully effaced cervix: 100%. The cervical canal is now a part of the lower uterine segment. (From Fraser D, Cooper M: *Myles' textbook for midwives,* ed 14, Edinburgh, 2003, Churchill Livingstone.)

Stage One: Active Phase

There is a marked change in the labor pattern and emotional response when latent labor ends and active labor begins. The contractions, which can last a minute or more, are more painful but still manageable. The contractions also come closer together—about 3 to 5 minutes apart. At this point, the laboring woman goes to the hospital or to a birthing center.

During the active and the transition phases of labor, there is more progress in dilation of the cervix and increased rate of descent.[5] This rapid change in contraction pattern may be more uncomfortable, but each contraction is more productive. The cervix is dilating from 4 or 5 cm to 7, 8, or even 9 cm. This should give the laboring woman more confidence to get through the hardest phase (Figure 16-8).

Relaxation is important at this time. Slow breathing may help some women relax, along with specific massage strokes, counter pressures, and mobility. Lying down will slow labor and cause more pain.[15,16]

Multigravida

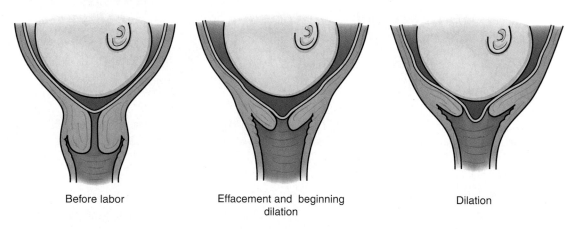

Before labor | Effacement and beginning dilation | Dilation

Primigravida

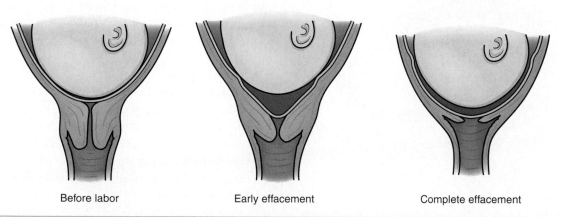

Before labor | Early effacement | Complete effacement

FIGURE 16-4 ■ A comparison of effacement and dilation between a woman who has had a previous birth *(top)* and a first time mother *(bottom)*.

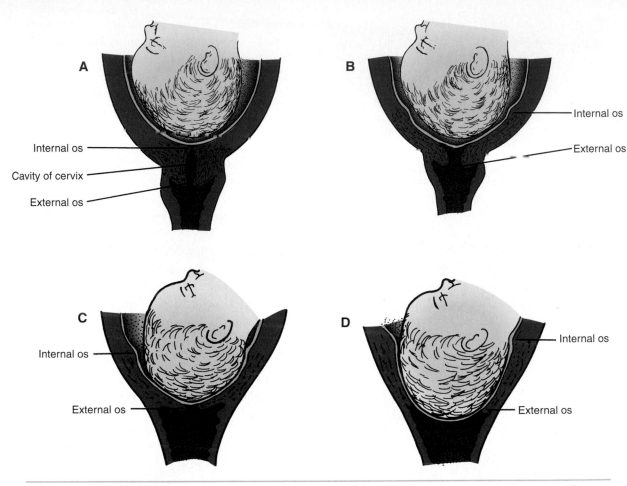

FIGURE 16-5 ■ The cervix opens, or dilates, from 0 to 10 cm. **A**, Before labor begins; **B**, early effacement; **C**, complete (100%) effacement; **D**, complete dilation: 10 cm. (From Lowdermilk DL, Perry SE: *Maternity & women's health care*, ed 8, St. Louis, 2004, Mosby.)

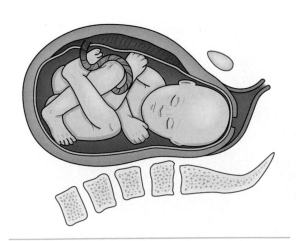

FIGURE 16-6 ■ The cervix is beginning to efface and dilate. The fetus descends in the vertex position facing mother's side.

Once labor has been firmly established, many women request epidural analgesia to control the pain. This is a personal decision based on many factors, but clients should learn about the advantages and disadvantages of a medicated birth to make an informed decision. Chapters 17 to 19 include pain control techniques without medication.

Epidural Anesthesia

Epidural anesthesia is a regional anesthesia within the epidural space. Many women decide that they want to receive pain medication for labor during their pregnancy long before labor begins. For others, the decision comes during labor when they feel incapable of continuing without pain relief.

There are different types of anesthetic that offer high levels of pain relief. Pain is controlled by blocking the conduction of impulses along

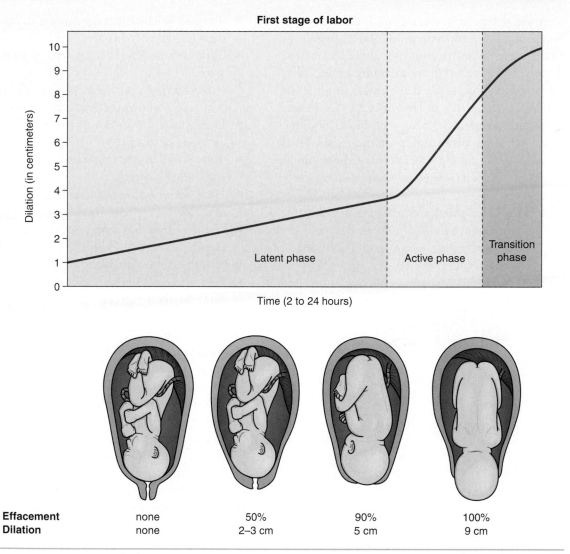

First stage of labor

| Effacement | none | 50% | 90% | 100% |
| Dilation | none | 2–3 cm | 5 cm | 9 cm |

FIGURE 16-7 ■ Women often become quiet, serious, and very focused on their labor during the latent phase. For some, it feels as if labor will never end and they feel trapped. During the active and the transition phases of labor, there is more progress in dilation of the cervix.

the sensory nerves as they enter the spinal cord. The epidural block was introduced for use during labor in the 1970s. Most of the concern was focused on application rather than problems the epidural block might create in a normal birth.[4] During this time, the epidural contained pain sensations, but it also caused the loss of bladder sensation and function and extreme relaxation of the pelvic floor, provided complete numbness of the lower extremities, resulted in significant hypotension, and thwarted the expulsive contractions during the second stage of labor.[4]

A standard epidural block, the most expensive of all pain relief medications, is administered by injecting a local anesthetic (i.e., mepivacaine

[Carbocaine], chloroprocaine [Nesacaine], bupivacaine [Marcaine], or lidocaine [Xylocaine]) in the epidural space between L1 and L2, L2 or L3, or L3 and L4 (Figure 16-9).[4,17] To receive this injection, the laboring woman must bend forward and remain very still so that to widen the space between the lumbar vertebrae. Any movement on her part may cause the needle to puncture the meninges (the subarachnoid space) and cause a dural tap, or leakage, of cerebral spinal fluid.[4] Once the needle is safely within the epidural space, a catheter is threaded through the needle for continuous infusion. An antibacterial filter is attached to the end of the catheter, which is then strapped to the woman's back. A syringe pump is set-up for continuous infusion.[4]

Another type of epidural block is the segmental block with lower concentrations of the same drugs administered after the mother's cervix has dilated 5 cm.[17] Other forms of medications are intrathecal narcotics, administered as a single injection in the lower back that can last from 2 to 24 hours, and epidural narcotics that will allow mobility. These have the advantage of offering pain relief without the numbing side effects of the epidural blocks.[17] The advantages of these pain medications are as follows:

- They often provide excellent pain relief.
- They can lower blood pressure that can be helpful in cases of pregnancy-induced hypertension (PIH).

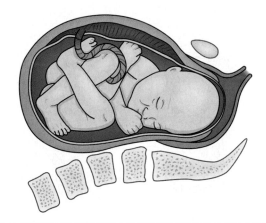

FIGURE 16-8 ■ The cervix is completely thinned out, or effaced, and opened to 6 centimeters. The fetus begins to turn to face the mother's sacrum. This position aligns the widest part of the fetal head with the widest part of the mother's pelvis, facilitating easy passage.

- The pain relief allows the mother to rest in cases of prolonged labors.
- They have no effect on the fetal respiratory system.[4]

The disadvantages of these pain medications may include the following effects on the woman:

- Dural puncture and consequent migraines or severe headaches.
- Total spinal block, may cause maternal respiratory distress.
- Local anesthetic toxicity resulting in cardiac arrest.
- Catheterization as a result of the loss of bladder sensation and function; up to 68% of women were unable to urinate.[18]
- Assisted vaginal birth and instrumentation; the use of epidural anesthesia requires constant intravenous fluids and electronic fetal monitoring.
- Neurological weakness and sensory loss[4]; the woman has little control over her body.[19]
- Immobility; the women must remain in bed on her side with her head at the same level throughout the labor, and many hospitals restrict movement after an epidural has been administered.
- Higher risk of cesarean section (C-section).
- Slowed labor; cervical dilation takes longer in a medicated birth[20]; 10 studies showed that labors were 0.9 to 5.1 hours longer with epidural anesthesia.[21]
- Postpartum backaches.

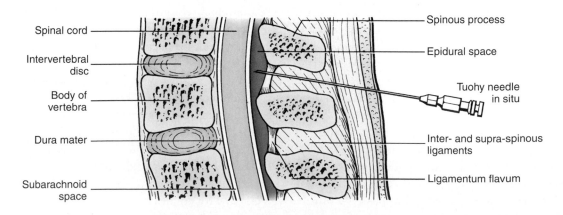

FIGURE 16-9 ■ The Tuohy needle is inserted into the epidural space during the administration of an epidural (regional) block. (From Fraser D, Cooper M: *Myles' textbook for midwives*, ed 14, Edinburgh, 2003, Churchill Livingstone.)

- Interference with woman's natural tendency and ability to find a birth position that encourages easy passage.
- Inhibited beta-endorphin production and suppresses the shift in awareness that is a normal part of labor. Oxytocin peaks just before birth, triggered by the stretch receptors in the lower vagina. These receptors are numbed as a result of epidural anesthesia, and this numbness lasts after the drug has worn off.[22,23]
- Causes the woman to miss the **fetal ejection reflex** (the secretion of catecholamines during labor to help push the baby through the birth canal) so she has to push, often against gravity because she cannot use her legs to stand or squat to overcome this loss of sensation. This prolongs stage two of labor and increases the chance of a need for forceps.[24]
- Suppression of catecholamine release, which is essential for fetal ejection reflex.[25]
- Inhibited release of uterine-stimulating hormone, prostaglandin F_2 (PGF_2), thereby prolonging labor.[26]
- Inadequate pain relief in up to 25% of women.[27]
- Pruritus or itchy skin; when opioids are included in the medication, up to 68% of women reported skin itching.[18]
- Perineal lacerations occurred slightly more with an epidural. Third- and fourth-degree tears were reported in 5% to 37% of women who had epidurals as compared with 3% to 34% of women who were not medicated.[18]
- Postpartum hemorrhage is twice as likely to occur.[21]
- Urinary retention and incontinence during postpartum recovery is twice as likely, even up to one year, with an epidural.[21]
- Chronic headaches were developed by 23% of women.[20]
- Increased use of **Pitocin,** which is synthetic oxytocin, to hasten labor in 27% to 78% of women who received epidurals and in 11% to 64% of women who received narcotic analgesia.[18]

- Women with a fever greater than 100.4° F are three times more likely to have antibiotics.[20,21,28-30] One study indicated that women with temperatures greater than 99.5° F were three times more likely to have a C-section and three times more likely to have instrument delivery.[21] The maternal fever also affects the newborn by lowering apgar scores and causing a tenfold increase in hypotension, a fourfold increase in bag and mask resuscitation, and a sixfold increase in oxygenation.[18]

Fetal complications and compromise also occur with the use of these drugs because they go directly to the fetus at equal or even greater levels than the mother. Some drugs are absorbed in the fetal brain, and almost all medications will take longer to be eliminated from the baby after the umbilical cord is cut.[31-33] There is a more difficult postpartum recovery period, with women who took pain medication citing fussy babies 1 month after birth.[34,35]

Other complications to the fetus include the following:

- May decrease the neonate's coordination for the first few weeks of life and increase colic and fussiness.[36]
- Decreased oxygen flow to the fetus and subsequent decreased fetal heart rate.[18,37]
- Fetal malpresentations occurred in 16% to 22% of women who received epidurals as compared with 4% to 18%. The study did not explain whether epidurals caused the malpresentation or whether the existing malpresentation caused more pain.[21]
- Jaundice in the newborn is 1½ to 2 times more likely.[21]

In addition, babies whose mothers were given these drugs are less likely to breastfeed at 6 months.[21] More serious risks, such as paralysis and death, from the use of these drugs are exceedingly rare.

In 2003, almost 60% of laboring women in the United States received epidural anesthesia.[38] In large city hospitals, this number can be as high as 90%.[39] The decision to have an epidural anesthesia is a personal one that may be based on information practitioners are not aware of or privileged to know. Practitioners can inform their clients of the advantages and disadvantages and provide them with useful information that can help them make educated choices.

Stage One: Transition Phase

The third phase of stage one, transition, is the hardest and most painful phase but also the shortest, averaging 5 to 25 contractions.[14] Transition is considered to be the peak of difficulty and intensity for most women because the contractions last longer and are closer together, not because the pain has increased. Contractions may last 90 to 120 seconds, some with double peaks, with only 30 seconds of rest before the next contraction begins. Laboring women feel more pressure in the pelvis as the cervix fully opens to 10 cm and the fetus' head presses down in the birth canal.

As a precursor to **bearing down,** the woman's diaphragm may be irritated by involuntary spasms resulting in hiccups, grunting or belching. Nausea and vomiting are often the harbingers of stage two of labor. The fetus' head presses against the vaginal wall and compresses the lower colon, which feels like a bowel movement. Backaches, aching and trembling legs, and a heavy mucus discharge are caused by the downward pressure of the descending fetus.[14]

Most women feel frightened, dependent, or even panicky by the intensity of transition. Others will cry and request anesthesia at this point. All these feelings are normal. The woman who is prepared and understands how labor progresses physically and how she might feel emotionally will have an easier time during transition. The hardest part is also the shortest. Pain medication can be avoided with proper preparation, good support, understanding of the process, changing birthing positions, comfort measures, and relaxation techniques.

Stage Two

Stage two, like stage one, is made up of three phases: latent, active, and transition. Stage two begins when the cervix fully dilates, which signals a change in activity as the fetus leaves the uterus, rotates within the pelvis, and passes through the birth canal (Box 16-2). The urge to push is an overriding sensation that often corresponds

---

> **BOX 16-2** *Signs of Stage Two of Labor*
>
> The shift from stage one to stage two is not always clinically clear. Some signs that stage two has begun are the following:
>
> - The woman has expulsive uterine contractions and has the urge to push.
> - The membranes rupture, although this can occur before labor or any time during labor.
> - The anus dilates and gapes. Deep placement of the presenting part may also create this sign in the latter part of stage one.
> - An anal cleft line appears as a purple pigmented mark in the cleft of the buttocks that moves up the anal cleft as labor progresses.*
> - The rhomboid of Michaelis appears. When a woman is in a position where her back is visible, a dome-shaped curve in the lower back indicates the posterior displacement of the sacrum and coccyx as the fetal occiput descends into the maternal sacral curve.† The laboring women tends to arch her back and push her buttocks forward, creating a lengthening and straightening of the pelvic canal that eases fetal passage.
> - Upper abdominal pressure and discomfort under the ribs is felt as the fetus uncurls. This seems to occur at the same time as full cervical dilation.
> - Blood-stained mucus, or bloody show, often appears at the end of the first stage.
> - The presenting part is seen at the perineum.‡
> - Sensations of transition are relieved.§
> - Complete dilation occurs.

*Data from Hobbs L: *Pract Midwife* 1(11):34-35, 1998.
†Data from Sutton J, Scott P: *Understanding and teaching optimal fetal positioning,* ed 2, Tauranga, New Zealand, 1996, Birth Concepts.
‡Data from Fraser D, Cooper M: *Myles' textbook for midwives,* ed 14, Edinburgh, 2003, Churchill Livingstone.
§Data from Simkin P, Whalley J, Keppler A: *Pregnancy, childbirth and the newborn,* Minnetonka, MN, 1991, Meadowbrook Press.

---

with full dilation. Some women may experience this urge before complete dilation, whereas other women do not feel the urge to push until after the cervix is completely dilated.[14]

There appears to be a transitional period between full dilation and when the urge to push actually begins. This period is sometimes described as a time of maternal restlessness, discomfort, need for pain relief, and feelings of helplessness and that labor will never end (Figure 16-10).[4]

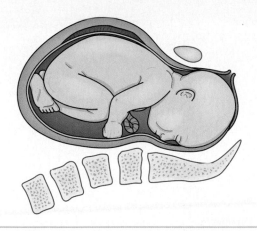

FIGURE 16-10 ■ The cervix is completely dilated, and the fetus has finished turning to face the mother's back. In this position, the fetus will be expelled from the uterus.

The second stage can last from 20 to 50 minutes, although a labor of 2 hours for stage two is still considered normal.[5] Medication will slow down stage two, and ethnicity may also be a contributing factor, with shorter second-stage labor for African-Americans and Puerto Rican women.[40,41]

The contractions of stage two become stronger and longer but less frequent, which provides both mother and fetus with a chance to rest. The amniotic membranes rupture spontaneously at the end of stage one or during the transition to stage two. This fluid drainage permits the fetal head to press directly on the vaginal tissues, assisting in distension. The pressure of the fetal axis increases the flexion of the head, creating smaller presenting diameters, enhanced progress, and less trauma to mother and fetus. An upright birthing position optimizes these changes.[4]

As the fetus continues its descent, the contractions become expulsive. The urge to push is stimulated by pressure on the nerve receptors in the pelvic floor ("Ferguson reflex"). The woman can contract her abdominal muscles and diaphragm, which are the secondary powers of expulsion, and help with each contraction.

As the fetal head descends, the soft tissues of the pelvis are displaced.[4] The bladder is pushed into the abdomen to avoid injury or trauma and the rectum flattens into the sacral curve. Any fecal matter left in the rectum will be expelled. The levator ani muscles dilate and are displaced laterally. The perineum is flattened, stretched, and thinned.

Stage Two: Latent Phase

The latent phase of labor is also referred to as the resting phase. There is a relief from the pain of transition, and women become calmer, more aware of their surroundings, and feel happier. The uterus rests, and those contractions that women experience are weak and farther apart for approximately 15 to 20 minutes. The urge to push also diminishes or weakens. At this point, the fetal head has passed through the cervix and the uterus slackens (Figure 16-11)

Stage Two: Active Phase

After the temporary rest, strong contractions resume and the urge to push becomes involuntary and compelling. Bearing down relieves a lot of pressure for her, and she feels she is making progress. The fetal head distends the vagina and presses against the wall of the rectum. The most efficient way to permit passage is to relax the muscles of the pelvic floor and then let the perineum bulge. At this point, the care provider should be doing perineal massage to support the stretching of the perineal tissues. This is also the time some care providers will perform an episiotomy. Towels or other compresses placed against the perineum will support the pelvic floor and help the laboring woman focus on her bearing-down efforts. Relaxation is important now as any physical tension could increase pain and slow down the progress of labor.

Episiotomy

As the perineum distends during stage two of active labor, an episiotomy may be performed to enlarge the vulval outlet. Minimizing the risk of severe maternal trauma, preventing a tear, and speeding up delivery when there is evidence of fetal compromise are often cited as rationales for this surgical procedure. During a normal birth, however, the indications for this incision are few.[4,42]

The episiotomy is an incision into the superficial muscles and skin of the perineum and the posterior vaginal wall. It can only speed up the birthing process when the presenting part is directly applied to these tissues.[4] If the incision is performed too early, it will not release the presenting part, which may cause hemorrhaging, and

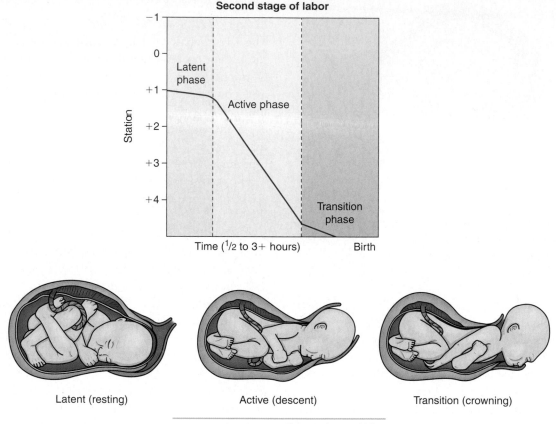

Second stage of labor

Latent phase

Active phase

Transition phase

Station

Time (¹/₂ to 3+ hours)   Birth

Latent (resting)   Active (descent)   Transition (crowning)

FIGURE 16–11 ■ The second stage of labor.

the levator ani muscles may be cut because they have not displaced laterally. A late incision will not permit enough time to anesthetize the area. If a tear has already begun, an episiotomy would be unnecessary. The surgery is performed with straight-bladed, blunt-ended Mayo scissors.[4]

Recent studies eschew the routine use of this procedure, which is performed 39.2% of the time in 1998 in the United States, down from 63.9% in 1980.[42] In the United States, the rate of this procedure is higher than any other country.[43] Researchers from the Johns Hopkins School of Medicine released a study in October 2004 that claimed that episiotomies performed in cases of shoulder dystocia, the fetal shoulder blocking passage through the birth canal, caused more injuries than they prevent. When the fetus was manually manipulated, only 35% of the newborns had arm injuries as compared with 60% who were delivered by episiotomy and 58% using both methods. The women who had an episiotomy also suffered from more anal tearing.[44] For shoulder dystocia,

turning the mother to a hands and knees position can often allow the birth of the baby without further trauma to the baby's shoulder.

The assumption that surgically incising the perineum will prevent a tear is erroneous and illogical. Almost half of all women who have no episiotomies will not tear, and the more serious third- and fourth-degree tears are more likely with an episiotomy.[14] Many doctors maintain that it is easier for them to suture a surgical incision than a natural erratic tear. However, when the tissue does tear, jagged healing allows for more elasticity and less collagenous scarring in the perineum.

Postpartum recovery is more uncomfortable with an episiotomy. It may delay immediate mother-infant interaction as the incision is sutured, the site of the incision may become infected, intercourse may be painful for several months, and the perineum is more apt to tear more seriously when an episiotomy is performed.[14]

The accumulated facts against routine episiotomies are forcing care providers to use other

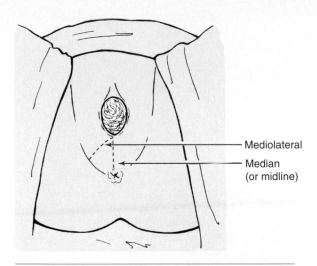

Mediolateral

Median
(or midline)

FIGURE 16-12 ■ Types of episiotomies. (From Lowdermilk DL, Perry SE: *Maternity & women's health care,* ed 8, St. Louis, 2004, Mosby.)

techniques to support the perineum and to suggest favorable birthing positions, such as squatting, to keep the perineum intact (Figure 16-12).

As the active phase advances, the perineum bulges, the labia separate, and the vagina opens as the fetal head moves further down. At this point, the head is visible and the mother can feel the baby coming out (Figures 16-13 and 16-14).

Stage Two: Transition (Crowning) Phase

Crowning occurs when the top of the fetal head can be seen at the vaginal opening. The crowning phase starts as the baby's head crowns and no longer retracts between pushing and bearing-down efforts. As the baby's head stretches the vaginal tissues, women often feel a burning sensation referred to as the "rim of fire."[13] This is the time when women should stop pushing and let their bodies open naturally to prevent tearing. Perineal support with hot compresses or massage will slowly permit the vaginal widening, preventing the baby from being born too quickly and tearing the perineum.

The top of the baby's head to the ears is born first (looking wet, wrinkled, and bluish), followed by the face. Once the head is out, it rotates to face the mother's side. One shoulder passes through the pelvis, followed by the other, and the rest of the baby emerges easily (Figure 16-15).

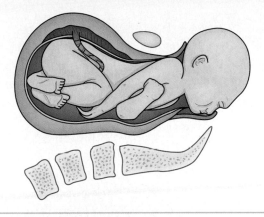

FIGURE 16-13 ■ The fetal head is now visible, and its body begins to elongate.

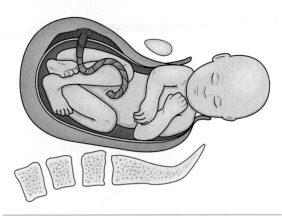

FIGURE 16-14 ■ Once the baby's head is born, it will rotate toward the mother's side again. This allows the shoulders to align with the widest part of the mother's pelvis.

During the actual birth, the mother is working hard to push the baby down and out. She might have a resurgence of energy as she recognizes the tremendous progress she has made and knows that the birth of her baby is only minutes away. Her limbs may be shaking with the effort and back pressure may be uncomfortable, but she knows this will be over soon.[45] Transition and second stage labor can be very intense for many women, both physically and emotionally. The better prepared she (and her partner) are, the easier this process will be for all concerned. Nonjudgmental, unobtrusive support following the mother's signals and needs where the mother is the primary participant are paramount to ensuring a positive birth outcome and experience.

Once the baby is born, the mother's (and partner's) mood dramatically changes to a myriad of

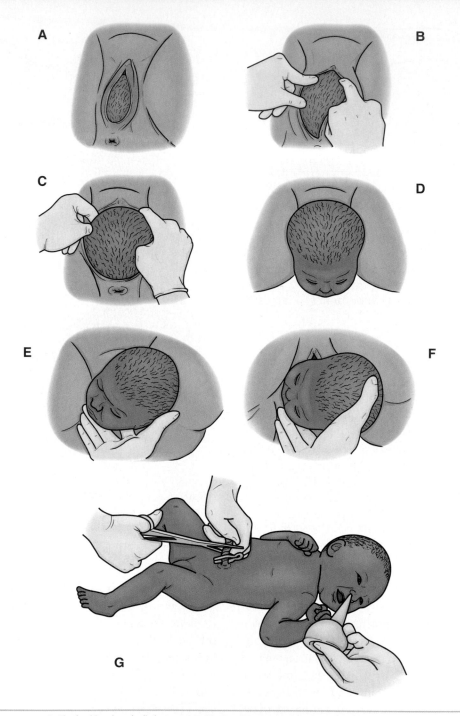

FIGURE 16–15 ■ **A**, The fetal head gradually becoming visible; **B**, emerging; **C**, crowning; **D**, head is born; **E** and **F**, the baby rotates laterally, permitting the shoulders to be born. **G**, The newborn with a clamped umbilical cord being suctioned.

emotions—relief, amazement, satisfaction, pride in a job well-done, with tears of joy, awe, exhaustion, love, giddiness, and elation. There is no right or wrong way to feel, and women should be supported and respected in their unique expressions.

Stage Three

Stage three labor begins with the birth of the baby and ends with the expulsion of the placenta. The placenta is attached to the decidual layer of the endometrium by many fibrous anchor villi. Immediately after the baby's birth, there is a lull

Touch Points

In my opinion, I think there should be a different vocabulary and attitude for labor. Instead of "contractions," women should experience "releases" or "power surges." Instead of trying to convince women to anesthetize against pain, they should be allowed to be ambulatory and change positions whenever they feel like it. They should be allowed to have as many people supporting them as they want. They should be allowed access to bath tubs and showers, massage, and acupuncture and as many comfort measures as they need, in whatever form they need.

Women need to be respected, honored, and allowed to be dignified during labor because what we are capable of doing deserves that kind of treatment. If all the little girls in the world grew up watching their mothers, sisters, cousins, and friends give birth, they would understand the process and embrace it instead of fearing it. They would see the beauty and glory of womanhood and be empowered by it.

The media is also responsible for scaring women. Most representations of labor feature women screaming for drugs. Rarely, if ever do you see a water birth on television (other than the nature channels) or a woman employing hypnotherapy techniques to control the pain. Have you ever witnessed a scene in the movies where a massage practitioner or doula attended the birth? This is an egregious disservice to women because it reiterates the negative images of childbirth without exploring the many magnificent options women can successfully employ.

Massage practitioners can provide positive information to pregnant clients and disabuse them of the conventional attitudes about childbirth.

BOX 16-3 Indicators of Placental Separation and Expulsion

- A strong contracting fundus
- A change in uterine shape and position as the placenta moves into the lower uterine segment
- A gush of dark blood
- Lengthening of the umbilical cord as the placenta descends into the introitus
- Vaginal fullness or fetal membranes at the introitus

From Lowdermilk DL, Perry SE: *Maternity & women's health care,* ed 8, St. Louis, 2004, Mosby.

in uterine activity. Strong uterine contractions resume, causing the placental site to shrink appreciably. These contractions cause the anchor villi to detach and the placenta to separate from its attachments. This process takes about 5 to 7 minutes but is considered within normal range up to 1 hour[5] (Box 16-3).

There are several methods that can be employed to encourage the expulsion of the placenta. Many caregivers prefer watchful waiting, also referred to as expectant management, allowing the natural, spontaneous separation and expulsion through maternal efforts. Skin-to-skin contact between mother and child (Kangaroo care) or nipple stimulation promote the release of endogenous oxytocin that encourages placental expulsion. Gravity-friendly positions also facilitate separation. Active management is the

administration of uterotonic (oxytocic) medications to promote the expulsion of the placenta and prevent hemorrhages[5,46] (Figures 16-16, 16-17, and 16-18).

Once the placenta has separated, powerful uterine contractions force the placenta and membranes to fall into the lower segment of the uterus and out through the vagina[4] (Figure 16-19 and Box 16-4). If the placenta is retained, allowing the mother to shift into a squatting position almost always allows the placenta to quickly detach.

Stage Four

As soon as the placenta has been delivered, the fourth stage begins and lasts until maternal metabolic signs are stable. Blood pressure, **lochia** (normal postpartum vaginal discharge), uterine tone, blood pressure, heart rate, and temperature are all examined over a period of 1 to 2 hours. With a medicated birth, a prolonged difficult labor, or if the delivery was surgical, the fourth stage may last longer.

Immediately after birth, the fundus should remain as firm as a grapefruit. If it appears to be soft, fundal massage can aid in involution (Box 16-5). Right after the birth, the new mother may experience trembling in her legs, uterine pain as it starts to contract and shrink, and swelling and discomfort in the perineum, especially if she had an episiotomy. Warm blankets should be placed on her legs, which can control the shaking, and a cold compress on the perineum will reduce swelling and pain.[13]

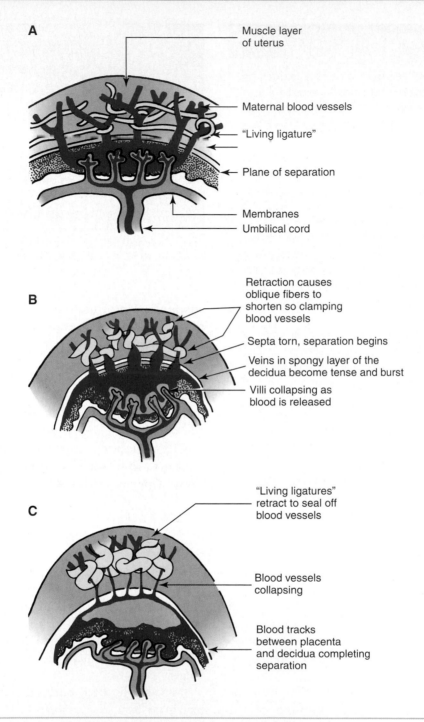

FIGURE 16-16 ■ The placental site during separation. **A,** The top picture shows the uterus and placenta before separation; **B,** the beginning of placental separation; **C,** the separation nearly complete. (From Fraser D, Cooper, M: *Myles' textbook for midwives,* ed 14, Edinburgh, 2003, Churchill Livingstone.)

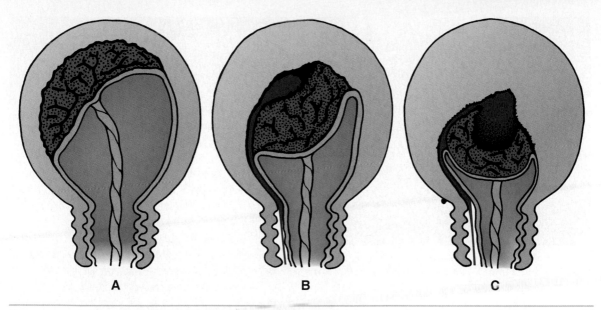

FIGURE 16-17 ■ **A,** The uterine wall is partially retracted, but not sufficiently to cause placental separation. **B,** Further contractions and retraction thicken the uterine wall, reduce the placental site and aid in separation. **C,** Complete separation and formation of the retroplacental clot. (From Fraser D, Cooper M: *Myles' textbook for midwives,* ed 14, Edinburgh, 2003, Churchill Livingstone.)

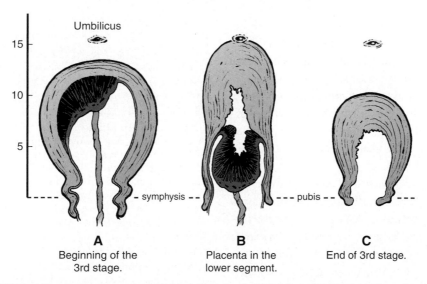

FIGURE 16-18 ■ Fundal height relative to the umbilicus and pubic symphysis during the third stage of labor. **A,** Beginning of stage 3; **B,** placenta in lower uterine segment; **C,** expulsion of placenta and end of stage 3. (From Fraser D, Cooper M: *Myles' textbook for midwives,* ed 14, Edinburgh, 2003, Churchill Livingstone.)

Maternal Physiological Adaptations During Labor

During **parturition** (the process of birthing), the woman's body undergoes many physiological adaptations.

Cardiovascular System

With each contraction, 300 to 500 ml of blood is pumped out of the uterus through the uterine artery and into the mother's vascular system and peripheral vessels. This increases cardiac output by 10% to 15% during the first stage of labor and

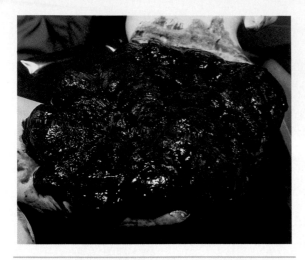

FIGURE 16-19 ■ The placenta. (From Lowdermilk DL, Perry, SE: *Maternity & women's health care,* ed 8, St. Louis, 2004, Mosby.)

30% to 50% in the second stage. Her heart rate increases only slightly.[5] The mother's blood pressure may increase as peripheral vessel resistance increases.[47] During the first stage of labor, contractions cause the systolic readings to increase by 10 mm Hg. During stage two, systolic readings may increase by 30 mm Hg and diastolic readings by 25 mm Hg. These levels remain somewhat elevated between contractions.[5]

Fibrinogenic activity increases, clotting time shortens, and fibrinolytic activity decreases on completion of the third stage of labor. About 10% to 15% of the total body fibrin covers the site of the placental attachment.[48]

When a woman lies on her back during labor (the **lithotomy** position), the weight of the uterus compresses the ascending vena cava and descending aorta, causing supine hypotension (Figure 16-20). Other possible risk factors for supine hypotension are a multiples pregnancy, obesity, hydramnios, dehydration, or hypovolemia (hemorrhagic shock). Anxiety, stress, pain, and certain medications may also contribute to the dangerous condition.

Women should avoid using the **Valsalva maneuver** for pushing during the second stage of labor. Holding her breath and tightening the abdominal muscles increases intrathoracic pressure, reduces venous return, and increases venous pressure. Cardiac output and blood pressure increase while the maternal pulse temporary slows down. Fetal

---

BOX 16-4   *Cultural Views Regarding the Placenta*

Most tribal peoples were aware of the serious sequelae of retention of the placenta and used innovative techniques to support the delivery of the placenta. The most common method was massage.*

A United States Army surgeon, describing the labor of a Sioux woman he had helped during childbirth, mentioned the use of an abdominal belt to facilitate expulsion of the placenta:

"The moment I cut the cord she jumped to her feet, and, standing erect, seized the squaw-belt, a leather belt about four inches wide, which she buckled over her hips and abdomen, drawing it as tightly as her strength would permit. During this time the hemorrhage was very abundant; within a minute, however, the placenta dropped on the floor, bleeding ceased the womb becoming firmly contracted, and she sat down on a stool looking as if nothing unusual had happened. The belt was removed the next morning, and she remained up and went about the house as usual."†

A hot compress on the abdomen was also a very common and effective way of expelling the placenta. (This is not a recommended practice.)

Some cultures have ceremonies regarding the burying or storing of the placenta, whereas some new mothers eat their placentas, finding it natural and nutritious.‡ In Chinese medicine, the placenta is made into a medicine the new mother takes for the first few days postpartum.§

---

*Data from Jocano LF: *Sulod society,* Queen City, Philippines, 1968, University of the Philippines Press; Hogbin IH: *Kinship and marriage in a New Guinea village,* London, 1963, The Athlone Press; Blackwood B: *Both sides of Buka passage,* Oxford, 1935, Clarendon Press; Mead M: *Growing up in New Guinea,* New York, 1930, William Morrow.
†Data from Ray VF: *Primitive pragmatists: the Medoc of Northern California,* Seattle, 1963, University of Washington Press.
‡Data from April E: *Mothering* 28:76, 1983.
§Data from Romm AJ: *Natural health after birth: the complete guide to postpartum wellness,* Rochester, VT, 2002, Healing Arts Press.

hypoxia may result but reverses as soon as the woman inhales[5,46,49] (Box 16-6).

During labor, white blood cell (WBC) count may increase, although the reason is unclear. Labor is hard work, and physical exercise can increase WBC levels.[50] Other cardiovascular changes are flushed cheeks, hot or cold hands or feet, and hemorrhoids.[5]

BOX 16-5	*Fundal Massage (Uterine Involution Massage)*

After the birth, the fundus of the uterus should be firm. If it is relaxed, a fundal massage will cause it to contract and begin the process of involution. This massage is very important because there may be excessive bleeding if the uterus is not firm. It can be self-administered, done by a care provider, or by a massage practitioner. The pressure should be firm, and the desired effect is a tightened uterus.

The woman can be lying on her back with her knees bent, or sitting, supported comfortably by pillows with her knees bent. With both hands slightly cupped, the woman deeply and firmly massages the abdomen with small circular movements (circular pétrissage), using the fingertips. The contractions may hurt. If the uterus does not harden after this massage, then someone needs to contact her care provider.

This massage can be repeated every couple of hours during the first week postpartum to encourage uterine involution. The discomfort will diminish with each massage. Women with cesarean scars should perform the massage but should avoid direct contact with the incision, taking care not to pull on it.

Respiratory System

Oxygen consumption almost doubles for nonmedicated women during the second stage of labor. Some women may hyperventilate, causing hypoxia and hypocapnia. Nervousness and anxiety can be contributing factors to hyperventilation.[5]

Renal System

There is a slight increase in proteinuria levels during labor, which may be a response to the normal muscle tissue breakdown from the arduous work of labor. Urination is somewhat suppressed during labor because of tissue edema from the pressure of the presenting fetal part, discomfort and pain, analgesia, or embarrassment.[5] Levels of renin and angiotensinogen increase, which is necessary to maintain blood flow.

Metabolic Rate

Maternal glucose consumption increases during labor to provide much needed energy by the uterus and skeletal muscles. About 15 minutes after the birth, the woman may feel a transient postpartum chill, and a slightly elevated temperature for the first 24 hours postpartum is not uncommon.[51]

Integumentary System

Skin changes are easy to notice, especially in areas of greatest stretching. In spite of the perineal region's ability to stretch, minute tears in the skin surrounding the vaginal introitus often occur.[5]

Musculoskeletal System

The musculoskeletal system undergoes tremendous stress during labor. Profuse sweating, fatigue, increased proteinuria, and elevated body temperature accompany the increase in muscular activity. Backaches and joint aches are common as a result of the increased joint laxity at term and labor positions. Leg cramps and trembling legs are common during the second stage of labor.[5]

Nervous System

A woman's pain perception and sensorial experiences change as labor progresses through each stage. As labor commences, she may feel happy and excited. These feelings cede to more intense, serious feelings during the second stage of labor. Endogenous endorphins raise her pain threshold, and physiological anesthesia of the perineal tissue, caused by the pressure of the presenting part, will decrease her perception of pain.[5] Noradrenaline increases uterine contractions, and adrenaline causes relaxation. Neural influence of parturition is dominated, however, by hormonal control.[51]

Gastrointestinal System

Motility and absorption of solids foods decrease during labor, and the time it takes to empty the stomach also slows down. Women are often nauseous or vomit any undigested food. Belching is a normal reflex response to full cervical dilation. Loose bowels or diarrhea often precede early labor.

Endocrine System

The maternal endocrine system is the arbiter of parturition. Decreasing levels of progesterone with increasing levels of estrogen, prostaglandins, and oxytocin may trigger the onset of labor. Metabolism increases, and blood glucose levels may drop as labor progresses.

Oxytocin is stored in the posterior pituitary and is released from there. It is one of the most important hormones of labor and stimulates the

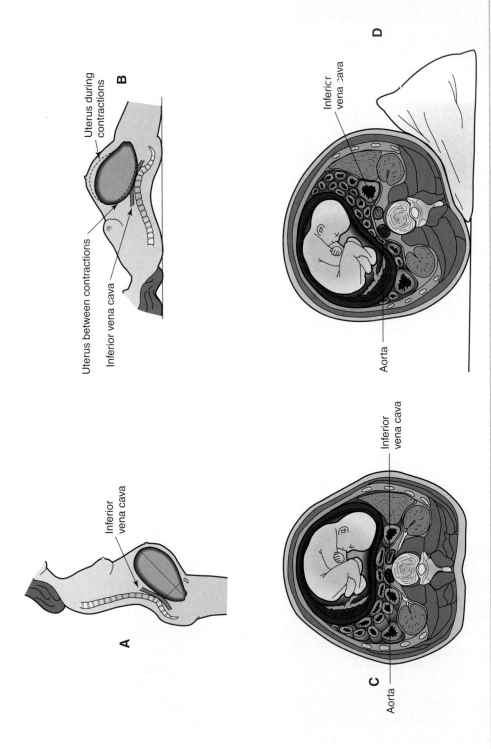

FIGURE 16-20 ■ Supine hypotension. **A,** Relation of the uterus to the ascending vena cava with woman standing. **B,** Compression of the inferior vena cava in a supine position. **C,** Compression of aorta and inferior vena cava in a maternal supine position. **D,** Pillow wedge, or bolster placed under the woman's right side relieves the compression. (From Lowdermilk DL, Perry, SE: *Maternity & women's health care,* ed 8, St. Louis, 2004, Mosby.)

BOX 16-6 *Pushing*

During labor, a woman should follow her own needs and inclinations about breathing during pushing. The need to push is so powerful and compelling that the woman can regulate her own breathing patterns with great success. Few women need instructions on pushing unless they have received an epidural anesthesia and cannot feel the uterine contractions.

The laboring woman generally establishes a rhythmic breathing pattern after only a few contractions. This results in the most pressure being exerted at the contractions' peaks, permitting the vaginal muscles to become taut and preventing bladder ligaments and transverse cervical ligaments from bring pushed in front of the fetus' head.

Some women vocalize or grunt loudly while pushing and should be encouraged to express themselves as they need.

Exhalation pushing involves taking a deep abdominal breath and then pulling the abdominal (transverse) muscles in while exhaling. This maintains normal blood pressure and intracranial pressure and is much easier and safer to do than the Valsalva maneuver.

From Tupler J: *Maternal fitness*, New York, 1996, Simon & Schuster.

ejection reflexes.[52] Oxytocin has also been associated with sexual activity, orgasm, and feelings of love and altruism. "Whatever the facet of love we consider, oxytocin is involved."[53]

Oxytocin causes the rhythmic contractions of labor (in addition to being present in large amounts during pregnancy to reduce stress, enhance nutrient absorption, and keep the expectant woman calm) through stimulation of the stretch receptors in the lower vagina that continue through the birth of the placenta. The fetus also produces oxytocin during labor. During breast-feeding, oxytocin mediates the let-down reflex as the baby nurses.

Maternal levels of oxytocin increase during the first stage of labor. However, the concentration of oxytocin receptors in the uterus (the myometrium and decidua) is greatest during later pregnancy. This explains why the uterus in late pregnancy can be stimulated by low levels of oxytocin but not in early pregnancy. In other words, this is why orgasms and other oxytocin-producing activities do not initiate labor during early pregnancy but may do so in late pregnancy.[54]

Beta-endorphins, the feel-good compounds, are naturally occurring opiates secreted by the pituitary gland, with properties similar to morphine and heroin, such as its ability to control pain, suppress the immune system, and contain stress. Beta-endorphins, like their opiate counterparts, induce feelings of pleasure and euphoria and levels are high in pregnancy and increase throughout labor. These heightened levels permit the unmedicated women to tolerate the pain and allow some to enter an altered state of consciousness during labor.[55]

The catecholamines, epinephrine and norepinephrine, are the fight-or-flight stress compounds that are secreted by the adrenal glands. During the first stage of labor, high catecholamine levels inhibit oxytocin production, thereby slowing labor. Once birth is imminent, however, a sudden increase in CA levels, especially norepinephrine, activates the fetal ejection reflex.[55] **Prolactin,** the breast-feeding and mothering hormone, levels increase during pregnancy and labor and peak at birth. Milk production is inhibited until the placenta is delivered.

Labor, whether spontaneous or induced, does cause varying degrees of stress. Consequently, maternal cortisol levels rise, and this stress compound can cross the placenta, although it is unlikely that cortisol is important in initiating labor.[51] Dehydroepiandrosterone sulphate (DHEA) is the fetal precursor for placental estradiol and estrone synthesis and has been implicated in labor.[51]

Progesterone levels stay the same before labor, although increases in free estriol levels have been recognized in 70% of women just before parturition.[56] The change in ratio of estrogen to progesterone may augment uterine contractions but appears not to initiate labor.[47] The production of estrogen by the placenta increases through labor, as well as in late pregnancy. Women with low levels of estrogen tend to have longer pregnancies, especially if it is their first pregnancy.[57]

Prostaglandins are a major factor in the progress of labor; the two most important are $PGF_{2\alpha}$ and PGE_2, but it is unknown what their role is in initiating parturition. During pregnancy, levels of prostaglandins are rather low but increase dramatically after 36 weeks' gestation.[58] There is some evidence that PGE_2 levels within the fetal circulation increase 48 to 72 hours before the onset of labor.[59] This may be duplicated by the local increase in PGE_2 concentration in uterine tissue that stimulates the onset of labor.

Relaxin has been found to promote cervical ripening during labor. Until late pregnancy, relaxin inhibits uterine contractions and promotes vasodilation. Relaxin supports PGE_2 production during labor.[51]

Levels of corticotropin-releasing hormone (CRH) increase steadily from midpregnancy to about 35 weeks when levels spike. Women who have preterm labor have extremely elevated levels of CRH.[60] CRH also increases the production of prostaglandins.[61]

The use of any kind of drugs or **interventions** interferes with the secretion of these essential hormones. Epidural anesthesia interferes with beta-endorphin production and oxytocin levels. The laboring woman misses out on the fetal ejection reflex because she cannot feel the stretch receptors in the lower vagina. **Induction,** or the artificial stimulation of labor, and **augmentation,** artificially speeding up labor, also thwart the natural hormonal response to labor.

Labor Induction and Augmentation

Initiating uterine contractions and labor with chemical or mechanical methods is called *induction* and promoting a labor that has slowed or stopped is called *augmentation*. In 2000, 20% of women had their labors induced.[62] Reasons for induction include the following:
- Postterm pregnancy
- Rupture of membranes without commencement of labor
- Diabetes, PIH, preeclampsia, or serious kidney disease
- Fetal distress
- Fetal or maternal health problem
- Convenience

Labor is chemically or mechanically induced in several ways, including the following:
- Stripping membranes
- Rupturing the membranes, or amniotomy.
- Cervical ripening with prostaglandin gel or Cytotec.
- Administering Pitocin, synthetic oxytocin, which is given intravenously and may cause

hypertonia or very long contractions that may cause fetal hypoxia.

Labor is naturally induced in several ways (see Chapter 17), including the following:
- Nipple stimulation
- Acupuncture
- Herbal preparations
- Strong laxatives such as castor oil[5]

Reasons for augmentation include the following:
- Slow or stopped labor[63]
- Fetal distress
- Hypotonic uterine dysfunction

Methods of augmentation include the following:
- Pitocin infusion
- Amniotomy
- Position changes
- Nipple stimulation
- Relaxation techniques
- Nourishment and hydration
- Hydrotherapy[5]

Cesarean Section

C-section is the surgical delivery of the baby through an incision made in the abdominal wall and uterus (Figure 16-21). More than any other major surgical procedure, the C-section has the potential to preserve life and health.[46] During the nineteenth century, maternal mortality from C-sections was 85% or more with the procedure performed only under dire circumstances.[64,65] Maternal mortality was reduced by the introduction of several important innovations: aseptic technique, reliable anesthesia, proper suturing to control hemorrhaging, ligation of severed blood vessels, blood transfusions, antibiotic therapy, and the introduction of the low-segment incision, which dramatically decreased the risk of peritonitis.[66]

Before 1960, C-sections constituted less than 5% of births in the United States and were primarily performed for maternal indications such as placenta previa and preeclampsia.[65] By 1988, the rate in the United States rose to 23.5% of births; maternal indications were dystocia, breech presentation, fetal distress, and repeat C-section.[68,69]

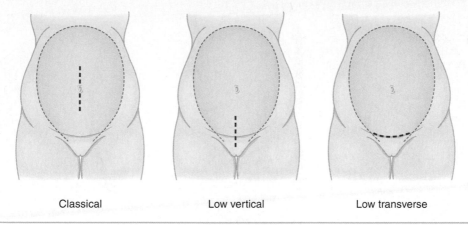

Classical   Low vertical   Low transverse

FIGURE 16-21 ■ Uterine incisions for cesarean section. Classical *(left)*, low vertical *(middle)*, low transverse *(right)*.

The rates for C-section continue to rise in the United States, Canada, Australia, and developing countries, but this rise has not resulted in improved newborn and maternal outcomes.[14] Many leading public and professional organizations, physicians, nurses, midwives childbirth educators, hospitals, and review boards recognize that the incidence of C-section can be safely reduced to about 12% to 15%.[70]

Reasons for a C-section include the following:

- Cephalopelvic disproportion that occurs when the baby's head is too large to pass through the pelvis or the pelvis itself is too small
- Malpresentation or malposition that occurs when the presentation is not favorable for a vaginal birth
- Prolonged labor or failure to progress
- Fetal distress
- Prolapsed cord
- Placenta previa
- Abruptio placentae
- Maternal disease
- Repeat cesarean
- Convenience with elective cesarean[14]

The Cesarean Procedure

With an epidural anesthesia in place, the woman lies on her back with a wedge under one hip to decompress the greater blood vessels. Her abdomen is washed with an antiseptic, and a sterile sheet is draped over her body. A screen is positioned between her head and abdomen to block her view of the procedure and to prevent her from touching the area.

Two incisions are made during the surgery. One is through the abdominal wall: skin, fat and connective tissue (the abdominal muscles are not cut, they are spread apart), and the other incision cuts through the uterus. Both incisions may be horizontal (transverse) or vertical, or one may be vertical and the other transverse. There are three types of uterine incisions: classical, low transverse, which is the most common, or lower segment vertical. The procedure lasts about an hour, but the baby is usually born 10 to 15 minutes after the operation begins.[14]

Women have a wide variety of reactions to the C-section. If it is planned, there is more opportunity to educate herself about the procedure and longer recovery time. Some women might feel ecstatic that it is over and went well, whereas others might feel cheated out of the vaginal birth they wanted.

An emergency C-section leaves the woman unprepared and often shocked and disappointed. Her dreams and fantasies about a vaginal birth have been shattered, and many women feel guilty, angry, sad, and depressed about the surgery.

Massage practitioners can offer help by listening to her talk about her feelings and her experience. Reviewing the reasons behind the decision might help her realize that she has done nothing wrong and the surgery was necessary for her and her baby.

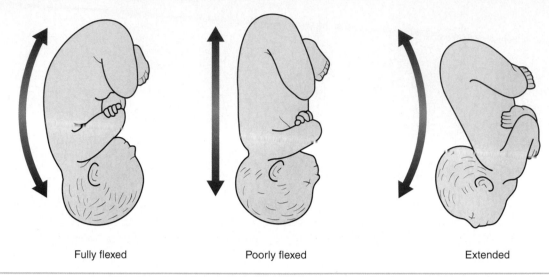

Fully flexed   Poorly flexed   Extended

FIGURE 16-22 ■ Fetal head attitudes. *Left,* Head is fully flexed. *Middle,* Head is poorly flexed. *Right,* Fetal head attitude is extended. (From Coad J: *Anatomy and physiology for midwives,* ed 2, London, 2005, Churchill Livingstone.)

Reducing Cesarean Sections

There are many programs underway to try and reduce the rising number of surgical births in this country. In Chicago, a teaching hospital serving mostly inner city poor women instituted the following new policies that reduced the C-section rate[71]:

- Second opinion was sought for all nonemergency C-sections.
- Trial of labor for all women with previous C-sections led to a 86% trial of labor rate.
- The diagnosis of dystocia was made after 2 hours of no progress with adequate contractions.
- Breech fetuses were delivered vaginally except in instances of true neck hyperextension (Figure 16-22).
- A peer-review process was initiated.

When these doctors successfully reduced the number of C-sections from 17.5% to 11.5% over 2 years, the hospital lost $1 million in revenue.[72] In Florida, a teaching hospital serving poor women reduced their C-section rates from 19.5% to 7.2% by the following[70]:

- All women were considered candidates for trial of labor except for those with previous classic incision, more than two previous C-sections, or unknown scar.
- No elective C-sections were performed.
- Once contractions were adequate, a diagnosis of dystocia required arrest of dilation

for 2 hours or arrest for descent for 1 hour in primiparas and 30 minutes in multiparas.

- With weak contractions, the diagnosis required arrest of dilation for 4 hours on oxytocin.
- Cervical ripening with prostaglandin gel would precede induction of labor with an unripe cervix.
- Fetal distress had to be confirmed with fetal scalp blood sampling or acoustic stimulation.
- Breech presentation would be treated with external cephalic version, and vaginal birth was made possible in selected instances.

Vaginal Birth After Cesarean

Many women who have had surgical births can have vaginal births in the future. The benefits of **vaginal birth after cesarean** (VBAC) are numerous, including lower maternal and neonate mortality, no postoperative complications, less time in the hospital, easier postpartum recovery, and numerous emotional and psychological benefits.

The popular belief that "once a C-section, always a C-section" came from "Conservatism in Obstetrics," which was a paper printed in 1916 that cautioned doctors to avoid a primary C-section for fear that it would cause surgical deliveries in the

BOX 16-7 *Home Birth*

A North American study published in the June 18, 2005 *British Medical Journal* cited that there was no difference in mortality rate between planned home births with certified midwives in attendance and hospital births for women with low-risk pregnancies. Almost 5500 women participated in this study.

The rates of electronic fetal monitoring at home was 9.6% as compared with 84.3% in the hospital. The number of home births that had to be transferred for C-section was 3.7% as compared with 19.0% of the hospital low-risk births. At home, the episiotomy rate was 2.1% versus 33.0% in the hospital. Eighty-seven percent of the mothers and infants in the home births did not require transfer to the hospital. The study also noted that an uncomplicated birth in the hospital cost three times as much as a similar home birth with an attending midwife.

From Home births with certified midwives just as safe as hospitals, Chiropractic Research. Available at http://www.chiropracticresearch.org/NEWS_Home%20Births%20With%20Certified%20Midwives%20Just%20as%20Safe%20as%20Hospitals.htm.

future. At that time, the national C-section rate was 2%. Further support of VBAC came during the 1980s when studies at large university hospitals indicated that a vast majority, nearly 80% of women, can have safe VBACs.[46]

In the United States, the incidence of VBAC went from 19.9% to 28.3% in 1996. In Europe, the number was 50% in 1997.[46] In this country, government health experts supported VBAC as a way to control rising C-section rates that reached 24.4% in 2001. Instead of following these guidelines, the rates of VBACs dropped dramatically from 18.3% in 1999 to 10.6% in 2003. Today, at hundreds of small community hospitals across the country, women are refused VBACs because of the concern of uterine rupturing.

The rate of uterine rupturing occurs less than 2% during a VBAC, which is the same degree as in repeat C-sections. Data suggest the use of hormones to induce or augment labor increase the chances of rupture up to 15 times. Women attempting VBAC given Cytotec (misoprostol) for labor induction had a uterine rupture rate of 5.6% as compared with a rupture rate of 0.2% for those women not given the drug. This is a 28-fold increase in rupture rate.[73] In midwifery practices where labor is nonmedicated, VBACs are performed without any complications in the majority of cases.[74,75]

A woman considering a VBAC must discuss with her care provider methods used during labor to ensure a successful, safe, and preferred vaginal birth (Box 16-7).

In My Experience...

T was pregnant with her second child and was told that because her first child was delivered surgically, this birth would be a C-section. I asked her what medical risk factors she had during her first pregnancy and if these same risk factors were present now. She said no, but her doctor never discussed any other options with her. I gave her some information to read about VBAC and told her that if this was something she wanted to consider, she should have a conversation with her doctor.

The next time I saw her, she told me that she did discuss VBAC with her doctor and that he was willing to work with her. T delivered a beautiful baby girl vaginally and was thrilled with the birth outcome.

Providing useful information in a nonjudgmental way can impact a woman's experience of her pregnancy and labor.

Summary

Labor is a complex and interwoven physiological process between the fetus, the placenta, and the mother. Unfortunately, many pregnant women neither fully understand the process nor recognize how their bodies are designed to successfully cope with this intense event. Educating clients about labor is one way massage practitioners can help women respect the process of labor without the emotional and physiological complications that fear and anxiety can provoke.

There are four stages in normal labor. Stage one, the longest of the stages, has three phases. Phase one is also called the latent phase and it is the longest phase. The contractions are mild and short and the cervix dilates to about 3 or 4, sometimes 5 cm. Phase two, the active phase, is marked by a change in labor pattern and emotional response. The contractions come closer together, and the cervix dilates to 7, 8 or 9 cm. Transition, or phase three of stage one, is the hardest but the shortest. Phase three ends with the cervix completely dilated at 10 cm.

Before stage two, there is a lull in uterine activity and relief of the symptoms of transition. This is the resting, or latent phase, of stage two. The active phase resumes with strong contractions, and birth comes during the transition phase of stage two. Stage three is the expulsion of the placenta, and stage four is recovery.

A medicated birth has some advantages, such as pain relief, and several disadvantages, among which are a slower, prolonged labor; serious headaches; fetal hypoxia; newborn grogginess as the medications cross the placenta; increased risk of C-section; and patient immobility.

An episiotomy, performed to widen the vaginal outlet, also has more deleterious effects than advantages to the laboring woman. Women should practice perineal massage and openly discuss their care providers' routine practices.

C-sections are sometimes necessary to save the life of the mother or child, but this major surgical procedure can also be elective. Recovery takes longer than a vaginal birth. VBAC is usually safe for both mother and child. Women should speak with their care providers about their attitudes toward VBAC.

References

1. Declercq ER, Sakala C, Corry MP, et al: *Listening to mothers: report of the first national U.S. survey of women's childbearing experiences*, New York, 2002, Maternity Center Association and Harris Interactive.
2. Kirkman S: The educational perspective, *Practising Midwife* 4(6):14, 2001.
3. WHO Department of Reproductive Health and Research: *Care in normal labor: a practical guide*, Geneva, 1997, WHO.
4. Fraser D, Cooper M: *Myles' textbook for midwives*, ed 14, Edinburgh, 2003, Churchill Livingstone.
5. Lowdermilk DL, Perry SE: *Maternity & women's health care*, ed 8, St. Louis, 2004, Mosby.
6. VandeVusse L: The essential forces of labor revisited: 13 Ps reported in women's birth stories, *MCN Am J Matern Child Nurs* 24(4):176-184, 1999.
7. Albers L: The duration of labor in healthy women, *J Perinatol* 19(2):114-119, 1999.
8. Tortora G, Grabowski S: *Principles of anatomy and physiology*, ed 9, New York, 2000, John Wiley.
9. Cunningham FG, MacDonald PC, Gant NF, et al: *Williams obstetrics*, ed 21, New York, 2001, McGraw Hill.
10. O'Driscoll K, Meagher D: *Active management of labour*, ed 3, London, 1993, Mosby.
11. Beazley JM, Lobb MO: *Aspects of care in labour*, New York, 1983, Churchill Livingstone.
12. Ferguson JK: A study of the motility of the intact uterus at term, *Surg Gynecol Obstet* 73:359-366, 1941.
13. *Labor and delivery: activities of the pregnancy and perinatology branch*, Washington, DC, 1999, National Institute of Child Health and Human Development.
14. Simkin P, Whalley J, Keppler A: *Pregnancy, childbirth and the newborn*, Minnetonka, MN, 1991, Meadowbrook Press.
15. Carlson JM, Diehl JA, Sachtleben-Murray M, et al: Maternal position during parturition in normal labor, *Obstet Gynecol* 68:443, 1986.
16. Roberts J, Malasanos L, Mendez-Bauer C: Maternal positions in labor: analysis in relation to comfort and efficiency, *Birth Defects Orig Artic Ser* 17(6):97-128, 1981.
17. Simkin P: *Comfort measures for childbirth*, Waco, Tex, 1997, Childbirth Graphics.
18. Mayberry LJ, Clemmens D, De A: Epidural analgesia side effects, co-interventions, and care of women during childbirth: a systematic review, *Am J Obstet Gynecol* 186:S81-S93, 2002.
19. Simchak M: *Just the facts about epidural anesthesia for labor*, Minneapolis, 1996, ICEA.
20. Thorp JA, Breedlove G: Epidural analgesia in labor: an evaluation of risks and benefits, *Birth* 23(2):63-83, 1996.
21. Lieberman E, O'Donoghue C: Unintended effects of epidural anesthesia during labor: a systematic review, *Am J Obstet Gynecol* 186:S31-S68, 2002.
22. Bacigalupo G, Riese S, Rosendahl H, et al: Quantitative relationships between pain intensities during labor and beta-endorphin and cortisol concentrations in plasma.

Decline of the hormone concentrations in the early postpartum recovery period, *J Perinat Med* 18(4):289-296, 1990.

23. Goodfellow CF, Hull MG, Swaab DF, et al: Oxytocin deficiency at delivery with epidural analgesia, *Br J Obstet Gynaecol* 90:214-219, 1983.

24. McRae-Bergeron CE, Andrews CM, et al: The effect of epidural analgesia on the second stage of labor, *AANA J* 66(2):177-182, 1998.

25. Falconer AD, Powles AB: Plasma noradrenaline levels during labor. Influence of elective lumbar epidural blockade, *Anesthesia* 37:416-420, 1982.

26. Behrens O: Effects of lumbar epidural analgesia on prostaglandin F_2 alpha release and oxytocin secretion during labor, *Prostaglandins* 45(3):285-296, 1993.

27. Eldor J: Combined spinal-epidural anesthesia, CSEN, The Global Regional Anesthesia. Available at http://www.csen.com/anesthesia/book/#ch11. Accessed 1993.

28. Fusi L, Steer PJ, Maresh MJ, et al: Maternal pyrexia associated with the use of epidural anesthesia in labour, *Lancet* 1(8649):1250-1252, 1989.

29. Vinson DC, Thomas R, Kiser T: Association between epidural analgesia during labor and fever, *J Fam Pract* 36(6):617-622, 1993.

30. Ploeckinger B, Ulm MR, Chalubinski K, et al: Epidural anaesthesia in labour: influence on surgical delivery rates, intrapartum fever and blood loss, *Gynecol Obstet Invest* 39(1):24-27, 1995.

31. Fernando R, Bonello E: Placental and maternal plasma concentrations of fentanyl and bupivacaine after ambulatory combined spinal epidural analgesia during labor, *Int J Obstet Anesth* 4: 1995.

32. Brinsmead M: Fetal and neonatal effects of drugs administered in labor, *Med J Australia* 146:481-486, 1987.

33. Hale T: The effects on breastfeeding women of anesthetic medications used during labor, Paper presented at Passage to Motherhood Conference, Brisbane, 1998.

34. Sepkoski CB: The effects of maternal epidural anesthesia on neonatal behavior during the first month, *Dev Med Child Neurol* 34:1072-1080, 1992.

35. Murray AD, Dolby RM, Nation RL, et al: Effects of epidural anesthesia on newborns and their mothers, *Child Dev* 52:71-82, 1981.

36. Humenick SS: Your labor guide, *Lamaze Parents,* 1998.

37. Leighton BL, Halpern SH: The effects of epidural anesthesia on labor, maternal, and neonatal outcomes: a systematic review, *Am J Obstet Gynecol* 186:S69-S77, 2002.

38. Eltzschig H, Lieberman E, Camann W: Regional anesthesia and analgesia for labor and delivery, *N Engl J Med* 348:319-332, 2003.

39. Simkin P: Emotional support for the woman with an epidural, *Int J Childbirth Educ* 18(3):4-7, 2003.

40. Zhang J, Klebanoff M, DerSimonian R: Epidural analgesia in association with duration of labor and mode of delivery: a quantitative review, *Am J Obstet Gynecol* 180(4):970-977, 1999.

41. Diegmann E, Andrews C, Niemczura C: The length of the second stage of labor in uncomplicated, nulliparous African American and Puerto Rican women, *J Midwifery Women's Health* 45(1):67-71, 2000.

42. Livingston C: *Just the Facts About Episiotomy,* Minneapolis, ICEA, 1996.

43. Tarkan L: *In many delivery rooms, a routine becomes less routine,* The New York Times, February 26, 2002.

44. *Clearing the way for baby, safely,* The New York Times, October 2004.

45. Hassid P: *Textbook for childbirth educators,* Philadelphia, 1978, Harper and Row.

46. Enkin M, Keirse M, Neilson J, et al: *A guide to effective care in pregnancy and childbirth,* Oxford, 2000, Oxford University Press.

47. Chamberlain G, Brougton-Pipkin F: *Clinical physiology in obstetrics,* ed 3, Oxford, 1998, Blackwell Scientific.

48. Hathaway WE, Bonnar J: *Haemostatic disorders of the pregnant woman and newborn infant,* New York, 1987, Elsevier.

49. Aldrich CJ, D'Antona D, Spencer JA, et al: The effect of maternal pushing on fetal oxygenation and blood volume during the

second stage of labour, *Br J Obstet Gynaecol* 102(6):448-453, 1995.

50. Pagana K, Pagana T: *Mosby's manual of diagnostic and laboratory tests*, ed 2, St. Louis, 2002, Mosby.

51. Coad J: *Anatomy and physiology for midwives*, Edinburgh, 2002, Mosby.

52. Odent M: *The fetus ejection reflex. In Odent M: The nature of birth and breastfeeding*, Westport, CT, 1992, Bergin and Garvey.

53. Odent M: *The scientification of love*, London, 1999, Free Association Press.

54. Fuchs AR, Fuchs F, Husslein P, et al: Oxytocin receptors in the human uterus during pregnancy and parturition, *Am J Obstet Gynecol* 150:734-741, 1984.

55. Buckley SJ: Ecstatic birth, *Mothering* March-April, 2002.

56. Darne J, McGarrigle HHG, Lachelin GCL: Saliva oestriol, oestradiol, oestrone and progesterone levels in pregnancy; spontaneous labour at term is preceded by a rise in saliva oestriol:progesterone ratio, *Br J Obstet Gynecol* 94:227-235, 1987.

57. Oakey RE, Cawood ML, MacDonald MM: Biochemical and clinical observations on a pregnancy with placental sulfatase and other enzyme deficiencies, *Clin Endocrinol* 3:31, 1974.

58. Dray F, Frydman R: Primary prostaglandins in amniotic fluid in pregnancy and spontaneous labour, *Am J Obstet Gynecol* 126:13, 1976.

59. Thorburn GD: The placenta, PGE2 and parturition, *Early Hum Develop* 29:63-73, 1992.

60. Wolfe CDA, Petruckevitch A, Quartero R: The rate of rise of corticotrophin releasing-factor and endogenous digoxin-like immunoreactivity in normal and abnormal pregnancy, *Br J Obstet Gynecol* 97:832-837, 1990.

61. Petralgia F, Benedetto C, Florio P, et al: Effect of corticotrophin-releasing factor—binding protein on prostaglandin release from cultured maternal decidua and on contractile activity of human myometrium in-vitro, *J Clin Endocrinol Metab* 80:3073-3076, 1995.

62. Martin J, Hamilton BE, Sutton PD, et al: Births: final data for 2000, *Natl Vital Stat Rep* 50(5):1-102, 2002.

63. Eggers P: *Just the facts about inducing and augmenting labor*, Minneapolis, 1997, ICEA.

64. Creasy R, Resnik R: *Maternal-fetal medicine*, ed 5, Philadelphia, 2004, Saunders.

65. Eastman NJ: The role of frontier America in the development of cesarean section, *Am J Obstet Gynecol* 24:919, 1932.

66. Frank F: Suprasymphyseal delivery and its relation to other operations in the presence of contracted pelvis, *Arch Gynaecol* 81:46, 1997.

67. Smith EF, MacDonald FA: Cesarean section. An evaluation of current practice in the New York Lying-in Hospital, *Obstet Gynecol* 6:593, 1953.

68. Curtin SC, Kozak LJ, Gregor KD: U.S. cesarean and VBAC rates stalled in the mid-1990s, *Birth* 27:54-57, 2000.

69. Rosen MG: Consensus task force on cesarean childbirth, National Institutes of Health, *NIH Publications* 82:2067, 1981.

70. Sanchez-Ramos L, et al: Reducing cesarean sections at a teaching hospital, *Am J Obstet Gynecol* 163:1081, 1990.

71. Myers S, Gleicher NA: Successful program to lower cesarean section rates, *N Engl J Med* 391(23):1511-1516, 1994.

72. Goer H: *Obstetric myths versus research realities*, Westport, CT, 1994, Bergin & Garvey.

73. Schwartz PM, Lubarsky S: Uterine rupture associated with the use of misoprostol in the gravid patient with a previous cesarean section, *Am J Obstet Gynecol* 180:1535-1542, 1999.

74. National Center for Health Statistics: Birth statistics, USA 1999-2001, VBAC.com. Available at http://www.vbac.com/birthtrends.html. Accessed 2005.

75. Grady D: *Trying to avoid 2nd cesarean, many find choice isn't theirs*, The New York Times November 29, 2004.

REVIEW QUESTIONS

1   At what point during pregnancy can normal labor occur?

_____

_____

_____

_____

_____

_____

2   What are the 5 Ps of labor?

_____

_____

_____

_____

_____

_____

3   Labor is comprised of how many stages? How many stages are further subdivided into three phases?

_____

_____

_____

_____

_____

4   Describe stage one of labor. What are the three phases of stage one called and what happens during each phase?

_____

_____

_____

_____

_____

5   Describe the unique capabilities of the uterine muscle and how it favors the normal progress of labor.

_____

_____

_____

_____

_____

6   What is cervical effacement?

_____

_____

_____

_____

_____

_____

7   What is cervical dilation?

_____

_____

_____

_____

_____

_____

8   Which is the longest phase of stage one of labor? The shortest?

_____

_____

_____

_____

_____

_____

9   What are some of the advantages and disadvantages to the mother and baby of epidural anesthesia?

_____

_____

_____

_____

10   When does stage two of labor begin? What are some of the signs of stage two?

_____

_____

_____

_____

11   Describe the process of labor during each phase of stage two.

_____

_____

_____

_____

12   What is an episiotomy? Why are they performed? Why are perineal tears more serious after an episiotomy has been performed?

_____

_____

_____

_____

13   Describe what occurs during stage three of labor.

_____

_____

_____

_____

14   What is stage four?

_____

_____

_____

_____

15   What physiological changes may occur immediately after the birth?

_____

_____

_____

_____

16   What is the purpose of fundal or uterine involution massage? Who performs it and how soon after the birth?

_____

_____

_____

_____

17   What changes occur to the mother's cardiovascular system during labor?

_____

_____

_____

_____

18   What is supine hypotension and what risks does this potentially cause?

_____

_____

_____

_____

19 Do most women establish their own breathing patterns during labor?

_____

_____

_____

_____

_____

_____

20 What is exhalation pushing and how is it easier on the mother and fetus during labor than holding the breath and bearing down (the Valsalva maneuver)?

_____

_____

_____

_____

_____

_____

21 How is the maternal respiratory system affected by labor?

_____

_____

_____

_____

_____

22 What changes are occurring to the mother's renal system during childbirth?

_____

_____

_____

_____

_____

_____

23 Does the maternal metabolic rate change during labor? How does it change?

_____

_____

_____

_____

_____

_____

24 What changes occur to the woman's skin during childbirth?

_____

_____

_____

_____

_____

25 How is the maternal musculoskeletal system affected by labor?

_____

_____

_____

_____

_____

26 How is the maternal nervous system changed during childbirth?

_____

_____

_____

_____

_____

27   How is the maternal gastrointestinal system affected by labor?

_____

_____

_____

_____

_____

28   What part does the maternal endocrine system play in labor?

_____

_____

_____

_____

_____

29   When do maternal levels of oxytocin increase during labor?

_____

_____

_____

_____

_____

30   What other naturally-occurring pain relieving hormones are secreted during a nonmedicated labor?

_____

_____

_____

_____

_____

31   What are labor induction and augmentation? What are some of the medical indications for induction or augmentation?

_____

_____

_____

_____

_____

32   What are some of the reasons C-sections are performed?

_____

_____

_____

_____

_____

_____

33   What is VBAC? How safe are VBACs when the labor is nonmedicated?

_____

_____

_____

_____

_____

_____

_____

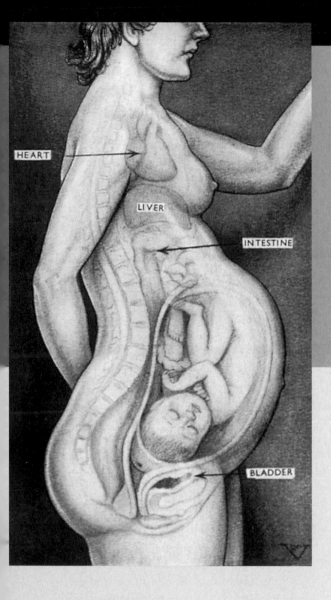

LIVER

INTESTINE

BLADDER

Stimulating Labor

Objectives

On completion of this chapter, the student will be able to do the following:

1 Explain natural, nonmedicated ways to start labor

2 Demonstrate techniques to speed up a prolonged or slowed labor

3 Compare and contrast natural techniques with medicated approaches

During the last few days of pregnancy, or when the pregnancy has passed the estimated due date for many days or weeks, it is not at all uncommon or unexpected for clients to want to start **stimulating labor** (initiating the onset of labor either naturally or medically). Sometimes there may be medical reasons such as pregnancy-induced hypertension (PIH), preeclampsia, fetal distress membranes that have been ruptured for an extended period of time, a fetus who is no longer thriving in utero, or maternal illness.[1] Other times, the mother is simply ready to be done with the pregnancy and is anxious to meet her baby.

Labor Stimulation

When a client requests a practitioner's help in this matter, it is important to make sure she is already exhibiting many of the prelabor physiological changes to ensure the best results (see Chapter 12). The following suggestions can be used by the woman and her partner:

- In the privacy of her home, the woman can have **orgasms** (sexual climaxes), clitoral stimulation, and sexual intercourse. During orgasms and the act of making love, oxytocin is secreted causing the uterus to contract. **Prostaglandins**, hormones that help ripen the cervix, are secreted into the maternal circulatory system and may act on the uterus and cervix. Semen also contains prostaglandins, and after intercourse semen can act directly to ripen the cervix. Clitoral stimulation, with or without orgasm, may also precipitate the onset of labor. It is important to recognize, however, that once the membranes have ruptured, intercourse and clitoral stimulation should be avoided. In addition, blowing into the vagina must always be avoided. Kissing and oral stimulation may work for some women.[2]

- **Nipple stimulation** also causes the release of oxytocin, which contracts the uterus. Nipple stimulation may have to be repeated every few hours to be effective. Self-stimulation, oral stimulation by the partner or a nursing infant, or the use of a breast pump may be effective. A word of caution about nipple stimulation: for some women, this form of stimulation may cause excessively long contractions (longer than 60 seconds) or strong painful contractions that may not be safe for the fetus. One way to avoid this is to time the contractions brought on by nipple stimulation. If they last longer than 1 minute or are painful, minimize the stimulation from both breasts to one or increase the time between stimulation.[1,3,4]

- The expectant woman can take long walks. Even though walking may be difficult because of joint laxity and hypermobility, walks that average 30 minutes or more may stimulate the onset of labor and will enhance labor once it has begun.

- **Herbal remedies**, such as teas or tinctures, may be used to induce labor under the strict guidance of an herbalist or naturopath. One of the most effective herbs, blue cohosh, stimulates the uterus to contract but may also elevate blood pressure to dangerous levels, so care must be taken when using this herb[8] (Box 17-1).

- Bowel stimulation may increase the secretion of prostaglandins to ripen the cervix. An enema may start labor by stimulating adequate intestinal activity to encourage uterine contractions.

- Another way to start labor through bowel stimulation is the use of **castor oil,** which is a very powerful laxative.[6] Castor oil can cause violent intestinal cramping and

Native Americans used many different herbs and substances to facilitate birth. Corn smut (*Ustilago zeae*) was used by the Zunis to stimulate uterine contractions. It was also used by Euro-American doctors in the 1880s and 1890s in problem births. Corn smut has similar properties as ergot, which was used for over 2000 years from the time of the Persians and Ancient Greeks, and controls postpartum bleeding.*

Another herb used by Native Americans is blue cohosh, also called squawroot or papoose root (*Caulophyllum thalictroides*).†‡§

In 1804, a famous remedy to speed up and ease labor used by Sacajawea is the decoction of pulverized rattles of a rattlesnake. This medicine was used throughout the Midwest with much success.‖¶

Black cohosh or squawroot (*Cimicifuga racemose*) was also used for its sedative qualities.§

*Data from Vogel VJ: American Indian foods as medicine. In Hand WD, ed: *American folk medicine: a symposium,* UCLA Conference on American Folk Medicine, Berkeley, 1976, University of California Press.
†Data from Hutchens AR: *Indian herbalogy of North America,* Boston, 1973, Shambala Publications.
‡Data from Kreig MB: *Green medicine,* New York, 1964, Rand McNally.
§Data from Lust J: *The herb book*, New York, 1974, Bantam.
‖Data from Stone E: *Medicine among the American Indians,* New York, 1962, Hafner.
¶Data from Vogel VJ: *American Indian Medicine,* Norman, OK, 1970, University of Oklahoma Press.

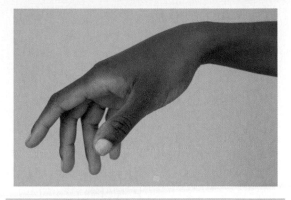

FIGURE 17-1 ■ Large intestine 4 on both hands can be stimulated at the same time for a count of 10, repeating a total of 10 times, to bring on and speed up prolonged labor.

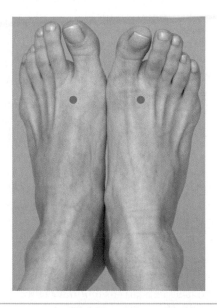

FIGURE 17-2 ■ Liver 3 on each foot can be stimulated for a count of 10, repeating a total of 10 times, to stimulate labor and speed up a prolonged labor.

diarrhea. Some care providers caution against using it, however, because of the concern of releasing meconium into the amniotic fluid and the inherent dangers involved with the fetus aspirating or ingesting this waste product.

■ The expectant mother can swing on a swing. Sometimes the gravitational pull from swinging can start labor contractions. Swinging is also a good way to turn the fetus, if the fetus is not in a vertex presentation.

■ Eating spicy foods can cause some women to go into labor.

The following suggestion can be used by the massage practitioner and the woman (and her partner): after a general massage, the practitioner can stimulate the acupuncture points on each side of the body: **large intestine**

4, which is located in the webbing of the thumbs (Figure 17-1); **liver 3,** which is found on the top of the foot between the big and second toes (Figure 17-2); **spleen 6,** which is the expression of female energy found above the ankles (Figure 17-3); and the reflex point for the uterus, which is located on the inside of the heels). Each point (i.e., both large intestine 4 points) should be held for a count of 10, repeating the process 10 times (Figure 17-4).

It is also possible that the general full-body massage will be enough to start labor in some cases.[5]

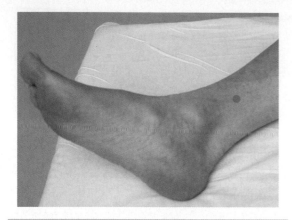

FIGURE 17-3 ■ Stimulating spleen 6 on both legs may help stimulate labor and encourage the progress of labor once it has been established. These points can be held for a count of 10, repeating a total of 10 times.

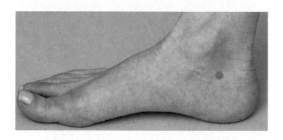

FIGURE 17-4 ■ The reflex point for the uterus is found on the inside of both heels. This point can be pressed for a count of 10, repeating a total of 10 times, to start or speed up labor. The practitioner can cross hands and turn palms up for stronger thumb pressure.

If all of these noninvasive, nonmedicated techniques fail to start labor, there might be a medical reason to use medications to induce labor. Induced labors are either elective or indicated for maternal or fetal complications. In the United States, between 1989 and 1998, the rate of induction rose from 9% to 19%.[8,9] The increase in necessary induction was significantly less that the overall increase, suggesting elective induction increased faster than indicated induction.

Labor Induction

Elective inductions are generally performed for the following reasons[10]:

1. To ensure that the preferred care provider is on call.
2. To ensure that labor will occur with maximum support personnel in case of an emergency.

Touch Points

I had a sign in my office that read, "You are not late!" Human gestation is 38 to 42 weeks. When a woman is given a "due date," she has to understand this is an arbitrary date and that 2 weeks on either side of that date is normal. So many women start to worry and panic when they "pass" their estimated due date. This worry and panic cannot help the situation.

Labor is a very complex physiological phenomenon and fretting about a few extra days can slow down the process even further. Practitioners should discuss this with the client to put her mind to rest. Her baby will come, when it is ready, in its own time.

3. To help the woman make arrangements for the care of other members of her household.

Indicated inductions are performed when there is a danger for the mother or fetus, such as the following[10]:

1. Severe PIH
2. Fetal death
3. Chorioamnionitis (intraamniotic infection)
4. Diabetes mellitus
5. Postterm pregnancy
6. Intrauterine growth restriction
7. Isoimmunization
8. Premature rupture of the membranes with established fetal maturity

Medical Induction

Medical induction of labor is done in a variety of ways.

- **Stripping the membranes**, or sweeping the membranes to soften the cervix, has a low success rate but may be tried if the client is postterm and the cervix is already ripe and dilated.
- **Artificial rupture of the membranes** (AROM), or amniotomy (the doctor ruptures membranes using an amniocentesis hook), only works if the cervix is ripened.
- The use of prostaglandin gels is more effective than AROM but is not available everywhere in the United States. However, this is a standard method of induction in Canada and Europe.

BOX 17-2   *"Laborade" to Fight Dehydration*

Dehydration during labor slows down the progress, depletes energy stores, alters physiological processes, and affects the muscles needed to support the client during labor. As labor begins, women should drink at least 8 oz of water each hour.

A wonderful "laborade" provides carbohydrates, electrolytes, and minerals to sustain the woman throughout labor is made of the following ingredients. She should sip this drink in between contractions.

⅓ cup lemon juice
⅓ cup of honey
¼-½ teaspoon salt
¼ teaspoon baking soda
1-2 calcium tablets, crushed
1 quart of water (juice can be added for additional flavor)

From Simkin P, Whalley J, Keppler A: *Pregnancy, childbirth and the newborn*, Minnetonka, MN, 1991, Meadowbrook Press.

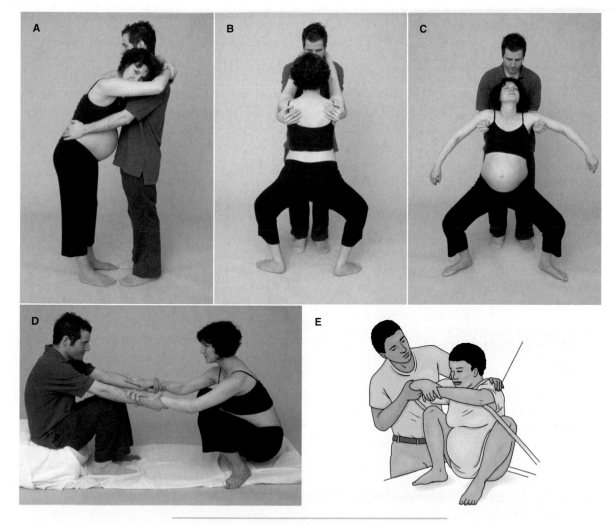

FIGURE 17-5 ■ Gravity-friendly positions to help speed labor.

- A pitocin infusion is the most common medical induction used in the United States. Intravenous Pitocin is often administered in concert with prostaglandin gel over a period of a few days.[1]

Speeding Up Labor

Once labor has established, the laboring woman has many viable choices to keep the labor moving at a progressive pace. One of the most important things the massage practitioner can remember is to help the woman stay focused and not become discouraged. The pace may pick up naturally if she remains calm and relaxed.

All of the techniques described to stimulate labor will also work to speed it up. Being ambulatory, upright, changing positions every 30 minutes or so, drinking fluids and staying hydrated, and nipple and oral stimulation are all effective during the first stage of labor (Box 17-2).

During the second stage of labor, the woman should find a comfortable, gravity-friendly position, such as squatting, a support squat, or dangling to enlarge the pelvic outlet.[11] Standing, semisitting, and hands and knees positions are also effective[1] (Figure 17-5). Stimulating the acupuncture points large intestine 4, liver 3, spleen 6, and the uterus reflex are extremely helpful in speeding up labor. Kissing and oral stimulation, vocal release through toning, positive visualization, and mental activity may facilitate a labor that has slowed.

In My Experience...

D received prenatal massages during both of her pregnancies. She had a preexisting condition similar to lupus that required daily baby aspirin to thin her blood. Two weeks before her first baby was born, she discontinued taking the baby aspirins to allow her blood to thicken (to prevent hemorrhaging during labor). Her doctor told her that after the 2 weeks, he would induce her, which is exactly what he did.

D decided she did not want the second pregnancy to be induced. She booked a massage appointment for the day she was supposed to check into the hospital and told me, "Do what you have to get this baby out!" She was determined to avoid the induction. I gave her a relaxing massage and ended it with deep stimulation of large intestine 4, liver 3, uterus reflex, and spleen 6 points. She said she felt great after the massage.

D never needed the induction. By the time she went to the hospital later that day, she was 5 cm dilated and in active labor.

Summary

In most cases, labor will start naturally without the need for intervention or induction. Sometimes, whether by elective choice or medical necessity, labor has to be coaxed. Natural methods include sexual activity and orgasms, nipple stimulation, walking or swinging, the use of herbs and tinctures or bowel stimulants, and eating spicy foods. After a general massage, the massage practitioner can also stimulate the large intestine 4, liver 3, spleen 6, and the uterus reflex acupuncture points. Medical interventions can include stripping of the membranes, AROM, and the use of drugs and medications to ripen the cervix.

Whenever possible, allowing the woman to control her body and establish her natural rhythms, as she stays calm and relaxed, will go a long way to promote a speedy labor and positive outcome.

References

1. Simkin P, Whalley J, Keppler A: *Pregnancy, childbirth and the newborn*, Minnetonka, MN, 1991, Meadowbrook Press.
2. Kavanagh J, Kelly AJ, Thomas J: Sexual intercourse for cervical ripening and induction of labour, *Cochrane Database Syst Rev* 2:CD003093, 2001.
3. Elliott JP, Flaherty JF: The use of breast stimulation to prevent postdate pregnancy, *Am J Obstet Gynecol* 149: 628-632, 1984.
4. Salmon YM, Kee WH, Tan SL, et al: Cervical ripening by breast stimulation, *Obstetrics and Gynecology* 67:21-24, 1986.
5. Kowalchik C, Hylton WH: *Rodale's illustrated encyclopedia of herbs*, Emmaus, PA, 1987, Rodale Press.

6. Davis L: The use of castor oil to stimulate labor in patients with premature rupture of the membranes, *J Nurse Midwifery* 29: 366-370, 1984.

7. Smith CA, Crowther CA: Acupuncture for induction of labour, *Cochrane Database Syst Rev* 1:CD002962, 2001.

8. Zhang J, Yancey MK, Henderson CE: US national trends in labor induction, 1989-1998, *J Reprod Med* 47:120-124, 2002.

9. MacDorman MF, Mathews TJ, Martin JA, et al: trends and characteristics of induced labor in the United States, 1989-98, *Paediatr Perinat Epidemiol* 16:263-270, 2002.

10. Creasy R, Resnik R: *Maternal-fetal medicine*, ed 5, Philadelphia, 2004, Saunders.

11. Russell JGB: The rationale of primitive delivery positions, *Br J Obstet Gynecol* 89:712-715, 1982.

12. Sears W, Sears M: *The pregnancy book*, Boston, 1997, Little Brown.

REVIEW QUESTIONS

1 What techniques can massage practitioners use to help initiate the onset of labor in a woman who is desirous and ready to be done with the pregnancy and meet her baby?

_____

_____

_____

_____

_____

2 Which acupuncture points can massage practitioners stimulate to potentially initiate the onset of labor?

_____

_____

_____

_____

_____

3 What other suggestions can massage practitioners offer their clients to stimulate the onset of labor?

_____

_____

_____

_____

_____

4 What may necessitate the medical induction of labor?

_____

_____

_____

_____

5 What are some of the ways medical induction of labor is performed?

_____

_____

_____

_____

6 Why do some women opt for an elective induction?

_____

_____

_____

_____

_____

7 What suggestions can massage practitioners offer their clients to speed up a labor once it has been established?

_____

_____

_____

_____

8 How can dehydration affect the progress of labor? What suggestions can massage practitioners make to help their laboring clients avoid dehydration?

_____

_____

_____

_____

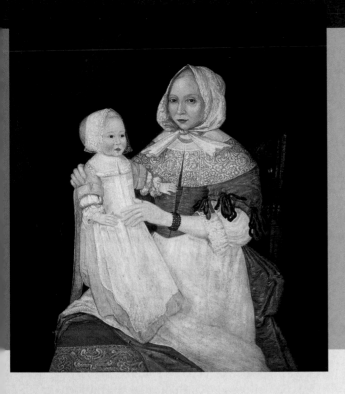

CHAPTER 18

Benefits of Touch during Labor and Other Pain Control Methods

Objectives

On completion of this chapter, the student will be able to do the following:

1 Explain the causes of pain and its perception during labor
2 Cite evidence-based research on the efficacy of touch during labor
3 Offer natural, alternative methods to reduce pain during labor

Key Terms

Analgesic	Environment	Narcotics
Anesthesia	Fetal monitoring	Pain control
Attention focusing	Focus	Relaxation techniques
Bath	Gate control theory	Shower
Breathing techniques	Hydrotherapy	Transcutaneous electrical nerve stimulation
Cold pack	Hypnotherapy	Tension-releasing scan
Counterpressure	Imagery	Visualizations
Doula	Intradermal water blocks	Warm pack
Emotional support	Mobility	

In many traditional cultures, birth was not considered a time of stress or major change.[1] In some societies, women gave birth by themselves.[2-4] Tribal people generally had a positive attitude about the birth process, and the mood at a birth was positive and encouraging[5] (Box 18-1). Since the pregnant woman was well acquainted with her environment and the people supporting her, birth was often a festive social event complete with laughing, ribald joking, and game playing.[6-8]

Pain

Although pain is a complex neurophysiological phenomenon, personal attitude, environment, medical interventions, personal control or lack thereof, psychological state and former traumatic events(such as sexual abuse), past experiences and preconceived beliefs, culture, education, support,

and acceptance can alter the perception or expectation of pain.[9] Many women today expect that labor will be painful or unbearable (Box 18-2). Pain is a "a complex, personal, subjective, multifactorial phenomenon which is influenced by psychological, biological, sociocultural and economic factors."[10]

Labor rarely occurs without some discomfort or pain, and sometimes, even under the best circumstances, the pain may be more than the mother anticipated. Some factors that affect the perception and experience of pain are as follows[11]:

- Immobility from **anesthesia** (pain medication) or **fetal monitoring** (a belt worn around the laboring woman's abdomen to monitor the fetal heart rate)
- Malposition or malpresentation of the fetus
- Rapid progress of labor
- Ruptured membranes, in which there is no fluid to absorb and mediate the contractions
- Tension, fear, anxiety, or posttraumatic stress disorder from previous abuse or trauma
- Induced or augmented labor

BOX 18-1   *Cultural Approaches to Controlling Labor Pain*

Traditional people use a variety of natural methods to control pain during childbirth. In India, placing a knife, a sickle, and a plough share under a woman's bed can "cut" the pain. In a Ga tribe in Africa, broom brushing the laboring woman chases away bad spirits. In a Bagos tribe in the Philippines, the midwife makes a lot of noise to force the baby out of the pregnant woman in a ritual called a *kistat*. In England, the pealing of church bells helps delivery by drowning out the mother's cries.

From Jackson D: With child: wisdom and traditions for pregnancy, birth and motherhood, San Francisco, 1999, Chronicle Books.

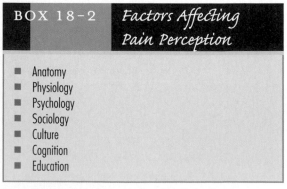

BOX 18-2   *Factors Affecting Pain Perception*

- Anatomy
- Physiology
- Psychology
- Sociology
- Culture
- Cognition
- Education

From Coad J: *Anatomy and physiology for midwives*, St. Louis, 2001, Mosby.

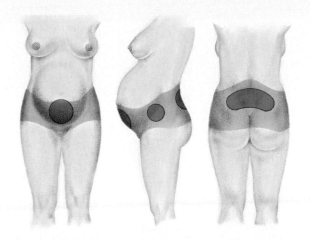

FIGURE 18-1 ■ Pattern of pain during the first stage of labor. Gray areas are mild discomfort levels of pain. Light orange are moderate, and bright orange are intense pain levels. (From Lowdermilk DL, Perry SE: *Maternity & women's health care*, ed 8, St. Louis, 2004, Mosby.)

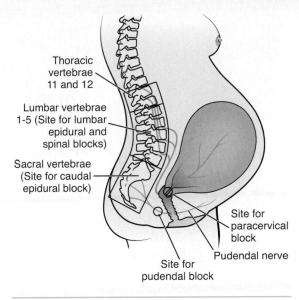

FIGURE 18-2 ■ Pain pathways in labor. (From Fraser D, Cooper, M: *Myles' textbook for midwives*, ed 14, Edinburgh, 2003, Churchill Livingstone.)

- Multiples pregnancy
- Dehydration
- Lack of preparation or understanding of the birth process
- Environment
- Perception and pain tolerance levels
- Coping skills
- Ability to communicate
- The individual meaning of pain

Pain and discomfort are generated from two sources—visceral and somatic.[12] During stage one of labor, the uterine contractions cause cervical dilation and effacement. Uterine ischemia results from compression of the arteries to the myometrium during each contraction. Pain impulses are transmitted along the lower thoracic spine (T11 and T12) and the accessory lower thoracic and upper lumbar sympathetic nerves. These nerves originate in the uterus and cervix.[13] Pain experienced during the first stage, brought on by cervical changes, uterine ischemia, and distension of the lower uterine segment, is visceral pain, and it is generally felt in the lower abdomen. Referred pain occurs when the pain from the uterus radiates to the abdominal wall, lumbosacral region, iliac crests, gluteals, and down the thighs[13] (Figures 18-1 and 18-2). Most of the discomforts of early labor occur only during a contraction, although some women do complain of contraction-related low back pain between contractions.[12]

As labor progresses, the pain pattern and intensity also changes. During stage two, the pain can be sharp, burning, and localized.[13] Stage two pain is created by the stretching and distension of the perineal tissues and the pelvic floor, distension and traction on the peritoneum, and uterocervical supports from lacerations to the soft tissue.[13] The expulsive nature of the contractions or the pressure on the bladder, bowel, or other pelvic structures increases the discomfort. Pain impulses during stage two are transmitted by way of the pudendal nerve through S2 and S4 and the parasympathetic system[12] (Figures 18-3 and 18-4).

The pain of the third stage of labor, in which the placenta is expelled, is similar to the first stage of labor; however, the intensity is somewhat less.

Several physiological adaptations occur in reaction to labor pain. There is an increased respiratory rate, which may correspondingly raise pH levels. The acid-base homeostasis can be adjusted by hyperventilation and breathing exercises. Alkalosis may interrupt the diffusion of oxygen across the placenta, causing fetal hypoxia.[11] The cardiac output increases during stages one and two, up to 20% and 50%, respectively.[11] Pain and fear may create a sympathetic response, increasing cardiac output. Fear also increases the release of

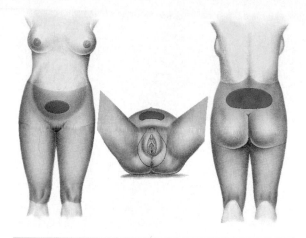

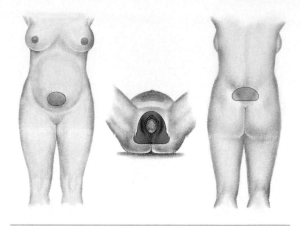

FIGURE 18-3 ■ Pattern of pain during the second stage of labor. (From Lowdermilk DL, Perry SE: *Maternity & women's health care,* ed 8, St. Louis, 2004, Mosby.)

FIGURE 18-4 ■ Pattern of pain during late second stage of labor. (From Lowdermilk DL, Perry SE: *Maternity & women's health care,* ed 8, St. Louis, 2004, Mosby.)

catecholamines during labor, 80% of which is epinephrine (adrenaline). This has a deleterious effect of reducing blood flow to the uterus, possibly leading to a reduction in uterine activity and slowing the progress of labor.[11]

Natural, alternative strategies for **pain control** (the ability to minimize the pain reaction) can be broken down into three categories: cutaneous stimulation, sensory stimulation, and cognitive strategies.

Cutaneous Stimulation Strategies

The Efficacy of Massage and Touch During Labor

Pain relief is a major concern for many pregnant and laboring women. Although analgesic medications offer good relief from labor pain, they also have many potentially harmful side effects (see Chapter 16). The massage practitioner can offer alternatives to **narcotics,** or pain medications, that work very well to control pain, keep the laboring woman calm, and speed up the progress of labor. One of the most effective and time-honored techniques is labor massage and **counterpressure**, or deep pressure against the painful area (see Chapter 19).

In many traditional societies, massage and touch are an intrinsic part of the care for the laboring mother. Family and neighbors who visited the laboring Semai women of Malaysia massaged the mother's belly to help.[11] Asian cultures employed acupuncture or acupressure points to stimulate contractions, calm the mother, and relieve her pain.[12] The use of massage and external pressure was a natural expression of the type of care provided for the laboring woman in all stages of birthing.[1,15] The honorable history of midwifery can trace the use of massage and touch throughout its practice to ease labor pain and to speed up the process.

In addition to stimulating uterine contractions, the labor support massage, which the practitioner can provide or teach to the partner, can alleviate pain, allay fear, reduce anxiety levels, and address musculoskeletal discomforts to encourage the progress of labor.

Most women perceive touch during labor as a positive, reassuring experience.[16] In addition, the presence and support of proactive partners, labor **doulas,** or coaches who touch a woman in labor has a direct correlation with less **analgesic** (medication or agent that relieves pain), short labors, fewer perinatal problems, and improved maternal and familial adjustment.[17-19]

There are many factors involved in a laboring woman's perception of touch. These include her cultural background, her feelings at the time she is being touched, and the type of relationship she has with the person touching her.[20] Other factors to consider are familial, regional, class, age, and

Touch Points

As labor progresses, a woman's desire to be touched will probably change, too. The best way to support her is to follow her verbal and nonverbal cues. Often, her needs are different than what she imagined they would be and there is no way to know this in advance.

Being prepared to support her in a number of ways is the best way massage practitioners can make sure she is kept calm and focused. This could mean a gentle touch in place of a massage, or simply physical closeness. Verbal encouragement, breathing techniques, and other supports can be interchanged as the need arises. Practitioners may have to improvise something as labor moves forward. Practitioners should remember to keep it simple, specific to her present needs, and loving.

BOX 18-3 *The Effects of Touch during Labor*

- Encourages a more progressive labor.
- Elevates the mood of the laboring woman and offers encouragement.
- Lowers stress levels and increases calmness and relaxation.
- Reduces pain and lowers the need for analgesic medicines.
- Provides enhanced emotional supported.
- Offers greater self-control.
- Is reality-orienting.
- Relieves musculoskeletal aches and pains.
- Increases feelings of reassurance, being cared for, and safety.
- Increases feelings of acceptance and respect.
- Improves trust between laboring woman and person touching her.
- Makes it easier to follow directions.
- Makes communication between laboring woman and care provider easier.

From Sears W, Sears M: *The pregnancy book*, Boston, 1997, Little, Brown.

gender.[21] The perception of touch can also be affected when she is in labor.

In a study performed in 1984 by a nurse-midwife, all 30 of her subjects felt the touch they received during labor was a positive experience. Ninety-seven percent averred that touch actually helped them cope with labor, and the touch of a partner was perceived as having the most therapeutic value.[22] These women described rubbing and massaging as having an active therapeutic value, whereas holding was more passive and emotionally supportive. This study also supported the reality-orienting effect of touch during labor, as well as for pain relief.[23,24]

A study done by the Touch Research Institute in 1997 found that women who were massaged during labor experienced less depression, lower stress levels, reduced pain, and faster progress than the control group that did not receive massage[25] (Box 18-3).

The **gate control theory,** proposed by Melzack and Wall in 1965,[26] also helps explain the mechanism of pain relief through massage. Small diameter nerve fibers carry pain stimuli through a "gate mechanism," but larger nerve fibers passing through the same gate can inhibit the transmission of the smaller nerves. By stimulating the periphery of the pain site, the signals of pain and the perception of pain can be altered. Massage techniques, such as rubbing and using ice packs, can shut the pain gate and inhibit the pain sensation by stimulating the touch signals that are larger myelinated fibers.

A painful stimulus feels more painful at certain times and under certain conditions. The awareness of the pain decreases when the brain receives input from other nonpainful, pleasant stimuli. During labor, the pain may not be totally eliminated, but sending pleasant messages to the brain can substantially reduce the perception of pain and make it more manageable.

The gate can also be closed by stimulating the release of endogenous opioids. Acupuncture and **transcutaneous electrical nerve stimulation** (TENS) increase opioid production, thereby inhibiting the pain signal.[22,26-28]

Light effleurage on the abdomen in rhythm with breathing during early labor contractions is often used to distract a pregnant woman from the pain. A **fetal monitor** may make this awkward or impossible. As labor progresses and pain becomes more intense, effleurage may become less effective or unwelcome by the laboring woman.

Counterpressure, or a steady pressure applied to a specific area such as the sacral area, addresses the sense of internal pressure and pain in the lower back. It is especially effective when the fetal head is occiput posterior and pressing against the maternal sacrum. The counterpressure and sacral lift actually moves the occiput off the nerves.

The pelvic squeeze is another form of counterpressure that reduces low back pain.[29]

Touch can be nothing more than holding hands. It is important that the laboring woman's touch preferences be respected as far as who can touch her, when to touch her during labor, and where on her body she can be touched.[30] Noninvasive techniques, such as therapeutic touch or healing touch, may be effective in aligning and balancing the body's energy and may prove more appropriate for some women than using deeper techniques.

Head, hand, back, and foot massages during labor will help relax the woman in early labor. As labor progresses, hand and foot massage may be the most effective because hyperesthesia limits her ability to tolerate touch on other parts of her body.[13]

Acupressure, or the stimulation of specific acupuncture points, can be effective in reducing the pain of labor. Pressure, heat, or cold can be applied to specific Tsubos that have increased density of neuroreceptors and electrical conductivity. Acupressure relief has been explained by the gate control theory of pain and attributed to heightened endorphin levels.[31] Pressure is applied with the hands, fists, thumbs, fingers, tennis balls, and other devices during contractions in early labor and then continually as labor progresses to transition. It is even more effective when pressure is synchronized with breathing.[13]

A recent study on the potential pain-relieving effects of an ice massage on large intestine 4, which is located on the hands, revealed that women felt a 19% reduction of pain when ice was applied to their right hands and a 50% reduction in pain when ice was applied to their left hands. The ice massage was administered for 20 minutes or until the fourth contraction, whichever came first[32] (Figure 18-5).

It is suggested that the client, her partner, and the massage practitioner experiment with various types of touch and massage to determine which is the most advantageous and comfortable during labor.

Labor Doulas

The presence of a skilled support person to guide and assist the laboring woman is not a new concept. In fact, since ancient times, doulas have

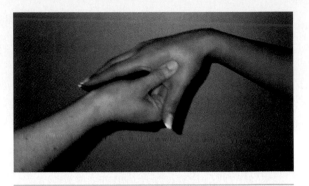

FIGURE 18-5 ■ When ice was applied to large intestine 4, the Ho-Ku point, during labor, pain was decreased by 19% on the right hand and 50% on the left hand. (From Lowdermilk DL, Perry SE: *Maternity & women's health care*, ed 8, St. Louis, 2004, Mosby.)

helped women during labor, delivery, and early infant care. Professional labor assistants (PLA), or monitrices, who are mostly women, provide **emotional support,** comfort, companionship, and technical knowledge and experience with childbirth. The doula is not a medical professional and is not part of the birthing team, but her knowledge of the process and her focused, undivided attention on the laboring woman make her an indispensable part of the team.[33]

In addition to the emotional, physical, and spiritual support they provide, doulas can counsel, advocate for the couple, and tend to her needs and comforts, while allowing the partner to **focus,** or concentrate on the labor. In a controlled study conducted at a public hospital affiliated with the Baylor College of Medicine, those women who had doulas during their labors had cesarean section (C-section) rates of 8% as compared to 18% for women without doulas. The need for epidural anesthesia dropped from 55% to 8%, the length of labor was shorter by 2 hours, and only half as many neonates required prolonged hospitalization.[34] In addition, doulas on average touch a laboring woman 95% of the time as compared with less than 20% by male partners.[34]

Five studies conducted in Guatemala, Canada, the United States, and South Africa proved that the continuous presence of a doula reduced the need for C-sections, shortened labor time, and reduced prenatal problems.[35] A metaanalysis of all five studies demonstrated the benefits of the

BOX 18-4   *Benefits of a Doula during Labor*

In a randomized controlled trial in 1993 at Jefferson Davis Hospital in Houston, Texas, 600 nulliparous women were divided into three groups: a control group, an observed group to measure the effect of a passive observer, and a group actively supported by a labor doula. The support group versus the control group had the following results:

- Cesarean section rates dropped 56%.
- Epidural anesthesia use dropped 85%.
- Forceps delivery declined 70%.
- The use of Pitocin to speed up labor dropped 61%.
- The duration of labor was shorted by 25%.
- The need for neonatal hospitalization dropped by 58%.

From Sobel DS: Mind/Body Health Special Report, 2004.

presence of a doula during labor (Box 18-4). Based on these findings, if each woman in the United States had a doula attending their labor, it is estimated that maternity health care costs might be reduced by as much as $2 billion annually.[36]

Mobility and Changing Birthing Positions

Having **mobility** or being ambulatory and changing positions every 30 minutes not only reduces labor pain but can also speed up the labor process by using gravity to expedite birth. Swaying or slow dancing from side to side, rocking, and other rhythmic movements offer effective pain relief for some women. The upright position increases the sense of control, or being proactive, and provides an overall sense of comfort when compared to the supine position. Being free to move around controls pain and muscle tension more effectively.[37]

Certain positions, such as upright positions, optimize uterine efficiency. The lithotomy and back-lying positions are advantageous only to those delivering the baby, and there are no physiological benefits of this position. Fetal alignment, pelvic diameter, and efficiency of contractions are deleteriously effected by the lithotomy position. In addition, maternal blood pressure decreases and the fetus is in danger of hypoxia.

Positions for the First Stage of Labor

King Louis XIV of France liked to watch his mistresses give birth, thus the lithotomy position, in which the woman is back-lying with her legs raised in stirrups and her hips over the edge of delivery table, became the fashion. Although it does not favor physiology, most medical practices used the lithotomy birthing position until recently. Other positions, such as hands and knees, kneeling, sitting, and sidelying, favor physiology (Figure 18-6). These positions have advantages, as well as disadvantages, and are as follows.

Standing
Advantages
- Uses gravity during and between contractions.
- Each contraction is less painful and more productive.
- Excellent fetal alignment with the angle of the pelvis.
- Relieves backaches.
- May speed up labor.
- Excellent oxygenation for the fetus.
- Helps create a good pushing urge.

Disadvantages
- May be tiring after a long period of time.
- Poor control at delivery.
- Difficult visibility for birth attendant.
- Cannot be used with anesthesia.

Leaning
Advantages
- Excellent for rotation of posterior presentation.
- Uses gravity.
- Contractions are less painful and more productive.
- Fetus is well aligned with the angle of the pelvis.
- Relieves backaches.
- Facilitates the use of more back counterpressure.
- Is more restful than standing.

Disadvantages
- The same as with standing.

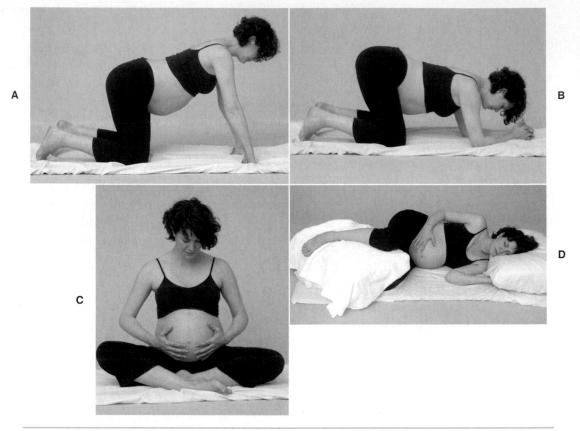

FIGURE 18-6 ■ Positions for the first stage of labor. **A**, Hands and knees; **B**, elbows and knees; **C**, sitting upright; **D**, side-lying.

Walking

Advantages
- Uses gravity.
- Contractions less painful.
- Encourages uterine contractibility.
- Encourages fetal descent.
- Fetus well aligned with angle of pelvis.
- May speed up labor.
- Reduces backaches.

Disadvantages
- Tiring for long periods of time.
- Cannot use if mother has high blood pressure.
- Cannot be used with continuous electronic fetal monitoring or anesthesia.

Sitting Upright

Advantages
- Good for resting.
- Uses gravity.
- Can be used with electronic fetal monitoring.

- Can be used with birth ball to encourage descent.

Disadvantages
- May not be used if mother has high blood pressure.
- May slow labor if used for a long period of time.

Semisitting

Advantages
- Same as sitting.
- Vaginal examinations may be possible.
- Comfortable for mother.
- Uses gravity.
- Works well with hospital beds.
- Good visibility for mother and others.
- Access to fetal heart tones is good.

Disadvantages
- Same as sitting.
- May increase backaches.

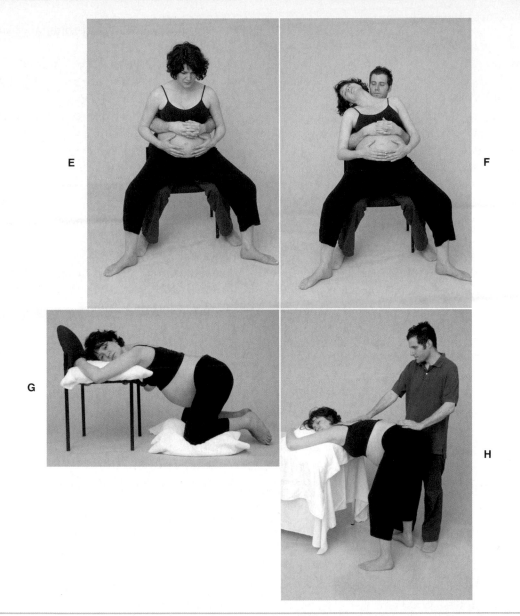

FIGURE 18-6—CONT'D ■ **E**, Sitting on partner; **F**, leaning on partner while sitting; **G**, on knees leaning on chair; **H**, upright, leaning on support with partner offering counterpressure.

- Poor access to perineum.
- Mobility of coccyx is impaired.
- Some stress on perineum.

Sitting and Leaning
Advantages
- Same as with sitting upright.
- Relieves back pain.
- Provides easy access for back massage.

Disadvantages
- Same as with sitting upright.

Sitting on Toilet
Advantages
- Relaxes perineum.
- Uses gravity.
- Mother is accustomed to open-leg position and pelvic pressure in this environment.

Disadvantages
- Pressure from toilet seat my cause pain after a long period of time.

Hands and Knees

Advantages

- Relieves backaches.
- Good for back labor.
- Reduces pressure on hemorrhoids.
- Helps with rotation of occiput posterior presentation.
- Allows for pelvic rocking.
- Assists when other positions create a drop in fetal heart rate.
- Useful with birth ball.
- Best position to avoid laceration or episiotomy.
- Good delivery position for large baby.
- Good delivery position for shoulder dystocia.

Disadvantages

- Vaginal examinations difficult for most care givers.
- Hands and knees may get sore.
- May be tiring over long periods of time.
- May interfere with external fetal monitor tracing.
- Hard to maintain eye contact with mother.
- Hard for mother to see.
- Baby must be passed through mother's legs.

Kneeling, Leaning Forward with Support

Advantages

- Helpful with posterior presentation.
- Assists in fetal rotation.
- Good for pelvic rocking.
- Good for use with birth ball.
- Less strain on hands and wrists.

Disadvantages

- May interfere with external fetal monitoring.
- May be tiring after a long period of time.

Side-Lying

Advantages

- Good for fetal oxygenation.
- Good resting position for mother.
- Helpful if mother has high blood pressure.

- Useful if mother has an epidural or any interventions.
- Makes contractions more effective.
- May encourage the progress of labor when alternated with walking.
- Easier to relax between contractions during second stage.
- Can slow precipitous (too fast) labor.
- Partner can assist in delivery.
- Decreases chances of lacerations or episiotomy.
- Access to perineum is good.

Disadvantages

- Contractions may be longer and less effective.
- Inconvenient for vaginal examinations.

Squatting

Advantages

- Uses gravity.
- Upper trunk presses on fundus to encourage rapid decent.
- May increase fetal rotation.
- Provides comfort and relief from backaches.
- Allows freedom to shift weight for comfort.
- Good access to perineum.
- Excellent for fetal circulation.
- May increase pelvic diameter by as much as 1 to 2 cm.
- Requires less bearing-down effort.
- Thighs keep fetus well aligned.

Disadvantages

- Tiring after a long period of time.
- Legs may go numb.
- May be hard for mother to assist delivery.
- May be hard to hear fetal heart tones.
- May not encourage descent if fetal station is high.

Lithotomy

Advantages

- Convenient for birth attendant.
- Easy access for vaginal examinations.
- Good for electronic fetal monitoring.
- May be restful.

Disadvantages

- May cause supine hypotension and fetal distress.
- Increases backaches.
- Makes the woman physically, emotionally, and psychologically vulnerable.
- Labor contractions take the longest, are least productive in this most painful of all positions.
- All major blood vessels are compressed.
- Laceration and need for episiotomy more likely.
- No use of gravity to aid delivery.
- Slows labor.
- Restricts free movement.

Positions for the Second Stage of Labor

Positions for the second stage of labor, such as semisitting, side-lying, or squatting, favor physiology (Figure 18-7). In the back-lying position, the woman's legs are pulled back and she raises her head to push. In the semilithotomy position, the woman is back-lying with head and shoulders elevated, legs in stirrups, and hips on edge of delivery table. These positions also have advantages, as well as disadvantages, and are as follows:

Semisitting
Advantages

- Convenient for birth attendant.
- Some gravity advantage.
- Easy to get into on bed or table.

Disadvantages

- Restricts free movement of sacrum.
- May slow passage of head under pubic bone.
- Aggravates hemorrhoids.

Side-Lying
Advantages

- Gravity-neutral.
- Easier to relax between contractions.
- Useful to slow a precipitous second stage.
- Favorable if mother has high blood pressure.

- Allows posterior sacral movement.
- Chances of intact perineum improved.
- Pressure relieved from hemorrhoids.

Disadvantages

- Unfavorable if second stage is too slow.

Hands and Knees
Advantages

- Gravity neutral.
- Helps assist rotation of occiput posterior presentation.
- Improves chances of intact perineum.
- Allows for pelvic rocking and pelvic tilting.
- May reduce backaches.

Disadvantages

- Same as for side-lying.
- Tiring for long periods of time.
- Cannot be used by women with hand or wrist problems.

Back-Lying
Advantages

- Widens pelvic outlet.
- Sometimes helps pass fetal head beneath pubic bone.

Disadvantages

- Supine hypotension.
- Does not use gravity.
- Increases pressure on hemorrhoids.
- Tiring after a long period of time.

Squatting
Advantages

- Uses gravity.
- Widens pelvic outlet 1 to 2 cm.
- Needs less bearing-down effort.
- May encourage fetal rotation and descent in difficult birth.
- Helpful if mother does not feel urge to push.

Disadvantages

- Difficult to do in an ordinary bed; bed with a squatting bar is needed.
- Hard for birth attendant to see perineum.

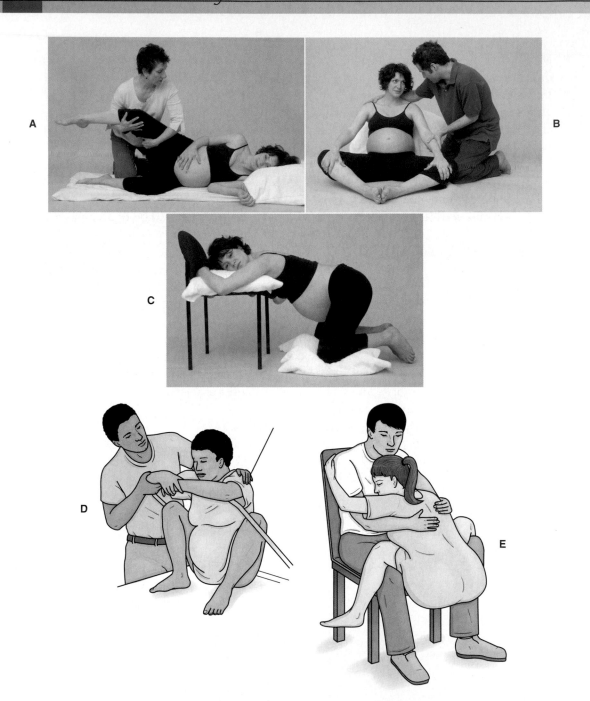

FIGURE 18-7 ■ Positions for the second stage of labor. **A**, Side-lying; **B**, sitting in tailor position; **C**, on knees, leaning on chair; **D**, using a squatting bar; **E**, sitting on partner, facing him.

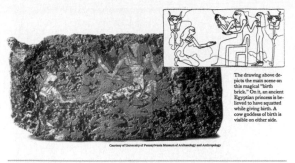

The drawing above depicts the main scene on this magical "birth brick." On it, an ancient Egyptian princess is believed to have squatted while giving birth. A cow goddess of birth is visible on either side.

Courtesy of University of Pennsylvania Museum of Archaeology and Anthropology

FIGURE 18-8 ■ In ancient Egypt, a woman in labor would squat on two large bricks, each colorfully decorated with a scene to invoke the magic of the gods for the well being of the mother and child. In 2001, an excavation at Abydos in southern Egypt uncovered one of these birth bricks from a 3700-year-old house. (Reprinted by permission of the *New York Times* and the University of Pennsylvania Museum of Archeology and Anthropology, Philadelphia.)

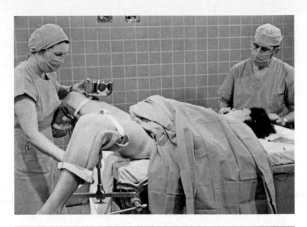

FIGURE 18-9 ■ The lithotomy position from a 1964 picture story book. The woman is flat on her back and her legs are strapped and placed in stirrups. (From Offen JA: *Adventure to motherhood*, New York, 1964, Simon and Schuster.)

- May cause precipitous second stage and lacerations.
- May be uncomfortable (Figure 18-8).

Sitting on Toilet
Advantages
- Relaxes perineum.
- Effective bearing-down.
- Uses gravity.

Disadvantages
- Mother has to move for actual birth.

Supported Squat or Dangle
Advantages
- Speeds descent in difficult birth.
- Relaxes pelvis.
- Improves chances of intact perineum.
- Uses gravity.

Disadvantages
- May be tiring for support person.
- May require changing positions for birth.

Semilithotomy
Advantages
- Mother able to view birth.
- Convenient for birth attendant.
- May be needed for interventions.
- Stirrups support mother's legs when anesthesia causes loss of muscle control.

Disadvantages
- Leg cramps common.
- May be unsettling and disturbing to give birth over the edge of a table.
- Inhibits sacral movement.
- Supine hypotension and fetal hypoxia.
- Restricts mother's efforts and prolongs labor.

Lithotomy
Advantages
- Convenient for birth attendant.
- Necessary for interventions.

Disadvantages
- Does not use gravity—works against gravity.
- May be unsettling and disturbing to give birth over the edge of a table.
- Leg cramps common.
- Difficult to view birth or birth attendant.
- Supine hypotension and fetal hypoxia.
- Restricts woman's movement and effort and slows progress of labor[37,38] (Figure 18-9).

Heat or Cold Compresses

A warm blanket or compress, hot water bottle, heated rice bag, warm **bath** or **shower,** or moist heating pad applied to the low abdomen, back, groin, or perineum can help reduce pain and promote relaxation during labor. Heat is effective for back pain caused by occiput posterior presentation or fatigue.[39]

If the laboring woman is feeling warm, then a **cold pack,** such as an ice bag, frozen wet wash cloth, a rubber glove filled with crushed ice, a bag of frozen peas, or a frozen gel pack, applied to the areas of pain may make her more comfortable. Cold relieves the pain by reducing muscle temperature and relieving spasms.[39] If she is cold, a **warm pack** might make her feel more comfortable.

Transcutaneous Electrical Nerve Stimulation

TENS was primarily used to treat chronic and postsurgical pain. Its use during labor is not widespread, but it has proved to be an effective treatment for backaches. Two pairs of flat electrodes are placed on either side of the woman's thoracic and sacral spine. These electrodes provide continuous low-intensity electrical impulses or stimuli. During a contraction, the woman can increase the level of stimulation from low to high intensity by adjusting the control dials.[40,41] To encourage the release of endorphins, high-intensity stimulation should be maintained for at least 1 minute (Figure 18-10).

Hydrotherapy

Hydrotherapy, or the use of baths, showers, and whirlpools baths at or below body temperature, has been an effective strategy to control pain and promote relaxation.[42] Sitting in a bath for 1 to 2 hours offers several immediate benefits. The buoyancy of the water assists with general relaxation and provides temporary relief from muscle spasms and joint aches and pains. Because stress is reduced, catecholamine secretions are inhibited and oxytocin and endorphin levels increase. The cervix has been observed to dilate 2 to 3 cm in 30 minutes of whirlpool therapy, and hydrotherapy has been associated with faster labor and lower incidence of genital tract trauma.[42] In addition, there is less need for augmentation, the mother is more relaxed and in control, and the use of analgesia and instrumentation is considerably lower with women who use hydrotherapy.[43-45]

If the laboring woman is experiencing back pain or back labor from an occiput posterior or

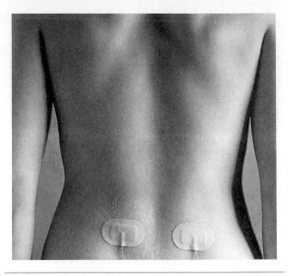

FIGURE 18-10 ■ Use of transcutaneous electrical nerve stimulation to treat pain during labor. (From Lowdermilk DL, Perry SE: *Maternity & women's health care*, ed 8, St. Louis, 2004, Mosby.)

transverse presentation, assuming the hands and knees or side-lying position while in the tub can ease her discomfort. These positions enable the fetus to rotate spontaneously to a preferred occiput anterior presentation, and it is easier to change positions in water than in a bed.[13]

Jet hydrotherapy is best suited for those women whose vital signs are normal and who are in the active phase of stage one. The cervix should be at least 5 cm dilated. If she is still in the latent phase, her contractions may slow.[46]

Another advantage of a bath or shower (a shower instead of a bath is often recommended for women whose membranes have ruptured) is that women can remain in the water as long as desired. Repeated baths with breaks from time to time may be more effective in relieving pain during long labors. The woman should stay hydrated and have a cool cloth placed over her face for additional comfort.[37,46] Most women use jet therapy for 30 to 60 minutes (Figure 18-11).

Intradermal Water Block

Intradermal water blocks are sometimes used to treat back pain. This involves four small injections beneath the skin of the lower back. The effectiveness maybe related to gate control theory, the mechanism of counter-irritation, or an increase in the level of endogenous opioids (endorphins).

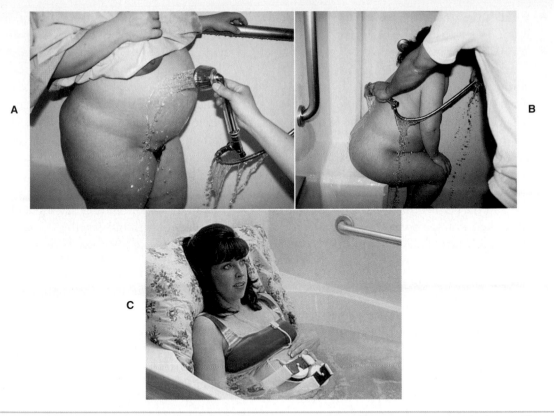

FIGURE 18-11 ■ Hydrotherapy during labor. **A**, The use of a shower during labor. **B**, A woman experiencing back labor feels relief from back pain as the partner sprays warm water down her back. **C**, A laboring woman wearing a fetal monitor enjoys a Jacuzzi. (From Lowdermilk DL, Perry SE: *Maternity & women's health care*, ed 8, St. Louis, 2004, Mosby.)

There is a stinging sensation that lasts for about 20 to 30 seconds after the injection, but the relief provided can last up to 2 hour. When the effects wear off, the process can be repeated (Figure 18-12).

Labor Equipment for Back Pain

During each stage of labor, various tools and physiotherapy equipment can be used to reduce back pain. Couples often have to provide these items themselves, although doulas may have some of them. These items include the following[48]:

- Large physical therapy birth ball (physioball) to relax the trunk and perineum by sitting and swaying or bouncing, or as a support for leaning and swaying while kneeling or standing. The birth ball can also be used in the shower or bath.
- A hollow rolling pin that can be filled with ice or hot water to roll over the woman's lower back.

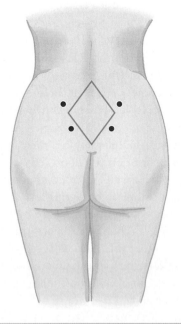

FIGURE 18-12 ■ Location of intradermal water block injections.

- Cold cans of soft drinks to roll over the lower back if the mother is warm.
- Tennis balls or other hard balls to press into the lower back or lean against while sitting.
- Massage tools and vibrators to press on trigger points anywhere the woman may feel discomfort.
- Hot packs to place over the lower abdomen, lower back, or shoulders. During the second stage of labor, hot packs can be used on the perineum to relax the tissues. A sock filled with uncooked rice microwaved on a high setting for 3 minutes stays warm for at least 30 minutes.
- Cold packs for the lower back or on the perineum after the birth.
- Hand-held fans and cool washcloths to keep the laboring woman cool during labor.

Sensory Stimulation Strategies

Relaxation Techniques

The ability to release muscle tension during labor can have a major impact on the woman's comfort level. Staying relaxed or calm can help her conserve energy and reduce fatigue, remain calm, reduce pain, maximize oxygen levels for her uterus, and shorten her labor.[49] There are several ways to encourage relaxation, and she should start learning **relaxation techniques** early in pregnancy so she can become proficient before the time of heightened stress levels. Some of theses relaxation techniques include the following:

- Tensing and releasing her muscles. Sitting in a chair or on the floor, the client should try to release all the muscles not involved with posture such as arms and shoulders.
- Tensing and releasing all the muscles of her body. While lying in a comfortable position, propped up with pillows, she should tighten all the muscles of her body for a count of five and then release all of the tension.
- Mind over matter. The brain and the consciousness mind play important parts in the perception of pain. Pain can be

overwhelming or your client can explore techniques to help her control the pain and panic. Attention focusing and distraction techniques are very helpful in relieving pain.[50] Concentrating on a favorite or familiar item helps some women cope, whereas others use imagery to focus attention on a pleasant scene or activity that is relaxing. Practicing these techniques early in pregnancy will increase their effectiveness during labor.[51]

- Passive relaxation. Sitting or lying and propped up with pillows, the woman can passively focus on her own body and locate areas of tension. Starting at the top of her head, she travels downward in her mind and breathes into each area, letting go of muscle tension. She can practice this easily before going to sleep and learn how deeply relaxing this technique can feel.
- **Tension-releasing scan** is a full body technique for deep relaxation. During late pregnancy, the partner works with the pregnant woman by touching each area of her body as she breathes deeply and releases the tension. She can be sitting or lying comfortably propped up with pillows. This is considered a more active form of relaxation. Starting at the top of her head, the partner touches the area and coaches her to release the tension through muscle release and breathing techniques. The partner works his or her way down the woman's body, touching her jaw, neck, shoulders, all the way to her feet. The more she practices this technique before labor, the more efficient she will be at letting go of physical tension that may slow down the progress of labor. This support, feedback, and touch enhances relaxation and reduces stress, thereby promoting the progress of labor[37,52] (Figure 18-13).

Imagery and Attention Focusing

Using **imagery, visualization,** or **attention focusing** as distraction techniques is considered helpful in relieving the pain of labor.[50] Some women bring favorite photographs or objects and focus their attention on that item during contractions. Others

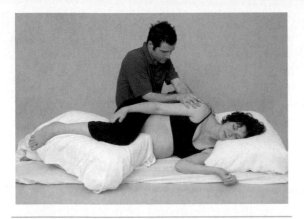

FIGURE 18-13 ■ The tension-releasing scan encourages relaxation during labor.

might focus on something in the room. Specific **breathing techniques** provide distraction and focusing to reduce the perception of pain.

With imagery, the woman imagines a favorite scene or activity during each contraction to take her mind off the pain. Both imagery and attention focusing require practice to master. Women should be advised to start using these techniques early in pregnancy to strengthen their effectiveness.[51]

Breathing Techniques

Specific breathing exercises provide distraction and focusing techniques for the laboring woman that help reduce the perception of pain and encourage greater control during contractions. During the first stage of labor, deep **breathing techniques** relax the abdominal muscles and increase the size of the abdominal cavity. This decreases the pain caused by the friction between the uterus and abdominal wall with each contraction. In addition, the muscles of the pelvic floor relax, permitting faster passage. During stage two, breathing is used to increase abdominal pressure, assisting in expelling the fetus.[37]

There are a number of different types of breathing patterns taught in childbirth education classes for each stage of labor. The woman will generally adapt the breathing pattern that works best for her.

All breathing patterns begin with a routine deep cleansing breath to "greet the contraction" and end with another deep breathe to "blow the contraction away."[13] The first stage of labor breathing pattern is slow breathing followed by light (accelerated) and variable (transition) breathing.[37] Slow breathing is used at the point in labor when it feels better to use this pattern than not. Light breathing is used when slow breathing is no longer relaxing or effective. Variable breathing is a variation of light breathing also called *pant, pant, blow.* It is often used when there is a need to change the breathing patterns, or when the laboring woman is experiencing fatigue, feels despair, or is overwhelmed.

Transition, when the cervix dilates from 8 to 10 cm, is the most difficult time for a woman to maintain control during contractions. A patterned-paced breathing technique is often used during this phase of stage one. It may be a 4:1 pattern (4 breaths and a gentle blow), 6:1, or 8:1. Hyperventilation is an undesirable side effect of this type of breathing, and the woman and her partner should be cognizant of the signs: light-headedness, dizziness, or tingling in the fingers. Breathing into a paper bag or with cupped hands held tightly around the mouth and nose can help eliminate the problem.

During the second stage of labor, women should follow whichever pattern of breathing that feels most comfortable and appropriate. Spontaneous bearing down is the overwhelming urge to push. The breathing pattern used with this urge is called *expulsion breathing.* The woman takes a deep, cleansing breath with the contraction, curls her body, and leans forward. As she bears down, she slowly releases the breath, often grunting or intoning to keep her throat relaxed, and retracts her abdominal muscles. All the while, her pelvic floor should remain relaxed. Some women hold their breaths and release after a few seconds. After the contraction subsides, she should take another deep, cleansing breath[37] (Box 18-5).

Music

The use of music enhances relaxation, reduces stress and anxiety, and can be used to promote the progress of labor during the first stage. In addition, music that is pleasing and personal can decrease tension and elevate the woman's mood.[47] A study comparing progressive relaxation tapes with music, noted that the Lamaze-trained women who listened to music demonstrated an improved relaxation response during labor.[53] Changing the music to correspond with the rhythm of labor and breathing patterns also helps maintain focus and control.[47]

BOX 18-5   *Directed Pushing*

Women who have anesthesia and cannot feel to push or those who have no urge to push are often directed when, how long, and how hard to push. The breathing pattern continues until the baby's head is almost out at which point the woman is told to stop pushing and avoid bearing down.

As the contraction begins, the woman takes two or three breaths and holds the last breath. She is told to push, tuck her chin to her chest, and bear down. She holds her breath for a count of 10 and releases the breath. She quickly takes another breath or two and repeats the process until the contraction subsides.

The Valsalva maneuver is the process of making a forceful bearing-down attempt while holding the breath with a closed glottis and tightened abdominal muscles.* This maneuver produces a vagal response and causes decreased maternal heart rate and blood pressure. Prolonged pushing using this technique can decrease placental profusion, alter maternal and fetal oxygenation, and increase the chances of fetal hypoxia.* More strain is placed on the perineum, and postpartum recovery is harder.

†Women should be urged to employ exhalation breathing when bearing down to avoid possible adverse consequences.

*Data from Lowdermilk DL, Perry SE: *Maternity & women's health care*, ed 8, St. Louis, 2004, Mosby.
†Data from Hansen S, Clark S, Foster J: *Obstet Gynecol* 99(1):29-34, 2002; Mayberry L, Hammer R, Kelly C, et al: *J Perinatol* 19(1):26-30, 1999; Sampselle C, Hines S: *J Nurse Midwifery* 44(1):36-39, 1999.

Aromatherapy

Some women respond very well to the use of aromatherapy during labor. A few drops of certain essential oils, such as lavender, Clary sage, and bergamot, can be added to a warm bath, the water used for compresses, or to a lamp to vaporize a room. These oils, which promote relaxation, can also be diluted in vegetable oil and used for a back massage. Essential oils should never be used full strength on the skin during pregnancy.[13]

Herbology

Practitioners are cautioned against making recommendations about the use of herbs during labor without first having the client consult with a naturopath, herbalist, or professional who can determine which herbs are safe and in what doses.

Herbs have been used to promote labor for centuries. Among those most often used are black cohosh (*Cimicifuga racemosa*), blue cohosh (*Caulophyllum thalictroides*), shepherd's purse (*Capsella bursa-pastoris*), motherwort (*Leonurus cardiaca*), trillium (*Trillium erectum*), valerian (*Valeriana officinalis*), and cranesbill (*Geranium maculatum*). These herbs should only be used once labor has been established.[53]

Cognitive Strategies

Biofeedback

Biofeedback theorizes that once a person can recognize the physical signals, certain internal reactions and physiological events can be changed. The pregnant woman has to learn to use her mind and mental processes to control body responses and functions. This work has to start in early pregnancy so she can become proficient with this strategy. Machines that measure skin temperature, blood flow, or muscle tension are used to provide the feedback and to help the laboring woman intensify their relaxation responses.[47,54]

Hypnotherapy

Hypnotherapy is associated with shorter labors and less pain.[47] When used for labor and birth, the emphasis is on relaxing the laboring the woman and containing her fears and anxieties, which gives her more confidence and control over her perception of pain. Self-hypnosis can be learned with audiotapes or indirect suggestions. As is the case with many of these techniques, it must be practiced and used during pregnancy to be most effective during labor.

Environmental Factors

The **environment** in which a woman labors and gives birth can contribute to her sense of well-being and control or have a negative impact on her experience. Some women choose to birth at home, at birthing centers, in hospitals, in tubs, and some with doctors and others with midwives. The more input a woman has on her environment, the easier it will be for her. Wearing her own clothes instead of a hospital gown and bringing familiar comforting items, such as her own pillow or pictures of her family, contribute to personalizing her birthing environment.

Childbirth Education Classes

Today, most women are expected to attend at least one type of childbirth education class before labor. In this country, however, only about one-third of first-time mothers follow-up on this suggestion. The major methods taught in the United States are Dick-Read, Lamaze, and Bradley, as well as more eclectic offerings from the International Childbirth Education Association and independent childbirth educators. These techniques all strive to give the laboring woman more control over her contractions and labor and to provide her with a variety of techniques to promote relaxation and have a positive birth outcome.

Until the late nineteenth century, childbirth was a social event in which women had their babies at home with the assistance of midwives and some of their friends. During the Industrial Revolution (1760-1840), crowded cities and associated health problems contributed to higher rates of maternal and fetal death from puerperal fever, sepsis, and infant diarrhea.[55] In addition, the patriarchal make-up of the medical establishment and advances in pain medication and infection control in birth moved childbirth from the hands of women to the control of the hospitals.[56]

In spite of these changes, women still sought to have a modicum of control in the management of birth. During the late nineteenth century, concerned women organized the National Twilight Sleep Association to promote the use of the new technique of morphine and scopolamine injections to treat labor pain. By the early twentieth century, most women had accepted the routine medicalization of birth in which they had little or no control or input. Energized by the woman's movement and consumer movement during the midtwentieth century and the increased number of certified nurse-midwives, women began to question these stern policies and the regimentation of birth by the medical establishment. Childbirth education classes began in the 1950s and are now recommended to all pregnant women.[57]

Dr. Grantly Dick-Read, an English physician, published two seminal books, *Natural Childbirth* (1933) and *Childbirth without Fear* (1944), in which he asserted that pain in childbirth is socially conditioned and caused by a fear-tension-pain syndrome. His work became the foundation for childbirth education programs and teacher trainings throughout the United Sates, Canada, Great Britain, and South Africa. In 1960, nurses and others trained in his theories organized the International Childbirth Education Association (ICEA).

Dr. Dick-Read proposed deep abdominal breathing during the early first stage of contractions, shallow breathing for later first stage, and sustained pushing with breath holding.[58] Women were taught relaxation exercises to consciously and progressively release tension, thus a high degree of relaxation was attained. This gave the women an opportunity to experience deep relaxation between contractions.

During the 1960s, the Lamaze method, originally called the psychoprophylactic method (PPM), gained tremendous popularity in the United States. This technique was brought to prominence by Marjorie Karmel's book *Thank You, Dr. Lamaze* (1959) and Elisabeth Bing's innovative teachings and emphasized control by using the mind and mental activities. Lamaze combined breathing techniques with muscular relaxation, with active relaxation as an integral part of the method. The woman learns to contract specific muscles while letting the rest of her body relax. Breathing patterns helped them through uterine contractions. In 1960, the American Society for Psychoprophylaxis in Obstetrics (ASPO) was established in New York and became the national organization promoting Dr. Lamaze's teachings. In 1998, the name of the organization was changed to Lamaze International.[59]

Another early advocate of childbirth preparation was Dr. Robert Bradley, an obstetrician from Denver. His book, *Husband-Coached Childbirth*, was published in 1965. He advanced the idea of natural childbirth, devoid of any analgesia, with the husband (partner) as labor coach and breathing techniques for labor. The American Academy of Husband-Coached Childbirth (AAHCC) was organized to teach the Bradley method and prepare teachers. This method of partner-coached childbirth incorporates breathing, relaxation, and abdominal breathing to foster working with the body's natural rhythms. The environment is an important component of the technique, and the birthing room should be dark and quite to make the process natural. Women using Bradley appear to be in a deep state of mental relaxation.[49]

A review of three studies conducted between 1995 and 2001 found positive changes in health behaviors among those couples that attended childbirth education classes. Communication with the partner, greater relaxation, interpersonal support, and health responsibility were all increased.[60] Another finding was more prenatal confidence in the ability to cope with labor by the end of the classes. The results of many of the studies published between 1960 and 1981 consistently showed that these classes contributed to birth satisfaction, building confidence, and strengthening relationships. Physiological components, such as the length of labor or the use of medical interventions, were less influenced by these classes.[56,61-63]

In My Experience...

It is not at all uncommon for many first time mothers to express their fears about the pain of labor. One client, V, came to see me for a series of prenatal massages and announced the day of her first massage that she intended to use drugs during labor because she did not think she "would be able to survive the pain."

Over the course of the massages, I explained the physiology of labor, which seemed to calm some of her concerns, and then I mentioned hypnotherapy as a way to stay profoundly relaxed and in control during labor without the need of pain medication. I referred her to a hypnotherapist, suggested she call and see if this was something that could work for her.

V made the call. She came back after the first class thrilled with the information and techniques she had learned. After the third session, she was positively gushing with excitement. She could not wait to use these techniques during labor.

V gave birth to a beautiful little girl without any medication at all and used the hypnotherapy (and massage) techniques to control her pain.

Summary

As labor approaches, many women express their concerns about the pain they may experience and their ability to cope with it. The perception of pain and the fears and anxieties that accompany it are mitigated by a number of factors, including personal attitude, environment, past experiences, medical interventions, education, personal control, culture, and support.

Although analgesic and anesthetic medications often relieve the pain and discomfort of labor, they also inhibit natural responses, can prolong the process, and can lead to many unintended medical interventions. There are many natural strategies and methods that can be safely and efficaciously substituted for drugs that can relieve pain, relax the laboring women, offer control, and speed the process without interfering with the delicate, harmonious balance of physiological factors that bring on labor. None of these strategies have harmful side effects and all promote a greater sense of personal control and confidence for the laboring women.

Massage is one of the most effective techniques to ease the pains of labor and help promote its progress. For centuries, the use of appropriate touch has been to support women during labor. Acupuncture and acupressure are also extremely beneficial in reducing pain and enhancing labor. The presence of a doula, or skilled labor assistant, can provide a myriad of support and shorten labor by as much as 25%. The presence of a labor doula has been shown to decrease the need for analgesia by 85%.

Mobility and changing laboring positions can also bring tremendous relief. Heat or cold compresses, TENS, hydrotherapy, intradermal water block, labor tools and equipment, active and passive relaxation techniques, breathing patterns, music therapy, aromatherapy, herbology, biofeedback, hypnotherapy, environmental comforts, and child birth education classes are all extremely helpful and natural techniques to reduce pain, promote greater self-assurance and confidence, enhance relaxation, and speed up labor.

Not all of these techniques are available in every home, birthing center, or hospital, but clients should choose among those strategies that are available to them. Most of these strategies require active participation and practice on the part of the client and her partner. This insures greater proficiency and skill when it is needed the most.

References

1. Goldsmith J: *Childbirth wisdom*, New York, 1984, Congdon & Weed.
2. Murdock GP: *Our primitive contemporaries*, New York, 1934, Macmillan.
3. Schapera I: *Married life in an African tribe*, Evanston, IL, 1966, Northwestern University Press.
4. Axtell J: *The native American people of the east*, West Haven, CT, 1973, Pendulum Press.
5. Jackson D: *With child: wisdom and traditions for pregnancy, birth and motherhood*, San Francisco, 1999, Chronicle Books.
6. Malefit ADW: *The Javanese of Surinam*, Assen Netherlands, 1963, Van Gorcum.
7. Mead M: *Coming of age in Samoa*, New York, 1928, William Morrow.
8. Basso EB: *The Kalapalo Indians of central Brazil*, New York, 1973, Holt, Rinehart & Winston.
9. Coad J: *Anatomy and physiology for midwives*, St. Louis, 2001, Mosby.
10. Telfer FM: Relief of pain in labour. In Sweet BR, Tiran D, eds: *Mayes' midwifery*, ed 12, London, 1997, Bailliere Tindall.
11. Fraser D, Cooper M: *Myles' textbook for midwives*, ed 14, Edinburgh, 2003, Churchill Livingstone.
12. Lowe N: The nature of pain, *Am J Obstet Gynecol* 186:S16-S24, 2002.
13. Lowdermilk DL, Perry SE: *Maternity & women's health care*, ed 8, St. Louis, 2004, Mosby.
14. Serizawa K: *Tsubo: vital points for Oriental therapy*, Tokyo, 1976, Japan Publications.
15. Hedstrom LW, Newton N: Touch in labor: a comparison of cultures and eras, *Birth Issues Perinat Care Educ* 13:181-186, 1986.
16. Stolte KM: *An exploratory study of patient perceptions of the touch they receive during labor*, Lawrence, KS, 1976, unpublished dissertation.
17. Sosa R, Kennell J, Klaus M, et al: The effect of a supportive companion on perinatal problems, length of labor and mother infant interaction, *N Engl J Med* 303:597-600, 1980.
18. Bertsch TD, Nagashima WL, Dykeman E, et al: Labor support by first-time fathers; direct observations, *J Psychosom Obstet Gynecol* 11:251-260, 1990.
19. Nagasihma L, Berschi T, Dykeman S, et al: Fathers during labor: do we expect too much? *Pediatr Res* 21:281, 1987.
20. Mercer LS: Touch: comfort or threat? *Perspec Psychiatr Care* 4(3):20-24, 1966.
21. Fuerst E, Wolff L, Weitzel M: *Fundamentals of nursing*, ed 5, Philadelphia, 1974, Lippincott.
22. Birch ER: The experience of touch received during labor, *J Nurse-Midwifery* 31(6): 270-276, 1986.
23. Cashar L, Dixon BK: The therapeutic use of touch, *J Psychiatr Nurs* 5(5):784-787, 1975.
24. Penny KS: Postpartum perceptions of touch received during labor, *Res Nurs Health* 2(1):9-16, 1979.
25. Field T, Hernandez-Reif M, Taylor S, et al: Labor pain is reduced by massage therapy, *J Psychosom Obstet Gynecol* 18:286-291, 1997.
26. Melzack R, Wall PD: *The challenge of pain*, ed 2, London, 1996, Penguin Books.
27. Taylor AG, West BA, Simon B, et al: How effective is TENS for acute pain? *Am J Nurs* 83:1171-1174, 1983.
28. Doody SB, Smith C, Webb J: Nonpharmacologic interventions for pain, *Critical Care Nursing Clinics of North America* 3(1):69-75, 1991.
29. Simkin P, Ancheta R: *The labor progress handbook: early interventions to prevent and treat dystocia*, Malden, MA, 2000, Blackwell Science.
30. Simkin P, O'Hara M: Nonpharmacologic relief of pain during labor: systemic reviews of five methods, *Am J Obstet Gynecol* 186(5):S131-S159, 2002.
31. Tiran D, Mack S: *Complimentary/alternative therapies for pregnancy and childbirth*, ed 2, Edinburgh, 2000, Bailliere-Tindalll.
32. Waters RL, Raisler J: Ice massage for the reduction of labor pain, *J Midwifery Women's Health* 48:317-321, 2003.
33. Turchaninov R: *Medical massage*, vol. 1, Phoenix, 1996, Aesculapius Books.
34. Sobel D, Ornstein R, eds: Emotional support eases labor, *The Mind/Body Health Newsletter* 1(1), 1992.

35. Klaus MK: Maternal assistance and support in labor: father, nurse, midwife or doula? *Clin Consult Obstet Gynecol* 4(4):211-217, 1992.

36. Sobel DS: Emotional support in labor reduces C-sections and shortens labor, *Mind/Body Health Special Report,* 2004.

37. Simkin P, Whalley J, Keppler A: *Pregnancy, childbirth and the newborn*, Minnetonka, MN, 1991, Meadowbrook Press.

38. Perez PG: Childbirth birthing positions, *Lamaze Parents,* 1998.

39. Simkin P: Reducing pain and enhancing progress in labor: a guide to nonpharmacologic methods of maternity caregivers, *Birth* 22(3):161-171, 1995.

40. Harrison RA, Woods T, Shore M, et al: Pain relief in labour using transcutaneous electrical nerve stimulation (TENS): a TENS/TENS placebo controlled study in two parity groups, *BJOG* 93:739-746, 1986.

41. Bundsen P, Peterson LE, Selstam U, et al: Pain relief in labor by transcutaneous electrical nerve stimulation: a prospective matched study, *Acta Obstet Gynecol Scand* 66:459-468, 1981.

42. Forde C, Creighton S: Labour and delivery in the birthing pool, *Br J Midwifery* 7(3):165-171, 1999.

43. Moore S: Psychological support during labour. In Henderson C, Jones K, eds: *Essential midwifery*, London, 1997, Mosby.

44. Cammu H, Clasen K, van Wettere L, et al: 'To bathe or not to bathe' during the first stage, *Acta Obstet Gynecol Scand* 73(6):468-472, 1994.

45. Downe S, McCormick C, Beech BL: Labour interventions associated with normal birth, *Br J Midwifery* 9(10):602-606, 2001.

46. Mackey M: Use of water in labor and birth, *Clin Obstet Gynecol* 44(4):733-749, 2001.

47. Gentz B: Alternative therapies for the management of pain in labor and delivery, *Clin Obstet Gynecol* 44(4):704-732, 2001.

48. Simkin P: *Comfort measures for childbirth*, Waco, TX, 1997, Childbirth Graphics.

49. Bradley R: *Husband-coached childbirth*, New York, 1965, Harper Collins.

50. Enkin M, Keirse M, Neilson J, et al: *A guide to effective care in pregnancy and childbirth*, Oxford, 2000, Oxford University Press.

51. Hoffart M, Pross-Keene E: The benefits of visualization, *Am J Nurs* 98(12):44-47, 1998.

52. Nichols F, Humenick S: *Childbirth education: practice, research, and theory*, ed 2, Philadelphia, 2000, Saunders.

53. Wiand N: Relaxation levels achieved by Lamaze-trained pregnant women listening to music and ocean sounds tapes, *J Perinat Educ* 6(4):1-8, 1997.

54. Clark D: What herbs are good for labor? The Birthkit issue 43, Midwifery Today. Available at www.midwfierytoday.com/enews/enews0706.asp. Accessed 2004.

55. In Snyder M, Lindquist R, eds: *Complimentary/alternative therapies in nursing*, ed 4, New York, 2000, Springer.

56. Wertz R, Wertz D: *Lying-in: a history of childbirth in America*, New York, 1979, Schocken Books.

57. Lindell S: Education for childbirth: a time for change, *J Obstet Gynecol Neonatl Nurs* 17(2):108-112, 1988.

58. United States Department of Health and Human Services (USDHHS): *Healthy People 2010: conference edition*, vol. II, Washington, DC, 2000, US Government Printing Office.

59. Dick-Read G: *Childbirth without fear*, ed 5, New York, 1987, Harper Collins.

60. Lamaze International: *Lamaze certified childbirth educator (ICCE) program*. Available at http://www.lamaze.org. Accessed September, 1999.

61. Koehn M: Childbirth education outcomes: an integrated review of literature, *J Perinat Educ* 11(3):10-19, 2002.

62. Hetherington S: A controlled study of the effect of prepared childbirth classes on obstetric outcome, *Birth* 17(2):86-90, 1990.

63. Slager-Ernest SE, Hoffman SJ, Beckman CJ: Effects of a specialized prenatal adolescent program on maternal and infant outcomes, *J Obstet Gynecol Neonat Nurs* 16(6):422-429, 1987.

64. Jones L: *A meta-analytic study of the effects of childbirth education research from 1960 to 1981*, Texas A&M University, 1983, unpublished doctoral dissertation.

REVIEW QUESTIONS

1 What are some of the contributing factors effecting pain perception during labor?

_____
_____
_____
_____

2 How does the sensation of pain change as labor progresses?

_____
_____
_____
_____

3 How does the laboring body react and adapt to these pain messages?

_____
_____
_____
_____

4 What are the three categories of natural and alternative coping strategies for pain control?

_____
_____
_____
_____

5 How does massage, or specifically touch, help ease the pain of labor?

_____
_____
_____
_____

6 What counterpressure techniques address lower back pain?

_____
_____
_____
_____

7 Explain the gate control theory and how it explains the mechanism of pain relief through massage or touch.

_____
_____
_____
_____
_____

8 List at least 10 benefits of touch during labor.

_____
_____
_____
_____

9 What other cutaneous stimulating strategies can be used during labor to minimize the pain sensations?

_____
_____
_____
_____

10 Describe the study that used ice massage on large intestine 4 to relieve the pain during labor.

_____
_____
_____
_____

11   What is a labor doula and how does she help control pain?

_____

_____

_____

_____

_____

12   Can being ambulatory and changing positions help with the pain of labor? How so?

_____

_____

_____

_____

_____

13   Describe the advantages and disadvantages of birthing positions during the first stage of labor.

_____

_____

_____

_____

_____

14   What is the lithotomy position and what are the physical reactions to this labor position?

_____

_____

_____

_____

_____

15   Describe the advantages and disadvantages of birthing positions for the second stage of labor.

_____

_____

_____

_____

_____

16   What other comfort measures can be used to minimize labor pain?

_____

_____

_____

_____

_____

17   What sensory stimulation strategies can be used during labor to keep the mother relaxed and calm?

_____

_____

_____

_____

_____

18   What is "directed pushing" and what are the disadvantages and sequelae of it?

_____

_____

_____

_____

_____

19   Explain the cognitive strategies that can be used during labor.

_____

_____

_____

_____

_____

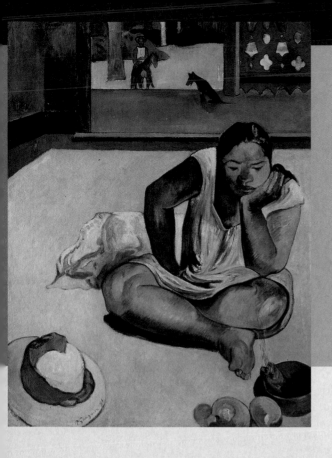

CHAPTER **19**

Labor Support Massage

Objectives

On completion of this chapter, the student will be able to do the following:

1. Use appropriate massage techniques for each stage of labor
2. Teach the woman's partner labor support massage
3. Work with laboring women who are survivors of physical or sexual abuse
4. Support a client who is having a cesarean section

"There is hardly a people, ancient or modern, that do not in some way resort to massage and expression in labor, even if it be a natural and easy one."[1]

Ales Hrdlicka, a physician and anthropologist, traveled throughout North America in 1908 and found that "The assistance given is everywhere substantially the same, consisting mainly of pressure or kneading with the hands or with a bandage about the abdomen, the object of which is to give direct aid in the expulsion of the child. The procedure, which is not always gentle, accomplishes very probably the same result as the kneading of the uterine fundus under similar conditions by the white physician, namely, more effective uterine contractions."[2]

No woman can really foresee how she will feel during labor or even if she will want to be touched at all. As her labor becomes more intense and her mood changes, the kind of touch that soothed her during early labor may irritate her in late labor. Therefore the practitioner or the woman's partner has to be sensitive to both verbal and nonverbal cues and flexible and creative to provide the most appropriate touch (or none at all) during labor.

Labor support massage follows the patterns and rhythms of the labor and therefore has no traditional sequence. In general, during a contraction in early labor, most women are comforted by counterpressure and localized stroking. When the contraction has subsided, light **effleurage,** which is the long, gliding Swedish massage stroke, can flush lactic acid and other waste materials from the muscles and joints, oxygenate the woman's muscles, and reduce the musculoskeletal discomforts that often accompany prolonged labor.

The tactile stimulation of stroking increases the input on the large-diameter nerve fibers and helps block the pain impulses. This is the action of the gate control theory of pain, which is also triggered by the dynamic activity of the mother's cerebral cortex that is additionally engaged in attention focusing or other mental activities for relaxation. The more proactive the laboring woman can be on breathing and relaxation strategies, the more her descending nerves fibers take priority within the central nervous system to override the pain signals.[3,4]

As the woman's partner prepares for labor or if the practitioner will be attending the birth, it is important to practice a variety of strokes and pressures to see which offer the most relief. Many women enjoy light effleurage during a contraction, especially on the abdomen.[5] Other useful massage techniques include firm effleurage (never on the legs because of fibrinogenic activity and the heightened lymph load), kneading, pelvic tilting, sacral lifts, hip squeezes, and acupressure. Many bodywork styles can be adapted or modified to support the laboring woman in early labor (Box 19-1).

Early Labor Massage

Most women are at home during the latent phase of stage one, thus massage can be provided easily, in a variety of positions, in familiar locations, and at her discretion. The massage practitioner accompanying a laboring woman needs to understand and respect a woman's unique response to labor and be ready to assist and support her appropriately. In early labor, the client is usually very happy about the onset of labor and rather excited. She may harbor some apprehension, but for the most part she is able to cope during this time.

The practitioner can massage her as frequently as she needs. Spot massages on tension areas are more easily tolerated by some women than an hour-long full body massage. Relaxation is an essential element to promote the progress of labor, and many strategies can be adapted throughout labor to ensure calmness and control (see Chapter 18). The tension-releasing scan that was practiced during late pregnancy can now be used to make

BOX 19–1 | *Appropriate Bodywork Techniques for Early Labor*

- Swedish massage may have to be modified to avoid deep pressure on the legs.
- **[DVD]** Manual lymphatic drainage (MLD) is the only appropriate massage technique for a pregnant woman's legs because of increased fibrinogenic activity and the increased amount of interstitial fluid. MLD is the safest and most comfortable massage for the laboring woman's legs. The pressure should be light and the direction of the stroke is always toward the woman's heart.
- Craniosacral therapy.
- Light myofascial release to reduce muscle spasms.
- Light foot and deep hand reflexology: pressure on the feet must remain light, whereas the pressure on the hands can be to the client's comfort level. It can often be rather deep as labor progresses.
- Esalen massage.
- Energy techniques.
- Counterpressures.
- Trigger point release.
- Specific acupuncture point stimulation.
- Relaxation strategies (see Chapter 18).
- **[DVD]** Sacral lifts, pelvic tilting, and hip squeezes.
- Passive and active stretching.

the woman aware of tension areas she needs to release. These areas may be muscles unrelated to the birthing process, such as the masseter and temporalis muscles of the jaw, muscles of the shoulder girdle and chest, muscles of the hands and feet, muscles of the thighs, and muscles of the lower back. Depending on the woman's reaction, a light touch or firm pressure using knuckles, fingertips, or elbows can bring her attention to the muscles she has to release.

During stage one of labor, pain impulses are transmitted along the lower thoracic spine (T11 and T12) and the accessory lower thoracic and upper lumbar sympathetic nerves. These nerves originate in the uterus and cervix.[6] Most of the pain and discomfort brought on by cervical changes is felt in the lower abdomen. Referred pain radiating from the uterus might be felt in the lumbosacral region, iliac crests, gluteal areas, and down the thighs.[6] Generally, the pain is present only during a contraction, although some women may experience contraction-related low back pain between contractions.[6] Light effleurage on her abdomen during a contraction can be very soothing.

Approximately 25% to 65% of women experience lower back pain during labor.[8] This pain is often referred to as **back labor** and can be ascribed to uterine changes, uterine ischemia, and distension or the fetal occiput posterior presentation as the fetal head stretches the ligaments of the sacroiliac (SI) joint. Most babies will rotate during birth and relieve the pressure on the lower back. Another cause of back pain occurs when the fetal head is too large for the pelvic outlet and pressure is exerted on the sacral nerves and other pelvic structures.

Massage is even more effective when the client is also using other pain-relieving strategies such as patterned breathing, attention focusing, active relaxation, imagery and visualization, and hypnotherapy.

Stage One Labor

Latent Phase

To treat the backache of early labor effectively, the practitioner (or partner) wants to override the pain signals with pleasure messages. This massage can be performed during a contraction with the woman lying prone (with the bodySupport system cushions and wedges correctly placed), propped with pillows, sitting and leaning, standing and leaning, or on her hands and knees. The client will offer the best feedback as to which techniques work most effectively. Practitioners should remember that labor is a dynamic process, and techniques she may not prefer at one point may be welcome at a later time. Practitioners can employ all or some of the following techniques:

- As the contraction starts, the client should take a deep cleansing breath, in through the nose and out through the mouth. (This deep cleansing breath will be repeated at the end of the contraction as well.) The practitioner starts with effleurage of the lower thoracic spine down to the sacrum longitudinally, in the direction of the muscle fibers. The pressure should be as deep or as light as the client prefers to distract from the pain. The pressure

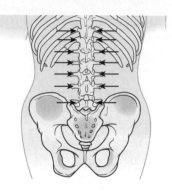

FIGURE 19-1 ■ Pressure across the direction of the muscle fibers from T11 to the sacrum can provide pain relief by overriding the neurological transmission of pain. (From Lowdermilk DL, Perry, SE: *Maternity & women's health care,* ed 8, St. Louis, 2004, Mosby).

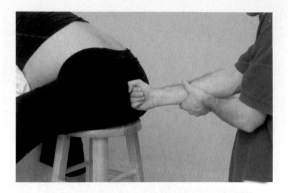

FIGURE 19-3 ■ Counterpressure using knuckles without pressing bone on bone.

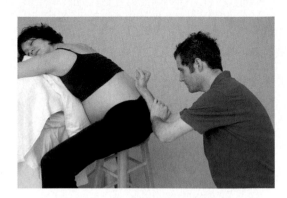

FIGURE 19-4 ■ Counterpressure using forearm.

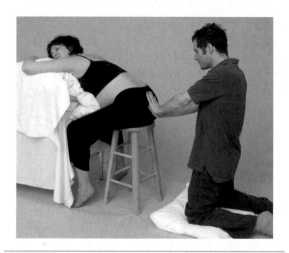

FIGURE 19-2 ■ Counterpressure with or without vibration, particularly on an identified tender region, helps provide relief from back pain. The practitioner pulls slightly inferior to provide a mild pelvic tilt and decompression of the lumbar spine.

will change as labor progresses, so practitioners should continue to look for feedback through verbal and nonverbal cues such as pulling away from touch if it is too deep, or arching into the practitioner's hands if the pressure is too light.

■ To work deeper into the lower erector spinae muscles from T11 to the sacrum, the practitioner uses fingertips, thumbs, pisiform bones, knuckles, or elbows across the muscle fibers from the lateral border of the erector spinae to the transverse processes of the spine and down to the lumbosacral joint (Figure 19-1).

■ The practitioner or partner applies counterpressure to the sacrum, with or without vibration, on a specific pain site. This area will change as the fetus continues to descend (Figure 19-2). This pressure has to be strong enough to override the pain messages, so the use of knuckles, elbows, or knees in alignment with the practitioner's body weight can be very powerful and easier to sustain throughout the contraction (Figures 19-3, 19-4, and 19-5).

■ Counterpressure should also be directed inferior to approximate a pelvic tilt in conjunction with the counterpressure. The pressure is sustained throughout the contraction.

■ The sacral lift can be performed to reduce the pressure of the fetal head on the spinal nerves (Figure 19-6). This technique offers tremendous relief from lower abdominal pressure and can be done in a number of ways to prevent hand fatigue. Practitioners can use their hands, knuckles (avoid direct bone-on-bone contact), forearm, shoulder, knee, hip, buttocks, and

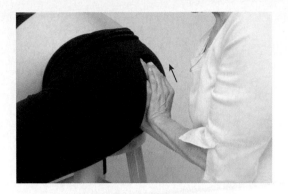

FIGURE 19-6 ■ Sacral lift.

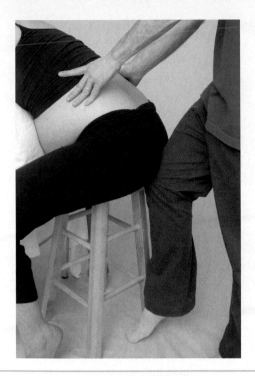

FIGURE 19-5 ■ Counterpressure using knee. This is strong pressure for a partner whose arms get tired.

foot for a very strong pressure that is easier to hold for the duration of the contraction (Figure 19-7). This technique should be held continuously throughout the contraction.

■ **[DVD]** Active or passive pelvic tilting (Figure 19-8).

■ Effleurage the entire back and across the shoulders with as much pressure as the client desires (Figure 19-9).

■ Acupuncture points **gall bladder 34,** located in the depression anterior and inferior to the small head of the fibula (Figure 19-10) and **bladder 67,** located on the lateral side of the top of the little toe, just posterior to the corner of the nail (Figure 19-11), can be pressed to treat lower back pain. Each point should be held bilaterally for a count of 10, repeating a total of 10 times.

■ When the contraction ends, the client takes another cleansing breath in through the nose and out the mouth as the practitioner performs effleurage on her back from the sacrum up and across her shoulders.

During the latent phase of stage one, the expectant mother can alternate normal activities with rest periods. She may need to be reminded to empty her bladder regularly. She can eat and drink small amounts of food and fluids according to her needs. Using the bath or shower can be an extremely relaxing activity that eases a great deal of the physical discomfort of early labor.[5] The practitioner and the woman's partner can help her pass the time with activities that are pleasant and distracting. The massages can be administered as often as the client desires (Box 19-2).

Active Phase

As labor progresses and moves into the active phase, there is a noticeable shift in contraction pattern and the woman's emotional response. This phase is usually the time the laboring woman goes to the hospital. As the contractions become more intense and closer together, the expectant mother may feel anxious or trapped. She becomes more dependent on those around her as she is less capable to meet her own needs. She may exhibit increased fatigue and restlessness. Some women cannot tolerate small talk or supercilious distractions.[5,9]

The practitioner's goals during the active phase are to keep mother calm, comfortable, and focused. It is essential that the practitioner meet her emotional needs with understanding, nurturing, and respect, which will give the laboring woman a greater sense of control over her labor that results in heightened self-esteem and a more satisfying, empowered experience.[10]

The bodywork techniques must now adapt to mother's emotional and physical changes (Box 19-3). Her breathing pattern will change during

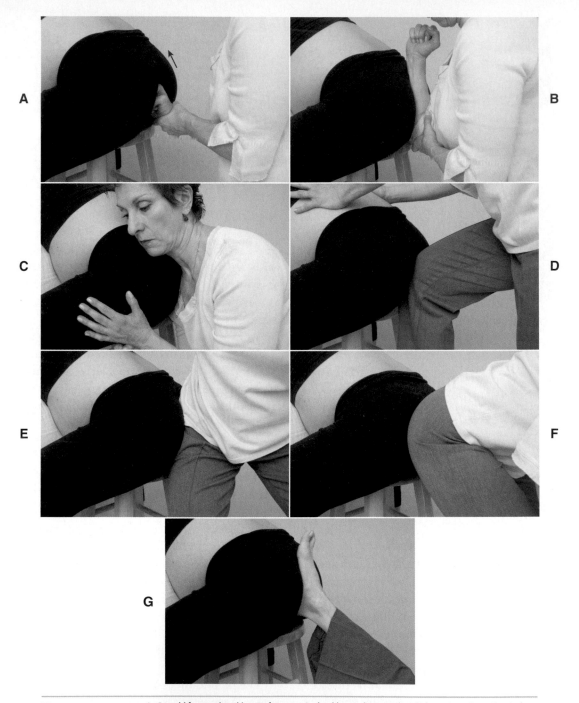

FIGURE 19-7 ■ **A**, Sacral lift using knuckles; **B**, forearm; **C**, shoulder; **D**, knee; **E**, hip; **F**, buttocks to buttocks; **G**, foot.

the active phases of stage one, and it is important to be mindful of these changes. The woman should change positions every 30 minutes to treat backache and speed up labor. Most women prefer an upright position during labor, such as standing, standing and leaning, walking, sitting upright, or squatting. These positions maximize gravity's pull

and can shorten the first stage of labor by one-third because vertical positions make the contractions more effective.[11] The following bodywork techniques can help keep the woman calm and comfortable:

■ **DVD**   Pelvic tilting is very effective in easing back labor during the active phase.

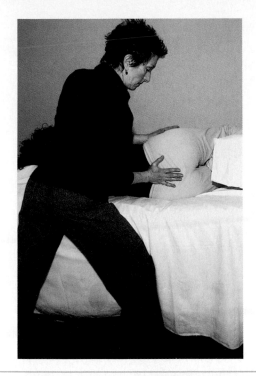

FIGURE 19-8 ■ The pelvic tilt during stage one of labor decompresses the lumbar spine and relieves the pressure from the lower back.

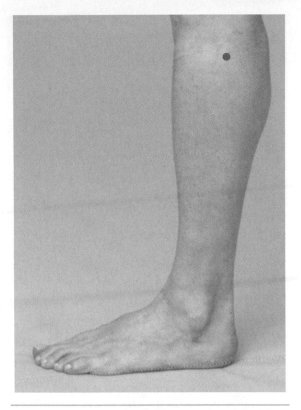

FIGURE 19-10 ■ Gall bladder 34 can be stimulated during labor to treat backache. Both legs should be pressed at the same time for a count of 10 repeating a total of 10 times.

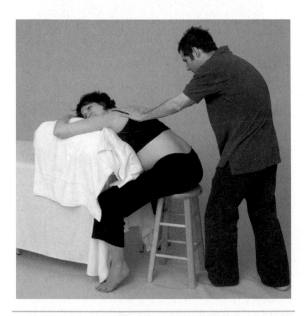

FIGURE 19-9 ■ Effleurage of the back between contractions rids the muscles of waste products and eases the pain of labor. The pressure can be as light or as deep as the client enjoys.

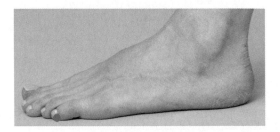

FIGURE 19-11 ■ Bladder 67 is located on the outside of the nail of the little toes. Bilateral pressure for a count of 10 repeating 10 times at any time during labor can reduce pain.

The position should be maintained throughout the contraction. The practitioner uses his or her forearm (instead of the hand) on the woman's anterior superior iliac spines (ASIS), with the practitioner's bottom hand on the woman's sacrum. This strengthens the pelvic tilt, saves the practitioner's hands, and makes it is easier to sustain this position for the duration of the contraction (Figure 19-12).

■ Hot or cold compresses, with or without rolling pressure on the woman's lower back, can be very effective in overriding the pain stimuli with pleasure messages.

■ The knee press is done with the client in a sitting or side-lying position, provides a slight

BOX 19-2 Techniques for Stage One: Latent Phases

- Cleansing breath as the contraction begins.
- Effleurage on the lower back from T11 to the sacrum.
- Fffleurage the lower back across the fibers of the erector spinae.
- Counterpressure with or without vibration for the duration of the contraction.
- **DVD** Sacral lift for the duration of the contraction.
- Active or passive pelvic tilting.
- Effleurage the entire back from the sacrum across and over the shoulders.
- Acupuncture points gall bladder 34 and bladder 67.
- Another cleansing breath as the contraction subsides.

BOX 19-3 Techniques for Stage One: Active Phase

- Cleansing breath as the contraction begins.
- **DVD** Pelvic tilt.
- Heat or cold compress with or without rolling pressure.
- Knee press.
- Pelvic squeeze.
- Relaxing throat and pelvic floor through use of deep toning, moaning, or vocalization.
- Holding, rocking, gentle stroking.
- **DVD** Acupuncture points large intestine 4, liver 3, spleen 6, and uterus reflex.
- Lymphatic drainage on the legs.
- Another cleansing breath as the contraction subsides.

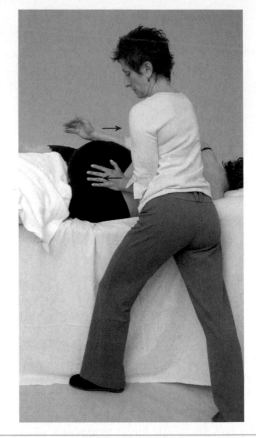

FIGURE 19-12 ■ Pelvic tilt using the forearm on the top hip is a stronger movement that can be sustained easily throughout the duration of a contraction.

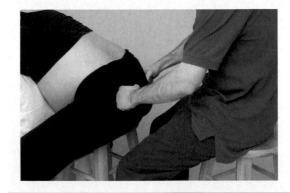

FIGURE 19-13 ■ The hip or pelvic squeeze using fists with the wrists stay in neutral position. The pressure is inward and slightly upward, bringing the SI joints together and providing tremendous relief to back labor.

pelvic tilt, and relieves the pain in the SI joint.[12]

- The pelvic squeeze is effective in replacing the ligaments of the SI joint that are being stretched by the fetus' head against the sacrum. This is often a major source of back pain and can be remedied with this effective technique. The practitioner or partner places his or her fists, with wrists in a neutral position, in the middle of the woman's gluteals, squeezes medially toward the sacrum, and superiorly provides a slight lift as if making an "X" (Figure 19-13). This hip squeeze is held for the duration. This squeeze can also be performed when the client is lying on her side.

- The seated knee press provides a slight posterior pelvic tilt and releases pressure on the SI joints. The practitioner or partner kneels before the woman and places his or her hands below the woman's knees on the

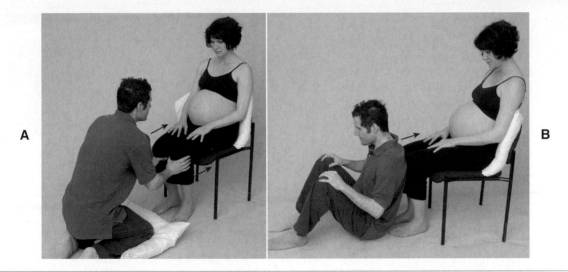

FIGURE 19-14 ■ **A,** The seated knee press can be done facing the sitting mother as shown, or **B,** facing away from her with the practitioner's or partner's back pressing against her knees. The latter is easier to hold for the duration of a contraction. Side-lying knee press can be done with a partner behind the mother, supporting her lower back. With her knees bent at a 90-degree angle, the partner leans over and pulls the woman's knees toward himself, creating a posterior pelvis tilt. He can also lean his body over her hips for addition pressure.

tibial tuberosities and presses (Figure 19-14, **A**). The knee press can be also be done with the practitioner's or partner's back against the woman's knees as she sits (Figure 19-14, **B**), or side-lying with one person pressing her knees and another supporting her lower back. The practitioner support the woman's lower back with his or her knee and lean over to pull the woman's knee into her acetabulum with the contraction. This movement repositions the SI joint and opens the pelvic outlet.

■ The woman should keep her pelvic floor relaxed during this trying phase. There is a correlation between the cervix and the cervical spine because both are necks and when one is relaxed, the other corresponds in kind.[13] A tension-releasing scan can draw her attention to any jaw clenching or tightening she may be doing. She should be encouraged to exhale through her mouth, and the practitioner should support any low vocalizations or toning that she may do. If her sounds become shrill and high-pitched, the practitioner should guide her back to deep belly breathing and a relaxed throat.

■ Massage may or may not be tolerated at this point. Care should be taken to not dislodge any monitors or intravenous lines that may be in place. Often, the laboring woman wants

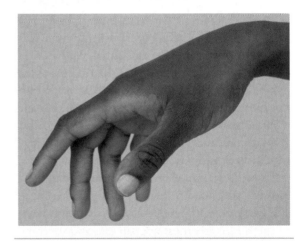

FIGURE 19-15 ■ Large intestine 4 ("The Great Eliminator") can be stimulated bilaterally to speed up labor. Each point is held for a count of 10 repeating 10 times. (Using ice on this point will also relieve some of the pain of labor.)

hand holding, rocking, or light therapeutic touch at this point. The presence of a loving, understanding support person can help her get through the active phase faster.

■ **DVD** Acupuncture points large intestine 4, liver 3, spleen 6, and the uterine reflex treated bilaterally during or between contractions can promote a speedier labor (Figures 19-15, 19-16, 19-17, and 19-18). The practitioner can apply ice on large intestine 4 for 20 minutes on the right or left

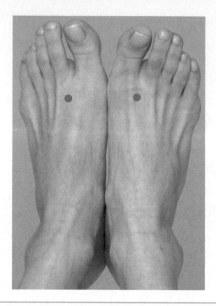

FIGURE 19-16 ■ Liver 3 can be bilaterally stimulated to enhance labor.

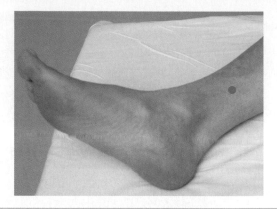

FIGURE 19-17 ■ Spleen 6 (Sanyinjiao) is the point where the three yin meridians of the leg come together. This is the manifestation of female energy and reflexes to the uterus. This point can be pressed bilaterally for a count of 10, repeating a total of 10 times, to initiate or stimulate uterine contractions.

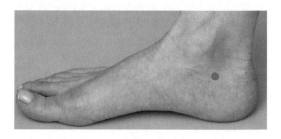

FIGURE 19-18 ■ The reflex point for the uterus is found on the inside of the heel of both feet. The practitioner crosses his or her arms and squeezes the points, cupping the woman's heels in the practitioner's palms.

hand. Applying ice reduces labor pain by 19% when applied to the right hand and 50% when applied to the left hand.[14]

■ A long and arduous labor, squatting for prolonged periods of time, and general fatigue can make a woman's legs particularly sore and tired. Because of increased fibrinogenic activity to prevent hemorrhaging at labor, the leg massage must follow lymphatic drainage protocol. Light pressure in the direction of the heart (starting at the knee to the hip, followed by the leg to the hip, followed by the foot to the hip) is the most appropriate and soothing massage for the legs. This will also help drain the excess fluid she is retaining.

During the active phase, the mother may express ill-defined fears and concerns and exhibit fatigue and restlessness. She may demonstrate a strong desire for company and support and may become unsure if she can cope with the contractions.[9] The goals of the practitioner are to help her remain calm through bodywork or emotional support, encourage her to continue using patterned breathing that supports the active phase, remain with her constantly, soothe her with a low, calm voice, help her move about, provide liquids and remind her to urinate, and match her mood.[5]

A prolonged active phase is more serious than a prolonged latent phase.[5] Labor that slows down during the second phase of stage one often results from inefficient uterine contractions, breech presentation or position, cephalopelvic disproportion, or a combination of these factors. Medical interventions, immobility, restriction to bed, a full bladder, fear, and anxiety also contribute to a prolonged active phase.

The resolution of slow labor depends on the etiology. If a full bladder is suspected, for example, reminding the woman to empty her bladder hourly can help. Medications that slow labor may have to wear off before labor progress can resume. Changing positions or favoring a gravity-friendly position can help. Nipple stimulation, the stimulation of the acupuncture points large intestine 4, liver 3, spleen 6, and the uterus reflex can promote a speedier labor. Fatigue can be treated and fears addressed with relaxing treatments such as a massage, bath or shower, and patterned breathing.[5]

It is usually during the active phase or transition that women request pain medication. Most of the nonpharmacological strategies are very helpful in reducing pain perception and keeping her comfortable and calm. If the client decides she needs the assistance of pain medication, it is essential that the practitioner respect her wishes and support her decision. Once she has received the medication and is restricted to bed, the practitioner can assist her with reminders to change positions often, pressing acupuncture points to speed up labor, and continuing to nurture her in any way that helps her.

Transition

The transition, or third phase, is marked by the lower uterine segment, the cervix, the pelvic floor, and the vulval outlet formed into a continuous dilated birth canal.[15] The forces necessary to expel the fetus come from uterine activity, as well as from the secondary muscles of the abdomen and diaphragm that enhance the uterine activity.[15] There are only brief pauses between contractions, perhaps 30 seconds, and the contractions are long, 90 to 120 seconds, some with double peaks, and painful. Transition is considered to be the peak of difficulty and intensity. Fortuitously, this phase is the shortest phase, averaging 5 to 25 contractions.[5] Backaches, aching and trembling legs, and heavy mucus discharge are caused by the downward pressure of the descending fetus.[5]

There is a noticeable almost palpable restlessness and irritability during transition. Hiccupping and belching are not uncommon, and many women experience nausea and vomiting. Uncontrollable sobbing is also a common reaction to this phase. Perspiration covers her face from all of her efforts.[9]

Many women feel that they cannot endure this pain, but the recognition that this is the shortest and hardest phase to get through can help tremendously. When a woman and her partner understand how far into labor they are and how close to the birth they are, it can be reassuring. The client should take one contraction at a time, changing positions as needed and using patterned breathing and relaxation techniques.

Touch Points

Supporting a woman during her labor is one of the most beautiful, awesome, and reverential work massage practitioners can ever expect to experience. Practitioners can provide help in many forms: healing touch, calming demeanor, a soothing breathing pattern, hand holding, or just the practitioner's presence. This bodywork follows the mother's needs as its guide. Whether the words are spoken or nonverbal, practitioners must be aware of the woman's cues and give her what she needs, when she needs it, and how she needs it.

Since no one knows how they will feel during labor, or how the labor will go, an attentive massage practitioner or partner should watch, listen, and respond to the mother-to-be in ways that support and enrich the dynamic process of labor.

BOX 19-4 *Techniques for Stage One: Transition*

- When the contractions come, the client should follow the patterned breathing that suits her best.
- Light stroking, gentle holding, or rocking for some women.
- Deep counterpressure on the sacrum, SI joints, muscles of the lower back for some women.
- **DVD** Sacral lift.
- Pelvic squeeze.
- Change positions as needed.
- Heat or cold packs.
- Encouragement, reassurance.
- Relaxation and calming strategies.
- Imagery and visualization.

SI, Sacroiliac.

Some women prefer not to be touched during transition. Hot or cold packs or ice chips might be welcomed. Holding and rocking with her may be all the support she needs. To relieve back pain, the practitioner can place his or her hand on an area of tension or firmly apply deep pressure on the woman's sacrum during a contraction.

Encouragement and reassurance are paramount during transition. The woman should be kept relaxed and calm so the natural rhythm of her labor can proceed smoothly and on course (Box 19-4).

BOX 19-5 | *Techniques for Stage Two: Latent (Resting) Phase*

- Allow the woman to rest, sleep, or move around.
- Help the woman change position.
- **DVD** Effleurage her lower back and sacrum as needed.
- Lymphatic drainage to her legs as needed.
- Tension-releasing scan to rid her body of tension areas.

BOX 19-6 | *Birth Assistants in Different Cultures*

In numerous tribal cultures, a birth assistant almost always sits, kneels, or stands behind the mother and puts her arms around her. Besides providing physical support, she presses downward on the fundus during the contractions. It was also common for the assistant to massage mother's back, legs, and thighs.

Data from Harley GW: *Native African Medicine*, Cambridge, 1941, Harvard University Press; Elwin V: Conception, pregnancy and birth among the tribesmen of the Maikal Hills, *Journal of the Royal Asiatic Society of Bengal* 4:1943; Best E: *The Maori*, Wellington, New Zealand, 1924; Tombs HH, Stein WW: *Hualcan: life in the Highlands of Peru*, New York, 1961, Cornell University Press.

Stage Two Labor

Latent (Resting) Phase

For approximately 15 to 20 minutes after the rigors of transition, there is a lull in uterine activity and a relief from the intensity of transition. The urge to push diminishes or weakens, and the woman becomes calmer and more aware of her surroundings. The contractions she does have are weak and farther apart.

Some women fall asleep during this resting phase. If she remains awake, there is a marked difference in her emotional state from one of self-doubt and near panic to cheerfulness and optimism. The practitioner or partner should help her change positions; remind her to relax her perineum, buttocks, and legs; and massage her as needed. During this resting phase of stage two, it is important to touch her with the intent to promote this state of calmness and relief (Box 19-5).

Active Phase

After the short resting phase, strong contractions resume and the urge to push becomes involuntary and compelling. Bearing down offers tremendous relief, and the perception of these contractions is different than in early labor. These contractions can last up to a minute and are only 3 to 5 minutes apart. By stage two, the uterus is clearly retracted and undergoing strong, regular, and repetitive contractions. As she inhales before pushing, the diaphragm lowers and the abdominal core muscles contract, increasing the contractile forces of the uterus. Bearing down helps to surmount the resistance of the soft tissues of the vagina and pelvic floor. Relaxation is vital to the conservation

of energy and smooth passage, particularly to her pelvic floor and adductors, because any physical tension could increase pain and slow labor. The pain of the second stage of labor is often decreased as cervical dilation is complete, and the woman can sense the rapid progress of labor.[15]

Encouragement, staying calm, and helping her follow her patterned breathing and **DVD** chosen relaxation strategies are helpful ways to support the expectant mother. Changing positions or standing upright often restarts the uterine contractions when she does not feel the urge to push. Stimulating the acupuncture points large intestine 4, liver 3, spleen 6, and the uterus reflex also helps initiate contractions.

The strokes of abdominal effleurage during the active phase begin at the fundus and move toward the pubic bone in tandem with the uterine contractions (Box 19-6). In between contractions, effleurage of her lower back or gentle pelvic or leg rocking may be welcome. Leg cramps or muscle spasms can be treated with active or passive stretching or appropriate massage technique. She will most likely need assistance straightening her legs after squatting to either an erect standing position or sitting down.

During contractions, the sacral lift, counterpressure, or hip squeeze are very helpful. Some women **DVD** become internalized during this stage and prefer not to be touched. Often the practitioner lends support by just holding the woman's hand, standing near her, or speaking calmly and directly to her. There is no right or

BOX 19-7	*Techniques for Stage Two: Active Phase*

- Relaxation strategies and energy conservation.
- Acupuncture points large intestine 4, liver 3, spleen 6, **DVD** and uterus reflex initiate the urge to push or expedite labor.
- Effleurage of the abdomen pressing from the fundus to the pubic bone during contractions.
- **DVD** Lower back massage between contractions.
- Active or passive stretching for leg cramps or muscle spasms.
- **DVD** Counterpressure, sacral lift, or hip squeeze for the duration of the contraction.
- Help the woman change positions.
- Visualization and imagery.
- Hold the woman's hand or offer physical support (leaning on practitioner).
- Stand nearby.
- Verbal encouragement and reassurance.

BOX 19-8	*Techniques for Stage Two: Transition (Crowning)*

- Relaxation strategies and energy conservation.
- Physical support and calm encouragement.
- Assist the woman in birthing positions.
- Perineal support (partner or medical professional ONLY).
- Counterpressure as needed.

wrong way to react, and the practitioner or partner must follow the verbal and nonverbal cues and respond accordingly (Box 19-7).

Transition (Crowning) Phase

As the baby's head crowns, a woman who had no medication may feel the stretching of the vaginal tissue that is called "the rim of fire." Endogenous endorphins and the pressure of the fetal head on the perineum will anesthetize this area within moments. This is when women should stop pushing and let their bodies open naturally to prevent tearing. Perineal support with hot compresses or massage to slowly allow the vaginal widening prevents the baby from being born too quickly and tearing the perineum.

The baby's head to the ears is born first followed by the face. Once the head is born, the baby rotates to face the mother's side. One shoulder passes through the pelvis followed by the other, and the rest of the baby is born easily.

During the birth, the expectant mother is pushing very hard and exerting a lot of energy. Her limbs may shake with the effort, and back pressure may be uncomfortable, but she is aware of the fact that she will soon be holding her baby. This can be a very emotional time with diametrically opposed feelings of laughter and sobbing, fear and joy, and exhaustion and exhilaration. Calm encouragement and physical support can promote relaxation and hasten the birth (Box 19-8).

Stage Three
Expulsion of the Placenta

After the birth of the baby, uterine contractions cease temporarily. After 10 to 30 minutes, there is an upward rise of the uterus in the abdomen, a visible lengthening of the umbilical cord, and a trickle or gush of blood as the uterus separates from the placenta. Two to three very powerful contractions expel the placenta, or afterbirth[9] (Figure 19-19 and Box 19-9). For some women, these painful contractions feel worse than labor pains. Other women are so involved with their baby they do not notice the third stage.

The umbilical cord is cut soon after the baby is born. Once the baby is born, the umbilical cord no longer contains oxygen, but the blood volume can be affected if the cord is cut too soon. Placental contractions squeeze more blood to the newborn. If the cord is clamped between contractions, the baby's blood volume is lower. Also, if the newborn is held below the placenta, more blood will flow from the placenta to the baby. Within a few minutes of exposure to the air, an expansion of Wharton's jelly (a substance contained in the cord) compresses of the blood vessels within the cord. From that point on, there is no circulation of blood either direction.[5]

During stage three, the woman should relax her perineum and pelvic floor to allow rapid expulsion of the placenta. Counterpressure against her sacrum to overcome the pain of these strong

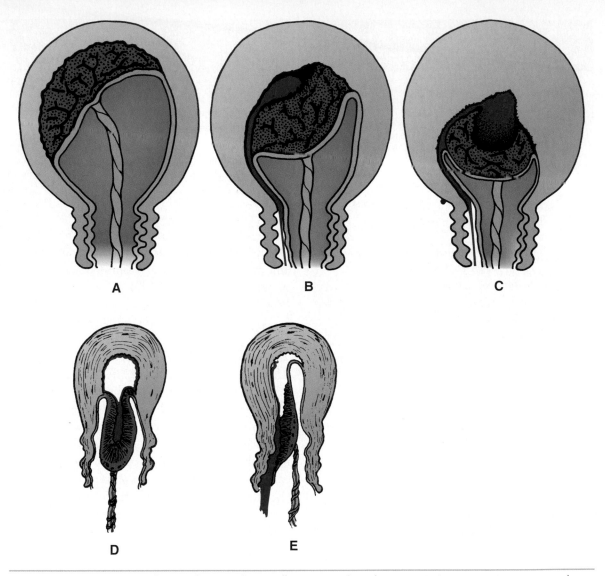

FIGURE 19-19 ■ **A**, Partially retracted uterine wall is not sufficient to cause placental separation. **B**, Continuing uterine contractions and retraction thicken the uterine wall, reduce the placenta site, and aid in separation. **C**, Complete separation with the formation of a retroplacental clot. **D**, Schultze method of expulsion with fundal site implantation. **E**, Matthew-Duncan expulsion with a lateral implantation. (From Fraser D, Cooper, M: *Myles' textbook for midwives,* ed 14, Edinburgh, 2003, Churchill Livingstone.)

contractions is very helpful. She should be reminded to keep breathing in a comfortable pattern and continue providing encouragement and support until stage three is over.

Abdominal massage from the fundus to the pubic bone can expedite expulsion of the placenta. Skin-to-skin contact between mother and baby, breastfeeding, nipple stimulation, and oral stimulation (by mother, baby, or partner only) promote the release of endogenous oxytocin that encourages the uterus to contract and expel the placenta. The practitioner can press

spleen 10 ("The Ocean of Blood"), which can help release the contents of the uterus (Figure 19-20). Other acupuncture points that are effective in stimulating the expulsion of the placenta are large intestine 4 or spleen 6. The use of any of these points is determined by where the practitioner or partner is standing in relation to the mother (Box 19-10).

Active management employs **uterotonic medications** (oxytocin [Syntometrine]) to promote the expulsion of the placenta and prevent hemorrhages.[6,15,16]

BOX 19-9 Delivering the Placenta

In 1861, a German obstetrician, Carl Siegmund Franz Crede, developed a new way to deliver the placenta. Before this time, mismanagement in this stage often led to hemorrhaging or internal infections and was a leading cause of death during childbirth in prehospital Europe. Midwives would tug on the cord, put their fingers inside the uterus, or shake the mother to deliver the placenta. Dr. Crede taught the midwives to press their hands on the fundus the moment the baby was born and not remove them until the placenta was expelled. They were to stimulate contractions by gently massaging the area while grasping firmly. This caused the uterus to contract and harden and after a few contractions, the placenta was expelled.*

Stage three, placental birth, was usually very fast in the tribal world because women were in good physical shape, and they used more efficient birthing positions. Standing and stretching can also expedite placental delivery.†

In tribal societies, massage was used almost exclusively to encourage expulsion of the placenta. Other procedures included contracting the abdominal muscles, having the woman sneeze, having the woman bite on something very hard, or asking her to blow into her hands or an empty bottle.†

Heat applications were also used to effectively expel the placenta. The women of Morocco soak the end of the severed umbilical cord in oil heated over hot coals. Within a few minutes of the treatment, the woman stands and the placenta falls out.‡ The Filipinos warm the handle of a wooden rice ladle and press it against the woman's navel. In Tepoztlan, Mexico, a hot tortilla is placed against the mother's right side.§ In India, the birth attendant oiled her head and rubbed it against the standing mother's belly until all the blood came out.‖ In Tahiti, the mother kneaded her own abdomen while bathing in the sea as her husband pressed his foot against her to stimulate further expulsion of fetal detritus.‖

In most of the tribal world, the umbilical cord was not cut until after the placenta was expelled.¶

*Data from Findley P: *The story of childbirth*, New York, 1933, Doubleday.
†Data from Sousa M: *Childbirth at home*, New York, 1976, Bantam.
‡Data from Boston Women's Health Book Collective: *Our bodies, ourselves*, New York, 1971, Simon & Schuster.
§Data from Lacey L: *Lunaception*, New York, 1975, Coward, McCann & Geoghegan.
‖Data from Hart DV: From pregnancy through birth in a Bisayan Filipino village. In *Southeast Asian birth customs*, New Haven, 1965, Human Relations Area Files Press.
¶Data from Coughlin RJ: Pregnancy and birth in Vietnam. In *Southeast Asian birth customs*, New Haven, 1965, Human Relations Area Files Press.

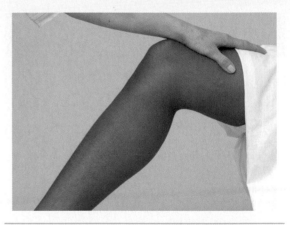

FIGURE 19-20 ■ Spleen 10 is located 2 cun above the superior border of the patella at the belly of the vastus medialis. An easy way to locate it is for the practitioner sits across from the client with his or her right palm over the woman's left patella. Spleen 10 is where the tip of the practitioner's thumb rests. Bilateral stimulation after the baby is born encourages functional uterine bleeding and release of the placenta.

BOX 19-10 Techniques for Stage Three: Expulsion of the Placenta

- Relaxation strategies and patterned breathing.
- Release of the perineum and pelvic floor muscles.
- Counterpressure on the sacrum as needed.
- Encouragement and calm support.
- Abdominal massage from the fundus to the pubic bone to stimulate uterine contractions.
- **DVD** Spleen 10 stimulation. Large intestine 4 or spleen 6 can also be used to encourage placental expulsion.
- Skin-to-skin contact of mother and baby, breastfeeding, or nipple or oral stimulation to encourage the secretion of endogenous oxytocin (NOT done by massage practitioner).

Stage Four

Recovery

After the placenta has been expelled, the fourth and final stage of labor is **recovery,** which lasts until all metabolic signs have stabilized (Box 19-11). For a vaginal birth, this usually takes about 1 hour. With the use of anesthesia or if delivery was by cesarean, the fourth stage will take longer.

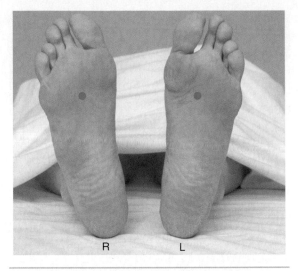

FIGURE 19-22 ■ Kidney 1 on both feet can be pressed for a count of 10 repeating 10 times to control trembling.

BOX 19-11   *Assessment of Metabolic Stability*

Every 15 minutes for the first hour after a vaginal birth, the new mother is assessed for the following:
- Prevention of hemorrhage
- Fundus location and consistency
- Amount of lochia discharge, color, and odor
- Vital signs: blood pressure, pulse, temperature
- Perineum: episiotomy for edema, hematoma
- Hydration
- Bladder for distention
- Fatigue and exhaustion
- Encouragement of breastfeeding and holding the baby

From Leifer G: *Maternity nursing: an introductory text*, ed 9, St. Louis, 2005, Saunders.

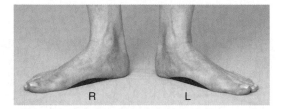

FIGURE 19-21 ■ Squeezing the arches of the woman's feet can help control trembling during or immediately after labor.

Women who want to breastfeed often do so within minutes of the birth. There are many advantages to this. First, if this was a nonmedicated birth, the newborn is very alert and its sucking reflex is strong. Evidence indicates that women who nurse soon after delivery continue to do so for longer periods of time.[17] In addition, nursing causes the pituitary to signal the release of oxytocin that causes the uterus to contract and shrink and promotes maternal feelings.

For the first few minutes after the birth, trembling of the legs, uterine pain, and perineum discomfort are quite common. A warm blanket can address the shaking, and an ice pack on the perineum reduces the pain and controls the swelling. If the practitioner is at the woman's feet, the arches of her feet can be squeezed to control the trembling (Figure 19-21), or acupuncture point kidney 1 can be pressed on both feet (Figure 19-22). If the practitioner is at the woman's side, pericardium 8 ("Palace of Anxiety") in the center of both

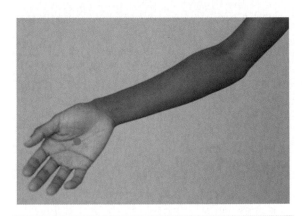

FIGURE 19-23 ■ Pericardium 8, also the hand reflex point for the solar plexus, is located in the middle of both palms. This point can be pressed for a count of 10, repeating a total of 10 times to treat labor trembling.

palms can be pressed to calm the woman (Figure 19-23). Afterpains, which are the postpartum uterine contractions, can be managed through slow breathing patterns. She may also experience difficulty with urination initially.[5]

Hunger, thirst, fatigue, exhilaration, exhaustion, and joy are some of the more common reactions to the end of labor and birth. After several hours, the newborn falls into a deep sleep and the mother's initial elation after the nonmedicated birth cedes to fatigue in the aftermath of labor. Women who received medication or had a surgical delivery often miss out on the initial

BOX 19-12 Techniques for Stage Four: Recovery

- Spot massage for tense areas.
- Provide fluids.
- Help client change positions.
- Warm blanket for the shivers.
- Grab the arches of the feet, kidney 1 or pericardium 8, to treat trembling.
- Ice pack for the perineum (placed by mother herself).
- Slow breathing patterns for afterpains.
- Discuss the labor and the baby with the new parents.
- Provide privacy.

postpartum exhilaration and are often very exhausted.

The support offered during recovery should be calm, nurturing, loving, and comforting. Spot massages for tense areas, providing fluids, helping her change positions, and discussing the birth and the baby if she desires are all appropriate. At this time, the practitioner can also give the mother, baby, and partner privacy, so they can begin the process of becoming a family (Box 19-12).

Working with women who are in labor is awe-inspiring and can be some of the most fulfilling, life-altering work bodyworkers can do. To be an effective massage practitioner for women in labor, it is strongly recommended that practitioners receive professional certification in a prenatal, labor, and postpartum massage class. Attending childbirth education classes and reading texts on the subject can enrich the practitioner's understanding and knowledge of the complex and dynamic physiology of labor.

The birth experience can be emotionally taxing for the massage practitioner. He or she should develop a professional but compassionate bedside manner that can be sustained throughout these long hours. Practitioners need to remain focused and nonjudgmental even when unexpected complications occur. It is a good idea that practitioners have their own support system to help them decompress after each birth.

Partner Labor Support Massage

Many partners want to be proactive and share the labor experience in any way they can (Box 19-13). Teaching them how to massage their loved ones during labor can be very rewarding. Many clients believe that this class was the most helpful and beneficial of all the classes they took together because it gave them concrete, hands-on techniques to treat the pain of labor.

Private lessons can be held in the last few weeks of pregnancy or classes may be conducted for several couples at one time. There are advantages and disadvantages to both, so practitioners have to see which works best for them (Box 19-14). Partners should be encouraged to practice on a regular basis so they can become fluent with each technique and use them spontaneously during labor to address the woman's changing needs (Box 19-15).

When the partner takes a proactive role and participates in the birth, the outcome is a more positive experience for both of them. Familial adjustments are easier, and self-confidence in parenting skills is buoyed. Laboring women have more of an emotional attachment with their partners and react with more self-assurance and heightened belief in their abilities to cope.

Supporting Survivors of Abuse

Although not all **survivors of abuse,** whether from physical, sexual, emotional, or psychological maltreatment, have direct memories of their experiences, they all share common characteristics.[18] Evidence indicates that as many as one third of women have been sexually abused, and many have present for prenatal care or in labor with no indications of this abuse.[19-21] However, certain behavioral patterns do emerge that can help practitioners understand survivors of abuse. Some behaviors are as follows:

- Some survivors engage in self-mutilation.[18,22]
- 97% of patients with multiple personality disorder have suffered childhood abuse.[23]

BOX 19-13 *Essentials for the Laboring Woman and New Mother*

The following list of items to bring for labor can be given to clients:

- A few plastic bags (in case of vomiting en route) should be kept handy.
- Travel size toothbrush, toothpaste, and mouth wash.
- A sealed plastic bag filled with a cut up lemon to help overcome nausea. "Seabands," which are sold at local pharmacies, are worn on both forearms at pericardium 6 also combats nausea.
- Bach flower, "rescue remedy," in tincture and cream form. As a tincture, a few drops on the tongue as needed when labor starts to keep calm during labor.
- Massage lotion or cream in a plastic container.
- Copy of partner labor support massage handouts.
- Extra underwear and one clean outfit to wear home.
- It is not necessary to bring a new or fancy nightgown for the postpartum period. The woman should be encouraged to wear the gowns provided, If she brings anything to wear, make sure it is made of natural fibers, such as cotton.

The following list of items that the new mother should have at home can be given to her before she has her baby:

- Fresh linens and a waterproof pad to protect the mattress from staining caused by night sweats.
- At least one extra box of large sanitary napkins or Depends for bleeding and incontinence.
- Stool softeners. Practitioners should encourage the woman to drink plenty of fluids and eat foods rich in digestive enzymes so she will not have to strain during a bowel movement. She can put her feet on a stool during a bowel movement to align her lower colon. She can be urged to use her transverse abdominis muscle during a bowel movement and keep her pelvic floor relaxed.
- Tucks or another medicated cleanser for cleaning after a bowel movement. Hemorrhoids are almost universal after birth. "Rescue remedy" cream, vitamin E, witch hazel, or calendula (a homeopathic remedy) can be applied topically on the hemorrhoids.
- Lansinoh can be purchased at local pharmacies to prevent and treat dry or sore nipples. If her baby latches on easily, she will not need this product; however, it can be used as a lip balm for the woman and the baby; skin protection for the baby in cold, windy weather; or as a wetness barrier on baby's bottom.

BOX 19-14 *Labor Support Classes*

Private Classes

Advantages

- Practitioner works closely with the couple and provides private tutoring.
- Practitioner is able to schedule the lesson during the last few weeks of pregnancy when stimulation of the labor points is safe.
- The client can be dressed or undressed as she sees fit.

Disadvantages

- Practitioner can only earn one fee for the session.

Group Classes

Advantages

- Practitioner earns more money by teaching a number of couples.
- Socialization between couples often occurs.

Disadvantages

- Not all clients can attend during the last weeks of pregnancy, and the labor stimulation points cannot be used for those who are earlier than 38 weeks.
- Clients have to wear bathing suits or leotards.
- The techniques have to be taught on the floor if there are not enough massage tables for the class.

- Many survivors come from foster homes, live with a step-father, and have run away from home.[24]
- A 1981 study reported that 60% to 70% of prostitutes were sexually abused as children.[25]
- Some survivors suffer from depression that manifests as lack of affect, poor hygiene, and sloppy personal appearance.[26]

Memories of childhood sexual abuse or spousal abuse may be triggered during labor by intrusive procedures like vaginal examinations; loss of control and being confined to bed, restrained by monitors and IV lines and epidurals; being examined and watched by a large medical team or unknown medical staff; and intense uterine and genital sensations.[6]

Survivors react in many differing ways. Some women may fight the labor process by panicking or exhibiting anger towards any care provider. Others may try to control the situation, because abuse was all about someone else's control. Others may surrender meekly and become submissive, whereas others may disassociate entirely[27] (Box 19-16).

BOX 19-15 *Partner Labor Massage Techniques*

- Body mechanics and leaning into the subject for maximum strength.
- Proper and relaxed use of hands, fingers, knuckles, elbows, and knees to save hands and to sustain specific techniques for the duration of a contraction.
- General effleurage of the back, shoulder, and neck in between contractions.
- Lower back massage during a contraction.
- **DVD** Sacral lift.
- Pelvic tilt.
- Hip squeeze.
- **DVD** Abdominal massage.
- Lymphatic drainage leg massage. (It is vital to explain the correct direction how consistently light the strokes must be.)
- **DVD** Acupuncture points and foot reflexes: large intestine 4, liver 3, spleen 6, gall bladder 34, bladder 67, uterus reflex can be pressed for a count of 10, repeating a total of 10 times. (These cannot be practiced on any woman prior to 38 weeks gestation.)
- Other comfort measures to practice before labor.

BOX 19-16 *Signs of Sexual Abuse Survivors in Labor*

- Little or no prenatal care.
- Several unplanned, unwanted pregnancies.
- Repeat abortions.
- History of STDs.
- Scars from self-mutilation.
- Excessive fears of needles and IV lines.
- Recoiling when touched.
- Insists on female medical staff (unless cultural).
- Obsessed with cleanliness.
- Extreme concern about bodily fluids.
- Cannot labor in a recumbent or lying down position.
- Concerns about exposure and nakedness.
- Refuses to breastfeed.
- Intense gag reflex.

From Burian J: Helping survivors of sexual abuse through labor. Grant sponsored by the Perinatal Foundation, Wisconsin Association for Perinatal Care, Madison, WI. Available at http://www.Gentlebirth.org/archives/abuselbr.html. *STDs,* Sexually transmitted diseases; *IV,* intravenous.

There are a number of ways to provide sensitive reassurance and care for survivors of abuse. The following are nursing guidelines that can be adapted for massage[18]:

- Practitioners can reassure the woman that the pain she is feeling is part of the process of childbirth and not past abuse.
- The laboring woman has to feel more in control of the situation by having all procedures explained to her before they are done, respecting and validating her needs, working at her pace, responding to her requests, asking for permission to touch her and letting her know where on her body she will be touched, offering nonjudgmental acceptance to her reactions, and respecting her privacy.[28,29]
- Practitioners can provide an emotionally and physically safe environment for survivors.
- Practitioners should be aware of their language and attitudes.

- The woman should be constantly reassured that she is safe and her hard work should be acknowledged with affirmations of her strength.
- The woman's feelings should be respected and honored.

Supporting the Client Having a Cesarean Section

Cesarean section (C-section) is the birth of a fetus through a transabdominal incision of the uterus (Figures 19-24 and 19-25). Before 1960, C-sections made up less than 5% of births in the United States. By 1988, the rate rose to 23.5%.[6,30-32] In 2000, the rate declined slightly to 22.9% but rose again to 24.4% in 2001.[6,33]

Reasons for C-sections vary from medically-established emergencies to elective surgical births. The large majority of C-sections performed in the United States are repeat C-sections. Cephalopelvic disproportion or failure to progress, maternal hemorrhaging, breech presentation, and fetal distress are other common reasons C-sections are performed.

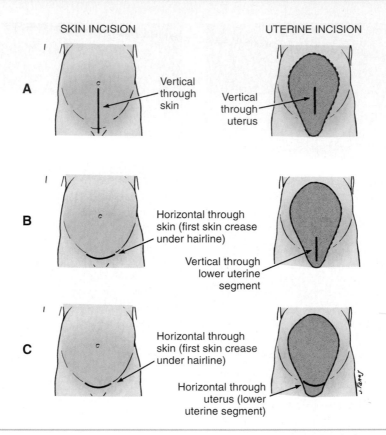

SKIN INCISION   UTERINE INCISION

A Vertical through skin — Vertical through uterus

B Horizontal through skin (first skin crease under hairline) — Vertical through lower uterine segment

C Horizontal through skin (first skin crease under hairline) — Horizontal through uterus (lower uterine segment)

FIGURE 19-24 ■ **A,** Classic incision: vertical incision of both skin and uterus. **B,** Low vertical incision: horizontal incision of the skin, vertical incision of the uterus. **C,** Low transverse: horizontal incision of both skin and uterus. (From Lowdermilk DL, Perry, SE: *Maternity & women's health care,* ed 8, St. Louis, 2004, Mosby.)

The remaining C-sections in this country are performed because of multiple gestation, advanced maternal age (in 2000, women over 35 years of age had a C-section birth rate of 30%, twice the rate for women under 20 years of age[34]), maternal disease, a failed elective induction, prolonged ruptured membranes, genital herpes, unusual indications (i.e., previous uterine, vaginal, bladder, or rectal surgery), postmaturity, and convenience.[5,35] Another possible reason for the increase in surgical births is the decline in vaginal births after cesarean (VBAC). After increasing from 18.9% in 1989 to 28.3% in 1996, the VBAC rate dropped to 20.6% in 2000.[22]

Women with private insurance, those in a higher socioeconomic level, or those who deliver in private (for-profit) hospitals are more likely to experience surgical births than women who have no insurance, are in lower income levels, are on public assistance, or give birth in public hospitals.[36]

Women generally do not go into labor when a C-section is planned, although many women do.

If a woman does experience labor contractions, the practitioner should work with her as if she was having a vaginal birth. For those women who intended a vaginal birth, the unexpected C-section can leave them desolate, guilty, angry, disfigured, disappointed, depressed, inadequate, feeling as if they have failed, and grieving for the loss of a desired birth experience.[37]

Massage practitioners are rarely permitted into the operating room during this abdominal surgery. Bodyworkers who do accompany the woman can help her by keeping her calm, encouraging her, helping her maintain breathing patterns, concentrate on a positive outcome, and perhaps stroke her hand or face as desired.

Maternal risks associated with C-sections are as follows:

■ Death
■ Emergency hysterectomy
■ Blood clots and stroke
■ Injuries and infections from the surgery

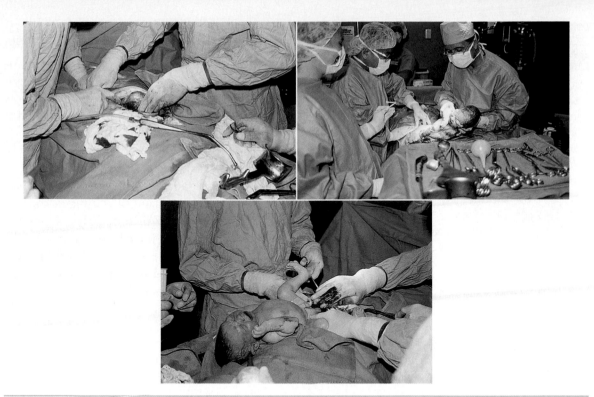

FIGURE 19-25 ■ An incision is made, and the muscle layer is separated *(top left)*. The abdomen is entered and the uterus is incised. Amniotic fluid is suctioned as the fetal head is brought up through the incision. Bleeding is contained. *Top right,* the newborn is pulled through the incision. *Bottom left,* Neonate assessment. Note the extreme head molding resulting from cephalopelvic disproportion. (From Lowdermilk DL, Perry, SE: *Maternity & women's health care,* ed 8, St. Louis, 2004, Mosby.)

- Prolonged hospital stay and longer recovery
- More pain in general and more pain at the site of the incision
- Poor birth experience
- Less early contact with the baby and an unfavorable reaction to the baby
- Depression or psychological trauma
- Poor overall mental health, self-esteem, and general functioning
- Ongoing pelvic and bowel obstruction
- Possible infertility
- Increased risk of future ectopic pregnancy, placenta previa, placenta accrete, abruptio placentae, rupture of the uterus

Fetal risks associated with C-sections are as follows:

- Accidental surgical cuts
- Respiratory difficulties and possible asthma during childhood and adulthood
- Difficulty breastfeeding

Risks for future pregnancies include stillbirth, low birth weight and preterm labor, malformation, and injury to the central nervous system[38] (Boxes 19-17 and 19-18).

In My Experience...

G, a triathlete, had her first labor contractions when she called me. She wanted to know if she could still keep her massage appointment even though she was in labor. My response was "Of course you can! Bring your husband along and we will work on you together!"

About a half hour later, they walked into my office and G got on the table. I proceeded to do the pelvic tilts and sacral lifts that offered her a great deal of relief from lower back pain. Her husband was rubbing her shoulders, kissing her, whispering in her ear, and stimulating the acupuncture points I showed him. Every so often, we would help her off the table and walk around with her. Because this was her first child, the labor could go on for quite some time.

After an hour, she dressed and left but they continued to walk around the neighborhood. About

Summary

Labor is a dynamic and progressive process. Although a woman can prepare and educate herself on how her body functions, she cannot know how she will feel and react when the time comes. Each woman and each labor is different.

Many helpful bodywork and massage techniques, as well as numerous comfort measures, can have a positive impact on the way a woman perceives her labor. Pain control is a major concern for most women, and these massage techniques have proved effective in reducing pain and the perception of pain, keeping her muscles relaxed and relieving tension, promoting a speedier labor, and providing more control.

A proactive partner who participates in the birth can help create a more positive birthing experience. Laboring women react with more self-assurance and heightened belief in their abilities to cope when the partner is present.

Survivors of physical or sexual abuse and those women who undergo C-sections need specialized care and encouragement to provide them with a fulfilling, satisfying birth experience.

BOX 19-17   *Avoiding a Cesarean Section*

During pregnancy or before becoming pregnant, women can be advised to avoid a C-section by doing the following:
- Work with a doctor or midwife with low rates of interventions.
- Discuss preferences with caregivers.
- Choose a birth setting with low rates of interventions.
- Establish and advise caregivers about the preferred birth plan.
- Work with a doula.
- Learn about pain control through natural comfort measures.
- Delay going to the hospital.
- Avoid continuous electronic fetal monitoring.
- Avoid using pain medications, interventions, and epidural anesthesia.
- If a C-section is proposed by the doctor or midwife, ask why it is recommended, the benefits and risks, and other possible solutions. Get a second opinion.
- Become informed about VBAC
- If fetus is breech at 37 weeks, try alternative ways to turn the fetus or suggest external manual (breech) version
- Consider hypnotherapy or psychotherapy to address fears of childbirth and pain.

From Maternity Center Association: *What every pregnant woman needs to know about cesarean section 2004,* New York, 2004, The Association.
VBAC, Vaginal birth after cesarean.

BOX 19-18   *Support Techniques for Cesarean Deliveries*

- Provide emotional support and encouragement.
- If labor is initiated, use appropriate labor techniques until the woman is prepared for surgery.
- Breathing patterns and visualization to keep her calm.
- Hold the woman's hand or stroke her face.
- Emphasize positive outcome.

an hour later, she called again. "Can I come back?" "Absolutely," I told her. This time the contractions were about 5 minutes apart, and I suggested that she notify her midwife before she even got on the table. I spent this mini-session stimulating the acupuncture points and concentrating on any areas that needed attention. After only about 10 minutes, she told me she had to leave and get to the hospital. It was a good thing the hospital was down the block. Two hours later, her daughter was born.

References

1. Englemann GJ: *Labor Among Primitive Peoples,* St. Louis, 1884, JH Chambers.
2. Hrdlicka A: *Physiological and medical observations among the Indians of southwestern United States and northern Mexico,* Washington, DC, 1908, Smithsonian Institute Bureau of American Ethnology.
3. Melzack R, Wall P: Pain mechanisms: a new theory, *Science* 150:971-978, 1965.
4. Sternbach RA: *Pain: a psychological analysis,* New York, 1968, Academic Press.
5. Simkin P, Whalley J, Keppler A: *Pregnancy, childbirth and the newborn,* Minnetonka, MN, 1991, Meadowbrook Press.
6. Lowdermilk DL, Perry SE: *Maternity & women's health care,* ed 8, St. Louis, 2004, Mosby.
7. Lowe N: The nature of pain, *Am J Obstet Gynecol* 186(5):S16-S24, 2002.
8. Cogin R: Backache in prepared childbirth, *Birth Fam J* 3(2):75, 1976.

9. Leifer G: *Maternity nursing: an introductory text*, ed 9, St. Louis, 2005, Saunders.

10. Olkin SK: *Positive pregnancy fitness*, New York, 1987, Avery Publishing Group.

11. Caldeyro-Barcia R: The effect of position changes on the intensity and frequency of uterine contractions during labor, *Am J Obstet Gynecol* 80:284, 1960.

12. Simkin P: Reducing pain and enhancing progress in labor: a guide to nonpharmacologic methods for maternity caregivers, *Birth* 22(3):162, 1995.

13. Harper B: *Gentle birth choices*, Rochester, VT, 1994, Healing Arts Press.

14. *J Midwifery Women's Health* 48:317-321, 2003.

15. Coad J: *Anatomy and physiology for midwives*, St. Louis, 2001, Mosby.

16. Enkin M, Keirse M, Neilson J, et al: *A guide to effective care in pregnancy and childbirth*, Oxford, 2000, Oxford University Press.

17. Salariya E, Easton P, Cater J: Early and often for best results, *Nursing Mirror* 148: 15-17, 1997.

18. Burian J: Helping survivors of sexual abuse through labor. Grant sponsored by the Perinatal Foundation, Wisconsin Association for Perinatal Care, Madison, Wisconsin. Available at http://www.Gentlebirth.org/archives/abuselbr.html.

19. Blume ES: *Secret survivors: uncovering incest and its after effects in women*, New York, 1989, Ballantine Books.

20. Morrison JA: *A safe place: beyond sexual abuse*, Wheaton, IL, 1990, H. Shaw Publishers.

21. Leventhal JM: Have there been changes in the epidemiology of sexual abuse of children during the 20th century? *Pediatrics* 82: 766-773, 1988.

22. Shapiro S: Self-mutilation and self-blame in incest victims, *Am J Psychother* 41:46-54, 1987.

23. Putnam FW, Guroff JJ, Silberman EK, et al: The clinical phenomenology of multiple personality disorder: review of 100 cases, *J Clin Psychiatr* 47:285-293, 1986.

24. Feldman W, Feldman E, Goodman JT, et al: Is childhood sexual abuse really increasing in prevalence? An analysis of the evidence, *Pediatrics* 88:29-33, 1991.

25. Silbert MH: Sexual child abuse as an antecedent to prostitution, *Child Abuse Neglect* 5:407-411, 1981.

26. Courtois CA: *Healing the incest wound: adult survivors in therapy*, New York, 1988, WW Norton.

27. Rhodes N, Hutchinson S: Labor experiences of childhood sexual abuse survivors, *Birth* 21(4):213-220, 1994.

28. Heritage C: Working with childhood sexual abuse survivors during pregnancy, labor, and birth, *J Perinat Neonat Nurs* 27(6):671-677, 1998.

29. Waymire V: A triggering time: childbirth may recall sexual abuse memories, *AWHONN Lifelines* 1(2):46-50, 1997.

30. Smith EF, MacDonald FA: Cesarean section: an evaluation of current practice in the New York Lying-In Hospital, *Obstet Gynecol* 6:593-602, 1953.

31. Curtin SC, Kozak LJ, Gregor KD: U.S. cesarean and VBAC rates stalled in the mid-1990s, *Birth* 27:54-57, 2000.

32. Rosen MG: Consensus task force on cesarean childbirth, *NIH Publications* 82:2067, 1981.

33. National Center for Health Statistics: Birth statistics, USA 1999-2001, VBAC.com. Available at http://www.vbac.com/birth-trends.html. Accessed 2001.

34. Hausknecht R, Heilman JR: *Having a cesarean baby*, New York, 1978, EP Dutton.

35. Martin J, Hamilton BE, Ventura SJ, et al: Births: Final data for 2000, *Natl Vital Stat Rep* 50(5):1-102, 2002.

36. Scott JR: Cesarean delivery. In Scott J, DiSaia PJ, Hammond CB, et al, eds: *Danforth's obstetrics and gynecology*, ed 8, Philadelphia, 1999, Lippincott, Williams & Wilkins.

37. Szczepaniak JC: *So You Have Just Had a Cesarean…*, Minneapolis, 1996, ICEA.

38. Maternity Center Association: *Vaginal birth and cesarean birth: how do the risks compare?* New York, 2004, The Association.

REVIEW QUESTIONS

1   During a labor contraction, what type of touch often comforts women?

_____

_____

_____

_____

2   Once the contraction has subsided, what type of massage stroke is most effective to flush waste products from her muscles and joints?

_____

_____

_____

_____

3   What influence does tactile stimulation have on the large-diameter nerve fibers?

_____

_____

_____

_____

4   Describe the massage support for early labor. What bodywork techniques are appropriate during the initial stage of labor?

_____

_____

_____

_____

5   What other coping strategies can a laboring woman employ to make the massage even more effective?

_____

_____

_____

_____

6   How common is back labor, and what are some possible causes?

_____

_____

_____

_____

7   What techniques can massage practitioners use, or teach the partners to use, to control back pain?

_____

_____

_____

_____

8   What are some stage one phase two (active) support techniques?

_____

_____

_____

_____

9   What are some of the goals for touch during the active phase of stage one?

_____

_____

_____

_____

10   What is physiologically happening during the transition phase of stage one, and what touch support can help the woman stay calm and focused?

_____

_____

_____

11 What is physically occurring during phase one of stage two?

_____
_____
_____
_____

12 What are some effective touch techniques for the resting phase of stage two?

_____
_____
_____
_____

13 What can the practitioner or partner do to help the laboring woman stay calm and focused during the transition or crowning phase of stage two?

_____
_____
_____
_____

14 What happens during stage three of labor? What massage techniques or acupuncture points can facilitate the expulsion of the placenta?

_____
_____
_____
_____

15 How long is the average recovery period for a woman who had a vaginal birth?

_____
_____
_____
_____

16 What are some of the advantages of nursing the baby immediately after the birth?

_____
_____
_____
_____

17 What techniques can be used during stage four to make the new mother more comfortable?

_____
_____
_____
_____

18 Describe the partner labor massage techniques.

_____
_____
_____
_____

19 Describe some of the common behavior patterns associated with childhood abuse that can help identify these women for practitioners who work with them.

_____
_____
_____
_____

20 How does the stress of labor trigger childhood abuse memories for some women?

_____
_____
_____
_____

21   What guidelines can be adapted for massage practitioners that can help survivors of abuse during labor?

_____

_____

_____

_____

22   What are some of the behaviors survivors of sexual abuse may exhibit during labor?

_____

_____

_____

_____

23   What can be done to help a client having a C-section?

_____

_____

_____

_____

24   What are some of the maternal risks associated with C-sections?

_____

_____

_____

_____

25   What are the fetal risks associated with C-sections?

_____

_____

_____

_____

26   What suggestions can help women avoid a C-section that is not medically necessary?

_____

_____

_____

_____

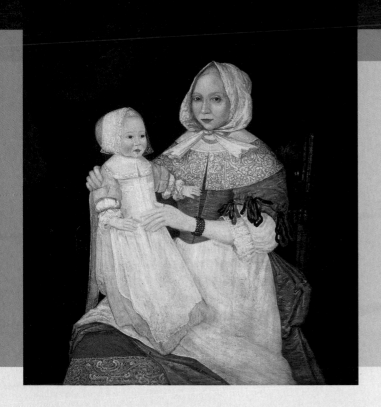

PART THREE

Postpartum Massage

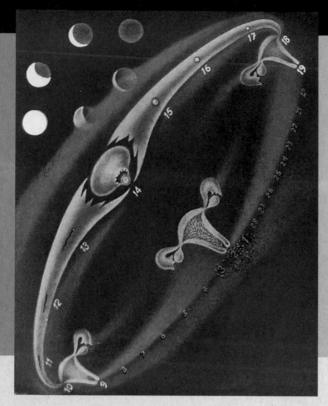

CHAPTER 20

Contraindications
to Postpartum
Massage

Objectives

On completion of this chapter, the student will be able to do the following:

1 Recognize the postpartum complications that indicate contraindications to massage

2 Assess clients for any possible postpartum complications

Postpartum Recovery

The **puerperium** recovery period, traditionally the 6-week period after childbirth, begins with the expulsion of the placenta and membranes from the uterus.[1] The recovery process actually takes much longer than 6 weeks because the woman's body undergoes metabolic and hormonal changes for several more months.

Postpartum Warning Signs

A new mother needs to learn to recognize the postpartum warning signs so she can differentiate between normal postpartum physiological changes and discomforts and serious medical complications. The bodyworker must also learn when to delay massaging the new mother in favor of immediate medical attention.

Hemorrhage

Postpartum hemorrhage is defined as a loss of more than 500 ml of blood after an uncomplicated vaginal birth and 1000 ml after a cesarean section.[2] Because of the increased blood volume during pregnancy, women can tolerate this blood loss without complication. Excessive bleeding is more dangerous if it occurs within the first 24 hours because of the large venous area exposed after placental separation, but hemorrhaging can also happen later—after 24 hours to less than 6 weeks.

Early hemorrhage is caused by uterine atony and lacerations from either vaginal, cervical, or perineal trauma. Late postpartum hemorrhage, or secondary postpartum hemorrhage, is a result of retained placenta fragments (placenta accrete) or subinvolution.

With reduced blood volume, or hypovolemia, the body reacts by elevating the heart and respiratory rates. Her skin becomes pale, cold, and

> **BOX 20-1** *Signs and Symptoms of Puerperal Infection*
>
> - Fever greater than 100.4° F or 38° C
> - Tachycardia and chills
> - Uterine tenderness
> - Localized reddened, warm (hot), and tender area
> - Purulent wound drainage
> - Abnormal lochia discharge (normal postpartum vaginal discharge)
> - Uterine **subinvolution** (when the uterus does not return to its prepregnant size, shape, tone, and position within the pelvis)
> - Malaise
>
> From Leifer G: *Maternity nursing: an introductory text,* ed 9, St. Louis, 2005, Saunders.

clammy. As blood loss continues, it affects her brain and she becomes restless, confused and lethargic. Prompt medical attention is essential before she goes into hypovolemic shock.

After the initial dangers of postpartum hemorrhage and shock are eliminated immediately on delivery, the primary concern is postpartum infection.[2]

Fever

Puerperal fever is suspected if the postpartum woman runs a fever more than 100.4° F (38° C) after the first 24 hours and if the fever is present for 2 days within the first 10 days postpartum. Temperature elevation could indicate the presence of an infection (Box 20-1) that may require immediate pharmacological treatment. Postpartum infection (postpartum sepsis) accounts for appreciable rates of postpartum maternal morbidity and mortality.

There are two categories of puerperal fever. The first category relates to infections of the reproductive system that are bacterial that arise in the genital tract after birth. The second category includes nonreproductive system infections that occur during postpartum recovery. These infections include mastitis and urinary tract infections that are indirectly related to the physiology of pregnancy, labor, birth, and lactation.[2]

If the woman's pulse rate indicates tachycardia or marked bradycardia, puerperal fever and possible infection may be indicated.[3]

Elevated Blood Pressure and Swelling

Postpartum hypertension and swelling are symptomatic of preeclampsia and need immediate medical attention.

Vaginal Discharge

The cleansing postpartum vaginal discharge, called *lochia*, is comprised of blood from the placental site, pieces of necrotic decidua, and mucus. Lochia has an earthy smell similar to menstrual bleeding. Lochia discharge is the heaviest during the first 1 to 2 hours after birth.

Lochia rubra is bright red and can last 1 to 3 days. It temporarily flows heavier when the new mother nurses or when she stands after sitting for a period of time. This lochia is initially sterile, and then the uterus begins to be colonized by normal vaginal flora.

After approximately 3 days, the red color starts to turn pale and becomes pink to brown. **Lochia serosa**, which has a slightly sweet odor, should no longer contain clots but is comprised of leukocytes, mucus, vaginal epithelial cells, necrotic decidua, and nonpathological bacteria. It generally lasts for 10 days, although this stage of the discharge can continue as long as 27 days.[4] By 10 days postpartum, the vaginal discharge becomes yellow, changes to white, and is called **lochia alba.** This lochia is made up of serous fluid and leukocytes, cervical mucus, and microorganisms, and it may continue to flow up to 6 weeks after the birth.[1,2]

Heavy bleeding with an offensive odor, maternal pyrexia, and a feeling of general malaise can be signs of an intrauterine infection.[1] Judging the amount of flow can be difficult (Box 20-2). Nurses often assess the amount of flow in terms of area soiled on a sanitary pad within 1 hour

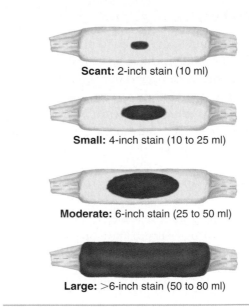

Scant: 2-inch stain (10 ml)

Small: 4-inch stain (10 to 25 ml)

Moderate: 6-inch stain (25 to 50 ml)

Large: >6-inch stain (50 to 80 ml)

FIGURE 20-1 ■ Estimating the amount of lochia on a perineal or sanitary pad. (From Leifer G: *Maternity nursing: an introductory text*, ed 9, St. Louis, 2005, Saunders.)

(Figure 20-1). The amount of lochia is less after a Cesarean delivery.

The vaginal discharge should follow the pattern of healing from bright red to pink to brown and then a pale flow. If the pattern reverts to an earlier stage of healing, or if the bleeding is accompanied by fever, pain, uterine tenderness, and a foul odor, the mother's caregiver should be notified.

Pain

If the woman experiences unremitting uterine or severe abdominal pain after 2 weeks postpartum, she should contact her caregiver. **Afterpains** are normal after childbirth and have been equated to the severity of moderate labor contractions.[5,6] Uterine contractions initiate the process of **involution** that restores the organ to its prepregnant size, shape, position, and tone. Afterpains can be

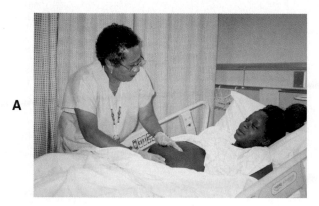

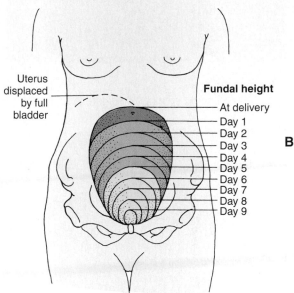

FIGURE 20-2 ■ **A,** A nurse measures postpartum fundal height. **B,** Involution of the uterus. The height of the fundus drops approximately 1 cm each day until it is no longer palpable after 10 days. (From Leifer G: *Maternity nursing: an introductory text,* ed 9, St. Louis, 2005, Saunders.)

felt when the woman nurses, and they generally diminish in intensity after a few days. If the pain persists or remains constant, she must contact her caregiver.

Incision Changes

If the woman notices any opening, swelling, pain, redness, bleeding, oozing, or foul odor from an incision, whether from a cesarean section (C-section) or episiotomy, she should contact her care provider. Foul odors accompanied by drainage indicate an infection.

Uterine Atony

Uterine atony occurs when the uterus remains boggy and flaccid after fundal massage and the expulsion of clots, remains above the umbilicus after 24 hours, and deviates from the midline.[3] Atony is a marked hypotonia of the uterus and is a leading cause of postpartum hemorrhage, complicating approximately 1 in 20 births.[3,7] It is associated with high parity, hydramnios, macrosomic fetus, uterine distention with clots, and multiple gestation.[3] The uterus is overstretched and does not contract well after the birth.

Subinvolution is the failure of the uterus to return to its prepregnant condition after 6 weeks.

This is usually the result of retained placental fragments or pelvic infection[2] (Figure 20-2). Signs of subinvolution include prolonged lochia discharge, irregular or excessive bleeding, and occasional hemorrhage.

Mood Disorders

Feeling depressed is quite normal after childbirth. The dramatic hormonal shifting, the arduous labor, and general fatigue all contribute to these fleeting feelings of sadness. Postpartum is a period with increased vulnerability to affective disorders. At least half to two-thirds of postpartum women experience transient emotional disorders at about day 3, which is known as the *baby blues*.[8] However, 10% to 20% of postpartum women become depressively ill with **postpartum depression** (depression occurring within 6 months of childbirth and lasting longer than postpartum blues) and 1% to 2% suffer from **postpartum psychosis.** These disorders can have long-term effects on maternal-newborn interaction. Postpartum depression and psychosis may have later onsets and delayed recoveries[1] (Box 20-3).

Postpartum psychosis is the rarest but most severe reaction to childbirth. There is a break with reality that may include hallucinations and

Signs of Postpartum Depression and Psychosis

- Depressed, hopeless mood
- Sleep disturbances; either sleeps too much or suffers from insomnia
- Unable to cope
- Feelings of guilt, inadequacy, worthlessness
- Thoughts of harming self or baby or acting on these feelings
- Rejection of baby and family
- Anxiety (postpartum anxiety disorder or panic disorder)
- Altered libido
- Weight loss
- Memory loss and confusion
- Uncontrollable crying and irritability
- Exaggerated highs and lows

From Coad J: *Anatomy and physiology for midwives*, St. Louis, 2001, Mosby; Leifer G: *Maternity nursing: an introductory text*, ed 9, St. Louis, 2005, Saunders; *Pregnancy and postpartum thought and mood disorders*, Belle Mead, NJ, 1996, Depression After Delivery, Inc.

Touch Points

Few childbirth education classes discuss the postpartum recovery period. Many first-time mothers do not understand how quickly their bodies change and are often scared and concerned about physical adaptations that are normal but rather dramatic. Practitioners can provide women with a clear guide to these warning signs so they can understand the difference between physical changes that might require immediate medical attention and those that are considered part of the normal, although sometimes awkward and embarrassing, process known as postpartum.

delusions. This is a serious emergency situation that requires immediate medical intervention.[9]

A woman who is lethargic and cannot rest or sleep should seek medical attention. These complications can be symptomatic of more serious postpartum complications.

Backaches and Headaches

Backaches and headaches are common discomforts during postpartum. Backaches that result from rectus abdominis diastasis can be treated with corrective exercises that recruit the transverse abdominis muscle.[10,11] However, when backaches persist

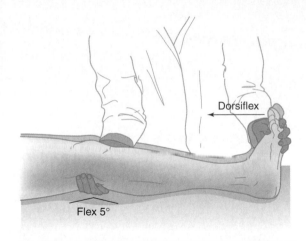

FIGURE 20-3 ■ Homan sign or check. If the new mother feels pain on sharp dorsiflexion of the foot, she must seek medical attention immediately. (From Leifer G: *Maternity nursing: an introductory text*, ed 9, St. Louis, 2005, Saunders.)

and headaches are frequent and severe (migraines), medical attention should be sought.

Backaches and headaches associated with spinal injections can be debilitating. Headaches or migraines from a dural tap that caused cerebral spinal fluid to leak affect women once they are mobile, are most severe when standing, and recede when lying down. They are often accompanied by a stiff neck, vomiting, and blurry vision. Symptoms are relieved with an injection of 10 to 20 ml of blood into the epidural space.[10]

Muscle Weakness or Numbness

If a client experiences muscle weakness or numbness in her face, legs, or anywhere in her body, she needs to seek medical attention immediately. These signs are symptomatic of a stroke and blood clots.

Thromboembolic Disorders

Before each postpartum treatment, practitioners should continue with pretreatment evaluations for up to 3 months postpartum (see Chapter 3), including the Homan check (Figure 20-3). If practitioners detect localized heat, swelling, redness, or pain in the woman's legs, particularly her calves, massage should be immediately stopped. The increase in fibrinogenic activity presents a disadvantage during pregnancy and postpartum recovery in that thrombi can form within the venous system. During the last trimester of pregnancy, the gravid woman develops a circulatory state of hypercoagulation to protect against hemorrhage. The risk of thromboembolic disorders increases about six times during pregnancy and even more in the puerperium.[1] This is further heightened by a decrease in fibrinolytic activity (the catabolism of clots) and raised concentration of clotting factors.

Thrombophlebitis is a clot in a superficial vein, most commonly the great saphenous vein supplying the calf (Figure 20-4). Symptoms include redness, tenderness, and possibly a slight increase in pulse and temperature over the thrombosed vein.[1]

Deep vein thrombosis (DVT) is less common but can be more serious because the clot can be dislodged, which can lead to a pulmonary embolism. Risk factors are hypercoagulability, increased maternal age, parity, dehydration after childbirth, and a surgical delivery.[1] Women are also at increased risk if they have a history of thromboembolic disorders, pregnancy-induced hypertension, anemia, or C-section.[12]

After a C-section, evidence indicates a greater chance of a DVT in the left leg because blood flow velocity is greatly reduced.[13] DVT is often asymptomatic, although there may be accompanying pain and swelling over the affected area with occasional pyrexia. Sometimes a difference in calf size is noticeable, or in extreme situations, circulation to the leg below the DVT is affected so the leg appears cold, white, and swollen. DVT is diagnosed through Doppler ultrasound or impedance plethysmography.

An obstetric emergency that may follow a DVT or happen without warning is a pulmonary embolism (PE). PE is a major factor in maternal mortality. If a fragment of a blood clot dislodges and enters the venous system (deep leg massage can be a contributing factor), it is circulated to the right side of the heart and the pulmonary circulation. As the pulmonary arteries get smaller, the thrombi may occlude arterial vessels within the lungs. Symptoms of a PE are sudden collapse, acute chest pain, dyspnea, cyanosis, and shock.[1]

Painful Urination

If a client complains about painful urination, sometimes accompanied by burning, or notices blood in the urine, she should contact her care provider. During pregnancy, the bladder loses some of its tone and as a result of the birth, the urethra,

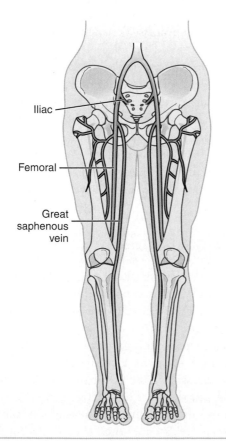

Iliac

Femoral

Great saphenous vein

FIGURE 20-4 ■ The great saphenous vein is a common site for a thromboembolism.

BOX 20-4 *Signs of Postpartum Urinary Tract Infection*

- Cystitis: inflammation of the urinary bladder
- Pyelonephritis: kidney inflammation
- Urinary urgency, frequency, and dysuria
- Suprapubic pain
- Fever and chills
- Costovertebral angle tenderness
- Leukocytosis
- Nausea and vomiting
- Laboratory results of white blood cells, red blood cells, protein, and bacteria in urine

From Leifer G: *Maternity nursing: an introductory text*, ed 9, St. Louis, 2005, Saunders.

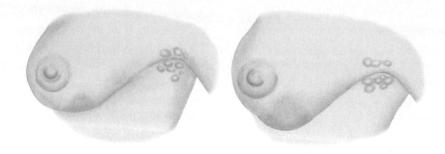

FIGURE 20-5 ■ *Left,* Early mastitis indicating enlarged and tender axillary lymph nodes. There is a red spot without swelling. *Right,* Acute mastitis with enlarged axillary lymph nodes and an inflamed area that is red, swollen, hot, and tender. (From Leifer G: *Maternity nursing: an introductory text,* ed 9, St. Louis, 2005, Saunders.)

bladder, and the tissue surrounding the urinary meatus may swell and suffer trauma. The urge to urinate is also suppressed by anesthetic drugs. Her lack of sensation may cause urine retention, which can have a direct influence on uterine contractions. When the bladder is distended, the uterus is displaced, usually to the right side, and its contractibility is weakened. As a result of the uterus failing to contract, blood vessels bleed freely.

Tenderness over the bladder, fever, urinary retention and dysuria with urinary frequency are signs are a urinary tract infection[4] (Box 20-4). Diarrhea, fecal incontinence, and constipation could also be potential complications warranting medical attention.

Mastitis

Mastitis is an infection of the breast and occurs approximately 2 to 3 weeks postpartum, although it may occur after 1 week. Symptoms are a painful localized hard mass and reddened area sometimes accompanied by enlarged axillary lymph glands. The woman may have a fever, chills, and general malaise, and if untreated, the infection can become an abscess (Figure 20-5). Prolonged symptoms require medical attention to rule out more serious complications, such as a tumor.

In My Experience...

Several years ago, perhaps in the early to mid 1980s, a client came to see me a few weeks after she had her baby. She described her labor in great detail (which is why I can still recall the story), told me about the birth, and then shared with me all her postpartum physical changes, leaving nothing to the imagination. Throughout this long list of symptoms, I often responded with, "This is normal during postpartum recovery." Over and over, I explained how her body was healing and that most of what she was going through was a natural cleansing and recovery process.

When I asked her if she had spoken with her doctor about this, or if she had ever learned about the recovery process in her childbirth education class, she responded, "No." This gave me the incentive to create a list of postpartum warning signs so that new mothers could refer to it if they had any concerns. As long as they were not experiencing any of the symptoms listed, they can assume that everything was normal—strange—but normal. They were also urged to ask their doctors or midwives any questions or speak about any apprehensions they might have about the recovery process.

Summary

Making a diagnosis about any of these postpartum complications is not within the scope of the bodyworker's practice. However, it is essential to recognize the warning signs of potentially dangerous postpartum complications to make the appropriate decisions about a client's care.

A client will be the best barometer of how she feels. A practitioner's knowledge and understanding of specific guidelines and precautions can help a woman feel secure when she is offering her a nurturing postpartum massage to help her on her road to recovery.

References

1. Coad J: *Anatomy and physiology for midwives*, St. Louis, 2001, Mosby.
2. Leifer G: *Maternity nursing: an introductory text*, ed 9, St. Louis, 2005, Saunders.
3. Lowdermilk DL, Perry SE: *Maternity & women's health care*, ed 8, St. Louis, 2004, Mosby.
4. Gabbe S, Niebyl J, Simpson J: *Obstetrics: normal and problem pregnancies*, ed 4, New York, 2002, Churchill Livingstone.
5. Mander R: Postnatal pain. In Mander R: *Pain in childbearing and its control*, Oxford, 1998, Blackwell Science.
6. Fraser D, Cooper M: *Myles' textbook for midwives*, ed 14, Edinburgh, 2003, Churchill Livingstone.
7. Gonik B: Intensive care monitoring of the critically ill pregnant patient. In Creasy R, Resnick R, eds: *Maternal-fetal medicine*, ed 4, Philadelphia, 1999, Saunders.
8. Kumar R: Pregnancy, childbirth and mental illness, *Prog Obstet Gynaecol* 5:146-159, 1985.
9. *Pregnancy and postpartum thought and mood disorders*, Belle Mead, NJ, 1996, Depression After Delivery, Inc.
10. Russell R, Dundas R, Reynolds F: Long-term backache after childbirth: prospective research for causative factors, *BMJ* 321:1384-1388, 1996.
11. Richardson CA, Jull GA: Muscle control–pain control. What exercises would you prescribe? *Man Ther* 1:2-10, 1995.
12. Weiner CP: Diagnosis and management of thromboembolic disorders of pregnancy, *Clin Obstet Gynecol* 28:107-118, 1985.
13. Macklon NS, Greer IA: The deep venous system in the puerperium: an ultrasound study, *Br J Obstet Gynaecol* 104:198-200, 1997.

REVIEW QUESTIONS

1   List the postpartum warning signs that necessitate medical intervention.

_____

_____

_____

_____

_____

_____

2   How much blood loss during labor is considered normal?

_____

_____

_____

_____

_____

_____

3   What are the signs of puerperal infection?

_____

_____

_____

_____

_____

_____

4   Can a postpartum woman develop preeclampsia? Is massage recommended or should she seek immediate medical attention?

_____

_____

_____

_____

_____

5   What is the cleansing vaginal discharge called? What phases does it pass through during the postpartum healing process?

_____

_____

_____

_____

_____

_____

6   What is uterine atony? Uterine subinvolution?

_____

_____

_____

_____

_____

_____

7   What are the "baby blues"? How long do they generally last?

_____

_____

_____

_____

_____

_____

8   What are some of the signs of postpartum depression or psychosis?

_____

_____

_____

_____

_____

9 What are some of the postpartum causes of back-aches or headaches? What can be done about them?

_____

_____

_____

_____

_____

10 For what period of time during the postpartum recovery process should the massage practitioner continue with the pretreatment evaluations?

_____

_____

_____

_____

_____

11 How long do the effects of increased fibrinogenic activity remain in a new mother's body?

_____

_____

_____

_____

_____

12 Which women are at increased risk for DVT?

_____

_____

_____

_____

_____

13 After a C-section, there is a greater chance of a DVT in which leg? Why?

_____

_____

_____

_____

_____

_____

14 What are the signs of a postpartum urinary tract infection?

_____

_____

_____

_____

_____

_____

15 What is mastitis? When does it generally occur during the postpartum period?

_____

_____

_____

_____

_____

_____

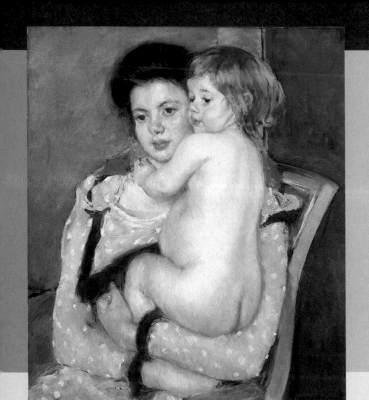

Immediate Postpartum Physiology and Treatment Goals

Objectives

On completion of this chapter, the student will be able to do the following:

1 Understand the dynamic physiological process that occurs within the first few hours and days of postpartum recovery

2 Understand the treatment goals of the immediate postpartum period and employ appropriate massage techniques to achieve these goals

3 Employ appropriate massage techniques to support breastfeeding

4 Recognize the differences between postpartum blues, depression, and psychosis

5 Understand maternal role adaptation

6 Understand the healing process for those women who had cesarean sections or were confined to bed rest and employ appropriate massage techniques

7 Use appropriate massage techniques for women who suffered miscarriages or stillbirths

8 Understand the process of grief and bereavement and what role the bodyworker plays in helping the client heal

Breastfeeding
Coccydynia
Diaphoresis
Diastasis
Diuresis
Endometrium

Episiotomy
Exfoliation
Hip displacement
Lactation
Let-down reflex
Letting-go phase

Maternal role adaptation
Milk ejection reflex
Postpartum blues
Sitz bath
Taking-hold phase
Taking-in phase

Puerperium is often referred to as the "Cinderella" period of midwifery and obstetrics because the excitement and thrill of birth is over. The challenges of parenting, maternal needs, and the dramatic postpartum physiological, emotional, and psychological changes receive little attention.[1] The traditional 6-week recovery period has its roots in the ritual of "churching," which is a medieval religious ceremony that accepted the new mother back into the church after a 40-day seclusion period, during which time they were considered unclean.[1]

In the United States, most childbirth education classes overlook or ignore the importance of teaching about postpartum recovery so many women go through this dynamic recuperative process without any understanding of normal physiological functions. The new mother sees her doctor again in 6 weeks and is expected to go back to work soon after that. About one-third of American women visiting their doctors for their postnatal checkup felt that their concerns about their health were not fully addressed.[2] As a matter of course, women in the United States do not consult their doctors about many postpartum health problems (Table 21-1).

The picture is quite different in other countries. In England, it is common for a midwife to visit a postpartum woman daily for the first week and provide a regular physical examination to assess the new mother's recovery.[3,4,6] In the Netherlands, a maternity aide, who has access to a midwife if necessary, undertakes most of the postnatal care at the mother's home.[6] Other European and Eastern countries offer long-term care and support to new families in contrast to the isolation and loneliness experienced by so many American new mothers.[6]

Bodyworkers are in a unique position to provide postnatal information to their clients during pregnancy visits. This information can include a list of warning signs for potential complications (see Chapter 20), as well as a general overview of the recuperative process. Learning how her body changes and what she should expect during this intense period of recovery will help a woman to be more accepting of herself and allay fears and concerns that something is wrong.

Another view regards the puerperium as a time of transition that begins with the birth of the baby and the expulsion of the placenta and ends with the return of fertility.[7-9] The exact reason for allocating 6 weeks time to heal relates to a range of cultural customs and traditions (such as "churching," as previously mentioned), as well as anatomical processes that occur during this time. The expectation that a woman would be completely recovered by 6 weeks is irrational, however, because some women have problems related to childbirth that continue well beyond this time and certain metabolic processes continue for several months after the birth.[8,10-14]

Learning about the postpartum recovery process can make some women uneasy and even upset. They have to be reminded that this is a necessary but temporary transition, and the unmitigated joys of motherhood will eclipse all of these annoyances and discomforts.

Postpartum Massage

Postpartum massage can be an emotional experience for some women. The safety of the nurturing environment and the supportive relationship established during pregnancy between the bodyworker and client could potentially make the sessions conducive for emotional release. This release should be protected, honored, understood, and supported as the combination of emotional

TABLE 21-1 *Physical Health Problems in First 2 Months after Birth and New-Onset Physical Problems*

Base: All Internet Respondents (Unless Otherwise Specified)	PROBLEMS AFTER BIRTH			"NEW" PROBLEMS AFTER BIRTH		
	Major (%)	Minor (%)	Major or Minor (%)	Experienced as New Problem (%)	Health Professional Never Consulted (%)	Persisting To at Least 6 Months Postpartum† (%)
Cesarean Births Only						
Pain at site of cesarean incision	25	58	83	79	72	7
Infection at site of cesarean incision	5	15	21	20	42	*
Vaginal Births Only						
Infections from cut or torn perineum	1	3	4	4	77	*
All Births						
Lack of sexual desire	24	35	59	33	88	16
Physical exhaustion	23	52	76	58	88	11
Sore nipples/breast tenderness	20	54	74	13	90	3
Backache	11	40	51	33	86	4
Painful intercourse	10	27	37	29	90	4
Painful perineum	9	35	44	43	89	2
Bowel problems	7	23	31	20	86	2
Frequent headaches	6	14	20	7	75	4
Urinary problems	5	22	27	18	82	7
Breast infection	4	5	9	9	49	*
Infection in uterus	1	1	2	2	76	-
Urinary tract infection	1	7	8	5	43	*

Reprinted with permission from Declercq ED, Sakala C, Corry MP, et al: *Listening to mothers II: Report of the Second National U.S. Survey of women's childbearing experiences*, New York, 2006, Childbirth Connection. Available at: http://www.childbirth-connection.org/listeningtomothers/

*Base, Those mothers for whom the problem did not exist prior to birth.

†Elapsed time between giving birth and participating in survey ranges from 0 to 24 months.

and physiological changes your client is undergoing. Touch can foster a cathartic response, especially during early recovery when hormonal shifting is extremely dramatic.

Clients can be comfortably positioned for a postpartum massage in the following ways:

- Sitting or semisitting
- Side-lying and bolstered with pillows
- Supine with legs elevated. (Practitioners should be aware of tenderness at the site of epidural injection.)
- Prone with special attention paid to the breasts. (Nursing pads should be placed under each breast while the client is in a prone position for leakage, and a contoured, recessed cushion or rolled towels should be used across her chest to avoid direct pressure on tender breasts.)
- Prone with special attention also paid to incisions. (A clean sanitary napkin can be placed over the site of a cesarean incision or a small pillow can be used for additional compression of the wound.)

The most relaxing sessions occur when the mother comes by herself, but it is not always possible for her to find someone to care for her child. While most babies sleep during the massage, mothers do not relax as much because they

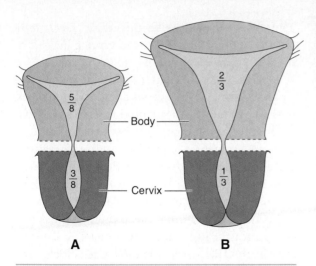

FIGURE 21–1 ■ Uterus involution. **A,** Nulliparous uterus. **B,** Parous uterus. (From Coad J, Dunstall M: *Anatomy and physiology for midwives,* ed 2, Edinburgh, 2006, Churchill Livingstone.)

From Leifer G: *Maternity nursing: an introductory text,* ed 9, St. Louis, 2005, Saunders.

BOX 21–1   *Uterine Involution*

Factors that Enhance Uterine Involution
- Uncomplicated labor and birth
- Nursing
- Early and frequent ambulation

Factors that Slow Uterine Involution
- Prolonged labor
- Incomplete expulsion of placenta and membranes
- Anesthesia or narcotic pain medications
- Previous labors
- A distended bladder

respond to every sigh, whimper, and noise from the baby. Some clients may want to hold their babies throughout the session. This can be accommodated by positioning the client in a semi-sitting positions with bolsters and pillows supporting her. Practitioners will need to be creative, spontaneous, and adaptable to satisfy the physical and emotional needs of a postpartum client.

Physiological changes in the Postpartum Woman

The postpartum woman's body is undergoing dramatic changes throughout every system in her body. These physiological changes start occurring immediately after the birth of the baby, and some of these adaptations overlap into later stages of recovery. Bodywork can begin as soon as the new mother desires.

Reproductive System
The Uterus

Immediately after the placenta is expelled, strong myometrial contractions cause the uterus to decrease in size (Figure 21-1). The enlarged uterine muscles are affected by the catabolic changes in protein cytoplasm that makes individual cells shrink. The products of this catabolic process are excreted into the urine as nitrogenous waste.[14] Within 24 hours the uterus becomes a round, hard mass and is about the same size it was at 20 weeks' gestation. Within 1 week postpartum, the uterus has involuted by 50%, from 1000 gm (2.2 lbs) after delivery to 500 gm (1.1 lbs).[15] After 2 weeks, the uterus weighs 340 gm (12 oz) because of normal involution and cannot be palpated by abdominal examination.[14,16,17] This rate can be affected by parity, the size of the newborn, and a multiple pregnancy (Box 21-1).

The placental site contracts immediately after birth to less than half its original diameter.[16] **Exfoliation** is a unique healing process that helps the placental site heal without scarring. This reparative process ensures future fertilized ova will implant in an unscarred uterus. The lining of the uterus, the **endometrium,** is completely healed and regenerated within 16 days except for the placental site, which takes 6 to 7 weeks postpartum to heal.[18] After 24 hours, the fundus descends by 1 cm per day (Figure 21-2).

Cervix

As soon as the baby is born, the cervix is flabby, amorphous, bruised and wide open.[14] Small tears or lacerations may be present, and the tissue is edematous. The cervix heals very quickly and by the end of the first week, it feels firm and the os is the width of one finger. The cervix never returns to its original condition and always shows evidence of birth by appearing slitlike rather than round (Figure 21-3).

Vagina

Once the baby is born, the vaginal rugae (folds) are smooth. The vagina is swollen and multiple tears or lacerations may be noticeable. The hymen is permanently torn, and small tags of tissue are visible at the vaginal introitus.

Within 3 weeks postpartum, the edema has decreased and the vaginal folds reappear. It takes 6 to 10 weeks for the vagina to completely involute and return to its normal appearance, size, and contour. The vagina, like the cervix, never fully regains its prepregnant size and varying degrees of mucosal or fascial atony may remain.[14,17,19]

During the postpartum period, the vaginal mucosa and vaginal walls atrophy and do not rethicken until the ovaries once again produce estrogen. Nursing mothers often complain about vaginal dryness because estrogen is suppressed during **lactation,** and dyspareunia, or discomfort during intercourse, may result.[14] Vaginal lubricants can restore moisture to make intercourse more pleasurable.

Lochia is the normal postpartum vaginal discharge. It is heaviest during the first 1 to 2 hours after birth. The first lochia discharge is lochia rubra and lasts 1 to 3 days. This bleeding may contain small clots along with other fetal, uterine, and placental waste products. The flow then pales, and the discharge is lochia serosa. This phase can last up to 27 days, although 10 days is more common. The final lochia discharge, lochia alba, is often yellow or white. This continues up to 6 weeks postpartum.

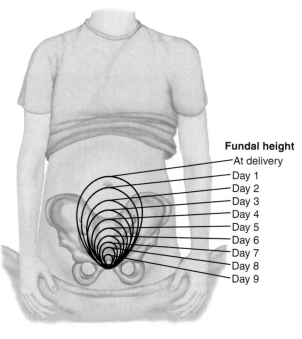

Fundal height
At delivery
Day 1
Day 2
Day 3
Day 4
Day 5
Day 6
Day 7
Day 8
Day 9

FIGURE 21-2 ■ Fundal height. The height of the fundus decreases about 1 cm per day. (From McKinney ES, James SR, Murray SS, et al: *Maternal-child nursing*, ed 2, St. Louis, 2005, Mosby.)

Perineum

The fetal head pressing against the pelvic floor during the second stage of labor caused the pubococcygeal muscles to stretch and weaken. This results in a bruised, edematous perineum. If an **episiotomy** was performed, healing may take up to 4 to 6 months.[20] Lacerations and tears of the perineum may also occur during labor (Boxes 21-2 and 21-3). An induced or augmented labor also can cause an extremely sore or bruised perineum.

The pelvic floor muscles are impaired to a greater extent as a result of a vaginal birth, particularly if there was more mechanical trauma (i.e., the use

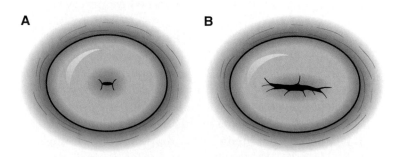

FIGURE 21-3 ■ **A**, The cervix of a nulliparous woman. **B**, Reformation of a parous cervix. (From McKinney ES, James SR, Murray SS, et al: *Maternal-child nursing*, ed 2, St. Louis, 2005, Mosby.)

BOX 21-2 *A Natural Alternative to Suturing*

"While on an Indian reservation, I had studied with a shaman and observed the use of seaweed to heal burns and deep lacerations. I suggested this alternative to a couple who refused suturing of a second-degree perineal tear. The couple agreed.

"I cut a piece of seaweed that was twice the length and the width of the tear, folded it in half and moistened it with sterile water. I placed it down the center of the tear and brought the edges of the tissue together, carefully aligning them. I also covered the entire length of the tear with a second patch of moistened seaweed. Before departing, I included in my postpartum care plan instructions to replace the outer patch of seaweed each time she used the bathroom. I also instructed her to keep her legs together and to stay in bed as much as possible, caring only for herself and the baby.

"Upon my arrival 24 hours later for the first postpartum check, all was well with mom and baby. When I examined the perineal area, I discovered the tissue had healed miraculously well. I could not even distinguish a separation of the tissue where the tear occurred. The mom also had virtually no pain in that area. She mentioned that the salt in the seaweed stung a little when first applied but quickly faded to a healing tingle.

"Ever since that birth in 1986, I have been using seaweed patches with great success as an alternative to suturing. I have taught this technique to other midwives and apprentices."

From Gilpin-Blake LM, Eliot S: *Midwifery Today* 60, 2001.

BOX 21-3 *Lacerations of the Perineum*

Lacerations of the perineum are classified by the following degrees to describe how much tissue is involved:

- First-degree tears involve the superficial vaginal mucosa or perineal skin
- Second-degree tears involve the vaginal mucosa, perineal skin and deeper tissue which may include perineal muscles
- Third-degree tears affect the same as the second degree tears but involves the anal sphincter
- Fourth-degree tears extend through the anal sphincter into the anal mucosa.

From McKinney ES, James SR, Murray SS, et al: *Maternal-child nursing*, ed 2, St. Louis, 2005, Mosby.

---

of instrumentation or augmentation). For these women, muscle strength and neuromuscular control are affected for the first week of puerperium.[21] It takes about 2 months for most women to have a complete recovery regarding strength and muscular tone of the pelvic floor muscles.

Hemorrhoids, which are distended rectal veins, may also occur during the second stage of labor. These, as well as lacerations of the perineum, can make many daily activities, such as walking, sitting, bending, squatting, defecating, and urinating, uncomfortable or painful.

Losing more than 500 ml of blood within 24 hours is considered to be a primary postpartum hemorrhage (PPH). It can be caused from uterine atony where the myometrium fails to contracts, failure of blood clotting mechanisms or both.[1] The risk of this excessive bleeding diminishes between 24 and 72 hours. A secondary postpartum hemorrhage may occur if the uterus fails to involute from an infection within the uterine cavity.

Bodyworkers can use the following massage techniques to facilitate healing of the reproductive system:

- Fundal massage to encourage involution.
- Spleen 10 pressed to encourage expulsion of placenta and functional bleeding (Figure 21-4). *DVD*
- Spleen 6 pressed to help tone the uterus (Figure 21-5).
- Uterine reflexes pressed to tone the uterus (Figure 21-6).
- Ice packs applied to the perineum for the first 24 hours to reduce swelling.
- Lymphatic drainage on legs to ease hemorrhoids. *DVD*
- Acupuncture point governing vessel 20 on top of head (Figure 21-7) and foot reflex point to ease hemorrhoids, similar to prenatal care.

Bodyworkers can make the following suggestions to help heal the reproductive system:

- Contract her gluteal muscles before sitting and lower her weight slowly onto her buttocks to prevent stretching of the perineal tissue.
- Avoid sudden impact to the traumatized area.
- Kegel exercises to restore functional integrity to the pelvic floor, control incontinence, and treat hemorrhoids.
- 15 drops of geranium oil and 5 drops of cypress oil diluted in 2 Tbsp oil placed

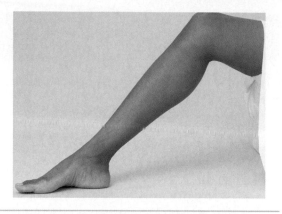

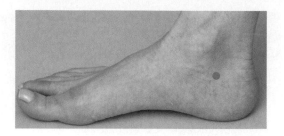

FIGURE 21-6 ■ The uterine reflex can be squeezed to help tone the uterus.

FIGURE 21-4 ■ Spleen 10 can be pressed to encourage expulsion of the placenta and functional uterine bleeding.

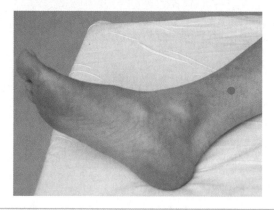

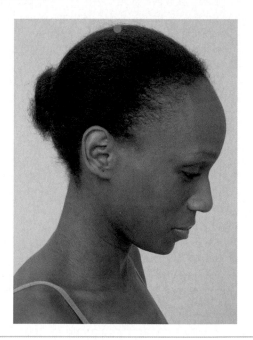

FIGURE 21-5 ■ Spleen 6 can be pressed to help tone the uterus.

topically on hemorrhoids to treat discomfort of hemorrhoids.
- Tucks, witch hazel, calendula, lemon to treat hemorrhoids.
- **Sitz bath** with 3 drops of lavender oil and 2 drops of cypress oil in the basin for perineal healing.
- Use of peri-bottle to dilute urine and cleanse after micturition.
- Slow breathing to ease afterpains.
- Arnica pills dissolved under the tongue (4 pills every 4 hours) or 1 to 2 droppers of tincture of Motherwort in a glass of water every 4 hours for the first week to treat afterpains.

Musculoskeletal System

Muscle fatigue and soreness are most common the first day or two after labor because of the extreme exertion of labor. Chronic compression of

FIGURE 21-7 ■ Acupuncture point on the top of the head (governing vessel 20).

the woman's lower spine and the anterior pelvic tilt of late pregnancy have shortened lumbar muscles, particularly the lower segment of the erector spinae, quadratus lumborum, and lumbosacral fascia (and corresponding neck muscles), and overstretched anterior hip flexors, in particular the psoas and iliacus. Lateral hip rotators, especially the piriformis, are tight. The function of the woman's sacroiliac (SI) joint can be affected by an imbalance of pelvic muscles. Triggers points are omnipresent in weakened muscles and around the SI and lumbosacral joints. The practitioner must also take care to avoid direct pressure on the site of the epidural injection.

Hip displacement, or symphysis pubis separation, may have occurred during labor from holding certain positions over a protracted period of time. When a hip is dislocated, the client should avoid hip medial rotation, adduction of the affected leg across the midline, and hip flexion above 90 degrees.

Another pelvic problem may be **coccydynia,** which is pain in the coccygeal region from damage to the coccygeal ligaments with or without coccyx displacement or fracture. For the woman whose coccyx angles upward, sacral lifts and counterpressures directly on the coccyx should be avoided.

During the first few days, levels of relaxin start to decrease, and the ligaments and cartilage of the pelvis slowly begin to return to their prepregnant position. This shifting can create hip or joint pain that may interfere with daily activities such as ambulation. Another contributing factor to gait instability is the prenatally weakened iliopsoas muscle.

Massage of the psoas in early recovery may prove too invasive for many women. Because of the intense nature of psoas release work and its proximity to the recuperating reproductive system, the practitioner should wait to work on this and other intrinsic musculature until later in the healing process when the client is feeling less vulnerable. However, because it is an important goal in early postpartum to stabilize the woman's pelvis

and hips, posterior pelvic tilts, positional release or the constructive rest position (see Chapter 10), and rocking in a chair can be effective ways to balance the psoas muscle in early recovery.

The longitudinal muscles of the rectus abdominis separate in late pregnancy, creating the diastasis recti (Figure 21-8). This separation can be small or severe, and exercises that recruit the transverse abdominis accompanied by abdominal binding in early postpartum are effective ways to treat the abdominal separation (Figure 21-9). The **diastasis** may have caused a displacement of the intestines, bladder, and other abdominal structures. Trigger points also develop along the attachments at the xiphoid process, costal edges, and pubic bone (Figure 21-10).

The woman's abdomen is quite distended, and she still looks pregnant. The abdomen feels doughy on palpation but once the placenta has been expelled, the effect of progesterone on the muscles is no longer present and muscle tone slowly starts to be restored. Her gait is further affected by the shift in her center of gravity. No longer pregnant, she may exhibit a lack of balance and still present the prenatal posture. One effective way to counteract this maladaptive stance is to remind her to use her abdominal core muscles throughout the day,

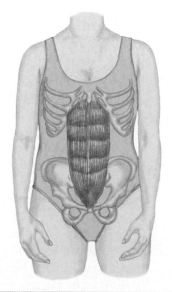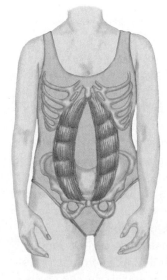

FIGURE 21-8 ■ *Left,* Normal position of rectus abdominis muscle. *Right,* Diastasis recti: the separation of the rectus muscles. (From McKinney ES, James SR, Murray SS, et al: *Maternal-child nursing,* ed 2, St. Louis, 2005, Mosby.)

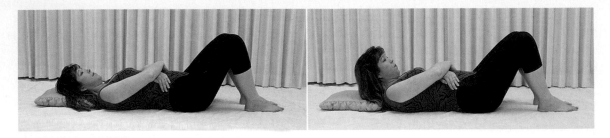

FIGURE 21-9 ■ Exercises that recruit the transverse abdominis by pulling the core muscles in will help to heal the diastasis and promote greater lumbar stability. In early postpartum, bringing the bellies of the rectus together with hands (as shown) or a splint (made from a long cloth wrapped around the midsection) also encourages abdominal integrity. (From McKinney ES, James SR, Murray SS, et al: *Maternal-child nursing*, ed 2, St. Louis, 2005, Mosby.)

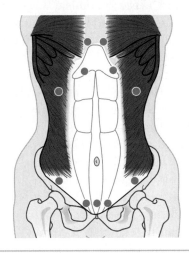

FIGURE 21-10 ■ Abdominal trigger points are located at muscle attachments.

especially when she lifts the baby, and to wear a splint for the first few weeks.

Carpal tunnel syndrome or de Quervain's syndrome can be potentially avoided if the new mother pays careful attention to body mechanics when she lifts and holds the baby and remembers to retract her cervical spine.

A generalized decrease in bone mineralization occurs after the baby is born and returns to normal within 18 months.[18]

Bodyworkers can use the following massage techniques and make the following suggestions to facilitate healing of the musculoskeletal system:

- Light Swedish massage to address muscle soreness and fatigue. Direct pressure is avoided to the site of the epidural injections or any intravenous (IV) bruising.

- Manual lymphatic drainage on the legs to treat muscle aches and reduce swelling.
- Gentle myofascial release to decompress the lumbar spine and corresponding neck, upper back, and shoulder tightness.
- Trigger point release along the sacroiliac and lumbosacral joints, hips, pelvis, and abdomen.
- Hip compression with fists behind the anterior superior iliac spines (ASIS) to restore placement of hips.
- **DVD** Pelvic tilt to decompress lumbar spine.
- Psoas release with pelvic tilt, positional release, or constructive rest position.
- Appropriate abdominal exercises that recruit the transverse abdominis to encourage healing of the diastasis recti.
- Treatment for carpal tunnel syndrome or de Quervain's syndrome.
- Strengthen and stabilize hip muscles from L1 to the greater trochanter to help realign the displaced hips or separation of the symphysis pubis.
- Strengthen and stabilize the psoas major and iliacus and use medial hip compression with fists directly behind the ASIS and avoid any hip or pelvic traction.
- To treat coccydynia, client rests with gentle hip and pelvic massage; avoid any sacral lifting or direct counterpressure to the coccygeal area.
- Internal osseous adjustment (not performed by massage practitioner) or therapeutic ultrasound.
- Pillows for sitting.[22]

Cardiovascular System

Cardiac output continues at an increased rate for at least 48 hours postpartum because of an increase in stroke volume despite a decrease in heart rate.[17] Two weeks after the birth, there is a 30% decrease in cardiac output as a result of decreased blood volume. The ability of the heart to contract that was enhanced during pregnancy returns to its prepregnant state by 6 weeks.[23,24] Stroke volume, cardiac output, end-diastolic volume, and systemic vascular resistance remain elevated up to 1-year postpartum.[25]

Blood volume decreases very quickly after birth. Blood loss of 500 ml is associated with an uncomplicated vaginal birth; blood loss during a surgical delivery is twice as high.[20,26] By day 3, blood volume has decreased by 16% of predelivery peak.[27] Plasma volume and interstitial fluid excesses and swelling from IV saline drips are disposed of through **diuresis,** excessive urination (as much as 3000 ml in a day), and **diaphoresis,** which is profuse perspiration mostly during the night.[16] Readjustments in heart rate, blood pressure, vasculature, consumption of oxygen, and total body fluid occur within a few days postpartum.

Some components of blood change during postnatal recovery. Leukocytosis occurs as the white blood cell count increases to 30,000/mm[3] and falls to normal 4 to 7 days after birth.[20,28] This increase is associated with elevated neutrophil levels that respond to inflammation, pain, and stress.

Fibrinolysis increases shortly after the birth, but elevation in clotting factors continues for several more days. It takes 8 to 10 weeks before blood clot formation risks decline to a prepregnant state.[29] New mothers are at an increased risk of thrombophlebitis; cesarean delivery is an even greater risk factor. Women with varicose veins or a history of venous obstruction should also be carefully monitored for evidence of a blood clot. The practitioner should continue the pretreatment evaluation for the presence of blood clots, particularly in the calves, for up to 10 weeks postpartum to be on the safe side. In addition, deep work on the legs during this period of time is not recommended. Instead, continue with manual lymphatic drainage. Antiembolism stockings or sequential compression devices are often provided to the woman

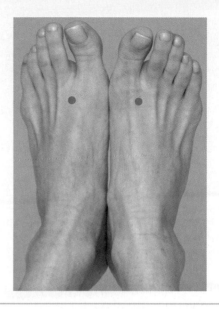

FIGURE 21-11 ■ Liver 3 can be pressed to expedite fluid waste removal and encourage fluid elimination.

who has had a cesarean section (C-section) or is at high risk for phlebitis.[14]

Bodyworkers can use the following massage techniques to facilitate healing of the cardiovascular system:

- Homan check and palpation to check for the presence of blood clots on the entire leg.
- Manual lymphatic drainage to protect against dislodging clots and to encourage reduction of interstitial fluid; also lymphatic compressions.
- Liver 3 pressed to treat diuresis and diaphoresis and to expedite fluid waste removal (Figure 21-11).

Bodyworkers can also make the following suggestions to the client to help heal the cardiovascular system:

- Drink 8 to 12 glasses of water daily.
- Wear natural fibers.
- Wear antiembolism hosiery or sequential compression devices to prevent thrombophlebitis.

Gastrointestinal System

A new mother's appetite and thirst return rapidly after childbirth, partly a result of the amount of energy she expended during labor, fluid restriction, fluid loss, and early diaphoresis.

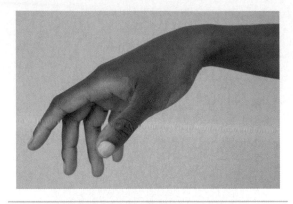

FIGURE 21-12 ■ Large intestine 4 can be pressed to treat constipation.

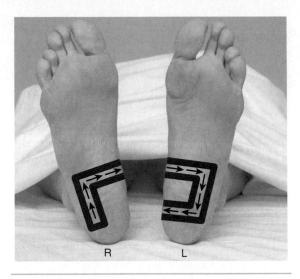

FIGURE 21-13 ■ Intestinal foot reflexes can be massaged to encourage peristalsis.

Constipation is a common problem in the early postpartum period for a number of reasons. Lax bowel tone, caused by the effects of progesterone, decreases peristalsis for the first few days. Restricted food and liquid intake often create small, hard stools. Weakened abdominal muscles make it more difficult to bear down to expel the stool. In addition, perineal trauma, episiotomy, and hemorrhoids are uncomfortable and can interfere with easy bowel elimination. Finally, some women anticipate pain when defecating and do not respond to their urge.

Temporary constipation is not serious but can lead to flatulence and bloating, which is uncomfortable. In addition to the helpful massage techniques and suggestions to treat constipation, stool softeners and laxatives are often prescribed. A bowel movement should occur by the third day, but it may take longer to establish a normal bowel pattern.[16,20]

Bodyworkers can use the following massage techniques to facilitate healing of the gastrointestinal system:

- Kenbiki for constipation
- **DVD** Large intestine 4 pressed to treat constipation (Figure 21-12)
- Massage the foot reflexes of the intestines to encourage peristalsis (Figure 21-13)
- **DVD** Lymphatic drainage of the leg.
- Gentle abdominal massage to encourage peristalsis (should not be performed on a woman who had a C-section until the scar has closed completely).

Bodyworkers can also make the following suggestions to the client to help heal the gastrointestinal system:

- Increase fluid consumption to 8 to 10 glasses of water daily.
- Eat foods rich in natural digestive enzymes,
- Exercise to encourage peristalsis.
- Elevate feet on a step stool when sitting on the toilet to place lower colon in postural alignment.
- Use stool softeners and laxatives initially but use judiciously to permit natural peristaltic activity to function.
- Do not strain while sitting on the toilet and void only when the feeling is there.

Urinary System

The urinary bladder has lost some of its tone, and the urethra, bladder, and tissue surrounding the urinary meatus might be traumatized and edematous from the birth. Urination may be blocked by anesthesia, and the mother has to be reminded to void. If she was given IV fluids during labor, her bladder will fill rapidly and her decreased sensitivity to fluid pressure might result in bladder distension. This in turn displaces the uterus (usually to the right side), and its ability to contract is decreased (Figure 21-14). Urinary retention and bladder distension can lead to urinary tract infections (UTIs) because urinary stasis

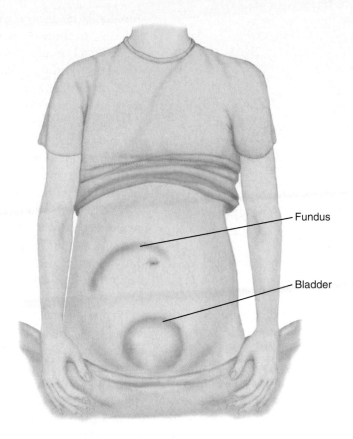

FIGURE 21-14 ■ A distended bladder displaces the uterus to the right and prevents contractions of the uterus. (From McKinney ES, James SR, Murray SS, et al: *Maternal-child nursing*, ed 2, St. Louis, 2005, Mosby.)

allows bacteria to multiply and to postpartum hemorrhage.

Urinary output in early recovery can be great (diuresis), whereas trauma to the perineum may result in urinary or fecal incontinence.

Bodyworkers can use the following massage techniques and make the following suggestions to facilitate healing of the urinary system:

- Bladder reflexes on the feet (Figure 21-15) pressed.
- Client can be reminded to void.
- Client can be reminded to increase fluid intake.

Integumentary System

The skin changes during pregnancy brought on by hormonal influences gradually decline after childbirth. Hyperpigmentation from melanocyte-stimulating hormone decreases very quickly and the skin starts to lighten. This is most apparent when chloasma and the linea nigra disappear.

The striae gravidarum, spider nevi, and palmar erythema eventually fade to silvery lines but do not disappear.[14] Hair growth slows, and hair loss may result in early months of postpartum but normalizes in time.

Neurological System

Headaches have to be carefully monitored in post-partum, particularly if they are accompanied by blurred vision, photophobia, abdominal pain, and proteinuria. This may indicate the development or worsening of gestational hypertension, or preeclampsia. Other headaches may be puncture headaches caused after regional anesthesia was administered. They are often worse in an upright position and are less severe when supine. These two types of headaches should be reported to the care provider for observation.

Fatigue, afterpains, discomforts, muscle aches, and breast tenderness may all contribute to sleeplessness and general malaise. If she received

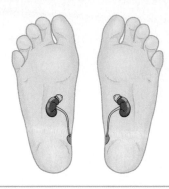

FIGURE 21-15 ■ The foot reflexology points for the bladder, ureters, and kidneys. Bladder points should be pressed for a count of 10, repeating a total of 10 times.

anesthesia, she may still be experiencing a lack of feeling in her legs or dizziness when she stands. The elimination of excess fluid through diuresis may relieve carpal tunnel syndrome by reducing the compression of the median nerve.[14,16]

Endocrine System

Once the placenta is expelled, levels of estrogen, progesterone, and human placental lactogen decrease by as much as 90% and fall to prepregnant levels within 72 hours.[14] This can account in part for the woman's emotional lability in early postpartum.[1] Placental protein hormones have a longer half-life so plasma levels drop off more slowly.[1] Human chorionic gonadotrophin levels may remain approximately 2 weeks as the adrenal hormones return to normal.[30]

If the new mother is not **breastfeeding,** it will take about 2 weeks for prolactin to return to prepregnant levels.[14] Estrogen begins to rise to follicular levels approximately 3 weeks after childbirth. This rise allows for the return of her menstrual cycle. Most nonnursing mothers resume their menses about 7 to 9 weeks postpartum, although it varies according to the woman.[20] If she is breastfeeding, she may resume her menstrual cycle as early as 12 weeks or as late as 18 months.[31] The first few cycles are often anovulatory for both lactating and nonlactating women, but ovulation may occur before the first menses, so couples should use contraception when resuming sexual relations.

The drastic drop in hormones levels readies the new mother's body for two significant purposes: lactation and the return of menses.[16] Decreased estrogen levels also contribute to excessive sweating, or diaphoresis (night sweats), that helps degrade and release the additional fluid that accumulated during pregnancy.

While pregnant, estrogen and progesterone prepared the woman's breasts for lactation. Prolactin levels are high in pregnancy, but increased estrogen and progesterone levels inhibited its function in milk production. Once the placenta is expelled and estrogen and progesterone levels drop dramatically, prolactin initiates milk production with 2 to 3 days postpartum (Figure 21-16). Once milk production has been firmly established, frequent feedings and suckling stimulate lactation. Levels of oxytocin are necessary to initiate the **milk ejection reflex** (the **let-down reflex**) and are also sensitive to lactation performance.

By day 3, the prolactin effects are evident within the breast tissue and engorgement may occur. The breasts become distended, firm, tender, heavy, warm, and painful (Figure 21-17). The milk, which is thin and bluish, replaces colostrum, or premilk (Box 21-4). Bodyworkers should urge clients to drink adequate amounts of water—8-12 glasses daily—to help encourage milk production.

Bodyworkers can use the following massage techniques to facilitate healing of the endocrine system:

- Spleen 3 pressed for hormone balancing (Figure 21-18).
- Spleen 6 (see Figure 21-5) and the uterine reflex pressed to tone the uterus (see Figure 21-6). **DVD**
- Liver 3 pressed to encourage fluid elimination (see Figure 21-11).
- Breast massage to treat engorgement and acupuncture points stomach 13 and 16, conception vessel 17, and breast reflex on the foot (Figure 21-19).
- Gall bladder 21 (Figure 21-20) to promote milk let-down. **DVD**
- Ginger compress to treat engorged breasts.
- Bruised cabbage leaves to treat engorged breasts or sore nipples.

The Benefits of Breastfeeding

"The newborn baby has only three demands. They are warmth in the arms of its mother, food from her breasts, and security in the knowledge

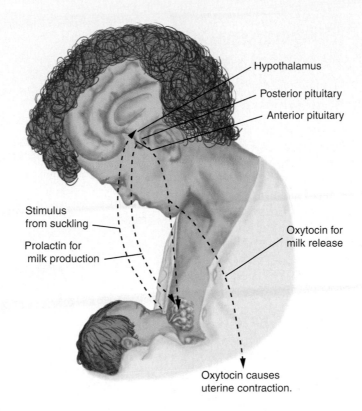

FIGURE 21-16 ■ The effect of prolactin and oxytocin on milk production. When the baby starts to suckle, nerve impulses travel to the hypothalamus that causes the anterior pituitary to secrete prolactin to increase milk production. Suckling encourages the posterior pituitary to secrete oxytocin, creating the let-down effect. (From McKinney ES, James SR, Murray SS, et al: *Maternal-child nursing*, ed 2, St. Louis, 2005, Mosby).

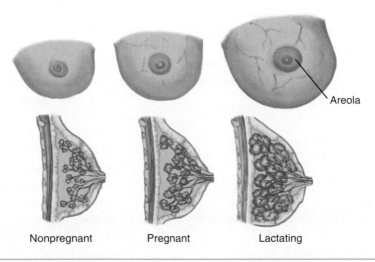

FIGURE 21-17 ■ Breast changes during pregnancy and lactation. (From McKinney ES, James SR, Murray SS, et al: *Maternal-child nursing*, ed 2, St. Louis, 2005, Mosby.)

How the Breasts Function and the Benefits of Breastfeeding

During pregnancy, the ducts, lobes, and alveoli of the breasts develop in response to estrogen, progesterone placental lactogen, prolactin, and chorionic gonadotrophin. Although prolactin levels are high, lactation is inhibited as a result of the heightened levels of estrogen, progesterone, and placental lactogen. The increase in breast size during pregnancy indicates that the breasts are responding to hormonal influences.

Milk is produced in the alveoli of the breasts via a complex process that removes necessary nutrients from maternal blood stream and reformulates it into milk. The milk is synthesized as the baby suckles. Milk is ejected as oxytocin levels elevate in response to nipple stimulation and cause the myoepithelial cells to squeeze the milk from the secretory cells of the alveoli into the alveolar lumen. The milk travels through the lactiferous ducts and empties into the lactiferous sinuses, which the newborn compresses during nursing to eject the milk through the pores in the nipple. This is called the *milk ejection reflex* or the *let-down reflex*.

From McKinney ES, James SR, Murray SS, et al: *Maternal-child nursing*, ed 2, St. Louis, 2005, Mosby.

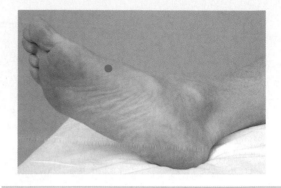

FIGURE 21-18 ■ Spleen 3 can be pressed for hormone balancing.

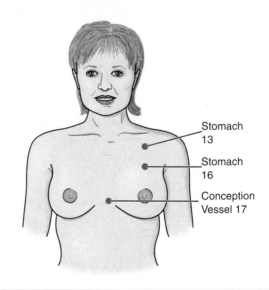

FIGURE 21-19 ■ Breast massage can treat engorgement and include acupuncture points: stomach 13, stomach 16, conception vessel 17, liver 3, and breast reflexes on the feet.

of her presence. Breastfeeding satisfies all three."[32]

"For if one places the nipple in the mouth of the newborn, they suck the milk and swallow it eagerly. And if they chance to be distressed or to cry, the best appeasement of their unhappiness is the mother's nipple put in their mouth. And whoever is able effectively to employ these arts will best develop both body and mind."—Galen of Rome, 180 AD.[32]

The numerous health and emotional benefits of breastfeeding for both mother and newborn are as follows[14]:

Maternal Benefits
- The release of oxytocin during nursing speeds up uterine involution.
- Mother loses less blood as a result of delayed menses.
- Mother is more likely to rest and relax during feeding.
- Maternal diet will be well-balanced.
- Bonding will be enhanced by frequent physical contact.

- Breast milk is the perfect temperature, always ready, convenient, and economical.
- Nursing may reduce the risk of certain cancers.

Newborn Benefits
- Baby is less likely to develop allergies.
- Breast milk has immunological properties that prevent frequent ear infections, respiratory problems, gastrointestinal infections, and less risk for sudden infant death syndrome (SIDS)
- Human breast milk is ideal for the human infant.

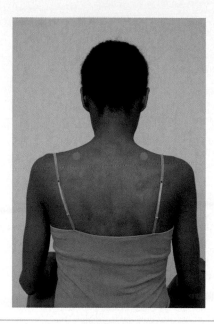

FIGURE 21-20 ■ Gall bladder 21, slightly inferior to the belly of the trapezius, can help stimulate milk let-down.

- Nutritional and immunological properties change with the growing baby.
- Easy to digest.
- Protein, fat, and carbohydrates are in correct proportions for the newborn's needs.
- Safer than formula (no improper dilution).
- Less likelihood of overfeeding.
- Baby is unlikely to be constipated (Figure 21-21).

Respiratory System

The drop in progesterone restores prepregnant sensitivity to carbon dioxide concentration so carbon dioxide pressures normalize. The respiratory diaphragm can increase its range since the uterus no longer impairs movement so the basal lobes of the lungs can fully ventilate. Chest wall compliance, tidal volume, and respiratory rate normalize within 1 to 3 weeks.[1]

Vital Signs

Immediate postpartum temperature may rise to 100.4° F (38° C) during the first 24 hours as a result of dehydration and exertion. After this initial period, the woman should be afebrile and any temperature greater than 100.4° F is a warning sign that infection may be present. Breast engorgement may contribute to a short-term increase in temperature on the second or third day postpartum.

It is quite normal for the pulse rate to drop to a rate of 50 to 60 beats per minute (bradycardia) for the first 6 to 8 days. An elevated heart rate may indicate hemorrhage, infection, pain, anxiety, or heart disease. Blood pressure readings should remain stable after birth. A drop in pressure may indicate a hemorrhage, whereas elevated pressure, especially when accompanied by a headache, could indicate gestational hypertension and require immediate medical attention.[16]

Immediately after delivery, the new mother loses about 10 to 12 lbs. This weight loss is a combination of the fetus, placenta, and amniotic fluid. Another 5 lbs or so is lost from diuresis and diaphoresis during the first few days postpartum. The woman's body stored about 5 to 7 lbs of fat during pregnancy for lactation needs, and breastfeeding will diminish this extra weight over a period of about 6 months. Her weight should normalize about 6 months after childbirth.[16]

This immediate loss of weight changes her center of gravity, although her sense of her body is still one that carries most of the weight in the anterior. She compensates with the same maladaptive posture of late pregnancy for the first few days.

Many women actually experience a weight gain in the first couple of days postpartum from increased adrenocorticotropic hormone (ACTH), antidiuretic hormone (ADH), and stress factors. These increase sodium and water retention which starts to diminish by the fourth day as diuresis increases. In general, weight loss is greater with lower parity, maternal age, and lower prepregnant weight. Postnatal weight loss is affected more by changes in lifestyle before and after pregnancy than by the pregnancy itself.[33]

Sleep

Disrupted sleep is associated with early postpartum. The first three days can be very exhausting and trying for the new mother. She may be unable to rest due to perineal pain or surgical discomforts and the fatigue from labor only compounds her sleeplessness. Euphoria, physical discomforts, and infant (and older sibling) disturbances (not to mention the constant traffic in a hospital setting) all lead to reduced and restless sleep.[34] This can

MOTHER'S MILK FOR TENDER INFANTS

WHEN a baby is prematurely born, or taken seriously ill, mothers' (human) milk is an absolute necessity; the weakened condition of the mother, as a rule, makes it impossible for her to feed her own child. Therefore, one of the first steps of the attending physician (as with the famous quintuplets) to secure a supply of mothers' milk. Of course, a "wet nurse" could often be obtained, but this method was not satisfactory, as the number was limited and their fees were very high. It was also known that "wet nurses" often neglect their own children in order to earn a few dollars. Physicians knew that many mothers had more milk than their own baby required and with the aid of baby health stations and hospitals, the Mothers' Milk Bureau of the Children's Welfare Federation of New York (established in 1921 by Dr. Henry Dwight Chapin) undertook to find these mothers and have them come daily to express (squeeze out) their excess milk for which they would be paid. These women, before being accepted, are subjected to a very rigid medical examination. Their own babies (whom they must nurse themselves) are kept under the supervision of a private physician

or Baby Health Station. A record is kept of the child's health and, if it should lose weight, the mother discontinues giving milk until the baby's doctor permits her to do so.

After the mothers express their milk, it is pooled, pasteurized, chilled and placed on ice. Milk is sold only when prescribed by a doctor. Those who cannot afford to pay for it are given the milk free; hospitals are charged 25¢ an ounce (the exact cost to the Bureau); private physicians 30¢. No request is ever refused because of inability to pay. (The demand for free milk is very great and the Bureau is seeking contributions in order to widen its scope. At present, between 35 and 45 infants are being supplied with mothers' milk.)

Any surplus milk, after all orders are filled is frozen by a special process into little wafers (as illustrated in a recent issue of YOUR BODY) and placed in a sterile container, which is placed on ice until the demand for mothers' milk is greater than the supply. In this way, the fluid can be kept indefinitely without losing any of its life-preserving qualities.

FIGURE 21-21 ■ "Mother's milk for tender infants." From *Your Body*, March, 1937.

have a tremendous impact on her mood, memory, and psychomotor tasks. Breastfeeding will also contribute to disrupted sleep patterns.[35]

Bodyworkers can use the following massage techniques to promote sleep:

- Light full body massage to reduce muscle soreness and pain.
- **DVD** Acupuncture points pericardium 8, pericardium 6, and heart 7 pressed (Figure 21-22).
- Kidney 1 pressed (Figure 21-23).
- Energy techniques such as Reiki.
- **DVD** Lymphatic drainage on the legs to ease fluid retention

Emotional and Psychological Changes

Mood disorders are interruptions in function, affect, or thought processes that can affect the entire family after childbirth as seriously as physiological problems.[14] Postpartum women have an increased vulnerability to mood disorders.

Touch Points

The extreme amount of sweating most new mothers experience often astounds and concerns many women. Physically, the suppression of ovarian function and decrease in estrogen levels causes these sweats, or diaphoresis. They regularly occur at night ("night sweats"), and women wake up and often remark that they are "half their size and have woken up in a pool of their own sweat." This is how her body rids itself of the additional interstitial fluid that accumulated during the pregnancy.

One way to prepare for this ahead of time is to suggest she make up her bed before going into labor with waterproof pads under her sheet. This will prevent her mattress from getting wet and stained. Linens can be easily laundered. Mattresses cannot. She can also cover her upholstered furniture and car seat with the pads to prevent staining the furniture. A little forethought and sensibility will make her and her family more comfortable.

Almost 50% to 70% of new mothers experience **postpartum blues**, also referred to as baby blues, within the first few days of childbirth.[36,37] This self-limiting period usually lasts no longer than 2 weeks and is characterized by weeping, insomnia,

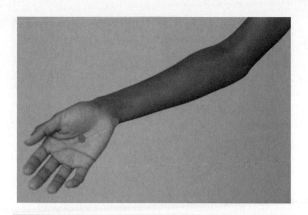

FIGURE 21-22 ■ Pericardium 8 is on the center of the palm, pericardium 6 is on the forearm, and heart 7 is on the ulnar side of the wrist. To treat fatigue and promote sleep, each point should be pressed bilaterally for a count of 10, repeating a total of 10 times.

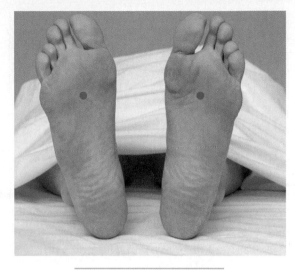

FIGURE 21-23 ■ Kidney 1.

fatigue, moodiness, and anxiety. This response is in part a result of the dramatic shift in hormone levels, the letdown that occurs after delivery, postpartum discomforts, concerns about her ability to care for her child, and concerns about how she looks.[14,28,38]

A more disabling mood disorder is postpartum depression (PPD) that affects approximately 15% to 20% of new mothers.[39] Postpartum depression has a later onset; it can occur anywhere from 1 to 2 weeks up to a year after the birth.[14] The etiology is unclear, but certain factors are suspected to contribute to the development of PPD (Box 21-5).

A woman with PPD often feels helpless, overwhelmed, anxious, and scared; has mood swings and sleep disturbances; fears losing control; is disconnected from the baby; may have suicidal thoughts; suffers from intrusive thoughts; and feels dependent on others. She may have intense feelings of guilt, shame, and worthlessness; suffer from headaches and palpitations; and show little interest food or exhibit binge eating.[14,38] Most of these symptoms persist intensely for at least a 2-week period. Puerperal depression is defined as a psychiatric illness, according to medical and psychology textbooks.[40-42]

PPD can have a tremendous effect on the family. Depressed mothers interact differently with their babies than those women who are not depressed. They often seem tense, express incompetence, and are more easily irritated. They may not pick up or hold their child as often and may not meet their child's emotional needs.[43] The babies tend to pick up on this lack of interaction and become fussier and discontented.

The partners of depressed mothers are also affected by this illness. They often report of a feeling of loss of their partner and former relationship and harbor feelings of anger, loss of control, and frustration. They may have to do more than their share of the childcare and may also suffer from depression[44] (Box 21-6).

Early recognition and treatment of PPD shortens the length of the syndrome. In most cases, doctors will recommend a combination of counseling, social support, and medication.

Postpartum psychosis affects 1 to 2 out of 1000 women, may occur more often in primiparas,[45] and is the most severe of the psychiatric disorders.[38] The onset is sudden and generally occurs within the first few days, although the mean onset is 2 to 3 weeks. The symptoms of postpartum psychosis are depression, delusions (present in 50% of women, usually of a religious nature), severe insomnia, emotional lability, hallucinations (25% of women), suicidal or infanticidal thoughts, grossly disorganized behavior, and a loss of reality.[38,46] Immediate medical and psychiatric interventions are vital.

Mood disorders are episodic, and the woman suffering from postpartum psychosis may undergo another episode of symptoms within a year or two after the birth. Antipsychotic medications, such as lithium, are the medications of choice. Women who are breastfeeding should avoid antipsychotics or lithium, but other mood stabilizers may be prescribed.[47]

Massage Techniques for Mood Disorders

The baby blues are short-lived, and women who suffer from them fare very well after a nurturing massage(s). In the case of the more serious PPD, the massage practitioner should work in tandem with a mental health professional to provide the most supportive environment for the client. It is vital that the practitioner recognizes the difference between maternal blues and the more serious PPD or postpartum psychosis. Bodyworkers can use the following massage techniques and make the following suggestions to help a client with PPD:

- Nurturing full body massage addressing muscle soreness and general tension areas.
- Spleen 3 pressed to help balance hormones (see Figure 21-18).
- Spleen 6 pressed to tone the uterus (see Figure 21-5).
- A nonjudgmental environment can provide a place for the client to feel safe when discussing her concerns or emotionally letting go.
- Clients should be urged to get out into the sunshine and take a walk, with or without the baby.
- Clients should be urged to resume exercising as soon as she feels up to it.
- Aromatherapy with jasmine, ylang ylang, rose, lavender
- Yoga
- Relaxation techniques
- Hypnotherapy

Maternal Role Adaptation

Maternal role adaptation is a behavioral process which the mother achieves comfort and readiness in her new role as mother. These three puerperal phases, taking-in, taking-hold, and letting-go, were first identified during the 1960s by Rubin to help anticipate maternal needs and appropriate interventions.[48]

During the **taking-in phase,** the new mother is still focusing on her own basic needs for fluid, food, and sleep. Although she is aware of her newborn, she appears to be passive and content with letting others make decisions for her and take care of her baby. A major task for the new mother is to accept the birth experience and integrate it into reality. The best way to do this is to discuss her labor and birth with friends, family, and her care team. This permits the mother to recognize the pregnancy is over, and her child is now separate from her.

The **taking-in phase** can last from less than a day to 2 days but may be prolonged with a C-section, especially if it was emergency surgery.

During the **taking-hold phase,** the new mother is more independent and shows concern about controlling her own bodily functions and self-care. As a result of being more comfortable with herself, she can now focus more attention on her child. During this phase, she may articulate concerns about her parenting abilities. Taking-hold lasts for a few days after the birth and is also called the *teachable, reachable, and referable moment.*

During the letting-go phase, the woman relinquishes her previous role as an independent individual and any preconceived notions of the child. There is a general acceptance of the child as he or she is, rather than how he or she was idealized. The new mother assumes her role as a parent. Mild depression may be a result of the demands placed on her. Verbalizing feelings is helpful for both parents during the letting-go phase.[14,52,53]

Healing After a Cesarean Section

C-sections are mostly safe surgical procedures. However, it is associated with higher risks of morbidity and mortality (seven times greater) than a vaginal delivery.[49] Serious intraoperative complications happen about 2% of the time and can include anesthesia accidents, hemorrhage, bowel or bladder injury, amniotic fluid embolism, or air embolism.[50] Postnatal deep vein thrombosis occurs in 1% to 2% of patients delivered surgically.[51] Special medical attention must be given to the mother who had a surgical delivery to assess pain, respiration (often affected by epidural narcotics for postoperative pain relief), gastrointestinal function, signs of edema, and urine output. Her stay in the hospital is generally 3 to 4 days, and the IV and Foley catheter remain in place for 12 to 24 hours after surgery.[14,52,53]

Possible long-term complications include C-sections for future births (over 75% of women in the United States have repeat C-sections), uterine rupture in future pregnancies, placenta previa and placenta accrete in subsequent pregnancies, ectopic pregnancies, infertility, and bowel obstruction from intraabdominal adhesions.[27]

Physical healing takes longer after this major abdominal surgery, and although the psychological responses to a scheduled Cesarean vary, a woman who undergoes an emergency C-section may experience more pronounced and negative feelings because she had no time to psychologically prepare.[54] The woman who has an emergency C-section faces the procedure tired and disheartened from a long, unproductive labor, and she may be anxious and fearful about the surgery. She may also be dehydrated with low glucose reserves, and her postpartum recovery is accompanied by fatigue and possible feelings of anger or guilt. Supportive care and patience are paramount to help these women come to terms with their labor and birth.

The sooner the client is up and walking, the faster she will heal.[55] Those initial steps, however, can be very uncomfortable. For the first few days postpartum, the women's physiological concerns may be dominated by pain at the incision site and pain from intestinal gas. Position changes, ambulation, rocking in a chair, splinting the incision with pillows, and deep breathing help relieve the pain from intestinal gas. Women are advised to cough to clear the lungs and encouraged to do deep breathing. Women who eat solid foods early are reported to require less pain medication and have fewer gastrointestinal discomforts than those who delay eating.[56]

The expressed needs of new mothers who underwent cesarean delivery were studied in 1998. The findings revealed that both the planned and unplanned surgery patients had the same three dominant needs: rest and sleep; relief of pain and discomfort; and help with child care, self care, and household chores.[57] Both groups verbalized the need for help with depression, socialization, and family closeness.[57]

Women who have C-sections lose about 1000 ml of blood as compared with 500 ml from a vaginal delivery. Women who have C-sections also experience vaginal discharge lochia and afterpains as the uterus contracts that often make the site of the incision more painful. Progressive scar massage should not begin until the wound is completely closed, which will be in about 2 to 3 weeks, although the sooner the work begins, the less likely it is for collagen fibers and restrictive scarring to develop (see Chapter 22).

Women recovering from a C-section need patience and understanding. It hurts them to lift anything over 5 lbs immediately after the surgery, so holding their child can be problematic. Milk let-down may be sabotaged from the anesthesia, which can frustrate the new mother. Using pillows to compress the incision and elevate the baby may help. Bringing the baby to her instead of to the new mother lean over and pick him or her up is thoughtful and considerate. Splinting her abdominals should wait until the incision has healed, or about 4 to 6 weeks.[51] The sooner she starts becoming active and taking care of herself and her baby, the faster she will recover.[55] The process should not be rushed, however. Supportive family and friends can make the healing much easier.

Techniques for Recovery After Cesarean Section

Practitioners should be aware of abdominal sensitivity and incision site pain when positioning postoperative clients. Pillows, clean sanitary pads, or towels can be placed against the incision for protection and support. The following list includes examples of where and how to massage safely:

- Light effleurage to reduce muscle soreness and fatigue.
- Pericardium 6, pericardium 8, heart 7, and governing vessel 20 pressed to treat fatigue (see Figure 21-22).
- **DVD** Lymphatic drainage of the legs to reduce edema (and avoid dislodging potential blood clots).
- Liver 3 pressed to encourage reduction of excess fluid (see Figure 21-11).
- **DVD** Large intestine 4 pressed to treat intestinal gas (see Figure 21-12).
- Foot reflexes of the intestines pressed to encourage peristalsis and reduce intestinal gas (see Figure 21-13).
- Light vibration can be done over the incision to initially reduce inflammation and swelling.

In addition, practitioners can make the following suggestions to help the client heal from a cesarean delivery:

- Encourage the woman to change positions and ambulate and raise her hips above her heart to eliminate intestinal gas.
- Encourage deep abdominal breathing, "huffing," and coughing.
- Suggest transcutaneous electrical nerve stimulation (TENS) to treat pain, gas, and flatulence.
- Urge the woman to recruit her transverse abdominis muscles for greater support of the core abdominal muscles when bending, lifting, getting out of bed, and standing.
- Suggest that the woman get help with daily activities and care of the child.
- Provide sympathetic listening and emotional support and referral to a mental health professional to help her understand and accept her delivery.

Postpartum recovery for women who were prescribed bed rest is commensurate with the amount of antepartum time spent inactive.[58] During bed rest, there is a reduction in cardiac stroke volume, output, and oxygen uptake, although bed rest alone does not appear to contribute to cardiac dysfunction. Muscle fatigue and stiffness is associated with reduced muscle blood flow, red cell volume, capillarization, and oxidative enzymes. Inactivity creates a loss of muscle mass, muscle strength, and bone density with a higher risk for injury to bones and joints. Cardiovascular and musculoskeletal deconditioning is associated with prolonged bed rest.[59,60] In addition, gastrointestinal function slows down, often resulting in constipation or sluggish bowel.

In addition to the physiological changes of bed rest, many pregnant women confined to bed report feelings of depression, anxiety, decreased self-esteem, body image problems, isolation, and disconnected.[60] Prolonged bed rest can also affect mental acuity, resulting in longer periods of time for verbal recall, verbal fluency, and concentration.

By 6 weeks postpartum, 40% of women screened reported that they were still experiencing fatigue, mood swings, and general tension; had difficulty concentrating; and suffered from back muscle soreness, headaches, and dry skin. Those women who had C-sections complained of significantly more symptoms than those who had vaginal deliveries. Although many of the symptoms decreased over time, there appears to be an underlying morbidity that goes beyond the 6-week puerperium recovery period.[61]

The rehabilitation after bed rest and childbirth can be particularly hard for some women, especially if there are older children to care for. Common short-term problems include difficulty walking and balancing, fatigue, dizziness, and depression. The recovery period is understandably longer. Women need to slowly increase their level of stimulation and activity to avoid overexertion.[62]

The massage should be light to avoid further exhausting the woman, and the amount of time spent with her during immediate recovery should be limited to less than 1 hour. Care must be taken to avoid all leg massage until she has become ambulatory. Massages can become gradually deeper as the woman's strength returns. Swedish pétrissage strokes can be incorporated to increase muscle tone, and passive then active resistant exercises can be introduced to restore muscle strength and function (Box 21-7).

Miscarriages or Stillbirths

Not every pregnancy results in a live birth. Whether the mother chooses to terminate her pregnancy, suffers a miscarriage, or has a stillborn, she still has to go through physical, emotional, and psychological healing. Perinatal loss can be emotionally devastating for the expectant couple. Almost 20% of known pregnancies end in miscarriage before 20 weeks and about 7 out of 1000 pregnancies from 20 weeks to term are lost. In addition, 5 out of 1000 babies die within the first 28 weeks of birth.[63]

The loss during early pregnancy is equally emotionally and psychologically significant as a loss in later pregnancy. Although a woman's physical adaptations may not be as exaggerated or pronounced as a later pregnancy, the loss of her hopes and dreams for a child is real and tangible. Women who miscarry or terminate their pregnancies in the first trimester are

---

BOX 21-7 | *Techniques for Postpartum Care of Women Confined to Bed Rest*

During immediate postpartum, it is advisable to limit massage to less than 1 hour and avoid massaging the woman's legs until after she has been up and about for a few days. At that point, the leg massage follows manual lymphatic protocol as follows:

- Light Swedish massage progressively using deeper strokes as she strengthens.
- Gentle myofascial stretching of her back to reduce muscle tension and fatigue.
- Pétrissage of her muscles to increase tone.
- Lymphatic drainage on her legs after she is ambulatory for a few days.
- Pericardium 6, pericardium 8, heart 7, and governing vessel 20 can be pressed to treat fatigue.
- Energy work to treat fatigue.
- Light abdominal massage to encourage peristalsis.
- Large intestine 4 pressed and intestinal foot reflexes massaged to encourage peristalsis.
- Passive exercises progressing to active resistant exercises to increase muscle tone and strength.

---

often overlooked and neglected, but these women need to feel acknowledged for their loss.[64]

Research on the mental health impact of miscarriage or stillbirth recognizes the increase in depressive symptoms in early weeks that can extend to several months.[65] Women may also blame themselves for having or not having done something to cause the miscarriage or stillbirth. Grieving can also occur when the labor or birth outcome was unexpected. A baby born with a medical condition or genetic defect can be devastating for his or her parents and family.

The loss of a pregnancy or a baby normally follows a bereavement sequence, although many phases may overlap or pass and then return. The initial phase is one of shock that includes feelings of numbness and denial. These are protective reactions to any trauma or tragedy. This phase is followed by acute grief as the reality of the loss sinks in. Physical and emotional despair may manifest as uncontrollable crying or with difficulties getting through the day. Acute grief cedes to grief work with feelings of blame, anger, and yearning.

Eventually, parents can accept or integrate the loss into their lives and although their lives have been changed, they can feel hopeful once again.

The best way to help a bereaved parent is to acknowledge the loss and the need to grieve. Practitioners may refer clients to a grief counselor to help them through the healing process. One of the best gifts a bodyworker can provide is to offer a safe haven where grieving woman can express her emotions.

Summary

Within the first few hours and days of childbirth, a woman goes through enormous physiological, emotional, and psychological changes. These dramatic changes occur in every system of her body and are mediated by major hormonal shifting.

Her uterus hardens at the site of the placental attachment to prevent hemorrhage and cleanses itself through the vaginal discharge lochia. Her muscles are stiff and sore and her abdominal wall is separated along the linea alba, thereby creating lumbar instability. She voids tremendous amounts of urine and endures night sweats that rid her body of excess fluid.

There is trauma in the pelvic floor, and her breasts are tender as they prepare for lactation. Emotionally there may be an immediate euphoria that gives way to fatigue and even a sense of loss.

More traumatic recoveries are experienced by women who had medicated labors, C-sections, or whose birth outcome was unexpected. Women who suffer loss are especially vulnerable to emotional and psychological duress in addition to the physical changes from which they must recover.

During this initial phase of recovery, the practitioner should employ techniques that encourage cleansing and elimination, address fatigue, treat muscle stiffness and soreness, enhance hormone balancing, and support the woman emotionally. Many reflexive techniques are helpful during early recovery to reach the deeper organs and muscles that cannot be palpated by hand.

If women are presented with realistic expectations of the immediate postpartum period and if they are taught that this process is initially extreme but short-lived, then they will be better prepared. These temporary discomforts indicate that they are healing and should be viewed as part of the normal recovery process.

References

1. Coad J: *Anatomy and physiology for midwives*, St. Louis, 2001, Mosby.
2. Maternity Center Association: *Listening to mothers: report of the first national U.S. survey of women's childbearing experiences*, New York, 2002, The Association.
3. Garcia J, Renfrew M, Marchant S: Postnatal home visiting by midwives, *Midwifery* 10(1):40-43, 1994.
4. Marsh J, Sargent E: Factors effecting the duration of postnatal visits, *Midwifery* 7:177-182, 1991.
5. Murphy-Black T: *Postnatal care at home: a descriptive study of mother's needs and the maternity services*, Edinburgh, 1989, University of Edinburgh.
6. van Teijlingen ER: The profession of maternity home care assistant and its significance for the Dutch midwifery profession, *Int J Nurs Stud* 27(4):355-366, 1990.
7. Kitzinger S: *Ourselves as mothers: the universal experience of motherhood*, New York, 1994, Addison-Wesley.
8. Ball J: *Reactions to motherhood*, ed 2, Cheshire, UK, 1994, Books For Midwives Press.
9. Hytten F: *The clinical physiology of the puerperium*, London, 1995, Farland Press.
10. Alexander J, Garcia J, Marchant S: The BLiPP study—final report for the South and West Research and Development Committee, IHCS, Dorset, UK, 1997, Bournemouth University.
11. Glazener C, Abdalla M, Stroud P, et al: Postnatal maternal morbidity: extent, causes, prevention and treatment, *Br J Obstet Gynaecol* 102(4):282-287, 1995.
12. Macarthur A, Lewis M, Knox G: Health after childbirth: an investigation of long term health problems beginning after childbirth in 11,701 women, London, 1991, HMSO.
13. Rome R: Secondary postpartum haemorrhage, *Br J Obstet Gynaecol* 82:289-292, 1975.

14. McKinney ES, James SR, Murray SS, et al: *Maternal-child nursing*, ed 2, St. Louis, 2005, Mosby.

15. Howie PW: The physiology of the puerperium and lactation. In Chamberlain G, ed: *Turnbull's obstetrics*, ed 2, New York, 1995, Churchill Livingstone.

16. Leifer G: *Maternity nursing: an introductory text*, ed 9, St. Louis, 2005, Saunders.

17. Creasy R, Resnick R, eds: *Maternal-fetal medicine*, ed 4, Philadelphia, 1999, Saunders.

18. Gabbe S, Niebyl J, Simpson J: *Obstetrics: normal and problem pregnancies*, ed 4, New York, 2002, Churchill Livingstone.

19. Kistner WR: Physiology of the vagina. In Haven ESE, Evans TN, eds: *The human vagina*, Amsterdam, 1978, North Holland.

20. Blackburn ST: *Maternal, fetal and neonatal physiology*, ed 2, Philadelphia, 2003, Saunders.

21. Peschers UM, Schaer GN, DeLancey JO, et al: Levator ani function before and after childbirth, *Br J Obstet Gynaecol* 104: 1004-1008, 1997.

22. Fraser D, Cooper M: *Myles' textbook for midwives*, ed 14, Edinburgh, 2003, Churchill Livingstone.

23. Robson SC, Dunlop W, Hunter S: Haemodynamic changes during the early puerperium, *BMJ* 294:106, 1987.

24. Gilson GJ, Samaan S, Crawford MH, et al: Changes in the hemodynamics, ventricular remodeling, and ventricular contractility during normal pregnancy: A longitudinal study, *Obstet Gynecol* 89: 957-962, 1997.

25. Capeless EL, Clapp JF: When do cardiovascular parameters return to their preconception values? *Am J Obstet Gynecol* 165: 883-886, 1991.

26. Pritchard JA: Changes in blood volume during pregnancy and delivery, *Anesthesiology* 26:393, 1965.

27. Ueland K: Maternal cardiac dynamics. VII. Intrapartum blood volume changes, *Am J Obstet Gynecol* 126:671-677, 1976.

28. Cunningham FG, Gant NF, Leveno KJ, et al: *Williams obstetrics*, ed 21, New York, 2001, McGraw Hill.

29. Jeffries J, Bochner F: Thromboembolism and its management in pregnancy, *Med J Austral* 155:253-258, 1991.

30. Reyes FI, Winter JSD, Faiman C: Postpartum disappearance of human chorionic gonadotrophin from the maternal and neonatal circulations, *Am J Obstet Gynecol* 153:486-489, 1985.

31. Scoggin J: Physical and psychological changes. In Mattson S, Smith JE, eds: *Core curriculum for maternal-newborn nursing*, ed 2, Philadelphia, 2000, Saunders.

32. La Leche League International: *The womanly art of breastfeeding*, ed 3, New York, 1981, New American Library.

33. Ohlin A, Rossner S: Trends in eating patterns, physical activity and sociodemographic factors in relation to postpartum body weight development, *Br J Nutr* 71: 457-470, 1994.

34. Swain AM, O'Hara M, Starr KR, et al: A prospective study of sleep, mood and cognitive function in postpartum and non-postpartum women, *Obstet Gynecol* 90: 381-386, 1997.

35. Quillan SL: Infant and mother sleep patterns during the 4th postpartum week, *Issues Comp Ped Nurs* 20:115-123, 1997.

36. American Academy of Pediatrics and American College of Obstetricians and Gynecologists: *Guidelines for perinatal care*, ed 5, Elk Grove Village, IL, 2002, AAP and ACOG.

37. Kumar R: Pregnancy, childbirth and mental illness, *Prog Obstet Gynaecol* 5:146-149, 1985.

38. *What are the postpartum psychiatric disorders?* Belle Mead, NJ, 1996, Depression After Delivery, Inc.

39. Hyash RH, Zettelmaier MA: Postpartum management. In Ransom SB, Dombrowski MP, McNeeley SG, et al, eds: *Practical strategies in obstetrics and gynecology*, Philadelphia, 2000, Saunders.

40. Kaij L, Nilsson A: Emotional psychotic illness following childbirth. In Howell SJ, ed: *Modern perspectives in psycho-obstetrics*, London, 1972, Oliver & Boyd.

41. Dalton K: *Depression after childbirth*, Oxford, 1980, Oxford University Press.

42. Cox JL: *Postnatal depression: a guide for health professionals*, Edinburgh, 1986, Churchill Livingstone.

43. Beck CT: The effects of postpartum depression on maternal-infant interaction: a meta-analysis, *Nurs Res* 44(5):298-304, 1995.

44. Meighan M, Davis MW, Thomas SP, et al: Living with postpartum depression: the father's experience, *MCN: Am J Matern Child Nurs* 24(4):202-208, 1999.

45. Kaplan H, Sadock B: *Synopsis of psychiatry*, ed 8, Baltimore, 2000, Williams & Wilkins.

46. American Psychiatric Association: *Diagnostic and statistical manual of mental disorders*, ed 4 revised, Washington, DC, 2000, The Association.

47. Stowe J: Psychopharmacology during pregnancy and lactation. In Schartzberg A, Nemeroff C, eds: *Essentials of clinical psychopharmacology*, Washington, DC, 2001, American Psychiatric Association.

48. Rubin R: Puerperal change, *Nurs Outl* 9(12):743-755, 1961.

49. Lilford RJ, van Coeverden de Groot HA, Moore PJ, et al: The relative risks of caesarean section (intrapartum and elective) and vaginal delivery: a detailed analysis to exclude the effects of medical disorders and other acute pre-existing physiological disturbance, *Br J Obstet Gynaecol* 97:883, 1990.

50. Neilsen TF, Hokengard KH: Cesarean section and intraoperative surgical complications, *Acta Obstet Gynecol Scand* 63:103-107, 1984.

51. Bergqvist A, Bergqvist D, Hallbooki T: Acute deep vein thrombosis (DVT) after cesarean section, *Acta Obstet Gynecol Scand* 58:473-477, 1979.

52. Pyle M: *Birth by cesarean and preventing unnecessary cesareans*, Costa Mesa, CA, 1994, Lifecircle.

53. Curtin S, Kozak L: Decline in US cesarean delivery rate appears to stall, *Birth* 25(4): 259-262, 1998.

54. DiMatteo M, Morton SC, Lepper HS, et al: Cesarean childbirth and psychosocial outcomes: A meta-analysis, *Health Psychol* 15(4):303-314, 1996.

55. Tupler J: *Lose your mummy tummy*, Cambridge, MA, 2005, Perseus.

56. Burrows W, Ginjo AJ, Jr. Rose SM, et al: Safety and efficacy of early postoperative solid food consumption after cesarean section, *J Reprod Med* 40(6):463-467, 1995.

57. Eakes M, Brown H: Home alone: meeting the needs of mothers after cesarean birth, *AWHONN Lifelines* 2(1):36-40, 1998.

58. Maloni JA, Chance B, Zhang C, et al: Physical and psychosocial side effects of antepartum hospital bed rest, *Nurs Res* 42(4): 197-203, 1993.

59. Convertino VA, Bloomfield SA, Greenleaf JE: Physiological effects of bed rest and restricted physical activity, *Med Sci Sports Exer* 29(2):187-190, 1997.

60. Isidro-Cloudas T: How to cope with pregnancy bed rest, Americanbaby.com. Available at http://www.americanbaby.com/ab/ story.jhtml?storyid=/templatedata/ab/story/ data/2099.xml. Accessed November, 2002.

61. Maloni JA, Park S: Postpartum symptoms after antepartum bed rest, *J Obstet Gynecol Neonatal Nurs* 34:163-171, 2005.

62. Maloni JA: *Postpartum rehabilitation*, Cleveland, 2004, Francis Payne Bolton School of Nursing, Case Western Reserve University.

63. National Share Office: *Pregnancy and infant loss support*, St. Charles, MO, 1997, National Share Office.

64. Luby E: Bereavement and grieving. In Schiff HS, ed: *The bereaved parent*, New York, 1977, Penguin Books.

65. Cordle CJ, Prettyman RJ: A 2-year follow-up of women who have experienced early miscarriage, *J Reprod Infant Psychol* 12: 37-43, 1994.

REVIEW QUESTIONS

1 What is puerperium?

_____

_____

_____

_____

_____

2 How can massage practitioners comfortably position their early postpartum clients on the massage table?

_____

_____

_____

_____

3 Describe the changes to the reproductive system in early postpartum—within the first few hours and days of the birth.

_____

_____

_____

_____

4 What is uterine involution? Describe the massage process that encourages uterine involution.

_____

_____

_____

_____

5 On average, how long does it take a postpartum woman to regain the strength and muscle tone in her pelvic floor muscles after a vaginal birth?

_____

_____

_____

_____

6 What massage techniques can body workers employ to facilitate healing of the reproductive system for a woman immediately after childbirth?

_____

_____

_____

_____

7 What are the changes to the new mother's musculoskeletal system immediately after birth?

_____

_____

_____

_____

8 What is the treatment for hip displacement or symphysis pubis separation? What is coccydynia and what is the treatment for it?

_____

_____

_____

_____

9 Right after birth, describe how the abdominal muscles feel. Where are the trigger points of the abdomen located?

_____

_____

_____

_____

10 Describe the massage techniques used to treat the musculoskeletal needs of a new mother.

_____

_____

_____

_____

11 How is the new mother's cardiovascular system changing? How long does testing continue for the presence of blood clots or pitting edema?

_____

_____

_____

_____

12 What changes are occurring to the gastrointestinal and urinary systems of a new mother?

_____

_____

_____

_____

_____

13 What is diuresis?

_____

_____

_____

_____

14 Explain the immediate postpartum changes to the new mother's skin and nervous systems? How can a massage help support these healing changes?

_____

_____

_____

_____

15 What changes occur in the woman's endocrine system after childbirth?

_____

_____

_____

_____

16 How does her body degrade and eliminate the excess interstitial fluid she accumulated during her pregnancy? What other techniques and acupuncture points can be stimulated to encourage the endocrine system to stabilize?

_____

_____

_____

_____

17 What are the benefits of breastfeeding to mother and newborn?

_____

_____

_____

_____

18 Describe the new mother's vital signs immediately after the birth.

_____

_____

_____

_____

19 How does her respiratory system adapt after childbirth?

_____

_____

_____

_____

20 What are some of the emotional and psychological changes that some women experience after childbirth?

_____

_____

_____

_____

21 Compare and contrast postpartum blues, postpartum depression, and postpartum psychosis. What massage techniques can work to treat mood disorders?

_____

_____

_____

_____

22 Describe the symptoms of postpartum depression in new fathers.

_____

_____

_____

_____

23 Explain what is meant by maternal role adaptation.

_____

_____

_____

_____

24 Describe the typical healing process after a C-section and the massage techniques that can help speed recovery.

_____

_____

_____

_____

25 What additional considerations are there for the new mother who was confined to bed during some of her pregnancy? What techniques can practitioners offer such a woman?

_____

_____

_____

_____

26 Explain the considerable reactions to a pregnancy loss, stillbirth, or neonatal death. How can massage practitioners help their clients deal with this tremendous loss?

_____

_____

_____

_____

_____

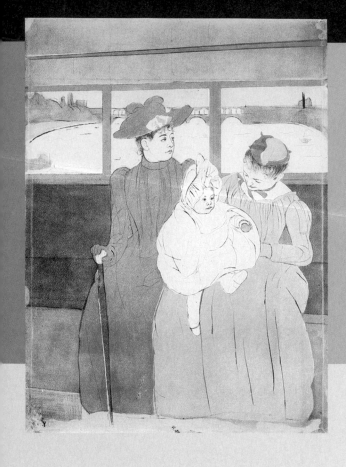

Puerperium Postpartum Physiology and Treatment Goals

Objectives

On completion of this chapter, the student will be able to do the following:

1 Understand the physiological process that occurs within the first 6 weeks of postpartum recovery

2 Understand the treatment goals of the 6-week puerperium recovery period

3 Use appropriate massage techniques to achieve these goals

4 Incorporate appropriate scar massage technique

5 Recognize the symptoms of postpartum depression

6 Recognize the emotional support needed for those mothers whose newborns remain in the hospital after the mothers are discharged

7 Understand the process of family adjustment

Key Terms

Dyspareunia
Engrossment

Latching-on
Premature infants

Scar massage

During the first 6 weeks of recovery, new mothers in the United States are generally expected to heal from the birth and adjust to motherhood before returning to work and normal activities. This traditional puerperium recovery period has its origins in a medieval ritual and ceremony (see Chapter 21) and is generally accepted to be the length of time it takes for the uterus to return to its prepregnant size, shape, position, and tone (involution) (Boxes 22-1 and 22-2).

Physiological changes in the Woman During the Puerperium

Many metabolic and physiological changes of the puerperium overlap and continue well past the 6-week mark, some as long as a year after childbirth, so it is an unfair deadline to expect the new mother to be fully recovered. It is important to explain this to the postpartum client so she can be patient with her recovery and not be so hard on herself about how long it takes to get back into her prepregnant shape and condition.

Reproductive System
The Uterus

After only 1 week postpartum, the uterus has involuted by 50% and weighs 500 gm (1.1 lbs) After 2 weeks postpartum, the uterus weighs 340 gm (12 oz) and cannot be palpated on abdominal examination.[1-3] This decrease in size can be affected by parity, the size of the newborn, and a multiple pregnancy.

The endometrium is completely healed and regenerated within 16 days; the placental site takes a full 6 to 7 weeks before completely healing.[4]

BOX 22-1 *The Trees of Children*

In early civilizations, trees were considered the children who grew between Mother Earth and Father Sky. All over the world, people plant trees to honor and celebrate the birth of a child. In Germany, fruit and nut trees are planted as a symbol of the fruit of the womb. (The German word for fruit is "obst," the etymological origin of "obstetrics.") In Nigeria, each banana tree is named after the child for whom it was planted. Ash trees signify long life, fig trees for wisdom, olive trees for peace, and maple trees for good luck.

From Jackson D: *With child: wisdom and traditions for pregnancy, birth and motherhood,* San Francisco, 1999, Chronicle Books.

BOX 22-2 *Butterflies*

According to English folklore, butterflies were symbolic of the souls of babies who were not yet named.

From Jackson D: *With child: wisdom and traditions for pregnancy, birth and motherhood,* San Francisco, 1999, Chronicle Books.

Cervix

The cervix never returns to its original condition and always shows evidence of birth by a change in appearance. After a birth, instead of returning to its prepregnancy round appearance, the cervix remains slitlike.

Vagina

Within 3 weeks postpartum, the edema of the vagina has decreased, and the rugae or vaginal folds reappear. It takes anywhere from 6 to 10 weeks for complete vaginal involution, and the vagina never fully regains its prepregnant size.[2,3,5]

Vaginal dryness may plague nursing women because estrogen levels are suppressed during lactation. Painful intercourse, or **dyspareunia**, may result. Vaginal lubricants can restore moisture and make intercourse more enjoyable.

Lochia serosa can continue for as long as 27 days and lochia alba for as long as 6 weeks.

Perineum

Healing from an episiotomy can take up to 4 to 6 months to completely heal.[6] It takes about 2 months for full recovery of strength and muscular tone of the pelvic floor muscles.[7] Postnatal perineal pain can have a negative impact on a new mother's functioning and early experience of motherhood.[8] After a spontaneous vaginal birth, 10 of 1000 women surveyed experienced pain for more than 2 months and the numbers increased to 30% with an instrumental vaginal delivery. Other studies showed pain and dyspareunia more than 1 year after childbirth.[10-12]

Menstrual Cycle

The return of the menstrual cycle can begin as early as 1 to 2 months postpartum for a nonnursing mother.[12] Hormone patterns in the postpartum period indicate low levels of gonadotrophins and sex steroids by elevated concentrations of prolactin. Therefore the return to ovulation and menstruation depends on whether and for how long lactation and nursing continue.[13] The mean average return of menses for nonnursing mothers is 10 weeks postpartum and 17 weeks for lactating women, although vaginal bleeding in breastfeeding women in the first 8 weeks does not represent a return to ovarian function.[14,15] The first menses is usually anovulatory, but subsequent periods are ovulatory.

Bodyworkers can use the following massage techniques to facilitate healing of the reproductive system at 6 weeks postpartum:

- Spleen 10 pressed to encourage functional bleeding and lochia discharge **DVD** (Figure 22-1).
- Spleen 6 pressed to help tone the uterus (Figure 22-2).
- **DVD** Uterine reflexes pressed on the feet to tone the uterus (Figure 22-3).
- Governing vessel 20 pressed (Figure 22-4)
- **DVD** Lymphatic drainage on the legs.

Bodyworkers can make the following suggestions to help heal the reproductive system at 6 weeks postpartum:

- Kegel exercises to restore functional integrity to the pelvic floor, control any remaining incontinence, and treat hemorrhoids.

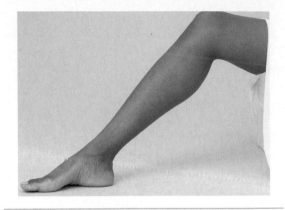

FIGURE 22-1 ■ Spleen 10 can be pressed to encourage functional bleeding and lochia discharge.

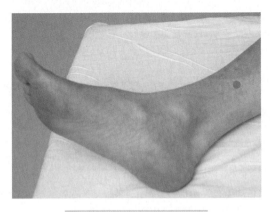

FIGURE 22-2 ■ Spleen 6.

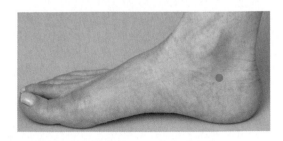

FIGURE 22-3 ■ Uterine reflex.

- 15 drops of geranium oil and 5 drops of cypress oil diluted in 2 tablespoons of oil placed topically on hemorrhoids.
- Tucks, witch hazel, calendula, lemon to treat hemorrhoids, if necessary.

Musculoskeletal System

During the first 6 weeks, there is a tremendous shift in the woman's center of gravity as her former pregnant posture starts to normalize. The diastasis

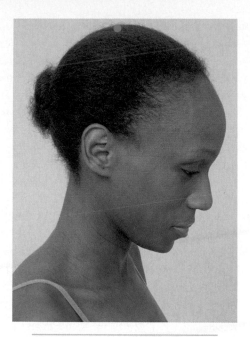

<FIGURE>FIGURE 22-4 ■ Governing vessel 20.</FIGURE>

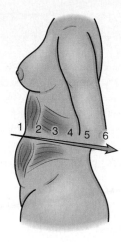

FIGURE 22-5 ■ The transverse abdominis drawn in can help heal the diastasis recti.

recti must be corrected with proper abdominal exercises that recruit the transverse abdominis muscle to prevent continued lumbar and pelvic instability. The following postpartum exercises can help heal the diastasis recti:

Seated Tupler Technique: Elevators

1. The client sits in a chair or cross-legged on the floor with her back against the wall and her shoulders aligned with her hips. When the client's abdomen is relaxed, the "elevator" is at the "first floor" and when her abdomen is squeezed all the way to her spine, it is at the "fifth floor."
2. The client then places both hands on her stomach and inhales deeply.
3. As she exhales, she brings her belly back toward her spine, or fifth floor.
4. As she holds that position, she counts to 30 out loud while breathing and holding the transverse at the spine.
5. She can try to bring the abdominals back even further to the "sixth floor" and repeat the same exercise to a count of 5.
6. She ends each elevator exercise with a deep breath.
7. Clients can perform 10 sets of these daily.

Transverse Contractions

1. The client sits in a chair or cross-legged on the floor with her back against the wall and her shoulders aligned with her hips. She places one hand below her navel and the other hand under her ribs.
2. Inhale and bring the abdominals to the "third floor" (halfway between first and fifth floors). This is the starting position.
3. While counting out loud (and breathing), she contracts her transverse back to the fifth floor. This is one repetition.
4. She returns to the third floor and squeezes back again to the fifth floor while counting out loud and breathing.
5. The client works up to 100 repetitions 5 times per day (Figure 22-5).[16]

Additional Techniques and Suggestions

Muscle balancing techniques on the extrinsic muscles can be introduced, although some women are unable to tolerate the deep work of intrinsic muscle release. This must be determined by the client because intrinsic muscle release might feel too invasive for some women during early recovery.

Relaxation and hypermobility of the joints are stabilized between weeks 8 to 10. Although her pelvis and other joints return to their prepregnant state, the joints of her feet do not and some

Touch Points

I tell my clients that the postpartum massage is going to be the best massage they have ever received. After pregnancy, labor, and childbirth, their bodies need the appropriate touch of a qualified massage practitioner. This work can speed up the recovery process and address any remaining issues from pregnancy and childbirth. It is also a wonderful time to honor these new mothers and provide them with the nurturing support and admiration they deserve.

women have a permanent increase in shoe size.[17] During this period of adjustment, while the effects of relaxin can still cause subluxations and instability, it is important to remind the client to use proper body mechanic while nursing, lifting, changing, carrying the baby, or performing any other childcare or household activities. In early recovery, splinting her abdomen will remind her to use her abdominals correctly and protect her lower back. In addition, carrying her child in an anterior baby carrier reintroduces the maladaptive posture of pregnancy. It is suggested that the newborn be carried in a sling across her body if she wants to keep the baby physically close.

Nursing postures, the weight of her breasts, and wearing an anterior baby carrier create additional tension in her cervical and thoracic spine. Recruiting the transverse abdominis muscle while nursing can help remedy these problems. Care must also be taken with hand positioning to avoid carpal tunnel syndrome or de Quervain's syndrome.

Trigger points are omnipresent in weakened muscles, particularly those of the hips, pelvis, lower back, and abdominals. In early recovery, practitioners must take care to avoid being too invasive with the depth of their massage pressure. A gentle vibration along with a lighter pressure can be effective and respectful of her physical and emotional needs. Some techniques that bodyworkers can use to facilitate healing of the musculoskeletal system at 6 weeks postpartum are the following:

- Swedish massage to address muscle soreness and fatigue. The area near injection sites may still be bruised or sensitive to touch, so care should be taken around those areas.
- Manual lymphatic drainage on the legs to reduce muscle aches and reduce swelling.

- Myofascial release to decompress the lumbar spine and relieve any muscle tightness.
- Trigger point release along the sacroiliac and lumbosacral joints, hips, pelvis, and abdomen.
- Hip compression with fists behind the anterior superior iliac spines (ASIS) to restore placement of hips.
- Pelvic tilt to decompress lumbar spine.
- Appropriate abdominal exercises that recruit the transverse abdominis to heal the diastasis recti.
- Treatment for carpal tunnel syndrome if necessary.
- For any residual discomfort from symphysis pubis separation or hip displacement, strengthen and stabilize muscles from L1 to the greater trochanter and iliopsoas. Hip or pelvic traction should be avoided.
- Extrinsic muscle balancing techniques to help restore function and strength to postural muscles. Techniques may include myofascial release, trigger point release, and proprioceptive work, such as neuromuscular spindle cell release (Figure 22-6) and Golgi tendon organ release (Figure 22-7).

Integumentary System
Cesarean Scar Massage

Cesarean **scar massage** is a technique to reduce scar tissue and improve skin elasticity. It is a progressive treatment, and if too much force is applied too quickly, the colloid gel within the connective tissue responds with increased resistance. Conversely, if not enough force is used, the pressure will not be sufficient to effect change.[18] During the first few weeks of recovery, a gentle vibration over the bandage is adequate enough to reduce some of the lymphatic congestion within the surrounding tissue and ease some of the discomfort the new mother is feeling. It also can help her recognize any emotions this surgery may have elicited.

Any incision causes trauma and edema to the surrounding tissues with accompanying emotional issues. A cesarean incision, in particular, can harbor a wide range of emotions because of its location on the vulnerable anterior of the body, its reproductive relationship (especially if it was an

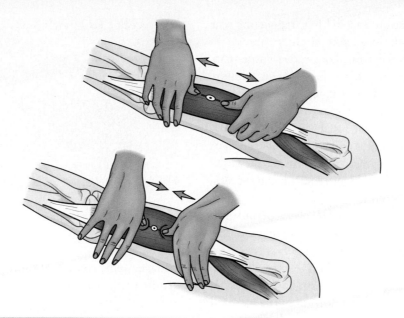

FIGURE 22-6 ■ *Top*, Digital pressure to strengthen a weak muscle from neuromuscular spindle cell malfunction. *Bottom*, Digital pressure at the ends of the neuromuscular spindle cell to weaken a hypertonic muscle.

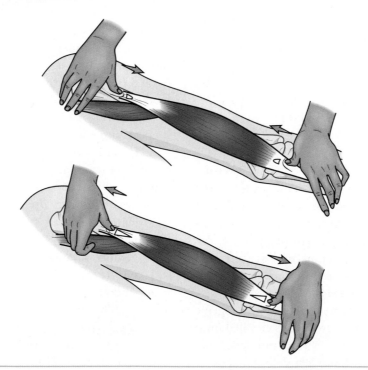

FIGURE 22-7 ■ *Top*, Direction of pressure of the Golgi tendon organs to strengthen a muscle. *Bottom*, Direction of pressure to weaken a hypertonic muscle with Golgi tendon organ technique.

emergency procedure), and its link to a woman's image of herself as a woman and a mother. With that in mind, the practitioner must proceed respectfully and at the client's pace when massaging the scar (see Chapter 23).

The goals in scar massage are to manage the development of scar tissue and keep the connective tissue as pliable and flexible as possible by reducing adhesions between the soft tissue layers. In addition, scar massage can render the scar stable, reduce discoloration and itching, reduce the scar to the normal skin level, and eliminate fibrosis.[19]

Scars are formed from connective tissue, particularly collagenous fibers, that provides support but little elasticity. When the repair reaction is excessive, the end result is a keloid scar. Keloid scars are dimensional, raised, often irregularly shaped, and contain more water and soluble collagen than normal scars.[19] The practitioner must avoid working directly on top of a keloid scar but can successfully work all around it.

During the first 6 week recovery period and with the client's permission, the light vibration can be continued as an introductory stroke and followed with lymphatic drainage. The drainage should be directed to the closest lymph nodes, so the edema from the upper portion of the scar will be directed to lymph nodes in the abdomen and the lower segment of the scar will be directed to the right or left inguinal lymph nodes. The pressure should be kept very light.

The practitioner uses very little lubrication and employs gentle myofascial stretching above and below the scar, both horizontally and vertically, pulling the tissue in opposite direction with the thumbs. Deeper scar massage can be performed when the client feels physically and emotionally ready.

Cardiovascular System

Two weeks after the birth, there is a 30% decrease in cardiac output as a result of decreased blood volume; however, the enhanced ability of the myocardium to contract does not return to its prepregnant state until 6 weeks postpartum.[20,21] Stroke volume, cardiac output, end-diastolic volume, and systemic vascular resistance remain elevated up to 1 year postpartum.[22]

Practitioners must remember that fibrinogenic activity, or the clotting factor, stays elevated until 8 to 10 weeks postpartum.[23] New mothers, especially those who had a surgical delivery, are at a higher risk for thrombophlebitis. Women with varicose veins or a history of venous obstruction should also be carefully monitored for evidence of a blood clot. The practitioner should continue the pretreatment evaluation for the presence of blood clots, especially on the calves (Homan check), for up to 10 weeks postpartum. Deep leg massage is not advised during this time. Lymphatic

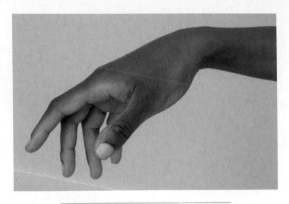

FIGURE 22-8 ■ Large intestine 4.

drainage can be continued through 10 weeks postpartum.

Gastrointestinal System

Constipation and gas may still be a problem during early puerperium for those who had a cesarean section (C-section). The sooner the surgical patient resumes normal activities, the sooner normal bowel patterns will be reestablished. Women should drink at least 8 to 12 glasses of water daily to help treat the dehydration of labor, and eating food rich in natural digestive enzymes can get the bowel functioning again. Exercise and ambulation can also encourage peristalsis. The client can also elevate her feet on a step stool when sitting on the toilet to place her lower colon in postural alignment.

Bodyworkers can use the following massage techniques to facilitate healing of the gastrointestinal system:

- Kenbiki on lower back and abdomen to encourage peristalsis.
- Abdominal massage to encourage peristalsis. **DVD** (Care should be taken to avoid a new cesarean incision.)
- Large intestine 4 pressed to treat constipation (Figure 22-8).
- Massage the intestinal reflexes on the feet and rub the tensor fascia lata that refers to the intestines (Figure 22-9).

Neurological System

In general, about one-third of postpartum women are affected by headaches within the first week after childbirth. They are usually mild and bifrontal

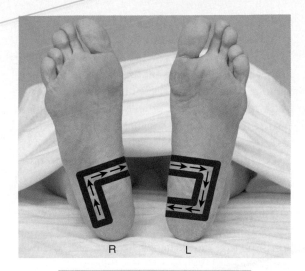

FIGURE 22-9 ■ Intestinal foot reflexes.

From Jackson D: *With child: wisdom and traditions for pregnancy, birth and motherhood*, San Francisco, 1999, Chronicle Books; Coad J: *Anatomy and physiology for midwives*, St. Louis, 2001, Mosby; Wharton BA, Balmer SE, Scott PH: *Adv Exper Med Biol* 357:91-98, 1994.

BOX 22-3 *Colostrum*

During the first 3 days, the mother produces from 2 to 10 ml of colostrum daily. If she has nursed before, she is more likely to produce more colostrum sooner. In some cultures, such as Bangladesh, Breton people of France, Japan and some southern African tribes, colostrum is thought to be old or bad milk and is not fed to infants.

Colostrum is transparent and yellow because it has high levels of beta-carotene. It contains more protein and vitamins A and K and less sugar and fat than the mother's milk that comes in later. Colostrum is easy to digest, is well absorbed, and is believed to facilitate the colonization of the intestines with lactobacillus bifidus. It also has a laxative effect, enabling the easy passage of meconium. Colostrum also contains an abundant number of antibodies to protect against infection.

Within the first 30 hours, there is a high protein to lactose ratio. During the following days, suckling stimulates production of the major whey protein and alpha-lactalbumin.

---

and respond well to simple analgesics or stress-reducing techniques. Headaches that persist should be carefully evaluated by a medical professional. Postpartum headaches can be brought on by many serious complications, including postpartum-onset preeclampsia, stress, and the leakage of cerebral spinal fluid into the extradural space from poorly administered epidural or spinal anesthesia.[17,24] Some of the women who suffer from migraines as a result of cerebral spinal fluid leakage can be plagued by them for many years.

Endocrine System

During puerperium, menstruation will return to nonlactating mothers about 7 to 9 weeks, although this varies according to each woman.[25] If the woman is breastfeeding, she may resume her cycle as early as 12 weeks or as late as 18 months.[25]

After birth, there is a dramatic reduction in all of the hormones that stimulated breasts development during pregnancy: estrogen, progesterone, human chorionic gonadotrophin (hCG), prolactin, cortisol, and insulin. The time it takes for these hormones to reach prepregnant levels is determined in part by whether the new mother nurses.[17]

The breasts of nonlactating mothers will feel nodular, and a yellowish fluid called *colostrum* will be expressed the first few days after birth (Box 22-3). The woman may experience tenderness the second and third day as milk production spontaneously begins and engorgement between days 3 and 4 as her breasts become distended, firm, tender, and warm. This distension is usually caused by the temporary congestion within the veins rather than from an accumulation of milk. Her milk should not be expressed, and the engorgement will resolve on its own within 24 to 36 hours. Ice packs can be used to relieve discomfort. If suckling was never begun or is discontinued, lactation will stop within a few days to a week.[17]

As lactation begins, women who choose to breastfeed will feel a mass in the breast tissue. This mass is usually a milk sac that changes position from day to day. Before lactation, her breasts are soft and colostrum can be expressed from her nipples.

Once lactation has begun, her breasts feel warm and firm and she may have slight tenderness for the first 48 hours after lactation has been established. True milk, a bluish-white milk (similar to skim milk) can be expressed from the nipples.

Feeding within the first 2 hours after birth increases the duration of breastfeeding when compared to a delay of even 4 hours or more.[8] Babies have a wide range of behaviors after birth and not all are ready to nurse immediately. Positioning of the baby at the breast is very important in the prevention of sore nipples (Box 22-4), pain-free nursing, and the successful establishment of nursing.[26] Breastfeeding is a learned skill that is generally acquired from observation and practice. In the United States, as well as in many industrialized nations, women rarely have the opportunity to watch other women breastfeeding.

When the baby is properly attached, the nipple, areola, and some of the surrounding breast tissue are drawn into a teat by the suction of the baby's mouth. This teat extends back into the junction of the baby's hard and soft palate. The teat is held between the baby's upper gum and the baby's tongue covers the lower gum. The breast tissue should be opposed to the baby's lower jaw and tongue milk can be transferred from breast to baby. The baby's tongue applies a force to the underside of the teat, and the hard palate provides resistance[8] (Figure 22-10).

As the mother nurses, she needs to remember proper body alignment and correct hand positioning. She can also try a variety of nursing positions to find which is most comfortable for her and her baby (Figure 22-11). Recruiting her transverse abdominis muscle, or wearing a splint in early recovery, can minimize upper and middle back discomfort. Placing her feet on a footstool or telephone book encourages a posterior pelvic tilt and acts as a gentle reminder to sit comfortably. Keeping her wrists neutral and bringing the baby to the breast rather than hunching over and bringing her breast to the baby reinforces good body mechanics (Figure 22-12). She should be aware of any extraneous tension areas and breathe deeply and slowly to stay relaxed.

Bodyworkers can use the following massage techniques to facilitate healing of the endocrine system:

- Spleen 3 pressed for hormone balancing (Figure 22-13).
- **DVD** Spleen 6 pressed to tone the uterus.
- Liver 3 pressed to encourage fluid elimination as necessary (Figure 22-14).
- Breast massage to treat engorgement and acupuncture points stomach 13, stomach 16, conception vessel 17, gall bladder 20, and breast reflexes on the feet (Figure 22-15).

Bodyworkers can also make the following suggestions to help heal the endocrine system:

- Ice packs to control pain and engorgement for nonlactating mothers.

BOX 22–4   *Care of Nipples*

If the nipples become sore, cracked, and tender, a major preventive of nipple trauma is good **latching-on**, or proper positioning of the baby at the breast.* Other remedies include the mother's own milk applied to the nipples; raw cabbage leaves, with the veins broken, placed in a bra against the nipples; Lansinoh (an over-the-counter lanolin product endorsed by La Leche League; this product cannot be used by anyone with a wool allergy); moist tea bags; and a drop of rose oil (must be removed before the baby nurses). In addition, the mother should avoid using soaps or perfumed lotions on her breasts.

*Data from Enkin M, Keirse M, Neilson J, et al: *A guide to effective care in pregnancy and childbirth*, Oxford, 2000, Oxford University Press.

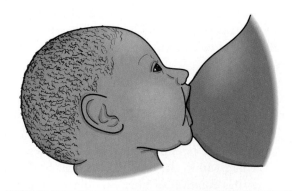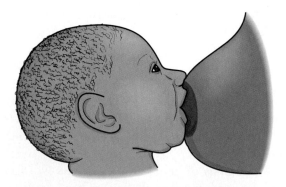

FIGURE 22-10 ■ *Left,* Correct positioning. When the teat is properly positioned in the infant's mouth, the gums compress the milk sinuses behind the areola. The tongue is between the lower gum and the breast and it moves over the sinuses like a peristaltic wave to bring milk forward into its mouth. *Right,* Incorrect positioning.

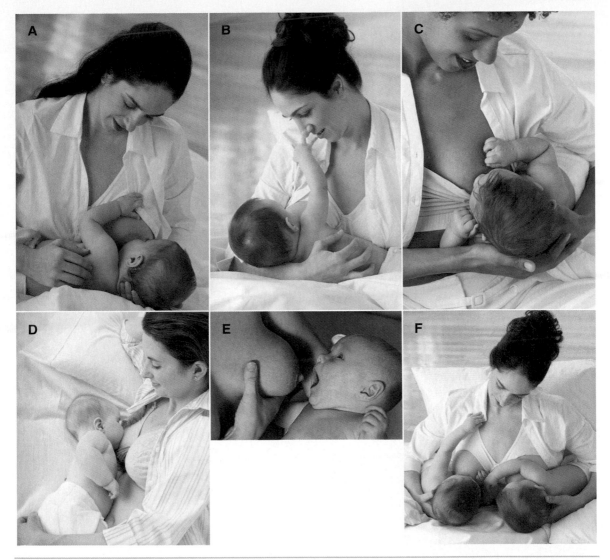

FIGURE 22-11 ■ **A**, The cradle hold. **B**, Cross-cradle hold. **C**, Football hold. **D**, Side-lying position, **E**, "C" position of hand on breast. **F**, Breast-feeding twins. (Courtesy Medela Inc., McHenry, IL.)

- Ginger compress for engorged breasts.
- Mother's milk, Lansinoh, bruised cabbage leaves, moist tea bags, or rose oil to treat sore nipples (see Box 22-4)
- Adequate amounts of water (8 to 10 glasses per day) to help encourage milk production.

Weight Loss

During pregnancy, the mother's body stored about 5 to 7 lbs of fat for lactation needs. Breastfeeding women lose this fat storage over a period of about 6 months, and they often return to their approximate prepregnant weight. Other women may have more difficulty shedding these excess pounds and are advised to increase their aerobic activity and incorporate strength training in their exercise regime. Aerobic activity has no adverse effects on nursing.[1,4]

Sleep

As long as a woman is nursing her infant, her sleep will be interrupted. Until such time that the baby starts to eat cereals (solid foods) and matures, most babies will wake up every 3 to 4 hours. Mother can express the milk and allow her partner to bottle-feed breast milk for a nighttime feeding to give her an opportunity to sleep, but

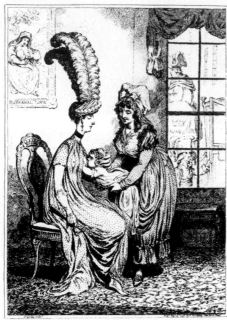

FIGURE 22-12 ■ "The Fashionable Mamma—or The Convenience of Modern Dress." 1793 woodcut. (From Smith L: *The mother book: a compendium of trivia and grandeur concerning mother, motherhood and maternity,* New York, 1978, Doubleday.)

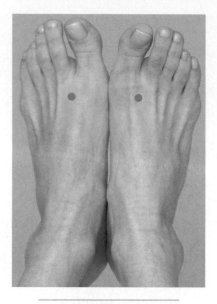

FIGURE 22-14 ■ Liver 3.

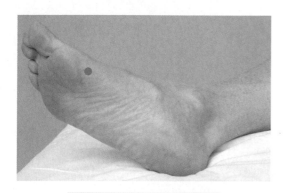

FIGURE 22-13 ■ Spleen 3.

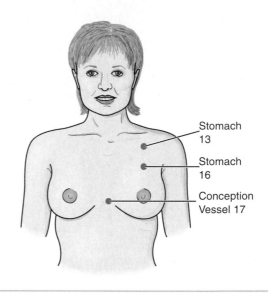

Stomach 13

Stomach 16

Conception Vessel 17

FIGURE 22-15 ■ Stomach 13, stomach 16, and conception vessel 17.

breast engorgement may still awaken her regardless of who is actually feeding the child.[27] Lack of sleep or interrupted sleep may contribute to the new mother's feelings of general malaise. Although nothing takes the place of an uninterrupted night's sleep, a full body massage can relax her and be appreciably restorative for those women who are sleep deprived. The practitioners should also incorporate all the acupuncture points used to treat fatigue.

Emotional and Psychological Changes

Anywhere from 1 to 2 weeks to 1 year, postpartum depression (PPD) can set in.[3] The symptoms are similar to symptoms of women who suffer from major depressive episodes unrelated to childbirth.[28] Symptoms include fatigue, sleep disturbance, and appetite and weight changes; these are all normal postpartum adaptations. However, these symptoms are also accompanied by feelings of anxiety, dysphoria, social withdrawal, cognitive disturbances, guilt, hopelessness, helplessness, a sense of worthlessness, or suicidal thoughts.

PPD is the most common complication of pregnancy, occurring in approximately 20% of new mothers.[29] In the United States, one-half million women suffer from this disorder yearly and most of these women have a previous history of a mood disorder.[8] The risk of recurrence in a subsequent pregnancy is 25%.[30]

It is important for the practitioner to be cognizant of the signs of depression. A client can benefit tremendously from a practitioner's concern and caring intervention with a referral to a mental health professional who can help her get through this difficult time.

Postpartum psychosis (PPP) is a clinical emergency requiring immediate intervention because of the risk of infanticide or suicide, especially with young mothers.[31,32] It differs from other psychotic manifestations, with the additional symptomology of sleep disturbances, even when the infant is sleeping, and depersonalization from people and the surrounding environment, and progresses quickly to confusion, extreme disorganization, bizarre behavior, delusions, and unusual visual, olfactory, or tactile hallucinations.[33] The symptoms could be an underlying manifestation of bipolar disorder that has a high frequency of occurrence during the postpartum period.[34]

PPP happens to 1% to 2% of the puerperal population. With subsequent deliveries, the risk predisposes a woman to a 33% to 40% chance of recurrence.[35] Practitioners are strongly advised to encourage these clients to seek immediate medical and counseling help. Early intervention dramatically improves the prognosis and prevention of a potentially devastating situation.

Emotional Support for Mothers Whose Babies Remain in the Hospital

Under certain circumstances, a new mother may be discharged from the hospital after a few days while her baby remains. When a baby is preterm or has a medical condition requiring hospitalization, the new mother has the burden of

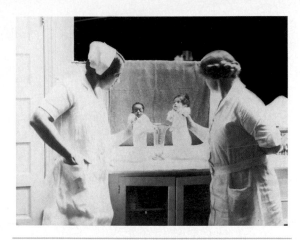

FIGURE 22-16 ■ "Nurses at the Atlantic City incubator are shown with two of the newest arrivals there—two tiny bits of humanity whose total weight is less than five pounds. Nurse E.C., at the left, is holding baby M.C., a negro child weighing but one pound six ounces. Nurse E.A.C., at the right, is holding baby V.L. of Brooklyn weighing three and a half pounds. Note their size compared to the graduate." (From International newsreel photo: "Tiny Humanity at the Atlantic City Incubator," August 17, 1931, Atlantic City, NJ.)

self-healing, as well as caring for her baby as best she can. Approximately 9% of all newborns are sick enough to require intensive care.[36]

Mothers who give birth to **premature babies**, or babies born between 20 and 37 weeks' gestation, produce milk that is unique in meeting the nutritional needs of the preterm baby. It is higher in protein, nitrogen, sodium, calcium, fat, and calories than the milk of full-term babies.[37] In addition, breast milk may increase the neonate's tolerance, reduce infections and later allergies, enhance neurological development, and help prevent intestinal complications.[3] Many women are encouraged to nurse or bottle-feed their baby breast milk to give their premature infant the best nutritional advantage. For the new mother, this could mean spending all day (and all night) in the hospital or making several trips throughout the day to feed her child (Figure 22-16).

Mothers who plan to breastfeed often require help in maintaining lactation until the infant is mature enough or able to nurse. In addition, these women require ongoing physical and emotional support. A breast pump can be used within the first 24 hours to provide breast milk for the neonate. The woman will also need to be shown

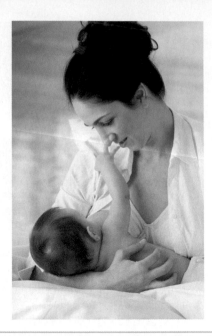

FIGURE 22-17 ■ The cross-cradle or modified cradle hold is especially helpful for premature babies or those with a fractured clavicle. The mother holds the infant's head in the hand opposite from the side the infant will feed, with the arm supporting the body across the mother's lap. The other hand holds the breast, and the mother can guide the baby's mouth to the breast. (Courtesy Medela Inc., McHenry, IL.)

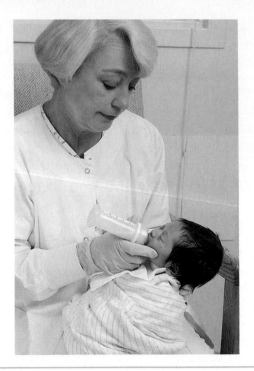

FIGURE 22-18 ■ Cheek and jaw support for feeding a preterm infant. (From McKinney ES, James SR, Murray SS, et al: *Maternal-child nursing*, ed 2, St. Louis, 2005, Mosby.)

how to hold her premature baby. Using the cross-cradle hold can enable her to see the baby latching on throughout the feeding (Figures 22-17 and 22-18). Kangaroo care can often be combined with breastfeeding to help maintain the infant's body temperature during feedings.

Extended hospitalization of a child separates parents from their newborn and can produce additional emotional trauma and a disruptive family life. Bonding and attachment can be seriously affected by this prolonged separation. It may interfere with the parents' ability to learn their baby's unique characteristics and raises doubts about their ability to care for their child. There might also be the additional burden of guilt and blame when a baby is too sick or immature to come home.

The practitioner should attempt to provide the bodywork the new mother needs for her physical and emotional recovery. Referral to a mental health professional can help her deal with her feelings when the birth outcome was unexpected or the baby has to remain hospitalized.

Family Adjustment

By the end of the traditional 6-weeks puerperium period, the family should have settled into some sort of routine. The roles and relationships within the family will adapt and reorganize with the birth of a baby. The new mother is particularly concerned about redefining her multiple roles as mother and partner. Conflicting demands between work and home can also add to her stresses.

There appear to be three continuous phases of maternal adjustment. The first phase is appreciating her body. This phase concentrates on how she feels and deals with her physical discomforts. It also deals with emotional lability and changes in the way she thinks. Phase two is called *settling-in*, and in this phase, the mother is becoming more comfortable with her baby. She begins to gain confidence with her parenting skills and finds ways to integrate the infant into daily routines. Finally, the woman works toward creating a family and learning to modify relationships with partners, other family members, and friends.[38]

The father's bonding process is called **engrossment,** and it is often characterized by an interest

BOX 22-5	*Factors Affecting Family Adaptation*

- Discomfort and fatigue
- Knowledge of infants needs
- Previous experience
- Expectations of the newborn
- Maternal age
- Maternal temperament
- Infant temperament
- Support system
- Cesarean birth
- Preterm or ill infant
- Multiples
- Cultural influences of communication, health beliefs, and dietary practices

From McKinney ES, James SR, Murray SS, et al: *Maternal-child nursing*, ed 2, St. Louis, 2005, Mosby.

BOX 22-6	*Statistics from the Guinness Book of World Records*

The world's tiniest surviving baby, a girl, was born in a Chicago hospital in December, 2004 at 28 weeks, weighing 8.6 oz.

The world's fattest baby was born in Italy to a mother who weighs 1230 pounds and a father who weighs 850 lbs. Their son, born by C-section on February 9, 2003, weighed 28 lbs, 4 oz.

The world's oldest mother is a 66-year-old Romanian woman who gave birth to twin girls in January, 2005. Before this birth, a 65-year-old retired teacher from India had the honors.

The world's youngest mother, a girl from Lima, Peru, with a rare syndrome called *precocious puberty*, got her first period at age 3 and had a baby when she was 5 years 7 months old. Lina Medina gave birth to a 6 ½-lb boy by C-section in 1939.

The world's tiniest mother is in a wheelchair and measures 3 feet tall and weighs 37 lbs. Her small stature is caused by type 3 osteogenesis imperfecta, which is a congenital condition. During her pregnancy, she gained 20 lbs and had a 3 lb 7 oz healthy boy by C-section at Stanford Hospital, Palo Alto, California in February, 2006.

In Provo, Utah, a 42-year-old woman and her 22-year-old daughter had babies 90 minutes apart, assisted by the same nursing team in the same room in February, 2006.

In 2006, in a suburb of St. Louis, Missouri, three babies were born to three sisters in three days.

From the *Guinness Book of World Records*, London, Guinness World Records.

in how the child looks with a strong desire to touch and hold the baby. Conversely, some fathers feel they do not have adequate parenting skills and he may need extra support to help him feel more confident and competent.[3,39]

Older sibling responses are determined by their age and developmental levels. Toddlers are generally not aware of the pregnancy but often feel as if they are being replaced by the newborn. Acting out, reverting to more infantile behavior, and attention-getting efforts are rather common for the young child. Preschool children like to spend some of their time close to the newborn and like to talk about their brother or sister with their mother. Older children are usually more willing to help out. At any age, attention should still be paid to the older siblings by their parents, families, and visitors.

Grandparents are often regarded as a major part of the support system that the new parents come to rely on. Proximity to their grandchild fosters a special relationship that brings additional love and security to the family members. Grandmothers in particular can be especially helpful with childcare activities.

There are a number of factors that can affect family adaptation. Some are expected, such as fatigue and physical discomfort, but others can be unanticipated events (Box 22-5). The family who works together and supports each other can make a smoother transition into the demands of parenthood.[3] (Box 22-6)

In My Experience...

H, a regular client during her pregnancy, came to see me 3 weeks after her baby was born. As soon as she walked into the office and saw me, she burst into tears.

"Do I look that bad?" I asked, trying to lighten the mood. "No, it's not that," she sobbed. "It's the first time I've left my baby at home." (The child was with her father and grandmother.)

I pointed to the phone and told her to call home and check up on her daughter. By the time I came back from washing my hands, H had calmed down and apologized for her outburst. "There is nothing to be sorry about," I assured her. "People look at me and cry all the time!"

She told me how hard it was to leave her child for the very first time and how lost she felt without her. I told her that was mother-love and it would only get deeper with time. But I promised her that she would eventually feel much stronger and more secure about taking some much-deserved time for herself.

Summary

Many physical and emotional adaptations continue for the new mother during the traditional 6-week puerperium recovery period. Many of these changes overlap from the earlier healing time frame, and some will continue into extended recovery.

The massage practitioner should continue providing physical and emotional support during this delicate period of adjustment. The bodywork should continue with cleansing and elimination support as needed and introduce extrinsic muscle balancing techniques, including medial compression and appropriate scar massage. Strengthening and supporting (splinting) the woman's abdominal core muscles will improve her body mechanics and postural alignment.

Hormones secreted by the endocrine system stimulate milk production and letdown. The bodyworker can help treat breast tenderness and engorgement and instruct the new mother in proper body mechanics while nursing.

The woman will experience three continuous phases of maternal adjustment throughout the puerperium recovery period. The new family generally settles into a routine and learns to adapt to the demands of parenthood.

References

1. Leifer G: *Maternity nursing: an introductory text*, ed 9, St. Louis, 2005, Saunders.
2. Creasy R, Resnick R, eds: *Maternal-fetal medicine*, ed 5, Philadelphia, 2004, Saunders.
3. McKinney ES, James SR, Murray SS, et al: *Maternal-child nursing*, ed 2, St. Louis, 2005, Mosby.
4. Gabbe S, Niebyl J, Simpson J: *Obstetrics: normal and problem pregnancies*, ed 4, New York, 2002, Churchill Livingstone.
5. Kistner WR: Physiology of the vagina. In Haven ESE, Evans TN, eds: *The human vagina*, Amsterdam, 1978, North Holland.
6. Blackburn ST: *Maternal, fetal and neonatal physiology*, ed 2, Philadelphia, 2003, Saunders.
7. Peschers UM, Schaer GN, DeLancey JO, et al: Levator ani function before and after childbirth, *Br J Obstet Gynaecol* 104: 1004-1008, 1997.
8. Enkin M, Keirse M, Neilson J, et al: *A guide to effective care in pregnancy and childbirth*, ed 3, Oxford, 2000, Oxford University Press.
9. Glazener C: Sexual function after childbirth: women's experiences, persistent morbidity and lack of professional recognition, *Br J Obstet Gynecol* 104:330-335, 1997.
10. Greenshields W, Hulme H: *The perineum in childbirth*, London, 1993, National Childbirth Trust.
11. Robson KM, Brant HA, Kumar R: Maternal sexuality during the first pregnancy and after childbirth, *Br J Obstet Gynecol* 88:882-889, 1981.
12. Hassid P: *Textbook for childbirth educators*, Philadelphia, 1978, Harper and Row.
13. Campbell OM, Gray RH: Characteristics and determination of postpartum ovarian function in women in the United States, *Am J Obstet Gynecol* 165:183, 1991.
14. Lyon RA, Stamm MJ: The onset of ovulation during the puerperium, *Cal Med* 65:99, 1946.
15. Visness CM, Kennedy KI, Gross BA, et al: Fertility of fully breast feeding women in the early postpartum period, *Obstet Gynecol* 89:164-167, 1997.
16. Tupler J: *Lose your mummy tummy*, Cambridge, MA, 2005, Perseus.
17. Lowdermilk DL, Perry SE: *Maternity & women's health care*, ed 8, St. Louis, 2004, Mosby.
18. Fritz S, Grosenbach JM: *Mosby's essential sciences for therapeutic massage*, ed 2, St. Louis, 2004, Mosby.
19. Wittlinger H, Wittlinger G: *Textbook of Dr. Vodder's manual lymph drainage*, ed 6, Heidelberg, 1998, Karl F. Haug Verlag.

20. Robson SC, Dunlop W, Hunter S: Haemodynamic changes during the early puerperium, *Br Med J* (Clin Res Ed) 294:1065, 1987.

21. Gilson GJ, Samaan S, Crawford MH, et al: Changes in the hemodynamics, ventricular remodeling, and ventricular contractility during normal pregnancy: A longitudinal study, *Obstet Gynecol* 89:957-962, 1997.

22. Capeless EL, Clapp JF: When do cardiovascular parameters return to their preconception values? *Am J Obstet Gynecol* 165:883-886, 1991.

23. Jeffreis J, Bochner F: Thromboembolism and its management in pregnancy, *Med J Australia* 155:253-258, 1991.

24. Stein GS: Headaches in the first postpartum week and their relationship to migraine, *Headache* 21:201-205, 1981.

25. Scoggin J: Physical and psychological changes. In Mattson S, Smith JE, eds: *Core curriculum for maternal-newborn nursing*, ed 2, Philadelphia, 2000, Saunders.

26. Coad J: *Anatomy and physiology for midwives*, St. Louis, 2001, Mosby.

27. Quillan SL: Infant and mother sleep patterns during the 4th postpartum week, *Issues Comp Ped Nurs* 20:115-123, 1997.

28. Wisner KL, Peindl KS, Hanusa BH: Symptomatology of affective and psychotic illnesses related to childbearing, *J Affect Disord* 30:77-87, 1994.

29. O'Hara MW, Swain AM: Rates and risks of postpartum depression: a meta-analysis, *Int Rev Psychiatry* 8:7, 1996.

30. Wisner KL, Perel JM, Peindl KS, et al: Prevention of recurrent postpartum depression: a randomized clinical trial, *J Clin Psychiatry* 62:82, 2001.

31. Davidson J, Robertson E: A follow-up study of postpartum illness, 1946-1978, *Acta Psychiatr Scand* 71:451-457, 1985.

32. Appleby L: Suicide during pregnancy and in the first postnatal year, *BMJ* 302:137-140, 1991.

33. Brockington IF, Meakin CJ: Clinical cues to the aetiology of puerperal psychosis, *Prog Neuropsychopharmacol Biol Psychiatry* 18:417-429, 1994.

34. Targum SD, Davenport YB, Webster MJ: Postpartum mania in bipolar manic-depressive patients withdrawn from lithium carbonate, *J Nerv Ment Dis* 167:572-574, 1979.

35. Kendell RE, Chalmers JC, Platz C: Epidemiology of puerperal psychoses, *Br J Psychiatry* 150:622, 1987.

36. Simkin P, Whalley J, Keppler A: *Pregnancy, childbirth and the newborn*, New York, 1991, Meadowbrook Press.

37. Stoll BJ, Kliegman RM: The high risk infant. In Behrman RE, Kliegman RM, Jenson HB, eds: *Nelson textbook of pediatrics*, ed 17, Philadelphia, 2004, Saunders.

38. Martell LK: Heading toward the new normal: a contemporary postpartum experience, *J Obstet Gynecol Neonatal Nurs* 30(5):496-506, 2000.

39. Matteson PS: *Women's health during the childbearing years: a community-based approach*, St. Louis, 2001, Mosby.

REVIEW QUESTIONS

1 How has the new mother's reproductive system adjusted during the 6-week puerperium recovery period?

_____

_____

_____

_____

_____

2 When does menstruation generally begin again?

_____

_____

_____

_____

_____

3 What adaptations is her musculoskeletal system making within the 6 weeks after childbirth? What massage techniques are beneficial to treat her musculoskeletal system?

_____

_____

_____

_____

_____

4 What exercises can be recommended to help close her diastasis recti?

_____

_____

_____

_____

_____

5 When does relaxation and hypermobility of the joints finally stabilize? Which hormone is responsible for these initial changes?

_____

_____

_____

_____

_____

6 Where can the massage practitioner find active trigger points within the soft tissues of new mothers?

_____

_____

_____

_____

_____

7 Describe scar massage.

_____

_____

_____

_____

_____

8 Describe the changes to a new mother's cardiovascular system and the massage protocol that supports it.

_____

_____

_____

_____

_____

9   How does the puerperium recovery period affect the gastrointestinal and neurological systems of the new mother?

_____

_____

_____

_____

_____

10 What hormones are being secreted by the endocrine system to stimulate milk production? What massage techniques can help treat breast tenderness and engorgement? What is colostrum?

_____

_____

_____

_____

_____

11 Proper body mechanics during nursing are important to prevent which syndromes from occurring?

_____

_____

_____

_____

_____

12 Describe some emotional and psychological changes women may expect to feel during puerperium.

_____

_____

_____

_____

_____

13 How can massage practitioners help support those mothers whose babies remain in the hospital?

_____

_____

_____

_____

_____

14 Describe the "typical" maternal adjustment process for the puerperium recovery.

_____

_____

_____

_____

_____

15 What are some factors that can affect family adaptation?

_____

_____

_____

_____

_____

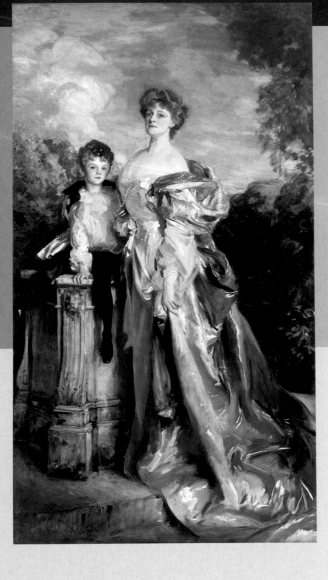

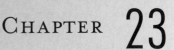

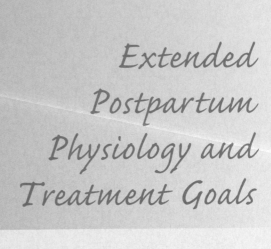

CHAPTER 23

Extended Postpartum Physiology and Treatment Goals

Objectives

On completion of this chapter, the student will be able to do the following:

1 Understand the physiological process of extended postpartum recovery

2 Understand the treatment goals for extended postpartum

3 Use appropriate massage techniques to achieve these goals

4 Incorporate cesarean scar massage technique for extended postpartum recovery

Libido
Thyroiditis

Extended postpartum is any time past the traditional 6-week puerperium recovery period. Unresolved physical discomforts and emotional issues can have far-reaching and long-lasting effects on a women's overall health for years after childbirth. Extended postpartum recovery begins at the end of puerperium and continues for months and years afterward. Table 23-1 illustrates the timeline of postpartum extended recovery, including emotional and physiological recovery from childbirth.

In this country, most women wait 6 weeks after childbirth before they see their doctors or midwives again for a check-up. Most women go through the postpartum period without sound counsel or advice about what is (or is not) normal physiological recovery. At this 6-week visit, the uterus is assessed for involution and other metabolic indicators are examined. Women are also told whether they can return to normal physical and sexual activity.

For those women who work outside of the home, most are back at their jobs soon after 6 weeks. Many women add vacation and personal days to their maternity leave to prolong their time at home with their baby. Unfortunately, their bodies are still undergoing many changes and adaptations and when the demands of work, coupled with a lack of sleep, are considered, returning to work too soon can take its toll.

Working mothers who breastfeed have to find a private place to pump and store their milk. Some nursing mothers decide to breastfeed at home and supplement with formula while they are at work. This flexible approach can remove the pressure to pump their breasts and help the woman enjoy the mutual benefits of nursing.

Physiological Changes in the Woman during the Extended Postpartum Period

Reproductive System

Menstrual Cycle

Menstruation can start as early as 1 to 2 months postpartum for a nonlactating mother.[1] The mean average is about 10 weeks for nonlactating women and 17 weeks for lactating women, although vaginal bleeding in breastfeeding women in the first 8 weeks is not an indication of menstruation.[2,3]

Perineum

Complete healing from an episiotomy can take as long as 4 to 6 months.[4] It takes almost 2 months for full recovery of strength and muscular tone of the pubococcygeal (pelvic floor) muscles.[5] Perineal pain plagues some women for more than 2 months after the birth of their babies, especially those women who had instrumental vaginal deliveries or episiotomies. (Natural tears will heal much faster and more easily than a surgical incision.) There is evidence that some women who had episiotomies experience dyspareunia for more than a year after childbirth.[6-8]

Cervix

The cervix never returns to its original condition and always shows evidence of birth by a change in appearance from round to slitlike.

Vagina

Vaginal involution is completed between weeks 6 to 10, but it never fully regains its prepregnant size.[9-11]

Uterus

By 5 to 6 weeks, the uterus has involuted and has returned to its prepregnant size (Figure 23-1).

TABLE 23-1	*Timeline of Postpartum Recovery*		
	IMMEDIATE	**PUERPERIUM**	**EXTENDED**
	Days 1 2 3 4 5 6 7	Weeks 1 2 3 4 5 6	Months 1 2 3 4 5 6+
Headaches	1-3 days +++++++++++	++++++++++++++++++	+++++++++++++++++++++
Puerperal fever	2-3 days		
Colostrum	3 days		
Estrogen and progesterone levels	3 days		
Bowel pattern	3 days		
Diuresis	3-4 days		
Postpartum blues onset	3-5 days		
Cessation of lactation for nonnursing mothers	4-7 days		
Diaphoresis	7 days		
Uterine lining		16 days	
Lochia serosa		10-27 days	
Gestational glucose intolerance reversal		1-2 weeks	
PPD onset		1-2 weeks +++++++++++	+++++++++++++++++++++
Skin lightening		1-2 weeks	
Edema		1-2 weeks	
Cardiac output 30% decrease		2 weeks	
hCG levels		2 weeks	
Prolactin		2 weeks +++	
Respiratory rates		1-3 weeks	
Cardiac contractibility		6 weeks	
Lochia alba		6 weeks	
Uterine involution		6 weeks	
Placental site		6-7 weeks	
Vaginal involution		6-10 weeks	
Fibrinogenic activity		8-10 weeks	
Evaluation for blood clots		10 weeks	
Pelvic floor			2 months
Menstruation begins (nonnursing)			2 months
Menstruation begins (nursing)			4-5 months
Episiotomy			4-6 months
Relaxin			4-6 months
Weight loss			6 months +
Disrupted sleep			6 months +++
Bone mineralization			+18 months
Stroke volume, cardiac output (100%), end-diastolic volume, systemic vascular resistance			+1 year
Perineal pain from episiotomy			+1 year
Dyspareunia			+1 year
Perineal pain			+1 year
Cervix			Permanent change
Vagina			Permanent change
PPP onset			+++++++++++++++++++++

PPD, Postpartum depression; *hCG,* human chorionic gonadotrophin; *PPP,* postpartum psychosis.

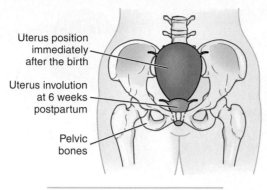

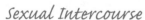

FIGURE 23-1 ■ Uterine involution.

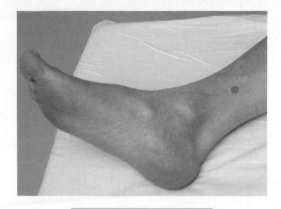

FIGURE 23-2 ■ Spleen 6.

Sexual Intercourse

Many postpartum women report a decline in sexual desire, or **libido**.[6,12,13] One study found 84% decrease in sexual activity at 4 months postpartum.[14] Another study found about two-thirds of the women surveyed enjoyed sex at 3 months postpartum, although 40% complained of some difficulties.[13] Studies suggest that the following six factors may be related to reduced sexual desire, frequency, and satisfaction[15-18]:

- Adjustment to changes in social role of women during the transition to motherhood
- Marital satisfaction
- Mood
- Fatigue
- Physical changes associated with birth
- Breastfeeding

Bodyworkers can use the following massage techniques to facilitate healing of the reproductive system during the extended postpartum period:

- Spleen 6 pressed to help tone the uterus (Figure 23-2)
- Uterine reflex points (Figure 23-3)

In addition, bodyworkers can suggest that clients do Kegel exercises to maintain strength and tone the muscles of the pelvic floor.

Musculoskeletal System

A diastasis recti that has not be corrected can contribute to chronic lower back pain and pelvic instability for as long as the separation exists. Regular recruitment of the transverse abdominis muscle to close the separation will remedy this situation. Care must be taken to employ the abdominal core

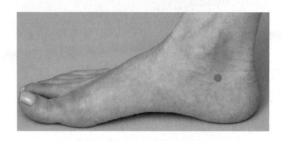

FIGURE 23-3 ■ Uterine reflex.

muscles correctly when lifting, nursing, or carrying the baby to avoid back pain. In addition, as the baby grows, slings should be substituted for anterior baby carriers to ensure a more appropriate postural alignment.

Practitioners can test for the presence of a diastasis by having the client lie flat on the massage table, without using any bolstering. She bends her knees and inhales deeply. As she exhales, she does a "crunch" by bringing her head and shoulders off the massage table. This will cause the rectus abdominis to bulge. The practitioner palpates with his or her hand across the linea alba from the top of the pubic bone to the xiphoid process. Any separation more than half a finger's width is a diastasis. Most of the separation will be palpable above and below the umbilicus (Figure 23-4).

Muscle balancing techniques on the intrinsic, as well as extrinsic, musculature can now be introduced. Special attention must be paid to the piriformis, iliopsoas, and paravertebral muscles to support pelvic stability and normalized gait.

Relaxation and hypermobility of the joints are stabilized between weeks 8 to 10. However, the effects of relaxin on the connective tissue can

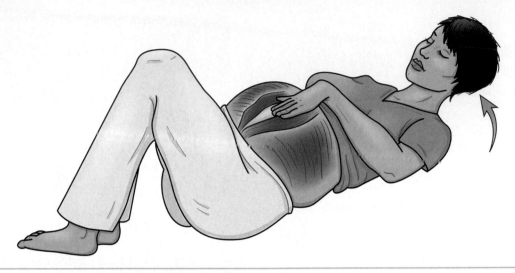

FIGURE 23-4 ■ Testing for a diastasis. In this illustration, the client is self-testing. When practitioners perform this test, they position themselves at the side of the table facing the client and palpate the linea alba from the pubic bone to the xiphoid process. Any separation more than a half finger's width is a diastasis that can be a contributing cause to chronic backaches.

remain in the woman's body for 4 to 6 months to permit her body to return to its prepregnant state over a period of time.

Trigger point work can now be performed using deeper pressure. After 6 weeks, most women can tolerate increased pressure during treatment, but client comfort and feedback is the defining element of how much pressure to use.

A symphysis pubis separation that does not heal in correct alignment will cause referred lower back and sciatic pain after the bones rejoin. This implies that chronic lower back pain during extended postpartum may originate from sources other than the lower back: a diastasis, symphysis pubis separation, and hypertonic hip muscles, especially the piriformis, should all be suspect in cases of chronic lower back pain, as well as the obvious lumbar and lumbosacral involvement.

Muscle Testing

During pregnancy, labor, birth, and postpartum, the client's body has undergone tremendous change and adaptations. This incredible metamorphosis, all within the course of 1 year, has put an extraordinary strain on her musculoskeletal system. How can a practitioner find the origin of the client's pain when her entire musculature was so dramatically affected?

One technique that is consistent and revealing is muscle testing. By "asking" the client's body "where it hurts," a practitioner can assess the origin(s) of her chronic pain. Practitioners should have the client lie comfortably on the table in a supine position, propped with pillows under her neck and legs. In this position, the strength of her pectoralis major, sternal division, will be tested, although any muscle can be used for the test. The client keeps one arm at her side and off her body and raises the other arm in medial rotation. The muscle is lightly tested by pushing her arm at the wrist in a linear direction with the muscle fibers (Figure 23-5).

The muscle has been tested "in the clear," and an arm that maintains the position is functioning correctly. Then the client holds her arm in this position and places her other hand where a suspected chronic problem may originate. For instance, if the practitioner suspects that the client has a misaligned symphysis pubis, the client places her hand directly on the site. The muscle is tested again with her hand on the symphysis pubis. If the client's arm moves or cannot sustain the position, it indicates potential problems with the symphysis pubis (or any other region of her body she palpates during the test.)

With the client in a prone position, practitioners may opt to test the hamstrings for suspected areas on her back (Figure 23-6).

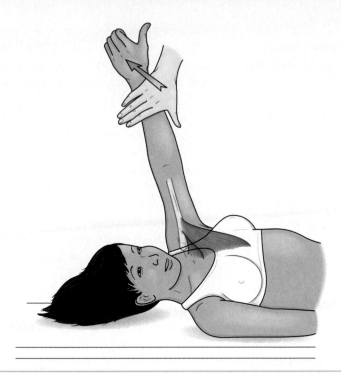

FIGURE 23-5 ■ To perform a muscle test on the sternal division of the pectoralis major, the client raises her arm and puts it in medial rotation. Her hand is placed as shown. The practitioner gently pushes in the direction of the fibers. A weak muscle cannot sustain the position, but a strong muscle will not move.

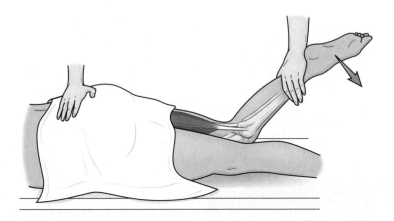

FIGURE 23-6 ■ General hamstring test. The practitioner applies pressure in the direction of the arrow to extend the knee from a flexed position.

In addition, much of a practitioner's corrective work will be discarded if the client reverts to poor body mechanics and postural shifting once she returns to normal daily activities. A concerted effort on her part must be made to employ proper body mechanics throughout the day to prevent injury and support postural integrity.

Bodyworkers can use the following massage techniques to facilitate healing of the musculo-

skeletal system during the extended postpartum period:

■ Test for the presence of a diastasis recti.
■ Muscle test to locate the origins of muscle weakness and referred pain, anterior and posterior.
■ Kenbiki along the erector spinae to assess muscle tension. (This muscle correlates with the bladder meridian whose

emotional expression is crying. It is not at all unusual for a new mother to have an emotional release during this soothing stroke.)

- Gentle rocking.
- **DVD** Swedish massage, using as much pressure as the client desires.
- Lymphatic drainage on the legs must continue as long as 10 weeks postpartum.
- Trigger point release on extrinsic and intrinsic muscles to support hip, pelvic and lower back stability, and postural alignment.
- Myofascial release.
- **DVD** Pelvic tilt.
- Muscle balancing techniques.
- Medial compression.

In addition, bodyworkers can explain the importance in recruiting the transverse abdominis muscle during daily activities and childcare and the correct way to exercise her abdominal core muscles. Practitioners should teach clients proper body mechanics to prevent injury or maladaptive posture.

Cesarean Scar Massage

At this point during recovery, it is important to work the cesarean scar as deeply as the client can tolerate (and show her how to work the scar) to restore pliability and flexibility to the soft tissues. If left untreated, the client will feel a "tugging" at the site of the incision whenever she bends over and will have a bulge of skin and soft tissue directly over the incision that dieting will not resolve. She also may develop additional myofascial restrictions created by the rigidity of collagenous scar tissue.

A wonderful lotion for scar work is made of equal parts of the tinctures of calendula, St. John's wort, comfrey, and arnica mixed in Shea butter. The following techniques can be used for scars anywhere on the body:

- Gentle vibration on top of the scar.
- Lymphatic drainage directing the edema towards the closest lymph nodes (Figure 23-7).
- Using a small amount of lubrication, the practitioner can perform a transverse friction in a vertical direction all around the scar using his or her thumbs. The practitioner should get as close to the scar as possible. The pressure needs to be adequate enough to gently tug at the skin and superficial fascia. In time, the practitioner can progress to deeper pressure to effect change within the deeper fascia and muscle layers.
- Transverse friction in a horizontal and slightly diagonal direction, first above the scar and then below it.
- Thumbs placed on either side of the scar and use a horizontal friction, stretching the tissues.
- Transverse friction directly over the incision can only be performed on the nonkeloid scar.
- Rolling the scar between the fingers and picking up the skin using a light vibration.
- Gently end the treatment with a gentle alternate thumb effleurage toward the scar.

Neurological System

Migraine headaches are a result of the leakage of cerebral spinal fluid into the extradural space from a poorly administered epidural or spinal anesthesia and can plague women for many years. Some women become highly sensitive to changes in barometric pressure and can sense when a storm is coming. General neck and scalp massage, as well as **DVD** pressing large intestine 4 (Figure 23-8), can alleviate and substantially reduce headache pain. Lack of sleep over protracted periods of time can also be debilitating, especially when the new mother has to return to work. Practitioners should treat her for fatigue

---

Touch Points

No matter how successful massages are, if clients resort to their bad postural habits (especially in the 4 to 6 month postpartum period when the effects of relaxin are still in their bodies), they will undermine all of the healing work. Clients have to do their homework: they have to learn, or relearn, proper body mechanics that use their muscles correctly and change habits that create misalignment.

This is especially important as the babies continue to grow and gain weight. Using their bodies correctly when they lift the babies, work out at the gym, do home chores, or perform daily living activities will ensure a faster, more constant recovery. If practitioners help them now, they will be in great shape when they decide to do this all over again.

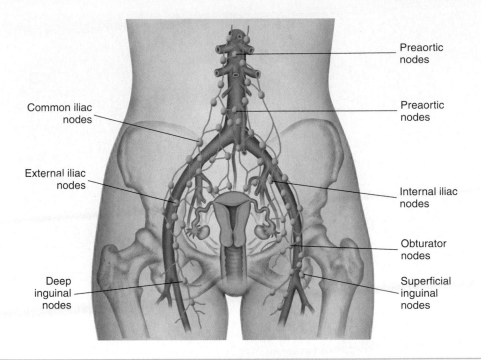

FIGURE 23-7 ■ Lymphatic drainage during scar massage directs the lymph toward the closest lymph nodes. The practitioner strokes lightly toward the external, internal, and common iliac nodes to reduce swelling on the top portion of the scar and strokes toward the obturator, deep, and superficial inguinal nodes for the bottom of the scar. The pressure is extremely light. (From Seidel HM: *Mosby's guide to physical examination*, ed 6, St. Louis, 2006, Mosby.)

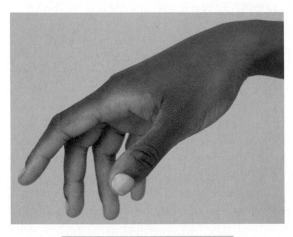

FIGURE 23-8 ■ Large intestine 4.

by including acupuncture points pericardium 8, pericardium 6, heart 7, governing vessel 20, and kidney 1 (Figure 23-9).

Endocrine System

The nursing mother must be aware of proper posture while breastfeeding. Her wrists should stay neutral, and her neck should remain retracted to avoid arm discomforts. Shin splints while using a rocking chair can be prevented by changing positions often or using a glider chair. Elevating her feet on a footstool or thick book prevents leg pain and has the additional benefit of providing a posterior pelvic tilt that will remind her to sit erect. Some women appreciate the additional comfort and support of nursing pillows. Continuing to press spleen 6 encourages continuous uterine support and tone. The effects of relaxin will leave the woman's body over an extended period of time, which can be as long as 4 to 6 months. This can affect her mental acuity and memory and can add to her sense of clumsiness as her joints are somewhat unstable for as long as a 6 months postpartum.

Weight Loss

Breastfeeding women lose their additional body fat over a longer period of time than nonlactating mothers. It can take as long as 6 months before nursing mothers return to their prepregnant weight. Others may be disheartened by the time it takes to lose those extra pounds and

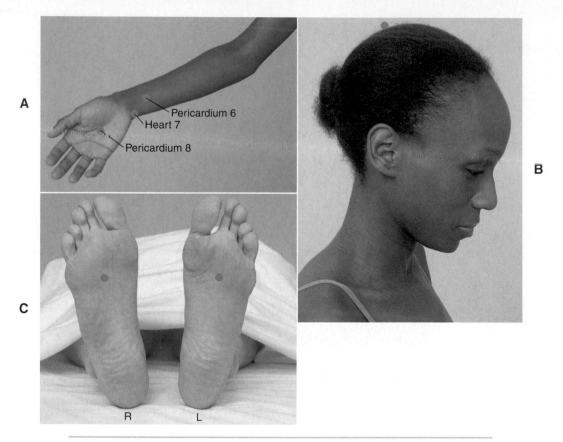

FIGURE 23-9 ■ **A**, Pericardium 6, pericardium 8, and heart 7. **B**, Governing vessel 20. **C**, Kidney 1.

should be encouraged to increase their aerobic activity and incorporate strength training in their exercise regime to stimulate their metabolic rates.[19,20]

Going Back to Work

Going back to work soon after the birth of her baby can take a physical and emotional toll on some women, but financial considerations, or any other personal reasons, may present the new mother with few options. Other women eagerly look forward to getting back to their jobs and careers as a way to engage with their contemporaries once again and continue on their career path.

Regardless of the reason for returning to work, it is often not an easy decision to make and many women feel pulled in opposing directions by their need to be with their child and the need to get back to work. Some women suffer guilt when they leave their children in the care of others but would feel equally as bad if they did not return to their careers.

Emotional and Psychological Changes

The onset of severe mood disorders, such as postpartum depression (PPD) or postpartum psychosis (PPP), can be delayed and occur as long as 1 year after childbirth (see Chapter 22).

The practitioner should understand that it is extremely common for new mothers to feel "blue" within a few days after the birth of the baby. These transient feelings, however, are short-lived and usually do not require intervention; however, the more severe and possibly life-threatening mood disorders require immediate medical intervention.

It is important to rule out postpartum metabolic disorders, such as thyroid disease, when assessing a woman for PPD or PPP because they share many symptoms. Autoimmune thyroid disease, affecting up to 10% of all women, is suppressed during pregnancy but is exacerbated during postpartum.[21] Postpartum **thyroiditis** (PPT) initially presents with a transient hyperthyroid phase 6 weeks to 6 months postpartum, followed by a hypothyroid phase that can last as long as 1 year. Approximately 6% to 9% of women develop PPT.[22,23] Symptoms include fatigue, hair loss, depression, impairment of concentration, inability to lose weight, and dry skin.

Depression and PPT are both common.[24] As many as 38% of women with PPT experience depression, so it is understandable how difficult it can be to determine the etiology of the depression.[25] Regardless of the cause, a client who presents with symptoms of depression should be referred to a doctor or mental health professional who can determine the best course of treatment for the new mother.

Memories of her pregnancy, labor, and birth may continue to haunt or delight the new mother for a long time. Childbirth is a major defining point for most women, and the way women experience and perceive this amazing period of their lives can have physical and emotional implications for many years to come.

In My Experience...

During one of my MotherMassage: Massage During Pregnancy professional certification workshops, I heard two similar versions of the same story from three different students. Each had completed the entire certification program of Dr. Vodder's manual lymphatic drainage.

They were all doing manual lymphatic drainage to treat old scars. One of the clients had a large thick, ropy, and red keloid "zipper" scar running down the center of her body from open-heart surgery 20 years prior when she was a young girl. Another client had a scar from a kidney operation that curved around her side. The third client had a severe leg injury that left a thick, deformed scar from the side of the client's thigh to the middle of his leg.

These practitioners were working very lightly to direct the edema (yes, even years later) to the closest lymph nodes. The work was slow, tedious, and specific. At some point, they all noticed the smell of anesthesia in the room and reported tasting it. The scars appreciably thinned and became whiter a short time after that.

Touch does not have to be deep to be profoundly effective.

Summary

Extended postpartum recovery begins at the end of the puerperium period and continues for months and years afterward. Some chronic conditions that clients present may be the result of a pregnancy, labor, or birth from many years ago. Conditions like a diastasis recti, misaligned symphysis pubis, or epidural migraine can plague clients for years after the birth.

Assessing and evaluating the origins of her chronic problems takes skill and practice. Palpation, muscle testing, and neuromuscular balancing techniques are effective tools that provide relief from chronic aches and pains and restore functional and postural integrity to a body that has been through so much change.

References

1. Hassid P: *Textbook for childbirth educators*, Philadelphia, 1978, Harper and Row.
2. Lyon RA, Stamm MJ: The onset of ovulation during the puerperium, *Cal Med* 65:99, 1946.
3. Visness CM, Kennedy KI, Gross BA, et al: Fertility of fully breast feeding women in the early postpartum period, *Obstet Gynecol* 89:164-167, 1997.
4. Blackburn ST: *Maternal, fetal and neonatal physiology*, ed 2, Philadelphia, 2003, Saunders.
5. Peschers UM, Schaer GN, DeLancey JO, et al: Levator ani function before and after childbirth, *Br J Obstet Gynaecol* 104: 1004-1008, 1997.
6. Glazener C: Sexual function after childbirth: women's experiences, persistent morbidity and lack of professional recognition, *Br J Obstet Gynecol* 104:330-335, 1997.
7. Greenshields W, Hulme H: *The perineum in childbirth*, London, 1993, National Childbirth Trust.
8. Robson KM, Brant HA, Kumar R: Maternal sexuality during the first pregnancy and after childbirth, *Br J Obstet Gynecol* 88:882-889, 1981.

9. Creasy R, Resnick R, eds: *Maternal-fetal medicine*, ed 5, Philadelphia, 2004, Saunders.

10. McKinney ES, James SR, Murray SS, et al: *Maternal-child nursing*, ed 2, St. Louis, 2005, Mosby.

11. Kistner WR: Physiology of the vagina. In Haven ESE, Evans TN, eds: *The human vagina*, Amsterdam, 1978, North Holland.

12. Fischman SH, Rankin EA, Soeken KL, et al: Changes in sexual relationships in postpartum couples, *J Obstet Gynecol Nurs* 15: 58-63, 1985.

13. Kumar R, Brant HA, Robson KM: Childbearing and maternal sexuality: a prospective survey of 119 primiparae, *J Psychosomatic Res* 25:373-383, 1981.

14. Hyde JS, DeLamater JD, Plant EA, et al: Sexuality during pregnancy and the year postpartum, *J Sex Research* 33:143-151, 1996.

15. DeJudicibus MA: *Psychological factors and the sexuality of pregnant and postpartum women*, Victoria, Australia, 2002, Society for the Scientific Study of Sexuality.

16. Terry DJ, McHugh TA, Noller P: Role dissatisfaction and the decline in marital quality across the transition to parenthood, *Aus J Psych* 43:129-132, 1991.

17. Snowden LR, Schott TL, Await SJ, et al: Marital satisfaction in pregnancy: stability and change, *J Marriage Fam* 50:325-333, 1988.

18. Miller BC, Sollie DL: Normal stresses during the transition to parenthood, *Family Relations* 29:459-465, 1980.

19. Leifer G: *Maternity nursing: an introductory text*, ed 9, St. Louis, 2005, Saunders.

20. Gabbe S, Niebyl J, Simpson J: *Obstetrics: normal and problem pregnancies*, ed 4, New York, 2002, Churchill Livingstone.

21. Davies TF: The thyroid immunology of the postpartum period, *Thyroid* 9:675, 1999.

22. Gerstein HC: Incidence of postpartum thyroid dysfunction in patients with type I diabetes mellitus, *Ann Intern Med* 188:419, 1993.

23. Alvarez-Marfany M, Roman SH, Drexler AJ, et al: Long-term prospective study of postpartum thyroid dysfunction in women with insulin dependent diabetes mellitus, *J Clin Endocrinol Metab* 79:10-16, 1994.

24. Pedersen CA: Postpartum mood and anxiety disorders. A guide for the non-psychiatric clinician with an aside on thyroid association with postpartum mood, *Thyroid* 9:691, 1999.

25. Pop VJM, de Rooy HAM, Vader HL, et al: Postpartum thyroid dysfunction and depression in an unselected population, *N Engl J Med* 324:1815, 1991.

REVIEW QUESTIONS

1   What is extended postpartum recovery?

_____

_____

_____

_____

_____

2   What are some of the physical changes that continue during the extended postpartum period?

_____

_____

_____

_____

3   When can menstruation begin for a nursing mother?

_____

_____

_____

_____

_____

4   How long can it take for full recovery of the perineum from an episiotomy?

_____

_____

_____

_____

_____

5   How long does it generally take for complete uterine involution?

_____

_____

_____

_____

6   If the diastasis recti is not corrected, what possible complications can a practitioner expect to treat in these clients?

_____

_____

_____

_____

_____

7   How does a practitioner test for the presence of a diastasis recti?

_____

_____

_____

_____

_____

8   When can trigger point therapy or muscle balancing techniques for the deeper, intrinsic muscles begin?

_____

_____

_____

_____

9   Which intrinsic muscles are important to secure pelvic stability and normalized gait?

_____

_____

_____

_____

_____

10   What symptoms can a woman experience if a symphysis pubis separation fails to heal correctly?

_____

_____

_____

_____

_____

_____

11   Explain the scar massage for extended postpartum recovery.

_____

_____

_____

_____

_____

_____

12   Describe the techniques for musculoskeletal balancing and support during extended postpartum recovery.

_____

_____

_____

_____

_____

13   How can muscle testing help in determining where a structural problem exists? How will the tested muscle respond to problem areas?

_____

_____

_____

_____

_____

14   What possible emotional reactions to the birth might emerge during extended postpartum? What can massage practitioners do to help their clients with these emotional challenges?

_____

_____

_____

_____

_____

15   What metabolic disorder can be mistaken for postpartum depression?

_____

_____

_____

_____

_____

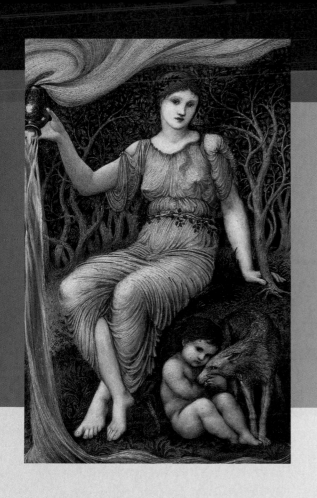

PART FOUR

Marketing
Strategies

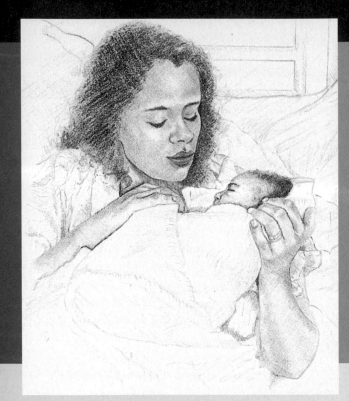

CHAPTER 24

Marketing Strategies

Objectives

On completion of this chapter, the student will be able to do the following:

1 Successfully market a prenatal massage business

2 Understand the importance of the resource list as a marketing tool

3 Learn the factors involved in offering services during labor

4 Have a successful initial contact with a potential client

5 Develop a client intake form

Marketing strategies are techniques to establish, grow and maintain a successful prenatal massage business and can be applied to a general massage practice as well. The marketing advice given here is intended to be used in conjunction with a hands-on, professional prenatal massage certification program, such as MotherMassage. Although there is unparalleled interest in the subject of pregnancy, labor, and postpartum massage, the lack of appropriate training and education should make a conscientious, responsible bodyworker pause before offering a massage to a pregnant woman. Although the intention to help is understandable, the lack of hands-on training and professional supervision represents a weak foundation for this specialized work.

Practitioners who are certified in this field must be wary of how the practice and the practitioner are advertised and described. Practitioners will need varying amounts of time before they have absorbed all of the science and are proficient in all bodywork techniques. Bodyworkers often like to use the words "specialist" or "expert" to describe themselves even after studying a new subject for a short period of time. It will take months or years of practice before practitioners should feel confident enough to rightfully call themselves experts.

All of the marketing strategies are taken directly from a lecture from the professional certification course, *MotherMassage: massage during pregnancy.*

Marketing Strategies

The good news about pregnancy is that it is not going to go away. There will always be an enormous supply of expectant women in need of nurturing attention.

Practitioners should remember that each pregnant woman knows several other women who are pregnant (e.g., coworkers, friends, sisters, sisters-in-law, and neighbors). Each new client can potentially refer the practitioner to all the other expectant women the client knows. A new client can also make referrals to her health care providers as well.

If a practitioner has a **private practice**, the growth of the business depends on the amount of time, energy, and creativity invested in it. Sole proprietors have to assume many roles in addition to being the massage practitioner. The sole proprietor is responsible for the public relations, advertising, bookkeeping, follow-ups, administrative work, and the expense and overhead of running a small business. The sole proprietor, however, is the sole beneficiary of the success of the practice.

Sole proprietors and health establishments can benefit from suggestions to increase their client base and establish successful practices. It is essential to be proactive about finding clientele but not aggressive. Massage practitioners should try as many of the following ideas as possible to increase their client base.

Business Cards

Bodyworkers never know when they will meet a pregnant woman or someone who knows one in need of a massage. A business card should list the types of services offered: prenatal, labor support, labor support classes, postpartum massage, infant

Touch Points

When it comes to marketing a practice, practitioners are limited only as far as their imagination limits them. Practitioners should think outside the box to develop and grow a successful prenatal/postpartum massage practice.

massage (infant massage classes), the name of the business, and complete contact information. Some business cards have appointment information printed on the back. An eye-catching logo that can be reproduced on all brochures and flyers can make a business card stand out from others.

Brochures and Pamphlets

The same logo used on the business card should be used on brochures and pamphlets so the business can be easily identified. A brochure should list and briefly describe the services; the benefits of prenatal, labor, and postpartum massage; a brief biography of the practitioner, and complete contact information. By mentioning the breadth of the prenatal practice, clients can start planning to work with the practitioner during pregnancy and well into postpartum recovery. If a brochure lists services with prices, the date when prices will change should be noted. Practitioners do not want someone to pick up an out-dated brochure and expect the service at the old rate.

Brochures should left in places that pregnant and postpartum women frequent, such as obstetricians' offices, midwifery practices, maternity clothing stores, prenatal yoga classes, and childbirth education classes. Practitioners should note where brochures were placed so the supply can be kept up-to-date. Bodyworkers should become familiar with doctors, nurses, and front desk staff and should ask for a brochure or pamphlet for their massage clientele.

Resource List

A **resource list** provides clients with a "yellow pages" of recommended pregnancy-related services (Box 24-1). The list should be dynamic and keep changing as names are added and subtracted. Each professional on the list should have a copy of the list, which indicates a willingness to refer clients to them and they can do likewise, but it also provides those on the list with a rich resource of professionals they may want to refer their clients to, with the massage practitioner as the main source.

Whenever anyone from the list sends a referral, the practitioner should take the time to write a hand-written thank you note and include no

---

BOX 24-1   *The Resource List*

A resource list should include health professionals, as well as ancillary services, that pregnant, laboring, and postpartum women use. Practitioners should be creative and think outside the box when developing this list. Some pregnancy-related categories that may be placed on a resource list are as follows:

Abuse hotline, acupuncture, Alexander technique, belly casting, belly dancing for pregnancy, birth announcements, birthing centers, breast pump rentals, cesarean section and vaginal birth after cesarean section (VBAC) information, childbirth educators, chiropractors, diaper services, doula services, exercise classes (only if they understand the importance of the transverse abdominis), furniture stores, herbalists, hospitals with birthing centers and water births, hypno-birthing, infant cardiopulmonary resuscitation (CPR) and first aid classes, grief counselors, lactation consultants, massage therapists, maternity clothing stores, mental health professionals, midwives, naturopaths, nursing bras, obstetricians, parenting newspapers, parenting support groups, physical therapists, prenatal yoga classes, prenatal swimming classes, and water birth locations and tub rentals.

Information can be added to this list on perineal massage and "Essentials for the Laboring Woman and New Mother" (see Box 19-13). Practitioners may have other categories for this list, but these are good starting points.

---

more than six business cards in the envelope. This thank you note can acknowledge the practitioner's appreciation for their support, and the extra business cards will most likely be given to the next few clients who walk in.

Client Referrals

A satisfied client is the best advertising. Clients should be encouraged to share their massage experiences with others who may be interested in booking an appointment.

In addition, practitioners should describe how beneficial prenatal massage is to the mother and the fetus, how labor support massage shortens labor and mediates pain, and how postpartum recovery is enhanced by appropriate massage techniques. This "word of mouth" can create an enormous amount of interest in people who may either be skeptical or scared or who were told it was unsafe to have a massage while pregnant. Practitioners need to educate people about the numerous benefits of massage during pregnancy and correct any

BOX 24-2 *Passive Income*

Passive income is additional income earned as a result of an investment of time or money. As long as practitioners are hourly wage earners, they earn only when they work. One way to generate more income is to devise ways to produce passive income, which is income produced without doing additional work. It may take a while to lay the foundation before this makes a significant change in annual income, but it is worth the investment of time and energy.

If practitioners continue as hourly wage earners, even as sole proprietors of their own businesses, any sick or vacation days are nonincome-producing days. Passive income can come in many forms: subrentals, selling products, or starting a parenting newspaper or a women's health co-op, but however it is done, passive income is a way to increase earnings.

BOX 24-3 *Passive Income: Dirty Diapers*

One of the first parenting newspapers and the paradigm for those that followed came about because of soiled diapers. In the late 1970s, two friends in New York City, one Australian and one American, were having lunch when they had to change their babies' diapers. As one of the young mothers came back from the bathroom, she remarked how large the space in the toilet was so she could easily lay her daughter down. They started comparing notes about which local restaurants and coffee houses had the best places for diaper changing.

This list grew and became the *Big Apple Parent Paper*. It started out as an over-sized newsletter and developed into a slick that was subsequently sold to a larger publishing house for a nice profit, which started from dirty diapers.

misconceptions and misinformation they may have been told.

Local Family or Parenting Newspapers

Family newspapers are grass-roots newspapers that address issues pertaining to young families that are free at local health food stores, maternity clothing stores, and obstetricians' offices. Practitioners can learn who advertises and gain other ideas about resources.

If there are no parenting newspapers in the area, one possibility is to start one. Someone could be hired on a commission basis to get advertisers, and it can be used as a regular forum for articles written about the benefits of prenatal massage. Other professionals can be invited to write about their practices. A parenting newspaper can provide **passive income** and become a major resource for new families and advertisers (Boxes 24-2 and 24-3).

Lectures and Demonstrations

Once practitioners have gained a modicum of proficiency in their work, they can give lectures and demonstrations and teach childbirth education classes and first-aid classes. Lectures can be tailored to the class (e.g., if it is an exercise class, talk about the core abdominals, and so on). Teachers are thrilled to have a speaker, and this can provide an opportunity to meet potential clients and clients have a chance to meet and speak with a practitioner. Bodyworkers should carry business cards and brochures to hand out. Even if only one person makes an appointment, she will go back to the class with a report about her massage, which may inspire others to make an appointment.

Women's Health Co-Op

A women's co-op may not be something a practitioner may want to do immediately, but a practitioner can grow in this direction. The adage "if you build it, they will come" has a lot of credence. A co-op can be a place for women to take classes, hear lectures, receive massages and other personal services during their pregnancies and recoveries, and meet other women. A co-op can be a very exciting suggestion for the right group of people.

Web Site

A **web site** can be an easy way to advertise a massage practice and to explain the scope of the practitioner's experience on the internet.

Advertising

Newspapers, local magazines, "penny savers," flyers, and brochures are effective ways of getting a massage practitioner's name out to the public. Advertising should be clear about who the target clientele is to avoid hearing from unwanted callers.

Networking Group

Networking groups (other professionals) and the local Chamber of Commerce have the same goals in mind: to establish and grow successful businesses. These people might not be involved with complimentary or holistic medicine, but the electrician and plumber may know someone who is pregnant and a practitioner or someone in the practice might need a good plumber.

Health Fair or Street Fair

During warmer months, street fairs or health fairs are usually well attended by local residents. Practitioners can rent a space or a table at a health or street fair. This is a wonderful way to sell products, advertise a practice, perhaps offer a quick example of bodywork, and make personal contact with prospective clients.

Day Care Centers and Nursery Schools

Practitioners can advise day care centers, nursery schools, and kindergarten teachers about available services. Where there are toddlers and young children, there is a very good chance that their families are growing. Practitioners can leave brochures, flyers, and business cards where the parents can see them when they come to pick up their children.

Baby Showers

Practitioners can speak at baby showers, which can also be a very entertaining way to communicate the benefits of prenatal massage by demonstrating a specific prenatal massage technique and then having the guests work on each other.

Birthing Centers/Maternity Units

Practitioners can take tours of **birthing centers** and hospital maternity floors and leave business cards and brochures where touring pregnant women can see them. This can help practitioners build a practice and learn about the local birthing centers and hospitals clients will be using.

Childbirth Education Classes

In addition to leaving business cards, brochures, and flyers, practitioners should attend a class or two to meet the childbirth educator and to provide an opportunity to meet potential clientele.

Practitioners can also gain first-hand experience of what is being taught, which can help them better address the clients' needs and concerns.

Media Event

Local newspapers often write about interesting and unique businesses. Practitioners can advise the local newspaper about the prenatal practice. To create a **media event,** practitioners should use their imaginations and tie-in the massage practice with something that is currently going on. Clippings can be mailed to other newspapers and local magazines, so the practitioner's name is on file for the next article on prenatal massage.

Written Articles

Practitioners can write articles for local newspapers and magazines describing the prenatal massage practice. Practitioners may decide to advertise in the same issue for additional coverage. Copies of these publications can be sent to other newspapers and magazines for their files.

Newsletters to Clients

Newsletters can keep clients in touch with the practitioner, and massage current in their minds. If they have not seen the practitioner in a while, a newsletter is a gentle way to urge them to call for an appointment.

Discounts

Practitioners can offer discounts for the first prenatal massage. This entices people to make that first appointment that will hopefully be followed by a second and third appointment.

Birthday and Holiday Cards

Practitioners should maintain a file and send birthday or holiday cards to clients. This is another wonderful way to gently remind someone to make an appointment. People feel good about treating themselves to a massage for a special occasion.

Gift Certificates

Special events, such as birthdays, anniversaries, seasonal holidays, Mother's day, baby showers, and giving birth are wonderful reasons for friends to provide a thoughtful gift for the expectant or new mother. During labor support classes, practitioners should remember to mention gift certificates so expectant fathers can treat their partners to a much-deserved postpartum massage.

If there is an expiration date on the gift certificate (many states do not allow expiration dates), or if a dollar value is cited, practitioners should keep track of the due date or when prices go up. On the certificate with a dollar value, practitioners can add the words "Prices subject to change." This will help avoid any discussion about higher pricing when the certificate is out-dated. As for expiration dates, it is a courtesy to contact the purchaser in advance of the deadline and advise them that the gift certificate will soon expire.

Practitioners may also want to consider adding the following on the gift certificate: "nontransferable" or "not redeemable for cash." These say that only the recipient of the certificate can use it and that in the event the massage is not desired, the cost of the certificate will not be refunded. These are optional additions to the gift certificate that serve to clarify business policies.

Massage Treatment Series

Clients appreciate having several appointments confirmed at a slightly discounted rate during their pregnancies. If a practitioner is thinking of expanding, renovating, or making a large purchase for his or her office, a **treatment series** is a wonderful way to raise capital without dipping into savings or seeking a bank loan. However, practitioners must remember that this initial check represents the entire series of massages. If a practice has budgeting difficulties, it may be hard to allocate and save this sum for bills and expenses.

Incentives

Loyalty should be rewarded, and long-term clients or those who make multiple referrals can be shown appreciation by giving them **client incentives** by charging them a reduced rate or thanking them with a thoughtful, personal gift at appropriate times during the year.

Massage during Labor

It is not at all uncommon for a pregnant woman to ask if a practitioner will be part of her labor team. This is one of the most complimentary and loving invitations a prenatal practitioner can receive. Practitioners should assist at labor at least once. Doing so will change a practitioner's attitude about massage work, will validate the reasons for doing prenatal massage, and will prove beyond any doubt how heroic, magnificent, and powerful women are.

However, there are certain considerations to discuss with the mother-to-be and her partner, if possible, before committing to attend a labor. These are seminal issues to agree on in writing to avoid any misunderstandings and to make sure the boundaries and expectations are understood and realistic (Box 24-4).

Making the Initial Client Contact

Client contact is the interaction and dialogue with clients. The first time a practitioner speaks with a potential new client, he or she should obtain some information from the client to help plan a treatment strategy. Practitioners should ask the following questions:

- What does the client need? Practitioners should not assume that they are pregnant until they tell you. It can be a devastating mistake if congratulations on her pregnancy are offered to a new client who is calling for care after a miscarriage. Practitioners should find out how the pregnancy or postpartum period is progressing and ask them what particular discomforts are bothering them.
- Who referred them? Practitioners should find out who referred them so a thank you note can be sent.
- Who is the client's obstetrician or midwife?
- What are the client's contact numbers? Home, work, and cell phone numbers should be obtained.
- Does the client have any preexisting conditions that might affect the pregnancy? These conditions include seizure disorders or diabetes mellitus.

Practitioners should then advise clients about the massage practice business policies. This includes telling the policy on arriving late, cancellations

BOX 24-4 — *Issues Regarding Attending a Labor*

Offering massage services to a client in labor is an opportunity to continue the nurturing work and loving support established with the client during pregnancy massage. Unlike obstetricians, midwives, or labor doulas whose 24-hours, 7-days a week availability is implicit in their work, a massage practitioner has to reorganize his or her schedule to accommodate the client. The following are some of the many considerations that should be contractually agreed to before attending the birth.

- Is the practitioner's participation approved by the facility or hospital?
- Will the practitioner be available at a moment's notice, 24/7? Or will the practitioner's hours be limited?
- Is a back-up system in place for the practitioner's practice? Is childcare available for the practitioner's family if needed?
- Where is the labor massage going to be done—at the client's home or at a facility?
- What are the arrangements for the practitioner's fees for services? Some people charge an hourly rate, others offer a flat fee, and some prefer a sliding scale. (Practitioners should be paid at least half the payment when the contract is signed, and the remaining fee can be remitted after the birth of the baby. The client can be sent an invoice with a self-addressed stamped envelop for her convenience.)
- What will happen if the practitioner gets to the birth and the laboring woman decides she does not want to be touched (which is not at all uncommon), and yet the practitioner's time has been allocated to be with her? Sometimes practitioners spend time running errands (or working with the partner) instead of massaging the mother. Conversely, what should the practitioner do if the contract was for a specific period of time and the client asks for more time?
- What if the birth outcome was unexpected (i.e., an emergency cesarean) and massage cannot be done? What happens if the medical team asks the massage practitioner to leave? (This is easy: the practitioner leaves graciously while offering best wishes to the mother.)

There are many factors to take into consideration when contracting to provide labor support because no one can ever know how labor will progress or how the laboring woman will feel. Whatever is agreed on, practitioners should get it in writing.

BOX 24-5 — *Charging for Services*

The amount practitioners charge should be commensurate with their experience, education, and skills. Where the work is being done (at the office or the client's home), the geographical location, what clients can afford, and what other practitioners within the area are charging should all be considered when setting fees.

Practitioners are being paid for the time allocated to a client, not necessarily what techniques are used during the hour. Clients should not be charged a premium just because they are pregnant.

After the appointment has been made, practitioners should confirm the correct date and time with the client. It is worthwhile to make the extra effort and call all the numbers the client has provided a day or two before the appointment to reconfirm. This way no-shows and misunderstandings about the appointment time can be avoided.

Practitioners can take this time to inform new client about the scope of their practice: pregnancy, labor support, and postpartum recovery, so she can start thinking about continuing with massage after the baby is born.

Client Intake Forms

Client intake forms include subjective, objective, assessment (analysis), and plan (SOAP) notes or other intake information. If a practitioner's place of business does not provide SOAP notes or a client intake form, one can be created (Figures 24-1 and 24-2).

This treatment plan can be customized to suit a practitioner's prenatal massage practice and should include the following elements:

1. Name
2. Address
3. Phone numbers
4. Occupation
5. Referred by…
6. Obstetrician or midwife's contact information
7. Maternal age
8. Gestational age and estimated due date
9. Previous pregnancies or miscarriages
10. Preexisting conditions
11. Any recent (within 5 years) surgeries, injuries, accidents, or traumas

(except when they are in labor!), price, and preferred method of payment (Box 24-5). Any other policies, such as no perfume, should be stated at this time. Practitioners can repeat this information on an out-going message so clients are alerted to these policies before arranging an appointment.

CLIENT INTAKE INFORMATION FORM

Name: _____ Date: _____

Address: _____ City: _____ State: _____ Zip: _____

Phone: (day) _____ (eve) _____ Date of Birth: _____

Occupation: _____ Employer: _____

Referred by: _____ Physician: _____

Previous experience with massage:

_____

Primary reason for appointment / areas of pain or tension:

_____

Emergency contact—name and number: _____

**Please mark (X) for all conditions that apply now. Put a (P) for past conditions,
an (F) for family history of illness.**

Pain Scale: minor-1   2   3   4   5   6   7   8   9   severe-10

_____ headaches, migraines	_____ chronic pain	_____ fatigue
_____ vision problems, contact lenses	_____ muscle or joint pain	_____ tension, stress
_____ hearing problems, deafness	_____ muscle, bone injuries	_____ depression
_____ injuries to face or head	_____ numbness or tingling	_____ sleep difficulties
_____ sinus problems	_____ sprains, strains	_____ allergies, sensitivities
_____ dental bridges, braces	_____ arthritis, tendonitis	_____ rashes, athletes foot
_____ jaw pain, TMJ problems	_____ cancer, tumors	_____ infectious diseases
_____ asthma or lung conditions	_____ spinal column disorders	_____ blood clots
_____ constipation, diarrhea	_____ diabetes	_____ varicose veins
_____ hernia	_____ pregnancy	_____ high/low blood pressure
_____ birth control, IUD	_____ heart, circulatory problems	
_____ abdominal or digestive problems	_____ other medical conditions not listed	

Explain any areas noted above:

_____

_____

Current medications, including aspirin, ibuprofen, herbs, supplements, etc.:

_____

_____

Surgeries: _____

Accidents: _____

Please list all forms and frequency of stress reduction activities, hobbies, exercise or sports participation:

_____

_____

FIGURE 24-1 ■ The standard client intake form for a prenatal practice. (From Fritz S, Grosenbach JM: *Mosby's essential sciences for therapeutic massage,* ed 2, St. Louis, 2004, Mosby.)

TREATMENT PLAN

Client Name:_____

Choose One: ☐ Original plan   ☐ Reassessment date_____

Short-term client goals:

_____

_____

Long-term client goals:

_____

_____

Therapist Objectives:

_____

_____

1) Frequency, 2) length, and 3) duration of visits:

1) _____   2) _____   3) _____

Progress "measurements" to be used: (Ex.— pain scale, range of motion, increased ability to perform function)

_____

_____

Dates of reassessment:

_____

Categories of massage methods to be used: (Ex.— relaxation, stress reduction, circulatory, lymphatic, neuromuscular, connective tissue, neurochemical, etc.)

_____

_____

Additional notes:

_____

_____

_____

Client Signature:_____   Date:_____

Therapist Signature:_____   Date:_____

FIGURE 24-2 ■ Treatment plan can be customized to suit a particular prenatal practice. (From Fritz S, Grosenbach JM: *Mosby's essential sciences for therapeutic massage,* ed 2, St. Louis, 2004, Mosby.)

12. Current medications
13. Pregnancy- or postpartum-related discomforts
14. Ask them to describe the pregnancy

When the massage is over, the practitioner can add any additional comments or treatment plans to the form. When the client's baby is born, the birth date, weight, gender, baby's name, and type of delivery can be added to the client's records.

In My Experience...

I received my New York state massage license in 1978. In 1979, I decided that I wanted to work exclusively with women and women's health issues. This was a year before my first pregnant client. I asked a client who her gynecologist was and made an appointment to meet him.

At the meeting, I brought a brochure I had printed called "Massage For Women" and left a few with him. Another patient came in for an examination and saw my flyer. Her cousin, a writer for the *New York Daily News,* was doing a feature article on massage therapy and was looking for a female practitioner to interview.

Within months of getting my license, I was featured in a 2-page article, complete with photos, in the *Sunday Daily News.* My phone rang off the hook, and my practice took off from there. When I sold my business in 2003, some of the same people from that article were still clients.

Follow your dreams, follow your heart, and success will follow you.

Summary

Establishing, growing, and maintaining a prenatal massage practice can be an exciting, creative, stimulating, and rewarding time for bodyworkers. The marketing ideas and suggestions in this chapter will work only if the practitioner is proactive. With imagination, determination, and a strong desire to succeed, the potential is limitless. Practitioners should also have the talent to support their claims of the value of prenatal massage.

REVIEW QUESTIONS

1 Describe at least a dozen marketing strategies.

_____

_____

_____

_____

_____

2 Why is a resource list such a valuable marketing tool?

_____

_____

_____

_____

_____

3 How does giving lectures enhance a profile as a prenatal practitioner?

_____

_____

_____

_____

4 What important information is needed from the initial client contact?

_____

_____

_____

_____

5 What are some of the questions that need to be discussed with a client about attending her labor?

_____

_____

_____

_____

_____

6 How is the decision made as to what to charge for massage services?

_____

_____

_____

_____

_____

7 What sort of client information should be contained in SOAP notes?

_____

_____

_____

_____

_____

Glossary

Abdominal muscles   Muscles that make up the core of the body: the rectus abdominis, external obliques, internal obliques. and the transverse abdominis.

Abdominal pressure   Uncomfortable feeling of pulling in the lower abdomen usually felt in the latter half of pregnancy as the uterus begins to get heavy.

Abortifacient   Herb capable of causing a miscarriage.

Abortion   Termination of pregnancy before the fetus is viable (i.e., 20 weeks' gestation).

Abruptio placentae   Premature separation of a normally implanted placenta from the uterine wall.

Acceptance   Emotional and psychological acknowledgement of the pregnancy.

Acroesthesia   Tingling or numbness in the hands.

Active exercise   Client putting her own limbs and joints through range of motion.

Active phase   Phase during the first stage of labor when the cervix dilates 4 to 7 cm.

Acupressure   A 4000-year-old Chinese massage system that treats points along meridians or energy channels.

Acupuncture points   Specific treatment points along a meridian or energy channel.

Acute   Condition that develops quickly, lasts a short time, and disappears.

Adaptations   Changes and modifications the body makes as a result of the pregnancy.

Adductor muscle   Thigh muscles that move toward the midline of the body. In applied kinesiology, the adductors reflex to the reproductive system.

Advertising   Marketing tool to grow and increase a massage practice.

Afebrile   Absence of a fever.

Afterbirth   Expulsion of the placenta and membranes after the birth of the newborn.

Afterpains   Uterine cramping after childbirth caused by alternating relaxation and contraction.

Aldosterone   Adrenal cortex hormone that controls reabsorption of sodium.

Alpha fetoprotein (AFP)   Fetal antigen; elevated levels of AFP in the amniotic fluid or adult serum during pregnancy are associated with neural tube defects.

Alkalosis   Increase above the normal pH range of the body.

Alveolar lumen   Secretory cells of the alveoli synthesize the milk and transfer it to the alveolar lumen of the breasts.

Amenorrhea   Absence of menstrual periods.

Amniocentesis   Prenatal test performed transabdominally in the second trimester for certain genetic disorders.

Amnion   Inner membrane of the two fetal membranes that form the sac and contain the fetus and the fluid that surrounds it.

Amniotic fluid   Fluid surrounding the fetus within the amniotic sac that allows fetal movement, prevents heat loss, and absorbs shocks.

Amniotic sac   Membrane that surrounds and protects the fetus.

Analgesia   Absence of pain without loss of consciousness.

Analgesic   Medication or agent that relieves pain.

Anemia   Condition caused by a decrease in erythrocytes, hemoglobin, or both.

Anencephaly   Absence of a cerebrum, cerebellum, and flat bones of the skull.

Anesthesia   Partial or complete absence of sensation with or without loss of consciousness.

Angiomas   Dilated blood vessels.

Anovulatory   Failure of the ovaries to produce, mature, or release eggs.

Anoxia   Absence of oxygen.

Antepartum   Before birth.

Anterior tilt   Displacement of the pelvis anterior caused by the forward shifting of the woman's center of gravity.

Antidepressants   Medicinal mood elevators for depression.

Anxiety   Feeling of uneasiness, distress, and tension often connected with sympathetic arousal response.

Apgar scores   Numeric rating of the condition of a newborn obtained at 1 and 5 minutes of age; developed by Dr. Virginia Apgar.

Applied kinesiology   System that evaluates the body's function through dynamic muscle testing.

Appropriate   Fitting, right, and supportive of the physical changes of pregnancy, labor and postpartum.

Areola   Pigmented ring of tissue surrounding the nipple.

Aromatherapy   Use of essential herbs during a massage.

Arrhythmias   Irregular heart action causing absence of rhythm.

Artificial reproductive technology (ART)   Use of fertility treatments and technology to conceive.

Artificial rupture of membranes (AROM)   Rupture of membranes using a plastic amniohook or surgical clamp.

Asynclitism   Oblique presentation of the fetal head at the superior strait of the pelvis.

Attention focusing   Comfort measure during labor that helps the laboring woman concentrate on something other than the pain.

Augmentation (of labor)   Stimulation of ineffective uterine contractions after labor has begun but not progressing satisfactorily

Back labor   Painful labor felt in the lower back often caused by a fetal occiput posterior position.

Backaches   Pain in the back muscles and joints.

Bag of waters   Lay term for amniotic sac containing amniotic fluid and fetus.

Ballottement   Movability of a floating object such as a fetus; diagnostic technique using palpation: a floating object when pushed moves away and returns to touch the examiner's hand.

Bath/shower   Comfort measure during labor using water that appreciably minimizes pain.

Bearing down   Pushing the baby down the birth canal during labor.

Bed rest   Confinement to bed for a period of time during pregnancy.

Bereavement   Feelings of loss, pain, desolation, and sadness after the death of a loved one.

Beta-endorphins   Endogenous opioids secreted by the pituitary gland that act on the central and peripheral nervous systems to reduce pain. Beta-endorphin is the most potent endorphin.

Bicornuate uterus   Structural abnormality of the uterus that may either be a double or single organ with two horns.

Binovular   Twins developed from two separate ova fertilizes by two separate sperm; fraternal twins.

Birth rate   Number of lives births per 1000 population per year.

Birthing centers   Women's centers that are family-centered where women can give birth without medication or interventions.

Bladder 67   Acupuncture point on the outside of the little toe nail that turns fetal presentation and draws energy downward; pressing is contraindicated during pregnancy but can be effective in turning a breech presentation (with moxibustion) in weeks 37 or 38 of pregnancy.

Blastocyst Stage of development of the embryo that follows the morula that consists of an outer layer and a hollow sphere of cells forming a cavity.

Blood clots Coagulation of blood to prevent hemorrhage.

Blood volume Amount of blood within the circulatory system.

Bloody show Operculum or mucous plug that fills the opening of the cervix.

Body image Person's subjective concept of his or her physical appearance.

Body mechanics Proper use of the body during daily activities or while doing a massage.

Bonding Process by which parents form an attachment and emotional relationship with their infant.

Bradley method Partner-coached childbirth using breathing techniques.

Bradycardia Slow heart rate.

Braxton Hicks contractions Intermittent, painless uterine contractions occurring during pregnancy; they become stronger and more apparent in the last trimester and are sometimes mistaken for true labor contractions.

Breakthrough bleeding Loss of blood between menstrual periods.

Breast feeding Nursing.

Breast soreness Tenderness and engorgement of the breasts.

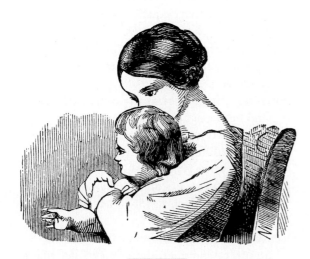

Our Little Ones.

Breathing techniques Comfort measures during labor that feature specific, rhythmic breathing techniques.

Breech presentation Nonvertex presentation; refers to the presentation of the buttocks or feet instead of the head.

Broad uterine ligament Posterior ligament attached to the internal pelvic cavity walls.

Brochures Marketing tool that may describe the kind of services offered by a practitioner; a pamphlet.

Buerger's disease Disorder affecting the muscles and blood vessels of the legs.

Business cards Small cards with business contact information.

Cardiac output Volume of blood ejected from the left ventricle in 1 minute.

Cardinal movements of labor Mechanism of labor in a vertex presentation; includes engagement, descend, flexion, internal rotation, extension, external rotation, and expulsion.

Cardiovascular system Circulatory system made up of the heart, veins, arteries, and blood.

Carpal tunnel syndrome Pressure and inflammation of the median nerve with subsequent swelling, pain and weakness of hand muscles.

Castor oil Powerful laxative sometimes used to stimulate labor.

Catecholamines Stress compounds (i.e., epinephrine, norepinephrine).

Caul Hood of fetal membranes covering the fetal head during birth.

Cephalic Pertaining to the head.

Cephalopelvic disproportion (CPD) Fetal head cannot fit through maternal pelvic out-let because of large size, shape, or position.

Cerclage Use of nonabsorbable stitches to keep a prematurely dilating cervix closed.

Cervical ripening Process of physical softening and distension of the cervix in preparation for labor and birth.

Cervix Lowest and most narrow ("neck") end of the uterus situated between the external os and the body (corpus) of the uterus and its lower end extends into the vagina.

Cesarean birth (section) Birth of the fetus, membranes, and placenta through an incision in the abdominal wall and uterus.

Childbirth education classes Classes that provide instruction on various birthing techniques, such as Lamaze or Bradley.

Chloasma Increased pigmentation on the face during pregnancy; the "mask of pregnancy."

Cholestasis Cessation of bile excretion.

Chorion Fetal membrane closest to the intrauterine wall that gives rise to the placenta and continues as the outer membrane surrounding the amnion.

Chorionic villi Small vascular protrusions on the chorion surface that project into the uterus.

Chorionic villi sampling (CVS) Removal of fetal tissue from placenta for genetic testing.

Cleft palate Congenital abnormality with an incomplete closure of the palate.

Client contact Interaction and dialoguing with clients.

Client incentives Special perks to encourage the clientele to refer other clients.

Client intake forms Forms that include SOAP notes or other intake information.

Climacteric Period of a woman's life when she passes from a reproductive to a nonreproductive state with regression of ovarian function; also called climacterium.

Clotting factor Coagulating factor or fibrinogenic activity to prevent hemorrhages at labor.

Coagulating factor Clotting factor or fibrinogenic activity.

Coccydynia Pain in the coccyx caused by either soft tissue damage or osseous dislocation.

Cold (hot) packs Comfort measure of heat or cold often used between contractions on the lower back or lower abdomen.

Colostrum Premilk rich in antibodies and high in fat and protein; it has a laxative effect that speeds the elimination of meconium.

Common discomforts Typical physical aches and pains of pregnancy.

Conception Union of sperm and egg resulting in fertilization; formation of the one-celled zygote.

Conception age In fetal development, the number of completed weeks since conception. Since the exact time of conception is usually difficult to ascertain, conception age is estimated at 2 weeks less than gestational age.

Conceptus Embryo or fetus, fetal membranes, amniotic fluid, and the fetal portion of the placenta.

Congenital Present at birth.

Constipation Difficulty or inability to have a bowel movement.

Constructive rest position Recumbent position with legs bent, feet wider than the shoulders, and placed 12 to 15 inches away from the hips to relax and shorten the overstretched psoas muscles.

Contraction (uterine) Tightening of uterine muscle; during labor, contractions dilate the cervix.

Contraindication Something to avoid.

Cornua Horn-shaped.

Corpus luteum Yellow body. After the follicle ruptures, it develops into a yellow structure that secretes progesterone and some estrogen in the second half of the menstrual cycle. If impregnation occurs, it continues to produce hormones until the placenta takes over this function.

Corticotrophin-releasing hormone Hypothalamus hormone that regulates the release of cortisol.

Cortisol Adrenal stress hormone.

Counterpressure Pressure to the sacral area during a uterine contraction.

Couvade syndrome Phenomenon of expectant fathers experiencing pregnancy-like symptoms.

Craniosacral therapy Gentle bodywork technique that provides balance to the craniosacral system.

Crowning Stage of birth when the top of the fetal head can be seen at the vagina.

Cultural differences Comparative distinctions between different ethnicities.

Cytomegalovirus (CMV) Cause of the most common cause of congenital viral infections in humans, affecting 1% of newborns. May result in birth defects.

Decidua Mucous membrane, lining of the uterus, or endometrium of pregnancy that is shed after birth.

Deep vein thrombosis (DVT) Thrombo-embolism in the deep veins of the legs.

Dehiscence Rupture of a surgical wound or scar.

Delivery (birth) Expulsion of the fetus with placenta and membranes by the mother or extraction by medical practitioner.

Depression Intensive and pervasive mood disorder with sadness and emotional ability.

De Quervain's syndrome Inflammation of the radial nerve resulting in pain and weakening in the thenar region.

Descent Movement down the birth canal.

Diabetes mellitus Systemic disorder of carbohydrate, protein, and fat metabolism; caused by deficient insulin production or ineffective use of insulin at a cellular level.

Diabetogenic Causing diabetes.

Diaphoresis Excessive sweating.

Diastasis recti abdominis Separation of the bellies of the rectus abdominis along the linea alba.

Dick-Read method Childbirth approach based on the premise that fear causes muscle tension, pain and greater fear. The technique includes teaching the physiological process of labor, exercises to improve muscle tone and techniques to reduce fear and assist in relaxation.

Diethylstilbestrol (DES) Drug given to pregnant women from the 1970s to 1990s to prevent miscarriages. Female fetuses are predisposed to reproductive tract malformations and dysplasia if their mothers ingested this drug during pregnancy.

Dilation Opening, stretching, or widening (of the cervix).

Discounts Charging less money for a service; a client incentive.

Diuresis Excessive urination.

Dizygotic Twins from two eggs and two sperm.

Dizziness Vertigo.

Domestic violence Abuse at home by the husband or domestic partner.

Doula Nonmedical labor or postpartum experienced assistant.

Down syndrome Genetic cause of mental impairment.

Draping Using sheets and towels to cover the client.

Due date Approximate date the baby will be born. See *Gestation.*

Dysfunctional labor Abnormal uterine contractions that prevent normal cervical effacement and dilation.

Dyspareunia Painful sexual intercourse.

Dysplasia Abnormal development of tissues or organs.

Dyspnea Difficult or labored breathing, snoring.

Dystocia Prolonged, painful, and difficult birth.

Dysuria Painful urination.

Eclampsia Severe form of gestational hypertension accompanied by convulsions and sometimes death.

Ectopic pregnancy Implantation of the fertilized ovum outside the uterine cavity, including the abdomen, fallopian tubes, or ovaries.

Edema Excessive interstitial fluid or swelling.

Effacement Thinning or shortening of the cervix during late pregnancy, labor, or both.

Effleurage Long, gliding stroke used in Swedish massage.

Electronic fetal monitoring (EFM) Electronic surveillance of the fetal heart rate by external and internal methods.

Embryo Conceptus from the second or third week of development until about the eighth week when mineralization of the skeleton begins.

Emmenagogue Herbs pertaining to menstruation.

Emotional adjustment Acceptance of the pregnancy or parenthood.

Emotional lability Rapid mood changes from sadness to joy and cheerfulness.

Emotional support Help of family, friends, and professionals on an emotional level.

Encephalocele Herniation of the brain and meninges through a defect in the skull.

Endocrine system Glandular system of the body responsible for the production and secretion of hormones.

Endogenous Made within one's own body.

Endometrium   Inner lining of the uterus that undergoes changes caused by hormones during menstruation or pregnancy.

Endorphins   See *Beta-endorphins*.

Energy work   Gentle techniques that work with the human energy biofield to encourage balance.

Engagement   Entrance of the fetal presenting part into the superior pelvic strait and the beginning of descent through the pelvic canal.

Engorgement   Distension or vascular congestion; the process of swelling of the breast tissue caused by an increase in blood and lymph supply to the breasts that precedes lactation.

Engrossment   Paternal bonding with the newborn; can be used to describe parental preoccupation, interest, and bonding.

Environmental factors   External influences, such as temperature, light, sound, air quality, and cleanliness.

Epidural (block)   Regional anesthesia produced by injection of a local anesthetic into the epidural (peridural) space.

Epinephrine   Stress compound produced by the adrenal glands; also known as adrenaline.

Episiotomy   Surgical incision of the perineum at the end of the second stage of labor to facilitate birth by widening the vaginal outlet.

Epistaxis   Nosebleeds.

Erythema   Inflammation of the skin or mucous membranes.

Esophageal reflux   Regurgitation of gastric acids, causing a burning sensation in the esophagus.

Essential oils   Pure plant and flower extracts made into oils used in aromatherapy.

Estradiol   An estrogen.

Estriol   Major metabolic of estrogen that increases during the second half of pregnancy.

Estrone   An estrogen.

Exfoliation   Process by which the uterus does not scar at the site of placental attachment.

Exhalation pushing   Bearing down and pushing using an exhalation breath.

External cephalic version (ECV)   Manual attempt to turn the fetus into vertex position.

External obliques   Abdominal muscles that facilitate forward flexion of the trunk and lateral flexion and rotation.

Failure to thrive   Condition where the neonate or infant's growth and development is below the norms for its age.

Fallopian tubes   Two oviducts that extend laterally from each side of the uterus through which the ovum travels; also called uterine tubes.

False labor   Uterine contractions that are irregular, do not result in cervical dilation, are felt anterior, do not become stronger, and last for only 20 seconds.

False pelvis   Part of the pelvis superior to a plane passing trough the brim or outlet.

Fatigue   Tiredness or exhaustion often caused by hormonal adjustments during pregnancy.

Femoral vein   Deep leg vein of the thigh where blood clots may aggregate.

Fertility   Ability to reproduce.

Fetus   Conceptus after 12 weeks' gestation.

Fetal ejection reflex   The secretion of catecholamines during labor to help push the baby through the birth canal.

Fetal monitoring   Technological system that records the fetal heart rate often used during labor to make sure the fetus is not in distress.

Fetal position   Relation of the designated part on the presenting fetal part to the front, sides, and back of the maternal pelvis.

Fetal presentation   Fetal body parts that enter the maternal pelvis first. Three possible presentations are cephalic (vertex), breech, or shoulder.

Fibrinogenic activity   Blood clotting activity, coagulation.

Fibrinolytic   Break down of blood clots.

First stage of labor   Stage of labor from the onset of regular uterine contractions through full dilation (10 cm) of the cervix.

First trimester   Period of time from conception to week 13 of pregnancy.

Focus   Comfort technique to help the laboring woman maintain concentration on her labor and what she needs to do to stay calm.

Folic acid anemia   Folic acid deficiency during conception and in early pregnancy increases the risk of birth defects such as neural tube defects, cleft lip, and cleft palate; second most common anemia of pregnancy.

Follicle-stimulating hormone (FSH)   Hormone produced by the anterior pituitary during the first half of the menstrual cycle; stimulates the development of the graafian follicle.

Footling (incomplete) breech presentation   - Presentation of one or both feet.

Forceps   Curve-bladed instrument used to apply traction and assist birth.

Fourth stage of labor   Initial period of postpartum recovery lasting the first 2 hours after expulsion of the placenta.

Fourth trimester   Puerperium.

Frank breech presentation   Presentation of buttocks with hips flexed so the thighs are against the abdomen.

Fundus   Dome-shaped upper portion of the uterus.

Gall bladder 34   Acupuncture point behind each fibular head to treat backaches.

Gamete intrafallopian transfer (GIFT)   Form of ART that transfers an ova and washed sperm into the fallopian tubes.

Gastrointestinal disturbances   Constipation, esophageal reflux, gas, and heartburn.

Gastrointestinal system   Digestive and elimination system of the body.

Gate control theory   Theory to explain the underlying perception of pain. The capacity of nerve pathways to transmit pain is reduced or completely blocked by using distraction techniques.

General   With regards to bodywork, in total or the whole body.

Gestation   Pregnancy, or period of intrauterine development from conception through birth. Human gestation is approximately 280 days, or 40 weeks, but birth within 2 weeks, either before or after 40 weeks, is normal.

Gestational age   In fetal development, the number of completed weeks counting from the first day of the last menstrual cycle.

Gestational glucose intolerance   Glucose intolerance first recognized during pregnancy; also known as gestational diabetes mellitus.

Gift certificates   Marketing tool bought by one person and given to another.

Glucose tolerance test   Test used to screen for gestational diabetes.

Gluteus maximus   Posterior pelvis muscles whose main function is trunk extension; in applied kinesiology, these muscles reflex to the reproductive system.

Glycosuria   Presence of glucose (sugar) in the urine.

Golgi tendon organs   Neuromuscular organs located within the tendons close to the musculotendinous junction; stimulation can tighten or relax a muscle.

Gonadotrophin-releasing hormone (GnRH)   Hypothalamus hormone that stimulates the pituitary gland to secrete FSH and LH.

Gravida   Pregnant woman.

Grief/grieving process   Complex emotional, physiological, social, and cognitive response to the death of a loved one.

Headaches   Pain in the head that can sometimes be severe or migraine.

Heartburn   Reflux of gastric acid or indigestion.

HELLP syndrome   Condition characterized by hemolysis, elevated liver enzymes, and low platelet count; a form of severe preeclampsia.

Hematocrit   Volume of red blood cells in circulating blood.

Hemoconcentration   Increase in the number of red blood cells in proportion to the volume.

Hemoglobin   Component of red blood cells consisting of globin, a protein, and an organic iron compound.

Hemolysis   Break down of blood cells and liberation of its hemoglobin.

Hemorrhage   Excessive bleeding.

Hemorrhoid   Varicosity of the anus.

Hematuria   Blood in urine.

Herbal remedies   Medicines made from plant, root, bark, flower, and leaf sources.

High risk   Increased possibility of suffering harm, damage, injury, loss, or death.

Hip displacement   Subluxation of the hip.

Homan sign (check)   Evaluation for presence of phlebothrombosis in the deep veins of the calf by dorsiflexing an extended leg.

Hormone   Chemical substance produced by an organ or gland to stimulate functional activity or secretion.

Hormonal imbalances   Chemical imbalances within the endocrine system.

Human chorionic gonadotrophin (hCG)   - Biological marker in pregnancy tests manufactured by the chorionic villi.

Human placental lactogen (HPL)   Hormone produced by the placenta.

Hydramnios   Excessive amounts of amniotic fluid; polyhydramnios.

Hyperemesis gravidarum   Excessive vomiting during pregnancy characterized by nausea, fluid loss, electrolyte imbalance, and weight loss.

Hyperplasia   Increase in new cells or tissue formation.

Hypertrophy   Enlargement of existing cells.

Hyperventilation   Rapid and shallow, or prolonged and deep, respiration.

Hypnobirthing   Use of hypnosis or hypnotherapy for pain control during labor.

Hypnosis   Induced state of deep relaxation.

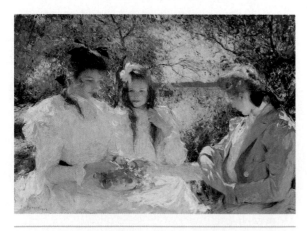

Portrait of My Daughters, 1907. Frank W. Benson, American (1862-1951). Courtesy Worcester Art Museum, Worcester, Mass.

Hypocapnia   Low levels of carbon dioxide.

Hypoperistalsis   Sluggish bowel.

Hypotension   Low muscle tone.

Hypovolemia   Low blood volume.

Hypoxia   Low levels of oxygen.

Iatrogenic   Caused by a health care professional.

Iliac vein   Deep vein of the thigh where blood clots may aggregate.

Iliopsoas (iliacus and psoas) muscle   Intrinsic pelvic muscle involved in leg flexion and minimal lateral rotation and abduction of the thigh; important muscle in gait mechanism.

Imagery   Comfort measure during labor that involves the mind in active visualization.

Implantation   Embedding of the fertilized ovum in the uterine mucosa.

Incompetent cervix   Cervix that is unable to remain closed during pregnancy.

Induction   Initiating labor by natural or pharmaceutical means.

Inferior vena cava   Major abdominal blood vessel.

Infertility   Inability or difficulty conceiving.

Insomnia   Inability to sleep.

Integumentary system   Skin system.

Internal obliques   Abdominal muscles, deep to the external obliques and the rectus abdominis, that assist with trunk flexion and lateral flexion and rotation.

Interstitial fluid   Fluid within the tissues or edema.

Interventions   Usually medical in nature, a way to speed up or enhance the rhythm of labor.

Intracytoplasmic sperm injection (ICSI)   ART that injects the sperm directly into the ovum.

Intradermal water blocks   Comfort measure during labor where water is injected into specific points in the lower back.

Intrapartum   During labor and birth.

Introitus   Entrance into a canal or cavity such as the vagina.

In utero   In the uterus.

In vitro fertilization (IVF)   ART using a technique that fertilizes the ovum in a glass tube.

Involuntary Primary uterine contractions of labor, called primary powers, that start labor.

Involution Rolling or turning inward; reduction in the size of the uterus after birth and its return to its prepregnant condition.

Ischemia/ischemic Local and temporary reduction or loss of blood.

Joint mobilization Putting each joint through its range of motion to locate resistance.

Kangaroo care Skin-to-skin contact with mother or father and newborn.

Kegel exercises Exercises to strengthen the pubococcygeal muscles.

Keloid Irregular, dimensional, raised scar tissue; overgrowth of connective tissue.

Kenbiki Rhythmic rocking stroke along a muscle for assessment and general relaxation.

Labor Process by which the fetus, membranes, and placenta are expelled.

Labor complications Difficulties that may occur during labor.

Lactation Function or period of milk secretion.

Lamaze method Type of childbirth preparation developed in the 1950s by French obstetrician, Fernand Lamaze, to minimize fear and the perception of pain by employing physical and mental preparation.

Lanugo Downy hair on the fetus and parts of the newborn after birth.

Large intestine 4 The acupuncture point found in the webbing of the thumbs that may initiate labor and speed up a prolonged labor; contraindicated during pregnancy but may be very effective in controlling pain and speeding up labor.

Latching-on Grasping the entire areola of the nipple into the newborn's mouth for effective nursing.

Latent phase Longest phase of the first stage of labor when the cervix dilates from 0 to 3 cm.

Leg cramps/Charley horse Spasms of the calf or leg.

Let-down reflex Milk ejection reflex.

Letting-go phase Interdependent phase after birth in which the new mother and family move forward with interacting members.

Leukorrhea White or yellow discharge from the cervical canal or vagina that can be either normal or caused by a pathological condition.

Libido Sexual desire.

Lightening Sensation of decreased abdominal distension produced by the uterine descent into the pelvic cavity as the fetus settles into the pelvis; usually occurs 2 weeks before the onset of labor in nulliparas.

Linea alba Perpendicular fascial sheath that provides a continuous, interconnected framework for the abdominal core muscles.

Linea nigra Dark line seen in some women that appears on the middle of the abdomen and extends from the symphysis pubis toward the umbilicus.

Lithotomy position Position where the pregnant woman lies on her back with her legs flexed and abducted thighs drawn to her chest.

Liver 3 Acupuncture point found bilaterally between the first and second toes that may initiate labor and speed up a prolonged labor, also has water influences and can be judiciously stimulated (a single count of 6) to treat common discomforts of pregnancy such as breast soreness, carpal tunnel syndrome, and edema, although generally contraindicated during pregnancy.

Lochia Normal postpartum vaginal discharge.

Lochia alba Lightest lochia that follows serosa from about the 10 days postpartum to 2 to 6 weeks after childbirth.

Lochia rubra Red, blood-tinged vaginal flow following birth and lasting 2 to 4 days.

Lochia serosa Serous, pink or brown watery vaginal flow that follows lochia rubra until about 10 days postpartum.

Lomilomi An ancient Hawaiian technique that uses rhythmic movements.

Luteinizing hormone (LH) Anterior pituitary hormone that stimulated ovulation and the development of the corpus luteum.

Lying-in Expression used for puerperium.

Macrosomia The condition in which a newborn has a large birth weight.

Manual lymphatic drainage Specific form of physiotherapy to empty and decompress lymph pathways supports the immune system and encourages toxin removal.

Manual version   Abdominal manipulation performed by a doctor or midwife to turn breech presentation into a vertex presentation; massage practitioners are strongly advised not to attempt this.

Marketing strategies   Techniques to establish, grow, and maintain a practice.

Mask of pregnancy   Chloasma.

Massage   Manipulation of the soft tissues of the body.

Massage during labor   Support during labor consisting of counterpressure techniques, stroking, relaxation techniques to speed up labor and keep the woman calm and focused.

Mastitis   Infection of the breast usually confined to a milk duct.

Maternal role adaption   Process a woman goes through in adjusting to motherhood; three phases are: taking-in, taking hold, and letting go.

Meatus   Opening from an internal structure to the outside.

Meconium   Neonate intestinal waste.

Media event   Organizing press, television, or radio coverage of a business event.

Melanocyte-stimulating hormone (MSH)   Hormone increased during pregnancy that results in hyperpigmentation.

Melasma gravidarum   Chloasma.

Metastatic   Spreading of cancer cells from site of original to other tissues and structures.

Micturition   Urination.

Midwife/midwifery   The art and practice of helping and assisting a woman in labor and giving birth.

Milk ejection reflex   Release of milk caused by contraction of myoepithelial cells within the milk glands in response to oxytocin.

Miscarriage   The loss of a fetus before the twentieth week; spontaneous abortion.

Mobility   The ability to move and walk around.

Monozygotic   Identical twin.

Mood disorders/mood swings   Disorders with an emotional state as primary feature.

Morbidity   Injury.

Morning sickness   Nausea and vomiting that affects many women during the first trimester of pregnancy.

Mortality   Death.

Morula   Solid mass of cells in the developmental stage of the fertilized egg.

Moxibustion   Use of a heated herb (mugwort) to treat acupuncture points.

Mucous plug   See *Operculum*.

Multiple pregnancy   Pregnancy with more than one fetus.

Multigravida   Woman who has been pregnant two or more times before.

Multipara   Woman who has carried two or more pregnancies to viability whether they ended in live births or stillbirths.

Muscle testing   Dynamic process of testing muscles to determine where a weakness may occur.

Musculoskeletal system   System of muscles, bones, and joints.

Myofascial release   Massage technique of the connective tissues that employs slow, stretching movements to evaluate and relieve fascial restrictions.

Myometrium   Muscle of the uterus.

Narcotics   Drugs or medication.

Nasal and sinus congestion   Stuffiness in the sinus cavities.

Natal   Pertaining to birth.

Nausea   Morning sickness with or without vomiting.

Neonate   Newborn.

Nesting instinct   Rush of energy before labor that lets the expectant mother clean and prepare her home for the baby's arrival.

Networking   Business tool to meet various people from all walks of life.

Neural tube   Tube formed from the fusion of the neural folds from which the brain and spinal cord develop.

Neural tube defect   Improper development of the neural tube resulting is malformation of brain or spinal cord.

Neurological system   The system of the body made up of the brain, spinal cord, and nerves.

Neurolymphatic reflexes   Specific points used in applied kinesiology that help strengthen their related muscles and organs.

Newsletters   Effective marketing tool to stay in contact with clients.

Nipple stimulation   Natural way to initiate labor.

Norepinephrine   Noradrenalin; a catecholamine.

Nulligravida   Woman who has never been pregnant.

Nullipara   Woman who has not yet carried a pregnancy to viability.

Nursing   Breastfeeding.

Obstetrics   The art and science of caring for a woman during pregnancy, labor, and puerperium.

Occiput   Back of the skull or head.

Occiput anterior   Back of the fetal head presented forward (face backward).

Occiput posterior   Back of the fetal head presented backward against the maternal sacrum.

Oligohydramnios   Small amount or absence of amniotic fluid.

Operculum   Mucous plug that fills the cervical canal during pregnancy.

Oral cavity   The mouth.

Orgasms   Sexual climaxes.

Os   Mouth or opening.

Ovum   Female sex cell.

Oxytocics   Drugs that cause uterine contractions, thereby accelerating childbirth and preventing postpartum hemorrhaging.

Oxytocin   Hormone produced by the posterior pituitary that stimulates uterine contractions and the release of milk (milk let-down).

Pain control   Ability to minimize the pain reaction.

Palmar erythema   Rash on the palms associated with pregnancy.

Palpation   Examination performed by touching and exploring with the hands.

Paracervical block   Regional anesthesia into the lower uterine segment.

Parental adjustment   Process a person goes through in adapting to the parental role; there are three sages: expectations, reality and transition to mastery.

Parenting newspapers   Local newspapers for families.

Parity (para)   Number of past pregnancies that have reached viability regardless of whether they were live births or stillbirths.

Partner/spouse   Domestic partner or husband.

Parturient   Woman giving birth.

Parturition   Process of birthing.

Passageway   Birth canal.

Passenger   Fetus during birth.

Passive exercise   Practitioner placing the client's joints through their range of motion.

Passive income   Additional income earned as a result of an investment of time or money.

Pelvic squeeze   Double hip squeeze or "clothes pin" to reposition the pelvic bones.

Pelvic station   Position of the fetal head within the pelvis; numbers start at -4 at the false pelvis, 0 at the true pelvis, and +4 at the perineum.

Pelvic tilt   Exercise to strengthen and shorten the abdominal muscles and elongate the lumbar spine.

Perinatal   Pertaining to the time and process of giving birth or being born.

Perineal massage   Massage of the vaginal region performed by the client on herself in preparation for labor.

Perineum   Area between the vagina and rectum on the female and between the scrotum and rectum on the male.

Peristalsis   Wavelike movements of muscular contraction and relaxation propelling contents through a tubular organ.

Phase   Three subdivisions of stages one and two of labor: latent, active, and transition phases.

Phlebitis   Inflammation of the veins with accompanying pain and tenderness along the course of the vein, inflammatory swelling and edema below the obstruction and discoloration of the skin because of injury or bruise.

Physiology   How the body functions.

Pica   Unusual cravings during pregnancy (clay, dirt, laundry starch).

Piriformis   Intrinsic muscle of the hips and a lateral rotator.

Pitocin   Synthetic oxytocin administered to initiate or speed up labor or expulsion of the placenta.

Pitting edema   Possible sign of preeclampsia or eclampsia when the impression made on the client's ankle fails to fill in after 10 to 30 seconds; massage is contraindicated with the presence of pitting edema.

Placenta   "Flat cake" in Latin; afterbirth; specialized vascular disk-shaped organ for maternal-fetal gas and nutrient exchange.

Placenta accrete   Invasion of the uterine muscle by the placenta making separation from the muscle difficult if not impossible.

Placenta previa   Placenta that is normally implanted in the lower segment of the uterus and is typed according to proximity to the cervical os: total: completely occludes the os; partial: does not occlude the os completely; marginal: placenta encroaches on the margin of the intern cervical os.

Plasma fibrinogen   Clot-making enzyme.

Polarity   Gentle energy technique that seeks to achieve energy balance.

Polyhydramnios   Excessive amounts of amniotic fluid.

Polyuria   Excessive secretion and discharge of urine from the kidneys.

Position   Relationship of a chosen fetal reference point, such as the occiput, on the presenting part of the fetus to its location in the front, back, or sides of the maternal pelvis.

Positive signs of pregnancy   Definite indicators of pregnancy (i.e., fetal heartbeat, fetal movement, and so on).

Posterior pelvic tilt   Preferred position of the pelvis that elongates the lumbar spine and shortens the overstretched abdominal muscles during pregnancy.

Postnatal   After the birth of the newborn.

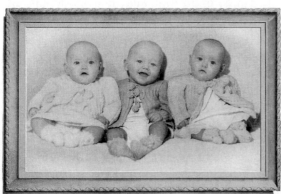

Triple Trouble?

Advertisement for FORMULAC. Life Magazine, September 13, 1948.

Postpartum blues   Transient feeling of sadness, let down, irritability, and anxiety that begins 2 to 3 days after the birth and lasts for a week or so; also called *baby blues*.

Postpartum depression   Depression occurring within 6 months of childbirth and lasting longer than postpartum blues, characterized by severe depression and symptoms that interfere with daily activities and childcare.

Postpartum hemorrhage   Excessive bleeding after childbirth defined as a loss of 500 ml or more of blood.

Postpartum psychosis   Clinical emergency: symptoms may begin as the blues or depression but are characterized by a break with reality, delusions, hallucinations, confusion, panic, and dangerous behavior.

Postterm (labor)   Labor past 42 weeks' gestation.

Powers   Primary and secondary.

Precautions   Taking special care to avoid doing something.

Precipitate labor   Rapid onset or sudden labor of less than 3 hours.

Preconception   Before pregnancy.

Preconception care   Care designed for health maintenance before becoming pregnant.

Preeclampsia   Hypertensive disease after 20 weeks' gestation characterized by elevated blood pressure, headaches, proteinuria, and hemoconcentration.

Pregnancy   Period between conception and birth, human pregnancy usually lasts 280 days, 9 calendar months, or 10 lunar phases.

Pregnancy-induced hypertension (PIH)   Hypertensive disorders of pregnancy including pre-eclampsia, eclampsia and transient hypertension.

Prelabor   Before labor begins.

Premature infant (prematurity)   Infant born before 37 weeks' gestation.

Premature rupture of the membranes (PROM)   Rupture of amniotic sac and leakage of amniotic fluid beginning at least 1 hour before the onset of labor at any gestational age.

Prenatal   Before birth.

Euphemisms for Pregnancy

With child
Brought-to-bed
Accouchement
Confined
Delivered
Enceinte
To be in an interesting state
Expectant
To be in the pudding club
Bow-windowed
Up the pole
In the family way
Knocked up
Irish toothache
Living in seduced circumstances
Infanticipating
Baby-bound
Caught with the goods
Belly up
Full of heir
Heir-conditioned
Past her time
Storked
Wearing a bustle wrong
Awaiting a bundle from heaven
Rehearsing lullabies
Blessed event
Declaring a dividend
Spawning
A bun in the oven

From Smith L: *The mother book: a compendium of trivia and grandeur concerning mother, motherhood and maternity,* New York, 1978, Doubleday.

Presentation   Part of the fetus that first enters the pelvis and lies over the inlet (i.e., head, breech, or shoulder).

Pressure (of the massage)   Amount of force used during the treatment.

Pressure edema   Edema of the lower extremities caused by pressure of the heavy pregnant uterus against the large veins.

Presumptive signs of pregnancy   Cessation of menses, morning sickness, and quickening, but these signs are not absolute.

Preterm labor   Labor occurring before 37 weeks' gestation.

Pretreatment evaluations   Tests performed before prenatal or postpartum massage to determine if the client should receive the treatment, including testing for the presence of blood clots in the legs, the Homan sign, and the test for pitting edema.

Primigravida   Woman who is pregnant for the first time.

Primipara   Woman who has carried a pregnancy to viability whether it was a live birth or stillbirth.

Private practice   Business run and owned by a sole proprietor.

Progesterone   Hormone manufactured by the corpus luteum and placenta that prepares the endometrium of the uterus for implantation, develops the mammary glands, and supports and maintains the pregnancy.

Prolactin   Pituitary hormone that stimulates milk production.

Prolapse of the umbilical cord   Protrusion of the umbilical cord in advance of the presenting part.

Prone   Lying face down.

Proprioceptor/proprioceptive work   Sensory receptors that detect joint and muscle movement; helps balance and strengthen the muscles by relaxing hypertonic muscles and strengthening hypotonic muscles.

Prostaglandin   Substance found in many body tissues that has a role in many reproductive tract functions; induces abortions, or is used for cervical ripening to induce labor.

Proteinuria   Presence of protein in the urine.

Pruritus   Itching.

Psychological adjustment   Period of time postpartum that it takes each individual to accept their new status as a parent.

Psychological response   Emotional reaction to learning about the pregnancy or being a parent that is unique to everyone.

Puerperal fever   Postpartum fever of 100.4° F (38° C) or higher on any 2 days of the first 10 days, excluding the first 24 hours.

Puerperal infection   Infection of the pelvic organs during postpartum.

Puerperium   Period after the third stage of labor and lasting through about 6 weeks postpartum.

Pruritic urticarial papules and plaques of pregnancy (PUPPP)   Lesions commonly begin in the abdominal striae with additional eruptions on the extremities.

Pyelonephritis   Urinary tract complication with symptoms of shaking, chills, flank pain, nausea and vomiting, urinary frequency and urgency, dysuria, and costovertebral angle tenderness.

Pyrexia   Abnormally high body temperature.

Pyrosis   Heartburn.

Ptyalism   Excessive salivation.

Quickening   First fetal movements felt by the mother usually between 16 and 20 weeks' gestation.

Recovery   Postpartum recovery.

Rectus abdominis   Most superficial abdominal muscle involved in flexion of the trunk.

Recumbent   Semisitting; during prenatal massage, the client's torso is at a 45- to 70-degree angle from her hips.

Referred pain   Discomfort originating in one part of the body but felt elsewhere on the body.

Reflexology   Bodywork technique that uses various methods of touch to stimulate specific points on the hands or feet that reflex to particular organs and body parts.

Regional   Local.

Reiki   Gentle but powerful form of energy work.

Relaxation techniques   Techniques to keep the laboring woman relaxed, calm, and focused, including massage, breathing exercises, imagery, meditation, attention focusing, and so on.

Relaxin   Hormone manufactured in the corpus luteum to relax the symphysis pubis and other pelvic joints and ripen or soften the cervix in preparation for labor.

Renin   Hormone manufactured in the kidneys that elevates blood pressure.

Reproductive system   System involved in becoming pregnant and childbirth.

Resource list   Marketing tool that lists medical and complimentary resources for clients.

Respiratory system   System involved with breathing.

Retraction   Bringing inward.

Retroversion of uterus   Displacement of the uterus where the organ is tipped backward and the cervix is pointed toward the symphysis pubis.

Rh factor   Inherited antigen present in red blood cells.

RhoGAM $Rh_0(D)$ immune globulin given after delivery to an Rh-negative mother of an Rh-positive fetus to prevent the maternal Rh immune response.

Rim (ring) of fire   Burning sensation as the vagina stretches and fetal head crowns.

Risk factors   Possible causes involved with miscarriage.

Rooting reflex   Normal response of a newborn to move toward whatever touches the area around the mouth and to attempt to suck; reflex usually disappears by 3 to 4 months of age.

Round uterine ligament   Pair of ligaments that originate at the anterior, superior surface of the uterus, pass through the inguinal region, and attach to the connective tissue of the pubic mons.

Rugae   Folds of mucous membranes on internal surfaces such as the vagina.

Sacral lift   Massage technique that lifts the pregnant uterus and gives relief to the pubo-coccygeal muscles and lower abdomen.

Sacrouterine ligaments   Pair of ligaments that originate at the posterior uterus and attach to the posterior pelvic cavity wall and anterior surface of the sacrum at S2 and S3.

Safe passage   Uneventful birth for mother and child.

Saphenous vein   Deep vein of the thigh where blood clots may aggregate.

Scar massage   Massage technique to reduce scar tissue and improve skin elasticity.

Sciatica   Inflammation of the sciatic nerve.

Second stage of labor   Stage of labor from full dilation (10 cm) to the birth of the baby.

Second trimester   Weeks 14 to 27 of pregnancy.

Serotonin   Neuroendocrine hormone that regulates mood and is calming and soothing.

Sexuality   Libido.

Sexual intercourse   The act of making love.

Shiatsu Oriental bodywork that uses finger pressure along energy channels called *meridians.*

Shortness of breath Inability to take deep breaths, panting, dyspnea.

Shoulder dystocia Failure of shoulders to spontaneously traverse the pelvis after delivery of the head.

Siblings Brothers or sisters.

Sickle cell anemia (hemoglobinopathy) Abnormal crescent-shaped red blood cells.

Side-lying Position of the client lying either on her right or left side on the massage table (or in bed).

Singleton Single fetus.

Sitting massage Treatment offered with the client sitting on a stool or chair.

Sitz bath Application of moist heat to the perineum by sitting in a tub or basin filled with warm water.

Somatic Of the body.

Sonogram Ultrasonography.

Spina bifida (occulta) Congenital malformation of the spine in which the posterior portions of the laminas fail to close, but there is no herniation or protrusion of the spinal cord or meninges.

Spindle cells Neuromuscular spindle cells are found within muscle tissue, generally near the belly of the muscle, and can be released to tighten or relax a muscle.

Spleen 6 Acupuncture point located on the lower leg that embodies female energy; pressing is contraindicated during pregnancy because deep stimulation may cause uterine contractions and initiate labor. Once labor has been established, stimulation of this point (bilaterally) may speed up a prolonged labor.

Spleen 10 Acupuncture point found on both thighs above the knee that releases the contents of the uterus; pressing is contraindicated during pregnancy. During postpartum, stimulation to this point may encourage expulsion of the placenta and uterine cleansing. Also called the *Ocean of Blood.*

Spontaneous abortion Miscarriage before the fetus is viable.

Spontaneous rupture of membranes (SROM) Natural rupture of the membranes.

Spontaneous abortion Miscarriage or the loss of the pregnancy prior to 20 weeks' gestation.

Spousal abuse Physical, emotional, or psychological mistreatment by the husband or domestic partner.

Stage Time delineations of labor: stage one is dilation and descent, stage two is descent and birth, stage three is the expulsion of the placenta, and stage four is recovery.

Station Relationship of the presenting fetal part to an imaginary line drawn between the ischial spines of the pelvis.

Sterility Complete inability to reproduce; state of being free from living microscopic organisms.

Stillbirth Birth of a baby after at least 20 weeks' gestation and 1 day or weighing 350 gm that shows no signs of life.

Stimulating labor Ways to initiate the onset of labor either naturally or medically.

Strain/counterstrain Bodywork technique designed to relieve muscle dysfunction and pain by locating a position of relief and holding it for 90 seconds; also called positional release.

Stress Undue emotional pressure.

Stress urinary incontinence (SUI) Loss of urine occurring with increased abdominal pressure (i.e., sneezing, coughing).

Stretch marks Loss of skin elasticity because of endocrine imbalance or adrenal cortex secretions; some women have a genetic predisposition for stretch marks.

Striae gravidarum Stretch marks.

Stripping the membranes Medical technique to encourage softening of the cervix.

Stroke volume Volume of blood rejected from the left ventricle during one cardiac cycle.

Subinvolution Uterine size appears larger than anticipated for days postpartum and may not contract strongly; uterus may be tender.

Substance abuse Use of drugs, cigarettes, or alcohol (during pregnancy).

Supine Lying on one's back.

Supine hypotension shock   Fall in blood pressure caused by impaired or blocked venous return when the pregnant uterus presses on the inferior vena cava; vena cava syndrome.

Support system   Network of family, friends, and professionals who help in times of crisis and need.

Survivors of abuse   Women who have been victims of sexual, physical, emotional, or psychological abuse by another person.

Swedish massage   Bodywork technique that manipulates the soft tissues of the body.

Symphysis pubis separation   Separation and shearing of the symphysis pubis caused by an accident during pregnancy or by maintaining certain positions during labor for a long period of time.

Taking-hold   Second phase of maternal adaptation during which the mother assumes some independence in control over her body and some responsibility for the newborn.

Taking-in   First phase of maternal adaptation during which the mother passively accepts care for herself and the newborn.

Tension-releasing scan   Full body technique for deep relaxation.

Term (newborn)   Newborn between 38 and 42 weeks' gestation.

Teratogen   Agent that can cause damage in the developing fetus.

Thalassemia   Form of anemia affecting Mediterranean and Southeast Asian populations where there is not enough globin to fill the red blood cells.

Third stage of labor   Stage of labor from the birth of the baby to the expulsion of the placenta.

Third trimester   Weeks 28-40 of gestation.

Thrombocytopenia   Abnormal hematological condition characterized by reduced platelet count.

Thromboembolism   Obstruction of a blood vessel by a clot that has become detached from its site of formation.

Thrombophlebitis   Inflammation of a vein related to the formation of a thrombus (clot).

Thrombus/thrombosis   Blood clot.

Thyroiditis   Postpartum complication involving inflammation of the thyroid gland.

Time allocation   Amount of time spent massaging a body part during the hour's massage.

Tocolytic   Drug that inhibits uterine contractions.

Toxemia   Term previously used to described hypertensive condition.

Toxic   Poisonous.

Toxoplasmosis   Parasitic infection transmitted through the placenta causing fetal abnormalities and acquired through cat feces and poorly prepared food.

Tragerwork   Gentle way to teach movement reeducation and neuromuscular release.

Transcutaneous electrical nerve stimulation (TENS)   Form of energy therapy that emits low-level current to a body area used to prevent nausea and control pain during labor.

Transition phase   Shortest but most intense phase in first stage of labor from a cervical dilation of 8 to 10 cm.

Transition to parenthood   Time from the preconception parenthood decision through the first months after the baby is born during which time parents adjust to their roles as parents.

Transverse abdominis muscle   Most intrinsic abdominal muscle that originates in the lateral one-third of the inguinal ligament, anterior three-fourths of the internal edge of the iliac crest, lumbodorsal fascia, and from the inner edges of the lower six costal cartilages.

Treatment room   Office or studio where the massage takes place.

Treatment series   Number of massages sold at a discount.

Trigger points   Specific sensitive areas within muscles, ligaments, tendons, and fascia that may cause referred pain elsewhere in the body.

Trimester   One of three segments of time of about 3 months each into which pregnancy is divided.

Trimester positioning   Appropriate placement of the pregnant client on the massage table (e.g., prone, supine, side-lying, recumbent, semisitting, or sitting).

Triple screen   Prenatal test that looks for genetic abnormalities in the fetus.

Triplets   Multiple pregnancy with three fetuses.

Tsubos   Japanese term for acupuncture points found along the meridians, or energy channels, that can be pressed, vibrated, or rubbed to release energy blockages and promote maximum health.

Tui-na   Oriental bodywork that uses a variety of techniques, such as grasping, rolling, pressing, or rubbing, to treat injuries of the soft and connective tissues and balance the body's energy.

Twins   Two neonates from the same pregnancy.

Ultrasound   Use of high-frequency waves directed through a transducer into the maternal abdomen to assess fetal development.

Umbilical cord   Cord containing two arteries and one vein that connects the fetus to the placenta.

Umbilicus   Navel.

Uniovular   Monozygotic.

Urethra   Small tubular structure that drains urine from the bladder.

Urinary frequency   Need to urinate often or at close intervals.

Urinary system   System involved with the production and excretion of urine.

Uterine atony   Low muscle tone of the uterus.

Uterine ligaments   Supporting ligaments of the uterus are a pair of round, a pair of broad, a pair of sacrouterine, and single attachments posterior and anterior.

Uterotonic   See *Oxytocic.*

Uterus   Womb; the organ of gestation.

Uterine reflex   Area on the foot or hand that reflexes to the uterus.

Vagina   Musculomembranous tube that forms the passageway between the uterus and external opening.

Vaginal adenosis   Vaginal disease.

Vaginal birth after cesarean section (VBAC)   Vaginal birth after a previous cesarean section.

Vaginismus   Painful spasm of the muscles surrounding the vagina.

Valsalva maneuver   Forced expiratory effort against a closed airway, such as holding one's breath and tightening abdominal muscles; sometimes used during the second stage of labor.

Varicose veins   Swollen, distended, and twisted veins commonly found in the legs; can also be found in the vagina during pregnancy.

Vernix caseosa   Protective, cheese-like, whitish coating that covers the fetal skin and newborn.

Version   Act of turning the fetus in utero to change the presenting part.

Vertex   Crown on top of head.

Viability   Capability to live.

Visceral organs   Organs within the abdominal cavity.

Visualization   Comfort measure during labor that involves mental activity in the form of imagery.

Voluntary   Secondary powers, or abdominal squeezing, that augment the force of the initial labor contractions.

Vulva   External female genitalia consisting of labia majora, labia minora, clitoris, urinary meatus, and vaginal introitus.

Weaning   Process of changing from breastfeeding to a bottle or cup.

Web site   Marketing tool to advertise massage services on the Internet.

Weight gain   Amount of additional weight put on during pregnancy.

Wharton's jelly   White gelatinous material surrounding the umbilical vessels within the cord.

Withdrawal   Painful and difficult reaction to the cessation of an addictive substance.

Womb   Uterus.

Word of mouth   Means by which clients tell each other about massage services.

Zygote   Fertilized ovum; cell produced by the fertilization of two gametes.

Zygote intrafallopian transfer (ZIFT)   ART method that transfers the zygote into the fallopian tubes.

Abuse

Family Violence Prevention Fund
383 Rhode Island Street, Suite 304
San Francisco, CA 94103-5133
www.fvpf.org
www.endabuse.org

The National Council for Research on Women
11 Hanover Square, 24th Floor
New York, NY 10005
212-674-8200
www.ncrw.org

National Child Abuse Hotline
800-422-4453
www.childhelpusa.org

National Coalition Against Domestic Violence
PO Box 34103
Washington, DC 20043-4301
202-638-8638
www.ncadv.org

National Coalition Against Sexual Assault
912 North 2nd Street
Harrisburg, PA 17102
717-232-6771

National Domestic Violence and Abuse Hotline
800-799-SAFE
www.ndvh.org

National Resource Center for Domestic Violence
800-537-2238
www.nrcdv.org

Rape Abuse and Incest National Network
www.rainn.org

Safe Horizon
2 Lafayette Street
New York, NY 10007
212-577-7700
www.safehorizon.org

Violence Against Women Office at the Department of Justice
810 7th Street
Washington, DC 20531
www.usdoj.gov/ovw

Bed rest

The Confinement Line
c/o Childbirth Education Association
PO Box 1609
Springfield, VA 22151
703-941-7183

A Free Home for Moms on Bedrest
www.momsonbedrest.com

High Risk Moms, Inc.
PO Box 4013
Naperville, IL 60567-4013
708-357-5048

Parent Care
101 ½ South Union Street
Alexandria, VA 22314
703-836-4678

Pregnancy Bedrest: A Reading Room
Amy E. Tracy
445C E. Cheyenne Mountain Boulevard, #194
Colorado Springs, CO 80906
www.pregnancybedrest.com

Pregnancy Bedrest Web
Judy Maloni, PhD, RN, FAAN
Case Western Reserve University Bolton School of Nursing
10900 Euclid Avenue
Cleveland, OH 44106
www.fpb.cwru.edu/bedrest

Sidelines National Support Network
PO Box 1808
Laguna Beach, CA 92652
888-447-4754
www.sidelines.org

Bereavement

The Compassionate Friends
PO Box 3696
Oak Brook, IL 60522
630-990-0010
www.compassionatefriends.org

Griefnet
www.griefnet.org

Growth House, Inc.
www.growthhouse.org

Hygeia
www.connix.com/~hygeia/

Miscarriage Support and Information Resources
www.pinelandpress.com/support/miscarriage.html

OBGYN.net
www.obgyn.net/woman/loss/loss.html
National Sudden Infant Death Syndrome Alliance
10500 Little Patuxent Parkway, Suite 420
Columbia, MD 21044
800-221-7437
www.babycenter.com

Parent Care, Inc.
101 ½ South Union Street
Alexandria, VA 22314-3323
703-836-4678

Pen-Parents
www.penparents.org

A Place to Remember
www.aplacetoremember.com

Pregnancy and Infant Loss Center
1421 E. Wayzata Boulevard, Suite 30
Wayzata, MN 55391
612-473-9372

RTS Bereavement Services
Lutheran Hospital La Crosse
1910 South Avenue
La Crosse, WI 54601
800-362-9567
www.bereavementprograms.com

SHARE
www.nationalshareoffice.com

Sudden Infant Death Syndrome Alliance
1314 Bedford Avenue, Suite 210
Baltimore, MD. 21208
800-221-7437
www.sidsalliance.org

SIDS Network
www.sids-network.org

Bodywork

American Association of Oriental Medicine
PO Box 162340
Sacramento, CA 95816
866-455-7999
www.aaom.org

American Massage Therapy Association
820 Davis Street, Suite 100
Evanston, IL 602-01-4464
847-864-0123
www.amtamassage.org

Applied Kinesiology
International College of Applied Kinesiology, USA
PO Box 905
Lawrence, KS 66044
913-542-1801
www.icak.com

Associated Bodywork and Massage Professionals
1271 Sugar Bush Drive
Evergreen, CO 80439
800-458-2267
www.abmp.com

Body Support Systems
1040 Benson Way
Ashland, OR 97520
800-448-2400
www.bodysupport.com

CranioSacral Therapy
Upledger Institute
11211 Prosperity Farms Road, D-325
Palm Beach Gardens, FL 33410-3487
800-233-5880
www.upledger.com

Diastasis Rehab
329 3rd Avenue
New York, NY 10010
212-388-1308
www.diastasisrehab.com

International Association of Infant Massage
www.iaim.net

Lymphatic Drainage
North American Vodder Association Lymphatic Therapy
PO Box 5701
Victoria, British Columbia, Canada V8R 6S8
250-598-9862
www.vodderschool.com

Massage Magazine
800-533-4263
www.massagemag.com

Myofascial Release
222 West Lancaster Avenue, Suite 100
Paoli, PA 19301
800-FASCIAL
www.myofascialrelease.com

T Spheres®
Aromatic massage balls.
www.MotherMassage.net

Touch Research Institute
University of Miami School of Medicine
PO Box 016820
Miami, FL 33101
305-243-6781
www6.miami.edu/touch-research/about.htm

Tuple Technique® Diastasis Repair
215 E 24th Street
New York, NY 10010
212-388-1308

Breastfeeding and Lactation

American Academy of Pediatrics
141 Northwest Point Boulevard
Elk Grove, IL 60007-10098
800-422-4784
www.aap.org

Breastfeeding Resources
www.parentsplace.com/expert/lactation

Bright Future Lactation Resource Centre
www.bflrc.com

International Lactation Consultant Association
1500 Sunday Drive, Suite 102
Raleigh, NC 27607
919-861-5577
www.ilca.org

Lact-Aid
PO Box 1066
Athens, TN 37303
614-744-9090

Lactation Education Resources
www.leron-line.com

La Leche League International
1400 N. Meecham Road
Schaumberg, IL 60173
800-LA-LECHE
www.lalecheleague.org

Cesarean and VBAC Information

American College of Obstetricians and Gynecologists (ACOG)
409 12th Street SW
PO Box 96920
Washington, DC 20090-6920
800-762-2264
www.acog.org

Cesarean Prevention Movement
PO Box 152
Syracuse, NY 13210
315-424-1942

C/SEC, Inc. (Cesarean/Support Education and Concern)
22 Forest Road
Framingham, MA 01701
508-877-8266
www.peacehealth.org

International Cesarean Awareness Network (ICAN)
1304 Kingsdale Avenue
Redondo Beach, CA 90278
www.ican-online.org

VBAC.com
Center for Family
24050 Madison Street, Suite 200
Torrance, CA 90505
310-375-3141
www.vbac.com

General Resources

Academy for Guided Imagery
PO Box 2070
Mill Valley, CA 94942
800-726-2070
www.healthy.net/agi/

American Cancer Society
1599 Clifton Road NE
Atlanta, GA 30329
800- ACS-2345
www.cancer.org

American Cleft Palate Craniofacial Association
1504 East Franklin Street
Suite 102
Chapel Hill, NC 27514-2820
800-24-CLEFT
www.acpa-cpf.org

American Diabetes Association
Diabetes Information Service Center
1660 Duke Street
Alexandria, VA 22314
800-342-2383
www.diabetes.org

American Fertility Foundation
2131 Magnolia Avenue, Suite 201
Birmingham, AL 35256
www.theafa.org

American Heart Association
Women's Heart Information: 1-888-MYHEART
www.americanheart.org

American Red Cross
430 17th Street, NW
Washington, DC 20006
202-737-8300
www.redcross.org

American Society for Reproductive Medicine
1209 Montgomery Highway
Birmingham, AL 35316
www.asrm.com

Association for Childbirth at Home, International
PO Box 39498
Los Angeles, CA 90039
213-667-0839

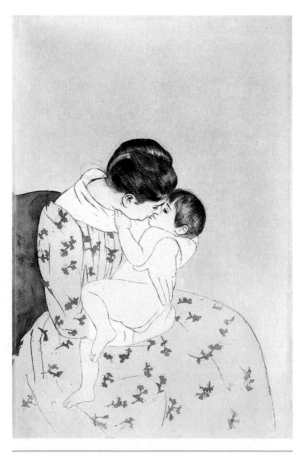

Mother's Kiss. Mary Cassatt (1844-1926). Reprinted by permission of the Worcester Art Museum, Worcester, Mass.

Baby Center
www.babycenter.com

Birth Trauma Association
www.birthtraumaassociation.org.uk

Bright Futures
www.brightfutures.org

Cancernet
www.cancernet.nei.nih.gov

Center for Sickle Cell Disease
2121 Georgia Avenue NW
Washington, DC 20059
202-636-7930

Centers for Disease Control and Prevention
1600 Clifton Road NE
Atlanta, GA 30333
404-329-1819
www.cdc.gov

COPE (Coping with the Overall Pregnancy/ Parenting Experience)
37 Clarendon Street
Boston, MA 02116
617-357-5588

Endometriosis Association
8585 North 76th Place
Milwaukee, WI 53223
800-992-3636
www.ivf.com/endohtml.html

Fraxa: Fragile X Research Foundation
45 Pleasant Street
Newburyport, MA 10950
978-462-1866
www.fraxa.org

Gynecologic Cancer Foundation
www.sgo.org/publications/gynecologic_cancer.cfm
Healthy Mothers, Healthy Babies Coalition
409 12th Street SW
Washington, DC 20024
202-863-2458
www.hmhb.org

Hysterectomy Education Resource and Services (HERS)
422 Bryn Mawr Avenue
Bala Cynwyd, PA 19004
215-667-7757
www.ccon.com/hers

March of Dimes Birth Defects Foundation
1275 Mamaroneck Avenue
White Plains, NY 10605
914-428-7100
www.modimes.org

National Abortion Federation Consumer Hotline
1156 15th Street NW, Suite 700
Washington, DC 20005
800-772-9100
www.healthfinder.gov

National Alliance of Breast Cancer Organization
9 East 37th Street, 10th floor
New York, NY 10016
800-719-0154
www.nabco.org

National Center for Education in Maternal and Child Health
www.ncemch.org

National Fragile X Foundation
PO Box 190488
San Francisco, CA 94119
800-688-8765
www.fragilex.org

National Healthy Mothers, Healthy Babies Coalition
2000 N. Beauregard Street
6th Floor
Alexandria, VA 22311
703-837-4792
www.hmhb.org

National Organization of Circumcision Information Resource Centers
PO Box 2512
San Anselmo, CA 94979
415-488-9883
www.nocirc.org

National Women's Health Network
514 10th Street NW
Washington, DC 20004
202-347-1140

National Down Syndrome Congress
1370 Center Drive, Suite 102
Atlanta, GA 30338
800-232-6372
www.ndsccenter.org

National Down Syndrome Society Hotline
666 Broadway
New York, NY 10012
800-221-4602
www.ndss.org

National Institute of Child Health and Human Development (NICHD)
National Institutes of Health
9000 Rockville Pike
Building 31, Room 2A32
Bethesda, MD 20892
301-496-4000
www.nih.gov

National Organization on Adolescent Pregnancy, Parenting and Prevention
2401 Pennsylvania Avenue, Suite 350
Washington, DC 20037
202-293-8370
www.healthyteennetwork.org

National Ovarian Cancer Coalition
2335 East Atlantic Boulevard #401
Pompano Beach, FL 33062
888-682-7426
www.ovarian.org

National Perinatal Association
101 ½ South Union Street
Alexandria, VA 22314-3323
703-549-5523

Parenthood After Thirty
451 Vermont Avenue
Berkeley, CA 94707
415 524 6635

Parents of Prematures
13613 NE 26th Place
Bellevue, WA 98005
206-883-6040

Planned Parenthood Federation of America
810 Seventh Avenue
New York, NY 100109
800-230-PLAN
www.plannedparenthood.org

Resolve, Inc.
1310 Broadway, Department GM
Summerville, MA 02144-1713
888-299-1585
www.resolve.org

Single Mothers By Choice
PO Box 1642
Gracie Square Station
New York, NY 10028
212-988-0993
www.mattes.home.pipeline.com

Spina Bifida Association of America
4590 McArthur Boulevard NW, Suite 250
Washington, DC 20007-4226
800-621-3141

Herbal Products and Mothering Supplies

Avena Botanicals
20 Mill Street
Rockland, ME 04841
207-594-0694
www.avenaherbs.com

Blessed Herbs
1090 Barre Plains Road
Oakham, MA 01068
800-489-4372
www.blessedherbs.com

Brushy Mountain Bee Company
800-BEESWAX
www.beeequipment.com

Cascade Health Care Products
141 Commercial Street NE
Salem, OR 97301
800-443-9942
www.1cascade.com

Frontier Cooperative Herbs
Box 299
Norway, IA 52318
800-669-3275
www.frontiercoop.com

Herb Pharm
PO Box 116
Williams, OR 97544
800-348-4372
www.herb-pharm.com

Herbalist and Alchemist
PO Box 553
Broadway, NJ 08808
908-689-9092
www.herbalist-alchemist.com

Mountain Rose Herbs
PO Box 2000
Redway, CA 95560
800-879-3337
www.mountainroseherbs.com

Sage Mountain
PO Box 420
East Barre, VT 05649
802-479-9825
www.sagemountain.com

Massage Supplies

Banner Therapy
891 Broadway Street
Asheville, NC
888-277-1188
www.bannertherapy.com

Body Support Systems
1040 Benson Way
Ashland, OR 97520
800-448-2400
www.bodysupport.com

Massage Warehouse
9005 N. Industrial Road
Peoria, IL 61615-1511
800-910-9955
www.massagewarehouse.com

Milk Banks

Lactation Support Services
Children's and Women's Milk Bank
British Columbia Children's Hospital
Vancouver, British Columbia,
Canada V6H 3V4
604-875-2345, ext. 7607

Mother's Milk Bank
Presbyterian/St. Luke's Medical Center
Denver, CO 80218
303-869-1888

Mother's Milk Bank
Valley Medical Center
San Jose, CA 95128
408-998-4550

Mother's Milk Bank
WakeMed
3000 New Bern Avenue
Raleigh, NC 276210
919-350-8599

Nursing Mothers Advisory Council
www.nursingmoms.net

Regional Milk Bank
The Medical Center of Central Massachusetts
Worcester, MA 01605
508-793-6005

Special Care Nursery Mother's Milk Bank
Christiana Care Health Services
4755 Ogletown Stanton Road
PO Box 6001
Newark, DE 19718
302-733-2340

**Special Supplemental Nutrition
Program for Women, Infants, and
Children (WIC)**
703-305-2286

Multiples

Mothers of Supertwins (MOST)
PO Box 951
Brentwood, NY 11717
631-859-1110
www.mostonline.org

**National Organization of Mothers
of Twins Club**
PO Box 438
Thompson Station, TN 37179-0438
615-595-0936
www.nomotc.org

The Triplet Connection
PO Box 429
Spring City, UT 84662
435-851-1105
www.tripletconnection.org

National Support and Resource Organizations

**American Academy of Husband-Coached
Childbirth (Bradley Method)**
PO Box 5224
Sherman Oaks, CA 91413
800-422-4784
www.BradleyBirth.com

American Association of Birth Centers
3123 Gottschall Road
Perkiomenville, PA 18074
215-234-8068
www.Birthcenters.org

American College of Nurse-Midwives (ACNM)
818 Connecticut Avenue NW
Suite 900
Washington, DC 20006
202-728-9860
www.ACNM.org

American Foundation for Maternal and Child Health
439 E. 51st Street
New York, NY 10022
212-759-5510

Association for Pre- and Perinatal Psychology and Health
1600 Prince Street, Suite 500
Alexandria, VA 22314
703-548-2808

Association of Labor Assistants and Childbirth Educators (ALACE)
PO Box 382724
Cambridge, MA 02238
617-441-2500
www.ALACE.org

Childbirth & Postpartum Professionals Association (CAPPA)
PO Box 491448
Lawrenceville, GA 30040
888-MY-CAPPA
www.CAPPA.net

Childbirth Connection
281 Park Avenue South
New York, NY 10010
212-777-5000
www.childbirthconnection.org

Childbirth Graphics
PO Box 21207
Waco, TX 76702
800-229-3366
www.Childbirthgraphics.com

Citizens for Midwifery
PO Box 82227
Athens, GA 30608-2227
316-267-7236
www.cfmidwifery.org

Doulas of North America (DONA)
1100 23rd Avenue East
Seattle, WA 98112
509-448-DONA
www.DONA.org

International Childbirth Education Association (ICEA)
1500 Sunday Drive
Suite 102
Raleigh, NC 27607
919-863-9487
www.ICEA.org

Lamaze International
1200 19th Street NW
Suite 300
Washington, DC 20036-2412
800-368-4404
www.Lamaze.org

Midwifery Today
PO Box 2672
Eugene, OR 97402
800-743-0974
www.midwiferytoday.com

Midwives' Alliance of North America (MANA)
375 Rockbridge Road, Suite 172-313
Lilburn, GA 30047
888-923-6262 (MANA)
www.MANA.org

National Association of Parents and Professionals for Safe Alternatives in Childbirth (NAPSAC)
PO Box 267
Marble Hill, MO 63764
314-238-2010
www.NAPSAC.org

Postpartum

Depression After Delivery (DAD)
PO Box 278
Belle Mead, NNJ 08502
www.depressionafterdelivery.org

National Association of Postpartum Care Services
PO Box 1020
Edmonds, VA. 98020
800-45-DOULA
www.napcs.org

Postpartum Support International
927 N. Kellogg Avenue
Santa Barbara, CA 93111
805-967-7636
www.postpartum.net

Prenatal Massage Education

Body Therapy Associates
11650 Iberia Place, #137
San Diego, CA 92128
800-586-8322
www.bodytherapyassociates.com

Bodywork for the Childbearing Year
8950 Villa La Jolla Drive, Suite A217
La Jolla, CA 92037
888-287-6860
www.katejordanseminars.com

MotherMassage: Massage During Pregnancy
Elaine Stillerman, LMT
PO Box 150337
Brooklyn, NY 11215-0337
estiller24@gmail.com
www.MotherMassage.net

Figure Credits

Chapter 1, p. 2; Chapter 13, p. 193
Astarte: The Phoenician Goddess of Love and Fertility. Reprinted by permission of JBL Statues, 1999.

Chapter 2, p. 20; Chapter 14, p. 199; Part 4, p. 399
Encaustic on mahogany. Earth Mother. Sir Edward Coley Burne-Jones (1833-1898). Reprinted by permission of the Worcester Art Museum, Worcester, Mass.

Chapter 3, p. 30; Chapter 15, p. 232
Oil on canvas. The Bath, 1891-1892. Mary Cassatt, American (1844-1926). Reprinted by permission of The Art Institute of Chicago.

Chapter 4, p. 49; Chapter 16, p. 239
From *Little Children: My Baby Brother*. New Pictures for Little Children, New York, ca 1800s, McLoughlin Brothers.

Chapter 5, p. 64; Chapter 17, p. 271
Picture of woman's body transparently revealing the end of pregnancy. From Willy A, Vander L, Fisher O: *The illustrated encyclopedia of sex*, New York, 1950, Cadillac Publishing.

Chapter 6, p. 102; Chapter 18, p. 279; Part 3, p. 329
Mrs. Elizabeth Freake and Baby Mary, circa 1671. Unknown 17th century American. Reprinted by permission of the Worcester Art Museum, Worcester, Mass.

Chapter 7, p. 111; Chapter 19, p. 303
The Brooding Woman. Paul Gauguin (1848-1903). Reprinted by permission of the Worcester Art Museum, Worcester, Mass.

Chapter 8, p. 129; Chapter 20, p. 330
This illustration is according to Professor Ogino's theory that there are a total of 7 to 11 fertile days. However, this is incorrect, as proved by exact scientific tests carried out by Professor Knaus, according to whom the total number of days on which fecundation might take place is only five. Reprinted from Willy A, Vander L, Fisher O: *The illustrated encyclopedia of sex*, New York, 1950, Cadillac Publishing.

Chapter 9, p. 139; Chapter 21, p. 340; Part 1, p. 1
Reine Lefebvre holding a nude baby, 1902. Mary Cassatt, American (1844-1926). Reprinted by permission of the Worcester Art Museum, Worcester, Mass.

Index

Note: Page numbers followed by "f" refer to illustrations; page numbers followed by "t" refer to table; page numbers followed by "b"refer to boxes.